THE PILL BOOK, 7th REVISED EDITION:
THE ILLUSTRATED GUIDE TO THE MOST PRESCRIBED DRUGS IN THE UNITED STATES
Illustrated with 32 pages of actual-size color photographs

With more than 8 million copies in print, THE PILL BOOK is the bestselling consumer drug reference ever, offering the most up-to-date, comprehensive information, now in a revised format designed for ease of use.

This new 7th edition of THE PILL BOOK is bigger than ever and contains more profiles of commonly prescribed drugs than any other consumer reference. Compiled by a team of eminent pharmacologists, it is based on official, FDA-approved information usually available only to doctors and pharmacists, plus the latest information gathered from computer databases and on-line resources. It synthesizes the most important facts about each drug in a concise, readable, easy-to-understand entry.

Here are complete profiles of more than 1,500 of the most commonly prescribed drugs, including:

- Generic and brand names
- What the drug is for and how it works
- Usual dosages, and what to do if a dose is skipped
- Side effects and possible adverse reactions, highlighted for quick reference
- Interactions with other drugs and foods
- Overdose and addiction potential
- Alcohol-free and sugar-free medications
- Information for seniors, pregnant and breast-feeding women, and others with special needs
- Cautions and warnings, and when to call your doctor

This completely revised and updated 7th edition contains over 150 new brand names and more than 80 important new drugs approved by the FDA in late 1995 that will go on sale for the first time in 1996. A 32-page insert provides actual-size full color photographs of the most-prescribed pills.

THE PILL BOOK
7th EDITION

Editor-in-Chief
HAROLD M. SILVERMAN, Pharm. D.

Production
CURRENT MEDICAL DIRECTIONS

Consultant
IAN GINSBERG, R.Ph.

Digital Photography and Color Separations
WACE, NEW YORK

Original Creators of THE PILL BOOK
LAWRENCE D. CHILNICK
BERT STERN
HAROLD M. SILVERMAN, Pharm. D.
GILBERT I. SIMON, Sc.D.

BANTAM BOOKS
NEW YORK • TORONTO • LONDON • SYDNEY • AUCKLAND

In Canada Aspirin *is a registered trademark owned by Sterling Winthrop Inc.*

THE PILL BOOK
A Bantam Book

PUBLISHING HISTORY

Bantam edition published June 1979
Bantam revised edition / October 1982
Bantam 3rd revised edition / March 1986
Bantam 4th revised edition / February 1990
Bantam 5th revised edition / May 1992
Bantam 6th revised edition / June 1994
Bantam 7th revised edition / June 1996
This revised edition was published simultaneously in trade paperback and mass market paperback.

ISBN: 0-553-57452-3

Published simultaneously in the United States and Canada

Bantam Books are published by Bantam Books, a division of Bantam Doubleday Dell Publishing Group, Inc. Its trademark, consisting of the words "Bantam Books" and the portrayal of a rooster, is Registered in U.S. Patent and Trademark Office and in other countries. Marca Registrada. Bantam Books, 1540 Broadway, New York, New York 10036.

PRINTED IN THE UNITED STATES OF AMERICA

OPM   19   18   17   16   15   14   13   12

Contents

The purpose of this book is to provide educational information to the public concerning the majority of various types of prescription drugs that are presently utilized by physicians. It is not intended to be complete or exhaustive or in any respect a substitute for personal medical care. *Only a physician may prescribe these drugs and their exact dosages.*

While every effort has been made to reproduce products on the cover and insert of this book in an exact fashion, certain variations of size or color may be expected as a result of the printing process. Furthermore, pictures identified as brand name drugs should not be confused with their generic counterparts, and vice versa. In any event, the reader should not rely solely upon the photographic image to identify any pills depicted herein, but should rely upon the physician's prescription as dispensed by the pharmacist.

How to Use This Book

The Pill Book, like pills themselves, should be taken with caution. Used properly, this book can save you money and, perhaps, your life. Our book contains life-size pictures of the drugs most often prescribed in the United States. *The Pill Book*'s product identification system is designed to help you check that the drug you're about to take is the one your doctor prescribed. The most prescribed brand name drugs are included, as are some of the more frequently prescribed generic (nonbrand) versions of those drugs. Although many dosage forms are included, not all available forms and strengths of every drug have been shown. While every effort has been made to create accurate photographic reproductions of the products, some variations in size or color may be expected as a result of the printing process. Don't rely solely on the photographic image to identify your pills; check with your pharmacist if you have any product identification questions.

Most, though not all, drugs in the color section can be matched with your pill by checking to see if:

- The imprinted company logos (e.g., "Roche") are the same.
- The product strengths (e.g., "250 mg"), frequently printed on the pills, are the same.
- Any product code numbers imprinted directly on the pill are the same.

To learn more about the pictured drugs, check the descriptive material in the text (page numbers are given).

Each pill profile in *The Pill Book* contains the following information:

Generic and Brand Name: The generic name is the common name of the drug approved by the Food and Drug Administration (FDA). It is listed along with the current brand names available for each generic drug.

Most prescription drugs are sold in more than one strength. Some drugs, such as the oral contraceptives, come in packages containing different numbers of pills. A few manufacturers reflect this fact by adding letters and/or numbers to the basic drug name; others do not. An example: Norlestrin 21 1/50, Norlestrin 21 2.5/50, Norlestrin 28 1/50, Norlestrin 28 2.5/50. (The numbers here refer to the number of tablets in each monthly packet, 28 or 21, and the amount of medication found in the tablets.) Other drugs come in different strengths: This is often indicated by a notation such as "DS" (double strength) or "Forte" (stronger).

The Pill Book lists generic and brand names (e.g., Norlestrin) together only where there are no differences in basic ingredients. However, the amount of the ingredient (strength) may vary from product to product. In most cases, the different brand names and generic versions listed for each generic drug product are interchangeable with one another; you can use any version of the drug and expect that it will work for you. *The Pill Book* identifies those drugs for which generic versions are not considered equivalent and which should not be interchanged with a brand-name product or another generic version of the same drug.

The Pill Book will also tell you which drugs are sugar free ⑤ or alcohol free Ⓐ . This is important information for people who must avoid these ingredients.

Type of Drug: Describes the general pharmacologic class of each drug: "antidepressant," "tranquilizer," "decongestant," "expectorant," and so on.

Prescribed for: Lists the conditions for which a drug is usually prescribed. All drugs are approved for some symptoms or conditions by federal authorities, but doctors also commonly prescribe drugs for other, as yet unapproved, reasons; these are also listed in *The Pill Book*. Check with your doctor if you are not sure why you have been given a certain pill.

General Information: Information on how the drug works, how long it takes for you to feel its effects, or a description of how this drug is similar to (or different from) other drugs.

Cautions and Warnings: Any drug can be harmful if you are sensitive to it. This information alerts you to possible important and more dangerous reactions and to physical conditions, such as heart disease, that can have serious consequences if the drug is prescribed for you.

Possible Side Effects: Side effects are generally divided into three categories—those that are most common, those that are less common, and those that occur only rarely—to help you better understand what to expect from your pills. If you are not sure whether you are experiencing a drug side effect, ask your doctor.

Drug Interactions: Describes what happens when you mix your medicine with other drugs and lists what should not be taken at the same time as your medicine. Drug interactions are more common than overdoses. Some interactions with other pills, alcohol, or other substances can be deadly. At every visit, be sure to inform your doctor of any medication you are already taking. Your pharmacist should also keep a record of all your prescription and nonprescription medicines. This listing, called a *Patient Drug Profile*, is used to check for potential problems. You may want to keep your own drug profile and take it to your pharmacist for review whenever a new medicine is added. You'd be surprised at how many drug interaction problems can develop.

Food Interactions: Provides information on foods to avoid while taking your medication, whether to take your medicine with meals, and other important facts.

Usual Dose: Tells you the largest and smallest doses usually prescribed. You may be given different dosage instructions by your doctor. Check with your doctor if you are confused about when and how often to take a pill, or why a dosage other than the one indicated in *The Pill Book* has been prescribed. Do not change the dose of ANY medicine you take without first calling your doctor. Drug doses often need to change with increasing age; this information is also given.

Overdosage: Describes overdose symptoms and what to do.

Special Information: Lists important facts to help you take your medicine more safely. Includes symptoms to watch for, when to call your doctor, what to do if you forget a dose of your medicine, and any special instructions.

Special Populations: *Pregnancy/Breast-feeding:* Women who are pregnant or nursing newborn infants need the latest information on how medicines can affect their babies. This section will help guide you on how to use medicines if you are or might be pregnant, and what to do if you must take a medicine during the time you are nursing your baby. *Seniors:* Our bodies change as we grow older. As an older adult, you want information about how each drug affects you and what kind of reactions to expect. This section presents the special facts you need to know about every drug and explains how your reactions may differ from those of a younger person. It describes symptoms you are more likely to develop just because you are older and how your doctor might adjust drug dosage to account for the changes in your body.

The Pill Book is a unique visual reference tool. It is intended not only to amplify the information given by your doctor and pharmacist but also to help you be a more informed consumer. If you read something in *The Pill Book* that does not agree with instructions you have received, call your doctor. Almost any drug can have serious side effects if abused or used improperly.

In an Emergency!

Each year some 1.5 million people are poisoned in the United States; about 70,000 of the poisonings are drug related, and about 7000 of those result in death. In fact, drug overdose is a leading cause of fatal poisoning in the United States. Sedatives, barbiturates, tranquilizers, and topically applied medicines are responsible for the bulk of the drug-related poisonings or overdoses.

Although each of the pill profiles in *The Pill Book* has specific information on drug overdose, there are a few general rules to remember if you are faced with an accidental poisoning.

1. Make sure the victim is breathing, and call for medical help immediately.
2. Call your local poison control center. The telephone number can be obtained from information; just ask for "poison control." When you call, be prepared to explain:

   - What was taken and how much.
   - What the victim is doing (conscious, sleeping, vomiting, having convulsions, etc).
   - The approximate age and weight of the victim.
   - Any chronic medical problems of the victim (such as diabetes, epilepsy, or high blood pressure), if you know them.
   - What medicines, if any, the victim takes regularly.

3. Remove anything that might interfere with breathing. A person who is not getting enough oxygen will turn blue

(the fingernails or tongue change color first). If this happens, lay the victim on his or her back, open the collar, place one hand under the neck, and lift, pull, or push the victim's jaw so that it juts outward. This will open the airway between the mouth and lungs as wide as possible. Begin mouth-to-mouth resuscitation ONLY if the victim is not breathing.

4. If the victim is unconscious or having convulsions, call for medical help immediately. While waiting for the ambulance, lay the victim on his or her stomach and turn the head to one side. Should the victim throw up, this will prevent inhalation of vomit. DO NOT give an unconscious victim anything by mouth. Keep the victim warm.

5. If the victim is conscious, call for medical help and give him or her an 8-ounce glass of water to drink. This will dilute the poison.

Only a small number of poisoning victims require hospitalization. Most can be treated with simple actions or need no treatment at all.

You may be told to make the patient vomit. The best way to do this is to use Syrup of Ipecac, which is available without a prescription at any pharmacy. Specific instructions on how much to give infants, children, or adults are printed on the label and will also be given by your poison control center. Remember, DO NOT make the victim vomit unless you have been instructed to do so. Never make the victim vomit if the victim is unconscious, is having a convulsion, has a painful, burning feeling in the mouth or throat, or has swallowed a corrosive poison (including bleach [liquid or powder], washing soda, drain cleaner, lye, oven cleaner, toilet bowl cleaner, or dishwasher detergent). If a corrosive poison has been taken and the victim can still swallow, give milk or water to dilute the poison. The poison control center will give you further instructions. If the victim has swallowed a petroleum derivative such as gasoline, kerosene, machine oil, lighter fluid, furniture polish, or cleaning fluids, do not do anything. Call the poison control center for instructions.

If the poison or chemical has spilled onto the skin, remove any clothing or jewelry that has been contaminated, and wash the area with plenty of warm water for at least 15 minutes. Then wash the area thoroughly with soap and water. The poison control center will give you more instructions.

Be Prepared

The best way to deal with a poisoning is to be prepared for it. Do the following now:

1. Get the telephone number of your local poison control center, and write it next to your other emergency phone numbers.
2. Decide which hospital you will go to, if necessary, and how you will get there.
3. Buy 1 ounce of Syrup of Ipecac from your pharmacy. The pharmacist will tell you how to use it. Remember, this is a potent drug to be used only if directed.
4. Learn to give mouth-to-mouth resuscitation. You may have to use this on a poisoning victim.

Do the following to reduce the risk of accidental poisoning:

1. Keep all medicine, household cleaners, disinfectants, insecticides, gardening products, and similar products out of the reach of young children, in a locked place.
2. Do not store poisonous materials in containers that once held food.
3. Do not remove the labels from bottles so that the contents are unknown.
4. Discard all medicines when you no longer need them.
5. Do not operate a car engine or other gasoline engine in an unventilated space. Do not use a propane heater indoors.
6. If you smell gas, call the gas company immediately.

Poison prevention is a matter of common sense. If you follow the simple advice given in this chapter, you will have taken a giant step toward ensuring household safety for you and your family.

The Most Commonly Prescribed Drugs in the United States, Generic and Brand Names, with Complete Descriptions of Drugs and Their Effects

Generic Name

Acarbose

Brand Name

Precose

Type of Drug

Antidiabetic.

Prescribed for

Non−insulin-dependent diabetes.

General Information

Acarbose works against diabetes in a way different from all other antidiabetes medicines. It interferes with enzymes in the intestine responsible for breaking the complex carbohydrates found in starchy foods down into simple sugars, including glucose, and lowers blood sugar by delaying the absorption of glucose into the blood. Because it works by a different method than the sulfonylurea-type oral antidiabetes drugs and Metformin, the blood-sugar-lowering effect of Acarbose is additive to that of other antidiabetes drugs. Acarbose may also be used by people who are unable to control their blood sugar by diet alone. Half of each dose of Acarbose remains unchanged in the intestines and passes out of the body in the stool; about 2 percent is absorbed into the blood, and the rest is broken down in the intestines. Most of Acarbose's side effects are directly related to the fact that it leaves undigested carbohydrates in the lower intestines. In studies of Acarbose, both black and white patients responded similarly, but a better response was seen in Hispanic patients.

Cautions and Warnings

Acarbose should not be used if you are **allergic** or **sensitive** to it. People should not use Acarbose if they have **diabetic ketoacidosis, cirrhosis, severe kidney disease, inflammatory bowel disease, ulcers of the colon, intestinal obstruction, severe digestive disease,** or **absorption diseases,** or if **intes-**

tinal gas will be a severe problem. Acarbose may lead to **liver inflammation**.

Possible Side Effects

▼ Most common: stomach gas (in ¾ of people who take it), abdominal pains, and diarrhea. These side effects tend to improve or go away after a few weeks.

▼ Other: liver irritation and some minor abnormalities in blood tests.

Drug Interactions

• Acarbose adds to the blood-sugar-lowering effect of sulfonylureas and other antidiabetes drugs.

• Like other antidiabetes agents, the effects of Acarbose will be countered by drugs that raise blood sugar, including diuretics, thyroid hormones, corticosteroids, Phenothiazines, Estrogens, oral contraceptives, Phenytoin, Nicotinic Acid, stimulants (and decongestants), calcium channel blockers, and Isoniazid.

• Activated charcoal, antacids, and other drugs intended to absorb stomach contents, and digestive enzyme preparations may reduce the effectiveness of Acarbose. Separate these drugs from Acarbose by at least 2 hours.

Food Interactions

Acarbose must be taken at the beginning (with the first bite) of each meal.

Usual Dose

Adult: 25 to 50 mg 3 times a day. Maximum dose is 100 mg 3 times a day in people weighing 132 pounds or more.

Child: not recommended.

Overdosage

There is no experience with Acarbose overdosage, but diarrhea, abdominal pains, and intestinal gas can be expected. Excess blood-sugar lowering should not occur. Call your local poison center for more information.

Special Information

It is essential to take each dose of Acarbose at the beginning of each meal. Since the drug works in the intestines, it has to be there at the same time as the food you are digesting.

As with all antidiabetes medicines, people taking Acarbose must follow their doctor's instructions for diet and exercise.

Read product labels carefully or check with your pharmacist before buying any nonprescription medicine to be sure it is safe for diabetics to take with Acarbose.

If you forget a dose of Acarbose, skip it and continue with your regular schedule. Taking a missed dose later on will not provide any benefit.

Special Populations

Pregnancy/Breast-feeding

Animal studies of Acarbose showed no effects on the developing fetus. There is no information available on the effect of Acarbose in pregnant women. As with all medicines, Acarbose should be taken during pregnancy only if absolutely necessary and only if the potential risks have been completely discussed with your doctor.

It is not known if Acarbose passes into breast milk. Nursing mothers who must take this medicine should consider bottle-feeding their babies.

Seniors

Blood levels of Acarbose are higher in older adults, but this is not considered important. Older adults with severe kidney disease should avoid this medicine.

Accupril

see **Quinapril Hydrochloride**, page 972

Generic Name

Acebutolol

Brand Name

Sectral

(Also available in generic form)

Type of Drug

Beta-adrenergic-blocking agent.

Prescribed for

High blood pressure and abnormal heart rhythms.

General Information

Acebutolol is one of 14 beta-adrenergic-blocking drugs that interfere with the action of a specific part of the nervous system. Beta receptors are found all over the body and affect many body functions. This accounts for the usefulness of beta blockers against a wide variety of conditions. The first member of this group, Propranolol, was found to affect the entire beta-adrenergic portion of the nervous system. Newer beta blockers have been refined to affect only a portion of that system, making them more useful in the treatment of cardiovascular disorders and less useful for other purposes. Other beta blockers are mild stimulants to the heart or have other characteristics that make them more useful for a specific purpose or better for certain people.

Cautions and Warnings

You should be **cautious about taking Acebutolol** if you have **asthma, severe heart failure, a very slow heart rate,** or **heart**

block because the drug may aggravate these conditions. Compared with the other beta blockers, Acebutolol has less of an effect on pulse and bronchial muscles (asthma), and less of a rebound effect when discontinued; it also produces less tiredness, depression, and intolerance to exercise.

People with **angina** taking Acebutolol for high blood pressure should have their **drug dosage reduced gradually** over 1 to 2 weeks rather than suddenly discontinued to avoid possible worsening of the angina.

Acebutolol should be used with caution if you have **liver or kidney disease** because your ability to eliminate this drug from your body may be impaired.

Acebutolol reduces the amount of blood pumped by the heart with each beat. This reduction in blood flow can aggravate or worsen the condition of people with **poor circulation** or **circulatory disease.**

If you are undergoing **major surgery,** your doctor may want you to stop taking Acebutolol at least 2 days before surgery to permit the heart to respond more acutely to things that happen during the surgery. This is still controversial and may not hold true for all people preparing for surgery.

Possible Side Effects

Side effects are usually mild, are relatively uncommon, develop early in the course of treatment, and are rarely a reason to stop taking Acebutolol.

▼ Most common: male impotence.

▼ Infrequent: unusual tiredness or weakness, slow heartbeat, heart failure (swelling of the legs, ankles, or feet), dizziness, breathing difficulty, bronchospasm, mental depression, confusion, anxiety, nervousness, sleeplessness, disorientation, short-term memory loss, emotional instability, cold hands and feet, constipation, diarrhea, nausea, vomiting, upset stomach, increased sweating, urinary difficulty, cramps, blurred vision, skin rash, hair loss, stuffy nose, facial swelling, aggravation of lupus erythematosus (a disease of the body's connective tissues), itching, chest pains, back or joint pains, colitis, drug allergy (fever, sore throat), and liver toxicity.

Drug Interactions

• Acebutolol may interact with surgical anesthetics to increase the risk of heart problems during surgery. Some anesthesiologists recommend gradually stopping your medicine 2 days before surgery.

• Acebutolol may interfere with the normal signs of low blood sugar and can interfere with the action of oral antidiabetes medicines.

• Acebutolol enhances the blood-pressure-lowering effects of other blood-pressure-reducing agents (including Clonidine, Guanabenz, and Reserpine) and calcium-channel-blocking drugs (such as Nifedipine).

• Aspirin-containing drugs, Indomethacin, Sulfinpyrazone, and estrogen drugs can interfere with the blood-pressure-lowering effect of Acebutolol.

• Cocaine may reduce the effects of all beta-blocking drugs.

• Acebutolol may worsen the condition of cold hands and feet associated with taking ergot alkaloids (for migraine headaches). Gangrene is a possibility in people taking an ergot and Acebutolol.

• Acebutolol will counteract the effects of thyroid-hormone-replacement medicines.

• Calcium channel blockers, Flecainide, Hydralazine, oral contraceptives, Propafenone, Haloperidol, phenothiazine tranquilizers (Molindone and others), quinolone antibacterials, and Quinidine may increase the amount of Acebutolol in the bloodstream and the effect of that drug on the body.

• Acebutolol should not be taken within 2 weeks of taking a monoamine oxidase (MAO) inhibitor antidepressant drug.

• Cimetidine increases the amount of Acebutolol absorbed into the bloodstream from oral tablets.

• Acebutolol may interfere with the effectiveness of Theophylline, Aminophylline, and some antiasthma drugs (especially Ephedrine and Isoproterenol).

• The combination of Acebutolol and Phenytoin or Digitalis drugs can result in excessive slowing of the heart, possibly causing heart block.

• If you stop smoking while taking Acebutolol, your dose may have to be reduced because your liver will break down the drug more slowly after you stop.

Food Interactions

Acebutolol may be taken without regard to food or meals.

Usual Dose

Adult: starting dose, 400 mg per day, taken all at once or in 2 divided doses. The daily dose may be gradually increased. Maintenance dose, 400 to 1200 mg per day.

Senior: older adults may respond to lower doses of this drug and should be treated more cautiously, beginning with 200 mg per day, increasing gradually to a maximum of 800 mg per day.

Overdosage

Symptoms of overdosage are changes in heartbeat (unusually slow, unusually fast, or irregular), severe dizziness or fainting, difficulty breathing, bluish-colored fingernails or palms, and seizures. The overdose victim should be taken to a hospital emergency room where proper therapy can be given. ALWAYS bring the medicine bottle with you.

Special Information

Acebutolol is meant to be taken continuously. Do not stop taking it unless directed to do so by your doctor; abrupt withdrawal may cause chest pain, difficulty breathing, increased sweating, and unusually fast or irregular heartbeat. The dose should be lowered gradually over a period of about 2 weeks.

Call your doctor at once if any of the following symptoms develop: back or joint pains, difficulty breathing, cold hands or feet, depression, skin rash, or changes in heartbeat. Acebutolol may produce an undesirable lowering of blood pressure, leading to dizziness or fainting. Call your doctor if this happens to you. Call your doctor about the following side effects only if they persist or are bothersome: anxiety, diarrhea, constipation, sexual impotence, headache, itching, nausea or vomiting, nightmares or vivid dreams, upset stomach, trouble sleeping, stuffy nose, frequent urination, unusual tiredness, or weakness.

Acebutolol can cause drowsiness, dizziness, lightheadedness, or blurred vision. Be careful when driving or performing complex tasks.

It is best to take your medicine at the same time each d~ If you forget a dose, take it as soon as you remem~

take your medicine once a day, and it is within 8 hours of your next dose, skip the forgotten tablet and continue with your regular schedule. If you take Acebutolol twice a day, and it is within 4 hours of your next dose, skip the missed dose and continue with your regular schedule. Do not take a double dose.

Special Populations

Pregnancy/Breast-feeding

Infants born to women who took a beta blocker weighed less at birth and had low blood pressure and reduced heart rate. Acebutolol should be avoided by pregnant women and those who might become pregnant while taking it. When the drug is considered essential by your doctor, its potential benefits must be carefully weighed against its risks.

Large amounts of Acebutolol pass into breast milk. Nursing mothers taking Acebutelol should bottle-feed their babies.

Seniors

Older adults may absorb and retain more Acebutolol, thus requiring less medicine to achieve the same results. Your doctor will need to adjust your dosage to meet your individual needs. Seniors taking this medicine may be more likely to suffer from cold hands and feet, reduced body temperature, chest pains, general feelings of ill health, sudden breathing difficulty, increased sweating, or changes in heartbeat.

Generic Name

Acetaminophen

Brand Names

Acephen	Arthritis Pain	Datril
Aceta	Formula,	Dolanex Elixir [S]
Anacin-3	Aspirin Free	Genapap
Anacin-3,	Aspirin Free Pain	Genapap,
Childrens [A]	Relief	Children's [A]
Anacin-3 Infants'	Banesin	Genapap Infants'
Drops [A]	Bromo Seltzer	Drops [A]
Apacet	Children's Feverall	Genebs
APAP	Dapa	Halenol

Halenol, [A]
 Children's [A]
Liquiprin
Liquiprin Infants'
 Drops [A]
Meda Cap/Tab
Myapap
Myapap
 Drops [S] [A]
Neopap
Oraphen-PD
Panadol
Panadol,
 Children's [S] [A]

Panadol Infants'
 Drops [S] [A]
Panex
Phenaphen
Sanplets-FR
 Granules
St Joseph Aspirin-
 Free Fever
 Reducer for
 Children [S] [A]
St Joseph Aspirin-
 Free Infant
 Drops [S] [A]

Suppap
Tapanol
Tempra
Tempra Drops [A]
Tempra Syrup [A]
Tylenol
Tylenol,
 Children's [A]
Tylenol Infants'
 Drops [A]
Uniserts

(Also available in generic form)

Type of Drug

Antipyretic and analgesic.

Prescribed for

Symptomatic relief of pain and fever for people who cannot or do not want to take Aspirin or a nonsteroidal anti-inflammatory drug (NSAID). Acetaminophen may be given to children about to receive a DTP vaccination to reduce the fever and pain that commonly follow the vaccination.

General Information

Acetaminophen is generally used to provide symptomatic relief from pain and fever associated with the common cold, flu, viral infections, or other disorders where pain or fever may occur. It is also used to relieve pain in people who are allergic to Aspirin, or those who cannot take Aspirin because of potential interactions with other drugs such as oral anticoagulants. It can be used to relieve pain from a variety of sources, including arthritis, headache, and tooth and periodontic pain, although it does not reduce inflammation.

Cautions and Warnings

Do not take Acetaminophen if you are **allergic** or **sensitive** to it. Do not take Acetaminophen for **more than 10 days** in a row unless directed by your doctor. Do not take more than is prescribed or recommended on the package.

Use this drug with extreme caution if you have **kidney or liver disease** or **viral infections of the liver**. Large amounts of alcohol increase the liver toxicity of large doses or overdoses of Acetaminophen. **Avoid alcohol** if you regularly use large doses of Acetaminophen.

Possible Side Effects

This drug is relatively free from side effects when taken in recommended doses. For this reason it has become extremely popular, especially among those who cannot take Aspirin.

▼ Rare: large doses or long-term use may cause liver damage, rash, itching, fever, lowered blood sugar, stimulation, yellowing of the skin or eyes, and/or a change in the composition of your blood.

Drug Interactions

• Acetaminophen's effects may be reduced by long-term use or large doses of barbiturate drugs, Carbamazepine, Phenytoin (and similar drugs), Rifampin, and Sulfinpyrazone. These drugs may also increase the chances of liver toxicity if taken with Acetaminophen.

• Alcoholic beverages increase the chances for liver toxicity and possible liver failure with Acetaminophen.

Food Interactions

Acetaminophen may be taken without regard to food.

Usual Dose

Adult and Adolescent (age 12 and older): 300 to 650 mg, 4 to 6 times per day, or 1000 mg, 3 or 4 times per day. Avoid taking more than 2.6 grams (8 325-mg tablets) per day for long periods of time.

Child (age 11): 480 mg, 4 to 5 times per day.

Child (age 9 to 10): 400 mg, 4 to 5 times per day.

Child (age 6 to 8): 320 mg, 4 to 5 times per day.
Child (age 4 to 5): 240 mg, 4 to 5 times per day.
Child (age 2 to 3): 160 mg, 4 to 5 times per day.
Child (age 1 to 2): 120 mg, 4 to 5 times per day.
Child (4 to 11 months): 80 mg, 4 to 5 times per day.
Child (birth to 3 months): 40 mg, 4 to 5 times per day.

Overdosage

Acute Acetaminophen overdose can cause nausea, vomiting, sweating, appetite loss, drowsiness, confusion, abdominal tenderness, low blood pressure, abnormal heart rhythms, yellowing of the skin and eyes, and liver and kidney failure. Liver damage has occurred after 12 extra-strength tablets or 18 regular-strength tablets, but most people need larger doses (20 extra-strength or 30 regular-strength tablets) to damage their livers. Regular use of large doses for long periods (i.e., 3000 to 4000 mg a day for a year) can also cause liver damage, especially if alcohol is involved. Acetaminophen overdose victims should be made to vomit as soon as possible by using Syrup of Ipecac (available at any pharmacy) or another method recommended by your poison control center. Then take the victim to a hospital emergency room for further evaluation and treatment. ALWAYS bring the medicine bottle.

Special Information

Unless abused, Acetaminophen is a beneficial, effective, and relatively nontoxic drug. Follow package directions and call your doctor if Acetaminophen does not work in 10 days for adults or 5 days for children.

Alcoholic beverages will worsen the liver damage that Acetaminophen can cause. People who take this medicine on a regular basis should limit their alcohol intake.

If you forget to take a dose of Acetaminophen, take it as soon as you remember. If it is within an hour of your next dose, skip the forgotten dose and continue with your regular schedule. Do not take a double dose.

Special Populations

Pregnancy/Breast-feeding

This drug is considered safe for use during pregnancy when taken in usual doses. Taking continuous high doses of the drug may cause birth defects or interfere with your baby's development. Three cases of congenital hip dislocation appear to have been associated with taking Acetaminophen. Check with your doctor before taking it if you are, or might be, pregnant.

Small amounts of Acetaminophen may pass into breast milk, but the drug is considered harmless to infants.

Seniors

Seniors may take Acetaminophen as directed by a doctor.

Acetaminophen with Codeine

see **Percocet**, page 877

Generic Name

Acetazolamide

Brand Names

Dazamide
Diamox
Diamox Sequels

(Also available in generic form)

Type of Drug

Carbonic-anhydrase inhibitor.

Prescribed for

Glaucoma and prevention or treatment of mountain sickness at high altitudes. This drug has also been used in treating epilepsy, including absence seizures, petit mal and grand mal epilepsy, tonic-clonic seizures, mixed seizures, and partial seizures.

General Information

Acetazolamide inhibits an enzyme in the body called *carbonic anhydrase.* This effect allows the drug to be used as a weak diuretic and as part of the treatment of glaucoma by helping to reduce pressure inside the eye. The same effect on carbonic anhydrase is thought to make Acetazolamide a useful drug in treating certain epileptic seizure disorders. The exact way in which the effect is produced is not understood.

Cautions and Warnings

Do not take Acetazolamide if you have serious **kidney, liver, or Addison's disease.** This drug should not be used by people with **low blood sodium** or **potassium.**

Possible Side Effects

Side effects of short-term Acetazolamide therapy are usually minimal.

▼ Most common: nausea or vomiting; tingling feeling in the arms, legs, lips, mouth, or anus; loss of appetite and weight loss; a metallic taste; increased frequency in urination (to be expected, since this drug has a weak diuretic effect); diarrhea; feelings of ill health; occasional drowsiness or weakness.

Since this drug is chemically considered to be a sulfa drug, it can have sulfa side effects, including rash, drug crystals in the urine, painful urination, low back pain, urinary difficulty, and low urine volumes.

▼ Rare: difficulty breathing, fever, sore throat, unusual bleeding or bruising, hives, itching, rash or sores, black or tarry stools, darkened urine, yellow skin or eyes, transient nearsightedness, clumsiness or unsteadiness, confusion, convulsions, ringing or buzzing in the ears, headache, sensitivity to bright light, increased blood sugar, weakness and trembling, nervousness, depression, dizziness, dry mouth, excessive thirst, abnormal heart rhythms, muscle cramps or pains, weak pulse, disorientation, muscle spasms, and loss of taste or smell.

Drug Interactions

• Avoid over-the-counter drug products that contain stimulants or anticholinergics, which tend to aggravate glaucoma or cardiac disease. Ask your pharmacist about ingredients contained in over-the-counter drugs.

• Acetazolamide may increase blood concentrations of Cyclosporine, used to prevent the rejection of transplanted organs and for other purposes.

• Acetazolamide may inhibit or delay the absorption of Primidone (for seizures) into the bloodstream.

• Avoid Aspirin while taking Acetazolamide, since Acetazolamide side effects can be enhanced by this combination.

• The combination of Diflunisal and Acetazolamide can result in an unusual lowering of eye pressure.

Food Interactions

Acetazolamide may be taken with food if it causes stomach upset. Because Acetazolamide can increase potassium loss, take this drug with foods that are rich in potassium, like apricots, bananas, orange juice, or raisins.

Usual Dose

250 mg to 1 gram per day, according to disease and patient's condition.

Overdosage

Symptoms of overdosage may include drowsiness, loss of appetite, nausea, vomiting, dizziness, tingling in the hands or feet, weakness, tremors, or ringing or buzzing in the ears. Overdose victims should be made to vomit as soon as possible with Syrup of Ipecac (available at any pharmacy), and taken to a hospital emergency room for further treatment. ALWAYS bring the medicine bottle.

Special Information

Acetazolamide may cause minor drowsiness and confusion, particularly during the first 2 weeks of therapy. Take care while performing tasks that require concentration, such as driving or operating appliances or machinery.

Call your doctor if you develop sore throat, fever, unusual bleeding or bruises, tingling in the hands or feet, rash, or unusual pains. These can be signs of drug side effects.

Acetazolamide can make you unusually sensitive to the sun. Avoid prolonged sun exposure and protect your eyes while taking this medicine.

If you forget a dose of Acetazolamide, take it as soon as you remember. If it is almost time for your next dose, skip the forgotten pill. Do not take a double dose.

Special Populations

Pregnancy/Breast-feeding
High doses of this drug may cause birth defects or interfere with your baby's development. Check with your doctor before taking it if you are, or might be, pregnant.

Small amounts of Acetazolamide may pass into breast milk, but it has not caused problems in breast-fed infants.

Seniors
Older adults are more likely to have age-related problems that could lead to problems with Acetazolamide. Take this medication according to your doctor's prescription.

Generic Name

Acyclovir

Brand Name

Zovirax Tablets/Capsules/Ointment/Suspension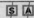

Type of Drug

Antiviral.

Prescribed for

Treatment and prevention of serious, frequently recurring herpes simplex infections of the genitals, mucous membrane tissues, and central nervous system. It also works against shingles (herpes zoster) and chickenpox (varicella). Other viral infections for which Acyclovir may be prescribed are nongenital herpes simplex infections, herpes simplex and cytomegalovirus (CMV) infections in immunocompromised patients, and varicella pneumonia.

General Information

Acyclovir is the only oral drug that can reduce the rate of growth of the herpes virus and its relatives, Epstein-Barr virus, CMV, and varicella. Both oral Acyclovir and oral Ganciclovir work against CMV; other drugs, given by intravenous injection, may be used for these infections, but they are usually reserved for patients with AIDS or cancer, or other immunocompromised patients. Acyclovir does not cure herpes, but it can reduce pain associated with the disease and may help herpes sores heal faster. It may also reduce the rate at which new herpes lesions form. Acyclovir does not affect common-cold viruses.

Acyclovir is selectively absorbed into cells that are infected with the herpes simplex virus. There, it is converted into its active form and works by interfering with the reproduction of viral DNA, slowing the growth of existing viruses. It has little effect on treating recurrent infections. The drug must be given by intravenous injection in a hospital or doctor's office or by mouth to treat both local and systemic symptoms. Local symptoms can be treated with the ointment alone. The capsules can be taken every day to reduce the number and severity of herpes attacks in people who usually suffer 10 or more attacks a year, and may be used to treat intermittent attacks as they occur, but the drug must be started as soon as possible to have the greatest effect.

Cautions and Warnings

Acyclovir ointment should not be applied to your skin if you have had an **allergic** reaction to it or to the major component of the ointment base, Polyethylene Glycol. Acyclovir ointment should not be used to treat a **herpes infection of the eye** because it is not specifically made for that purpose. Some people develop **tenderness, swelling,** or **bleeding** of the **gums** while taking Acyclovir. Regular brushing, flossing, and gum massage may help prevent these conditions.

Long-term high doses of Acyclovir have caused reduced sperm count in animals, but this effect has not yet been reported in men.

Do not apply inside the vagina because the Polyethylene ꞏꞏ꞉col base can irritate and cause swelling of those sensitive ꞏꞏꞏs.

Possible Side Effects

Ointment Form

▼ Most common: mild burning, irritation, rash, and itching. Women are 4 times more likely to experience burning than men, and it is more likely to occur when applied during an initial herpes attack than during a recurrent attack.

Tablets/Capsules/Suspension

▼ Most common: dizziness, headache, diarrhea, nausea, and vomiting.

▼ Less common: loss of appetite, stomach gas, constipation, fatigue, rash, feelings of ill health, leg pains, sore throat, a bad taste in the mouth, sleeplessness, and fever.

▼ Other: aching joints, weakness, and tingling in the hands or feet.

Intravenous Form

▼ Other: pain or inflammation at the injection site, liver inflammation, confusion, hallucinations, tremors, agitation, seizures, coma, anemia, kidney damage, blood in the urine, pain or pressure on urination, loss of bladder control, abdominal pains, fluid in the lungs, and fingertips turning blue.

Drug Interactions

• Do not apply Acyclovir together with any other ointment or topical medicine.

• Oral Probenecid may decrease the elimination of Acyclovir from your body, which increases Acyclovir's blood levels when it is taken by mouth or by injection, and thus increases the chance of side effects.

• Taking Acyclovir and Zidovudine (AZT) together may lead to severe drowsiness and lethargy.

Food Interactions

Acyclovir may be taken with food if it upsets your stomach.

Usual Dose

Tablets/Capsules/Suspension

For maximum benefit, treatment should be started as soon as possible. If you have kidney disease, your doctor should adjust your dose according to the degree of functional loss.

Adult: For a genital herpes attack: 200 mg every 4 hours, 5 times per day for 10 days. For recurrent infections: 400 mg twice a day or 200 mg 2 to 5 times per day. As suppressive therapy for people who suffer from chronic herpes infection: 400 to 800 mg per day, every day. For herpes zoster infections: 800 mg, 5 times per day for 7 to 10 days.

Child: Acyclovir is not recommended in children under age 2, but it has been given to children in daily doses as high as 36 mg per pound of body weight without any unusual side effects.

Ointment

Apply the ointment every 3 hours, 6 times per day for 7 days; apply enough to cover all visible lesions. About 1/2 inch of Acyclovir ointment should cover about 4 square inches of skin lesions. Your doctor may prescribe a longer course of treatment to prevent the delayed formation of new lesions during the duration of an attack.

Overdosage

Acyclovir overdose is likely to lead to kidney damage due to the deposition of drug crystals in the kidney. Divided oral doses of up to 4.8 grams per day for 5 days have been taken without serious adverse effects.

The chance of experiencing toxic side effects from swallowing Acyclovir ointment is quite small because there are only 50 mg of drug per gram of ointment.

Observe the overdose victim for side effects and call your poison control center for more detailed information.

Special Information

Women with genital herpes have an increased risk of cervical cancer. Check with your doctor about the need for an annual Pap smear.

Use a finger cot or rubber glove when applying the ointment to protect against inadvertently spreading the virus. Be sure to apply the medicine exactly as directed and to completely cover all lesions. If you skip several doses or a day or more of treatment, the therapy will not exert its maximum effect. Keep affected areas clean and dry. Loose-fitting clothing will help to avoid irritation of a healing herpes lesion.

Herpes can be transmitted even if you do not have symptoms of active disease. To avoid transmitting the condition to a sex partner, do not have intercourse while visible herpes lesions are present. A condom offers some protection against transmission of the virus, but spermicidal products and diaphragms will not. Acyclovir alone also does not protect against spreading the herpes virus.

Call your doctor if the drug does not relieve your condition, if side effects become severe or intolerable, or if you become pregnant or want to begin breast-feeding. Check with your dentist if you notice swelling or tenderness of the gums.

Special Populations

Pregnancy/Breast-feeding
Acyclovir crosses into the circulation of a developing fetus. Very small amounts of the drug are absorbed into the blood after application of the ointment. Animal studies have shown that large doses (up to 125 times the human dose) cause damage to both mother and developing fetus. While there is no information to indicate that Acyclovir affects a developing fetus, you should not use it during pregnancy unless it is specifically prescribed by your doctor and the possible benefit outweighs the possible risk of taking it.

Acyclovir passes into breast milk in concentrations up to 4 times the concentration in blood, and it has been found in the urine of a nursing infant. No drug side effects have been found in nursing babies, but mothers who must take this drug should consider bottle-feeding their infants.

Seniors
People over 50 years of age with shingles tend to have more severe attacks of shingles and may benefit more from Acyclovir treatment if the medicine is started within 48 to 72 hours of the appearance of the first rash. Seniors with reduced kidney function should be given a lower oral dose than younger adults to account for normal reductions in kidney function that occur with aging.

Adalat CC

*see **Nifedipine**, page 794*

Generic Name

Albuterol

Brand Names

Proventil Syrup ⑤/Inhalation Aerosol and Solution Ⓐ/
   Repetabs/Tablets
Ventolin Syrup ⑤/Inhalation Aerosol and Solution Ⓐ/
   Tablets

(Also available in generic form)

Type of Drug

Bronchodilator.

Prescribed for

Asthma and bronchial spasms.

General Information

Albuterol is similar to other bronchodilator drugs, such as
Metaproterenol and Isoetharine, but it has a weaker effect on
nerve receptors in the heart and blood vessels; therefore, it is
somewhat safer for people with heart conditions.

   Albuterol tablets and syrup begin to work within 30 minutes and continue working for up to 8 hours. There is also a
long-acting tablet preparation (Repetabs) that continues to
work for up to 12 hours. Albuterol inhalation begins working
within 5 minutes and continues for 3 to 8 hours.

Cautions and Warnings

Albuterol should be used with caution by people with a
history of **angina** (chest tightness/pain), **heart disease, high**
pressure, stroke or **seizure, diabetes, thyroid disease,**
ease, or **glaucoma.** Excessive use of Albuterol

inhalants can lead to **worsening of asthmatic** or other **respiratory conditions,** and can lead to increased breathing difficulty, instead of providing breathing relief. In the most extreme cases, people have had heart attacks after using excessive amounts of inhalant.

Animal studies with Albuterol have revealed a significant increase in certain kinds of tumors.

Possible Side Effects

Albuterol's side effects are similar to those of other bronchodilators, except that its effects on the heart and blood vessels are not as pronounced.

▼ Most common: restlessness, weakness, anxiety, fear, tension, sleeplessness, tremors, convulsions, dizziness, headache, flushing, appetite changes, pallor, sweating, nausea, vomiting, and muscle cramps.

▼ Less common: angina, abnormal heart rhythms, rapid heartbeat and heart palpitations, high blood pressure, feelings of ill health, irritability and emotional instability, nightmares, aggressive behavior, bronchitis, stuffed nose, nosebleeds, increased sputum, conjunctivitis ("pink-eye"), tooth discoloration, voice changes, hoarseness, and urinary difficulty.

Drug Interactions

• Albuterol's effects may be increased by monoamine oxidase (MAO) inhibitor drugs, tricyclic antidepressants, thyroid drugs, other bronchodilator drugs, and some antihistamines.

• The chance of cardiotoxicity may be increased in people taking Albuterol and Theophylline. Albuterol is antagonized by beta-blocking drugs (Propranolol and others). Albuterol may antagonize the effects of blood-pressure-lowering drugs, especially Reserpine, Methyldopa, and Guanethidine.

• Albuterol may reduce the amount of Digoxin in the blood of people taking both drugs. This could result in the need to adjust the Digoxin dose.

Food Interactions

Albuterol tablets are more effective when taken on an empty

stomach, or 1 hour before or 2 hours after meals, but can be taken with food if they upset your stomach. Do not inhale Albuterol if you have food or anything else in your mouth.

Usual Dose

Inhalation Aerosol
Adult and Adolescent (age 12 and older) (for Ventolin, Adult and Child age 4 and older): 1 or 2 puffs every 4 to 6 hours (each puff delivers 90 micrograms of Albuterol). Asthma brought on by exercise may be prevented by taking 2 puffs 15 minutes before exercising.

Inhalation Solution
Adult and Adolescent (age 12 and older): 2.5 mg 3 or 4 times per day. (Dilute 0.5 milliliters of the 0.5% solution with 2.5 milliliters of sterile saline.) Deliver over 5 to 15 minutes by nebulizer.

Inhalation Capsules
Adult and Child (age 4 and older): 200 to 400 micrograms inhaled every 4 to 6 hours using a special Rotahaler device. Adults and adolescents (age 12 and over) may prevent asthma brought on by exercise by inhaling a single 200-microgram dose 15 minutes before exercising.

Tablets
Adult and Adolescent (age 12 and older): 6 to 16 mg per day in divided doses to start; the dosage may be slowly increased until the asthma is controlled to a maximum of 32 mg per day.

Senior: 6 to 8 mg per day in divided doses to start, but increase to the maximum daily adult dosage, if tolerated.

Child (age 6 to 14 years): 6 to 8 mg a day in divided doses to start, up to a maximum daily dose of 24 mg.

Child (age 2 to 5 years): up to 4 mg, 3 times per day.

Extended-Release Tablets
Adult and Adolescent (age 12 and older): 4 to 8 mg every 12 hours. Dosage may be cautiously increased to a maximum of 32 mg a day. People being switched from regular to extended-release tablets generally take the same amount per day, but in fewer tablets, i.e., one 4-mg tablet every 12 hours (1 dose) instead of a 2-mg tablet every 6 hours (2 doses).

Overdosage

Overdose of Albuterol inhalation usually results in exaggerated side effects, including heart pains and high blood pressure, although the pressure may drop to a low level after a short period of elevation. People who inhale too much Albuterol should see a doctor, who may prescribe a beta-blocking drug (such as Metoprolol or Atenolol) to counteract the overdose effect.

Overdose of Albuterol tablets is more likely to lead to side effects: changes in heart rate, palpitations, unusual heart rhythms, heart pains, high blood pressure, fever, chills, cold sweats, nausea, vomiting, and dilation of the pupils. Convulsions, sleeplessness, anxiety, and tremors may also develop, and the victim may collapse.

If the overdose was taken within the past half hour, give the victim Syrup of Ipecac to induce vomiting. DO NOT GIVE SYRUP OF IPECAC IF THE VICTIM IS UNCONSCIOUS OR CONVULSING. If symptoms have begun to develop, the victim may need to be taken to a hospital emergency room (call for instructions). ALWAYS bring the prescription bottle.

Special Information

If you are inhaling Albuterol, be sure to follow the inhalation instructions that come with the product. The drug should be inhaled during the second half of your breath, allowing it to reach deeper into your lungs. Wait about 5 minutes between puffs, if you use more than 1 puff per dose.

Do not take more Albuterol than prescribed by your doctor. Taking more than you need could actually worsen your symptoms. If your condition worsens rather than improves after taking your dose, stop taking it and call your doctor at once.

Call your doctor immediately if you develop chest pains, palpitations, rapid heartbeat, muscle tremors, dizziness, headache, facial flushing, or urinary difficulty, or if you continue having breathing difficulty after taking the medicine.

If a dose of Albuterol is forgotten, take it as soon as you remember. If it is almost time for your next dose, skip the forgotten one. Do not take a double dose.

Special Populations

Pregnancy/Breast-feeding

When used during labor and delivery, Albuterol can slow or

delay natural labor. It can cause rapid heartbeat and high blood sugar in the mother and rapid heartbeat and low blood sugar in the baby.

It is not known if Albuterol causes birth defects in humans, but it has caused birth defects in animal studies. When it is deemed essential, the potential risks of taking Albuterol must be carefully weighed against any potential benefits.

It is not known if Albuterol passes into breast milk. Nursing mothers must look for any possible drug effect on their infants if taking this medication. You may want to consider bottle-feeding your infant.

Seniors
Older adults are more sensitive to the effects of Albuterol. Closely follow your doctor's directions and report any side effects at once.

Generic Name
Alendronate Sodium

Brand Name
Fosamax

Type of Drug
Biphosphonate.

Prescribed for
Osteoporosis (bone calcium depletion) in women who have gone through menopause. Alendronate is also used for Paget's disease of bone.

General Information
Alendronate is one of a group of drugs that has been used for many years to treat a variety of conditions in which bone mass (mostly calcium) is reabsorbed by the body. Alendronate is the first to be reviewed and approved specifically for osteoporosis, but Etidronate, another biphosphonate, has been used for this purpose for some time. Osteoporosis leads to weak and brittle bones in people who are affected by it.

After menopause, women lose their natural supply of estrogen, which provides a number of important benefits, including protection against osteoporosis. Biphosphonate drugs interfere with both normal and abnormal processes of bone resorption by a mechanism that is not well understood.

Cautions and Warnings

Do not use Alendronate if you are sensitive or allergic to it. People with **severe kidney disease** should not take Alendronate. People with active gastrointestinal disease such as **swallowing difficulty, ulcers,** and **stomach irritation** should use this drug with caution because of the chance that it could worsen the condition. It is not known if **men with osteoporosis** will benefit from taking Alendronate.

Possible Side Effects

The side effects of Alendronate are generally mild and are rarely serious enough to force people to stop taking the drug.

▼ Most common: abdominal pain and discomfort, upset stomach, nausea, breathing difficulty, constipation, diarrhea, stomach gas, and ulcers.

▼ Less common: swallowing difficulty, muscle pain, and headache.

▼ Rare: changes in taste perception and vomiting.

Drug Interactions

• Antacids, Calcium supplements, and some other oral medicines can interfere with the absorption of Alendronate into the blood. Separate doses of Alendronate from all other medicines by at least 30 minutes.

• Mixing aspirin, nonsteroidal anti-inflammatory drugs (NSAIDs) or other anti-inflammatory drugs with Alendronate can increase your chances of developing stomach or intestinal side effects.

Food Interactions

Food and drink (even mineral water, orange juice, and coffee) interfere with the absorption of Alendronate into the blood. Take this medicine at least 30 minutes before having any food or drink. Alendronate should be taken only with plain water.

Usual Dose

Adult: 10 to 40 mg a day.
Child: not recommended.

Overdosage

Very large doses of Alendronate are lethal to lab animals, but there is no experience with human overdose. The likely symptoms of Alendronate overdose are upset stomach, heartburn, irritation of the esophagus, ulcer, and very low blood-calcium and -phosphate levels. Taking milk or antacids will bind any Alendronate remaining in the stomach. Overdose victims should be taken to a hospital emergency room for treatment. ALWAYS bring the medicine bottle with you.

Special Information

Take Alendronate with plain water in the morning before any food, drink, or other medicine, and avoid lying down after you have taken your medicine. You must wait at least 30 minutes between taking Alendronate and anything else for the drug to be absorbed, but the longer you wait, the more drug will be absorbed into the blood.

Exercise, Calcium, and vitamin D contribute to the health of your bones. Your doctor will provide a treatment plan, but remember to take any other medicines at least 30 minutes after your Alendronate.

If you forget a dose of Alendronate, take it as soon as you remember. If it is almost time for your next dose, skip the forgotten dose and continue with your regular schedule. Remember, if you do forget your morning dose and take one later in the day, you must have an empty stomach (wait at least 2 hours after eating **anything** and then wait at least 30 minutes after Alendronate before taking any other medicines or food).

Special Populations

Pregnancy/Breast-feeding

Alendronate is not likely to be used by women who are

pregnant or nursing, because osteoporosis is common only after menopause. Alendronate affected bone formation in developing animal fetuses and was toxic to pregnant animals in laboratory studies. Pregnant women should take Alendronate only if the possible benefit outweighs its risks.

It is not known if Alendronate passes into breast milk. Since Alendronate affects bone formation, nursing mothers who must take this drug should bottle-feed their babies.

Seniors

Alendronate has been studied extensively in older adults. Seniors took the drug during its study phase without any unusual adverse effect.

Generic Name

Allopurinol

Brand Name

Zyloprim

(Also available in generic form)

Type of Drug

Antigout medication.

Prescribed for

Gout or gouty arthritis. Allopurinol is also useful for cancer and conditions that may be associated with too much uric acid in the body. Some studies have indicated that Allopurinol mixed into a mouthwash has been helpful for people taking Fluorouracil, an antineoplastic drug, in the prevention of ulcers of the mouth, stomach, and intestines.

General Information

Unlike other antigout drugs, which affect the elimination of uric acid from the body, Allopurinol acts on the system that manufactures uric acid in your body.

A high blood level of uric acid can mean that you have gout or that you have one of many other diseases, including various cancers and malignancies, or psoriasis. High uric acid levels can also be caused by taking some drugs, including diuretic medicines. However, a high blood level of uric acid does not point to a specific disease.

Cautions and Warnings

Do not take this medication if you have ever developed a **severe reaction** to it. If you develop a **rash** or any other **adverse effects** while taking Allopurinol, stop taking the medication immediately and contact your doctor.

Allopurinol should be used by **children** only if they have high uric acid levels due to neoplastic disease or very rare metabolic conditions where Allopurinol may be needed to correct the problem.

A few cases of **liver toxicity** have been associated with Allopurinol; they improved when the drug was stopped. Periodic liver and kidney tests should be performed while taking this medicine. People with severely **compromised kidney function** should take a reduced dose of this medicine.

Possible Side Effects

▼ Most common: rash, which has been associated with severe, allergic, or sensitivity reactions to Allopurinol. If you develop an unusual rash or other sign of drug toxicity, stop taking this medication and contact your doctor.

▼ Less common: nausea, vomiting, diarrhea, intermittent stomach pains, effects on blood components, and drowsiness or lack of ability to concentrate.

▼ Rare: effects on the eyes, loss of hair, fever, chills, difficulty breathing or asthma-like symptoms, arthritis-like symptoms, itching, loosening of the fingernails, pain in the lower back, unexplained nosebleeds, cataracts, conjunctivitis and other eye conditions, numbness, tingling or pain in the hands or feet, confusion, dizziness, fainting, depression, memory loss, ringing or buzzing in the ears, weakness, sleeplessness, and feelings of ill health.

Drug Interactions

- Large doses of drugs that make your urine more acid, like megadoses of vitamin C, may increase the possibility of kidney stone formation.
- Alcohol, Diazoxide, Mecamylamine, or Pyrazinamide can increase the amount of uric acid in your blood, requiring a possible increase in your Allopurinol dose.
- Allopurinol may increase the action of Azathioprine, Mercaptopurine, or Cyclophosphamide and other anticancer medicines, leading to possible bleeding or infection.
- Taking Allopurinol together with Dacarbazine, Probenecid, or Sulfinpyrazone may cause additive reductions in uric acid.
- Allopurinol may interact with anticoagulant (blood-thinning) medications, reducing the rate at which the antico-agulant is broken down in the body. Dosage reduction is necessary.
- Allopurinol can reduce the breakdown of Chlorpropa-mide (for diabetes), causing an increase in antidiabetic effect. Dosage adjustment may be necessary.
- People who are susceptible to Ampicillin, Amoxicillin, Bacampicillin, or Hetacillin rash are more likely to have that problem while also taking Allopurinol.
- Taking a thiazide diuretic with Allopurinol increases the chances of a drug-sensitivity reaction.
- Using Vidarabine and Allopurinol together can increase the risk of neurotoxic effects and anemia, nausea, pain, and itching.
- Large doses of Allopurinol (more than 600 mg per day) may increase the effects of and chances for toxic reactions to Theophylline by interfering with its clearance from the body.

Food Interactions

Take each dose with food or a full glass of water and drink 10 to 12 8-ounce glasses of water, juices, soda, or other liquids each day to avoid the formation of crystals in your urine and/or kidneys.

Usual Dose

Adult and Adolescent (age 11 and older): 100 to 800 mg per day, depending on disease and response.

Child (age 6 to 10): 300 to 600 mg per day.

Child (under age 6): 150 mg per day.

The dose should be reviewed periodically by your doctor to be sure that it is producing the desired therapeutic effect.

Overdosage

The expected symptoms of overdose are exaggerated side effects. Allopurinol overdose victims should be taken to a hospital. ALWAYS bring the medicine bottle.

Special Information

Allopurinol can make you drowsy or make it difficult for you to concentrate: Take care while driving a car or operating hazardous equipment.

Call your doctor at once if you develop rash, hives, itching, chills, fever, nausea, muscle aches, unusual tiredness, fever, yellowing of the eyes or skin, painful urination, blood in the urine, irritation of the eyes, or swelling of the lips and/or mouth.

Avoid large doses of vitamin C, which can cause the formation of kidney stones while you are taking this medicine. You should drink a lot of water (10 to 12 8-ounce glasses a day) while taking Allopurinol.

If you forget to take your regular dose of Allopurinol, take the missed dose as soon as possible. If it is time for your next regular dose, double this dose. For example, if your regular dose is 100 mg and you miss a dose, take 200 mg at the next usual dose time.

Special Populations

Pregnancy/Breast-feeding

This drug may cause birth defects or interfere with your baby's development. Check with your doctor before taking it if you are, or might be, pregnant.

A nursing mother should not take this medication, since it will pass through the mother's milk to the child.

Seniors

No special precautions are required. Be sure to follow your doctor's directions and report any side effects at once.

Generic Name

Alprazolam

Brand Name

Xanax

(Also available in generic form)

Type of Drug

Benzodiazepine tranquilizer.

Prescribed for

Relief of symptoms of anxiety, tension, fatigue, and agitation. Also prescribed for irritable bowel syndrome, panic attacks, depression, and premenstrual syndrome (PMS).

General Information

Alprazolam is a member of a group of drugs known as *benzodiazepines*, which work as either antianxiety agents, anticonvulsants, or sedatives. Benzodiazepines directly affect the brain. In doing so, they can relax you and make you either more tranquil or sleepier, or can slow nervous-system transmissions in such a way as to act as an anticonvulsant, depending on which drug you use and how much you take. Many doctors prefer benzodiazepines to other drugs that can be used for similar effects because they tend to be safer, have fewer side effects, and are usually as, if not more, effective.

Cautions and Warnings

Do not take Alprazolam if you know you are **sensitive** or **allergic** to it or another benzodiazepine drug, including Clonazepam.

Alprazolam can aggravate **narrow-angle glaucoma**. However, if you have open-angle glaucoma, you may take it. Check with your doctor.

Other **conditions where Alprazolam should be avoided** are severe depression, severe lung disease, sleep apnea (intermittent breathing during sleep), liver disease, drunkenness, and kidney disease. In all of these conditions, the depressive effects of Alprazolam may be enhanced and/or could be detrimental to your overall condition.

Alprazolam should **not be taken by psychotic patients,** because it doesn't work for those people and can cause unusual excitement, stimulation, and rage in them.

Alprazolam is **not meant to be used for more than 3 to 4 months in a row.** Your condition should be reassessed before continuing your medicine beyond that time.

Alprazolam **may be addictive,** and you can experience drug withdrawal symptoms if you suddenly stop taking your medicine after as little as 4 to 6 weeks of treatment. Withdrawal symptoms are more likely if this drug is taken for long periods. Withdrawal generally begins with increased feelings of anxiety, and continues with tingling in the extremities, sensitivity to bright lights or the sun, long periods of sleep or sleeplessness, a metallic taste, flulike illness, fatigue, difficulty concentrating, restlessness, loss of appetite, nausea, irritability, headache, dizziness, sweating, muscle tension or cramps, tremors, and feeling uncomfortable or ill at ease. Other major withdrawal symptoms include confusion, abnormal perception of movement, depersonalization, paranoid delusions, hallucinations, psychotic reactions, muscle twitching, seizures, and memory loss.

Possible Side Effects

Weakness and confusion may occur, especially in seniors and those who are more sickly.

▼ Most common: mild drowsiness during the first few days of therapy.

▼ Less common: depression, lethargy, disorientation, headache, inactivity, slurred speech, stupor, dizziness, tremors, constipation, dry mouth, nausea, inability to control urination, sexual difficulties, irregular menstrual cycle, changes in heart rhythm, lowered blood pressure, fluid retention, blurred or double vision, itching, rash, hiccups, nervousness, inability to fall asleep, and occasional liver dysfunction. If you experience any of these symptoms, stop taking the medicine and contact your doctor immediately.

▼ Rare: diarrhea, coated tongue, sore gums, vomiting,

Possible Side Effects *(continued)*

appetite changes, swallowing difficulty, increased salivation, upset stomach, incontinence, changes in sex drive,
urinary difficulties, changes in heart rate, palpitations,
swelling, stuffy nose, hearing difficulty, hair loss or gain,
sweating, fever, tingling in the hands or feet, breast pain,
muscle disturbances, breathing difficulty, changes in the
components of your blood, and joint pain.

Drug Interactions

• Alprazolam is a central-nervous-system depressant. Avoid
alcohol, other tranquilizers, narcotics, barbiturates, monoamine oxidase (MAO) inhibitors, antihistamines, and antidepressants. Taking Alprazolam with these drugs may result
in excessive depression, tiredness, sleepiness, difficulty breathing, or similar symptoms.

• Smoking may reduce the effectiveness of Alprazolam by
increasing the rate at which it is broken down by the body.

• The effects of Alprazolam may be prolonged when it is
taken together with Cimetidine, oral contraceptives, Disulfiram,
Fluoxetine, Isoniazid, Ketoconazole, Metoprolol, Probenecid,
Propoxyphene, Propranolol, Rifampin, or Valproic Acid.

• Theophylline may reduce Alprazolam's sedative effects.

• If you take antacids, separate them from your Alprazolam
dose by at least 1 hour to prevent them from interfering with
the absorption of Alprazolam into the bloodstream.

• Alprazolam may increase blood levels of Digoxin and the
chances for Digoxin toxicity.

• The effect of Levodopa may be decreased if it is taken
together with Alprazolam.

• Phenytoin blood concentrations may be increased if taken
with Alprazolam, resulting in possible Phenytoin toxicity.

Food Interactions

Alprazolam is best taken on an empty stomach but may be
taken with food if it upsets your stomach.

Usual Dose

Adult: 0.75 to 4 mg per day. The dose must be tailored to

your individual needs. Debilitated people will require less of the drug to control anxiety or tension.

Child: not recommended.

Overdosage

Symptoms of overdosage are confusion, sleepiness, poor coordination, lack of response to pain (such as a pin stick), loss of reflexes, shallow breathing, low blood pressure, and coma. The victim should be taken to a hospital emergency room. ALWAYS bring the medicine bottle with you.

Special Information

Alprazolam can cause tiredness, drowsiness, inability to concentrate, or similar symptoms. Be careful if you are driving, operating machinery, or performing other activities that require concentration.

Anyone taking Alprazolam for more than 3 or 4 months at a time may develop drug-withdrawal reactions if the medication is stopped suddenly (see *Cautions and Warnings*).

If you forget a dose of Alprazolam, take it as soon as you remember. If it is almost time for your next dose, skip the forgotten pill and continue with your regular schedule. Do not take a double dose.

Special Populations

Pregnancy/Breast-feeding

Alprazolam may cross into the developing fetal circulation and may cause birth defects if taken during the first 3 months of pregnancy. You should avoid Alprazolam while pregnant.

Alprazolam may pass into breast milk. Since infants break the drug down more slowly than adults, it is possible for it to accumulate and have an undesired effect. Tell your doctor if you become pregnant or are nursing an infant.

Seniors

Older adults, especially those with liver or kidney disease, are more sensitive to the effects of Alprazolam and generally require smaller doses to achieve the same effect. Follow your doctor's directions, and report any side effects at once.

Generic Name

Amantadine

Brand Name

Symmetrel

(Also available in generic form)

Type of Drug

Antiviral, antiparkinsonian.

Prescribed for

Prevention and treatment of some flu viruses; all varieties of
Parkinson's disease; uncontrolled muscle movements that
can be caused by phenothiazines and other psychoactive
drugs. Amantadine has also been used to treat fatigue associated with multiple sclerosis.

General Information

Amantadine appears to prevent the release of the infectious
part of some flu viruses into body cells and may also interfere
with the penetration of the virus into body cells, but its action
is not entirely known. It is 70 to 90 percent effective in preventing type A flu and reduces flu symptoms when taken
within 2 days after you get sick with type A flu. Amantadine
does not work for type B flu.

In Parkinson's disease, Amantadine has been shown to
increase the amount of dopamine released in the brain from
intact storage areas.

Cautions and Warnings

Do not take Amantadine if you are **sensitive** or **allergic** to it.
People with a history of **epilepsy** may experience increased
seizure activity. People have developed heart failure while
taking Amantadine; those who already have **heart failure**
should be carefully watched for signs that the disease is
worsening.

Amantadine is released unmetabolized from the body
through your kidneys. People with **kidney disease** must
receive lower doses.

Caution is also necessary in people with **liver disease**, a history of recurrent **eczema**, or **psychosis** or severe **psychoneurosis** not controlled by drug treatments.

Possible Side Effects

▼ Most common: nausea, dizziness, light-headedness, and sleeplessness.

▼ Less common: depression; anxiety; irritability; hallucinations; confusion; appetite loss; dry mouth; constipation; weakness; blue or purple discoloration of the skin (goes away 2 to 12 weeks after you stop taking the medicine); swelling in the arms, legs, or ankles; dizziness when rising suddenly from a sitting or lying position; low blood pressure; and headache.

▼ Infrequent: heart failure, psychotic reactions, urinary difficulty, breathing difficulty, fatigue, skin rash, vomiting, weakness, slurred speech, and visual disturbances.

▼ Rare: convulsions, increased white-blood-cell counts, eczema-type rash, and spasms of the eye muscles leading to uncontrollable rolling and movement of the eyes.

Drug Interactions

• Combining Amantadine with anticholinergic drugs like Benztropine produces increased drug side effects. Altering the dose of either drug will take care of this problem.

• Hydrochlorothiazide/Triamterene (a diuretic combination) interferes with Amantadine elimination through the kidneys.

• Alcohol may worsen some of the side effects of Amantadine, interfering with your ability to drive or concentrate.

Food Interactions

This drug may be taken without regard to food or meals.

Usual Dose

Adult and Child (age 10 and older): 100 to 300 mg daily.

Child (age 1 to 9): 2 to 4 mg per pound per day, up to 150 mg.

Senior (age 65 and older): 100 mg per day.

Overdosage

Symptoms are nausea, vomiting, appetite loss and nervous system side effects (excitability, tremors, weakness, tiredness, blurred vision, slurred speech, and convulsions). Possibly fatal abnormal heart rhythms can also occur with large doses. One person died after taking 2500 mg of Amantadine. Overdose victims should be taken to a hospital emergency room for treatment at once. ALWAYS bring the medicine bottle with you.

Special Information

Be careful while driving or operating any complex or hazardous equipment; avoid alcoholic beverages while taking this medicine.

Call your doctor *immediately* if any of the following occur: fainting; dizziness or light-headedness; visual difficulties; mood changes; swelling of the arms, legs, or ankles; or any other unusual or intolerable side effect.

Dry mouth, nose, or throat can be easily relieved with candy or gum. A stool softener (for example, Docusate) will usually relieve constipation. Dry mouth also leads to tooth and gum disease. Maintain good oral hygiene to prevent cavities and gum disease while taking Amantadine.

People taking Amantadine for Parkinson's disease may not see any effect for at least 2 weeks.

It is important to take Amantadine as your doctor has prescribed. If you are taking Amantadine syrup, be sure to use the measuring spoon supplied with your prescription.

If you forget to take a dose of Amantadine, take it as soon as possible. If it is almost time for your next dose, skip the missed dose and go back to your regular schedule. Do not take a double dose.

Special Populations

Pregnancy/Breast-feeding

In high doses, Amantadine can be toxic and cause malformations in animal fetuses. A cardiovascular malformation was reported in one infant exposed to this drug during the first 3 months of pregnancy. Pregnant women should take this drug only if it is absolutely necessary and all of the possible risks have been reviewed with their doctors.

Amantadine passes into breast milk. Since Amantadine may cause side effects in infants, nursing mothers should bottle-feed their babies.

Seniors

Older adults require dosage reduction because of normal losses of kidney function. Healthy people age 65 and older should receive half the dose prescribed for younger adults.

Ambien

see **Zolpidem**, page 1195

Generic Name

Amiodarone

Brand Name

Cordarone

Type of Drug

Antiarrhythmic.

Prescribed for

Abnormal heart rhythms.

General Information

Amiodarone should be prescribed only in situations where the abnormal rhythm is so severe as to be life-threatening and does not respond to other drug treatments. Amiodarone works by decreasing the sensitivity of heart tissue to nervous impulses within the heart. It has not been proven that people taking this drug will live longer than those with similar conditions who do not take it.

Amiodarone may exert its effects 2 to 5 days after you start taking it, but often takes 1 to 3 weeks to affect your heart.

Since Amiodarone therapy is often started while you are in the hospital, especially if you are being switched from another antiarrhythmic drug to Amiodarone, your doctor will be able to closely monitor how well the drug is working for you. Amiodarone's antiarrhythmic effects can persist for weeks or months after you stop taking it.

Cautions and Warnings

Do not take Amiodarone if you are **allergic** or **sensitive** to it or if you have **heart block**.

Amiodarone can cause potentially fatal drug side effects. At high doses, 10 percent or more of people taking this drug can develop **lung and respiratory effects**, beginning with cough and progressive difficulty breathing, that have the potential of being fatal. **Liver damage** caused by Amiodarone is usually mild. In rare cases, Amiodarone has been associated with liver failure that resulted in death.

Amiodarone can cause heart block, a drastic slowing of electrical impulse movement between major areas of the heart, or extreme slowing of the heart rate. Amiodarone heart block occurs about as often as heart block caused by some other antiarrhythmic drugs, but its effects may last longer than those of the other drugs. Amiodarone can also worsen existing **abnormal heart rhythms** in 2 to 5 percent of people who take the drug.

Most adults who take Amiodarone for 6 months or more develop tiny **deposits** in the **corneas** of their eyes. These deposits may cause blurred vision or halos in up to 10 percent of people taking Amiodarone. Some people develop **dry eyes** and **sensitivity to bright light**.

One-tenth of people taking Amiodarone can experience **unusual sensitivity to the sun**. Protect yourself by using an appropriate sunscreen product and reapplying it frequently.

Amiodarone can cause **thyroid abnormalities** because it interferes with normal thyroid hormone processing in your body. This can include worsening an already sluggish thyroid gland in 2 to 10 percent of people taking the drug and causing increased thyroid activity in 2 percent of people taking it.

Antiarrhythmic drugs are less effective and cause abnormal rhythms if **blood potassium** is low. Check with your doctor to see if you need extra potassium.

Possible Side Effects

About 75 percent of people taking 400 mg or more of Amiodarone every day develop some drug side effects. As many as 18 percent have to stop taking the drug because of a side effect. Side effects are more common in people taking Amiodarone for 6 months or more, but level off after 1 year.

▼ Most common: fatigue, a feeling of ill health, tremors, unusual involuntary movements, loss of coordination, an unusual walk, muscle weakness, dizziness, tingling in the hands or feet, reduced sex drive, sleeplessness or difficulty sleeping, headache, nervous system problems, nausea, vomiting, constipation, loss of appetite, abdominal pains, dry eyes, unusual sensitivity to bright light, and seeing halos around bright lights. Unusual sun sensitivity is the most common skin reaction to Amiodarone, but people taking this drug can develop a blue skin discoloration that may not go away completely when the drug is stopped. Other skin reactions are sun rashes, hair loss, and black-and-blue spots.

▼ Other: inflammation of the lung or fibrous deposits in the lungs, changes in thyroid function, changes in taste or smell, bloating, unusual salivation, and changes in blood clotting. Amiodarone can cause heart failure, reduced heart rate, and abnormal rhythms. Up to 9 percent of people taking Amiodarone develop abnormalities in liver function.

Drug Interactions

• Amiodarone increases the effects of Metoprolol and other beta blockers, Digoxin, Flecainide, Procainamide, Quinidine, Theophylline, and Warfarin and other anticoagulants. These interactions, which result from the interference of Amiodarone with the breakdown of these drugs in the liver, can take from 2 or 3 days to several weeks to develop. The dosage of these drugs must be reduced drastically to take the interaction into account.

• When Amiodarone and Phenytoin are taken together, both drugs can be affected. Amiodarone can be antagonized by Phenytoin and other Hydantoin anticonvulsants, and the effect of Phenytoin can be increased by Amiodarone, which interferes with its breakdown in the liver.

Food Interactions

Amiodarone is poorly absorbed into the blood and should be taken on an empty stomach. However, although food delays the absorption of Amiodarone into your bloodstream, the drug can be taken with food or meals if it upsets your stomach.

Usual Dose

The usual starting dose is 800 to 1600 mg per day, taken in 1 or 2 doses. Your dosage should be reduced to the lowest effective dose to minimize side effects. The usual maintenance dose is 400 mg per day.

Overdosage

There have been only a few reports of Amiodarone overdose: No one taking an overdose died because the drug usually takes several days or weeks to exert an effect on the body. All were effectively treated at a hospital emergency room. Anyone who has taken an overdose of Amiodarone should be taken to a hospital emergency room for treatment. ALWAYS bring the medicine bottle.

Special Information

Side effects are very common with Amiodarone. Three-fourths of people taking the drug will experience some drug-related problem. Call your doctor if you develop chest pains, difficulty in breathing or any other sign of changes in lung function, abnormal heartbeat, bloating in your feet or legs, tremors, fever, chills, sore throat, unusual bleeding or bruising, changes in skin color, unusual sunburn, or any other unusual side effect.

Amiodarone can make you dizzy or light-headed. Take care while driving a car or performing any complex tasks.

If you take Amiodarone once a day and forget to take a dose, but remember within 12 hours, take it as soon as possible. If you don't remember until later, skip the forgotten dose and continue with your regular schedule.

If you take Amiodarone twice a day and remember within 6 hours of your regular dose, take it as soon as you remember.

Call your doctor if you forget to take 2 or more doses in a row. Do not take a double dose.

Special Populations

Pregnancy/Breast-feeding

In animal studies, Amiodarone has been found to be toxic to a developing fetus when given at a dose 18 times the maximum adult human dose. Women of childbearing age should use contraceptives while taking Amiodarone, and women who become pregnant while taking this drug should carefully review with their doctors the possible effects on the fetus. Both the benefits to be obtained by taking this drug and the potential dangers should be discussed.

Amiodarone passes into breast milk. Nursing mothers who must take this drug should bottle-feed to avoid any complications.

Seniors

Amiodarone must be used with caution, regardless of your age. It is broken down in the liver, and dosage reduction may be needed if you have poor liver function. Kidney function is not a factor in determining Amiodarone dose.

Generic Name

Amitriptyline

Brand Names

Elavil
Endep

(Also available in generic form)

Combination Products

Amitriptyline + Perphenazine

Etrafon
Triavil

(Also available in generic form)

(The combination of Amitriptyline with Perphenazine, a tranquilizer, is prescribed for the relief of symptoms of anxiety or agitation and/or depression associated with chronic physical or psychiatric disease.)

Amitriptyline + Chlordiazepoxide

Limbitrol
Limbitrol DS

(The combination of Amitriptyline with Chlordiazepoxide, an antianxiety drug, is prescribed for the treatment of anxiety and depression.)

Type of Drug

Tricyclic antidepressant.

Prescribed for

Depression (with or without symptoms of anxiety or sleep disturbance), chronic pain (from migraines, tension headaches, diabetic disease, tic douloureux, cancer, herpes lesions, arthritis, and other sources), pathologic laughing or weeping caused by brain disease, and bulimia.

General Information

Amitriptyline and other tricyclic antidepressants block the movement of certain stimulant chemicals (norepinephrine or serotonin) in and out of nerve endings, having a sedative effect and counteracting the effects of a hormone called *acetylcholine* (making them anticholinergic drugs). One widely accepted theory of depression says that people with depression have a chemical imbalance in their brains and that drugs such as Amitriptyline work to reestablish a proper balance. It takes 2 to 4 weeks for Amitriptyline's clinical antidepressant effect to come into play. If symptoms are not affected after 6 to 8 weeks, contact your doctor. Tricyclics can also elevate mood, increase physical activity and mental alertness, and improve appetite and sleep patterns in depressed people. These drugs are mild sedatives and are useful in treating mild forms of depression associated with anxiety. Amitriptyline and other tricyclic antidepressants have been used in treating nighttime bed-wetting in young children, but they do not produce long-lasting relief. These drugs are broken down in the liver.

Cautions and Warnings

Do not take Amitriptyline if you are **allergic** or **sensitive** to it or any other tricyclic antidepressant. These drugs should not be used if you are recovering from a **heart attack**.

Amitriptyline may be taken with caution if you have a history of **epilepsy** (or other **convulsive disorders**), difficulty in **urination, glaucoma, heart disease, liver disease,** or **hyperthyroidism**. The condition of people who are **schizophrenic** or **paranoid** may worsen if they are given a tricyclic antidepressant. **Manic-depressive** people may switch phase; this can also happen if they are changing or stopping antidepressants. **Suicide** is always a possibility in severely depressed people, who should be allowed to have only minimal quantities of medication in their possession at one time.

Possible Side Effects

▼ Most common: sedation and anticholinergic effects (blurred vision, disorientation, confusion, hallucinations, muscle spasms or tremors, seizures and/or convulsions, dry mouth, constipation [especially in older adults], difficult urination, worsening glaucoma, and sensitivity to bright light or sunlight).

▼ Less common: blood-pressure changes, abnormal heart rates, heart attack, anxiety, restlessness, excitement, numbness and tingling in the extremities, poor coordination, rash, itching, retention of fluids, fever, allergy, changes in composition of blood, nausea, vomiting, loss of appetite, stomach upset, diarrhea, enlargement of the breasts in males and females, changes in sex drive, and blood-sugar changes.

▼ Rare: agitation, inability to sleep, nightmares, feelings of panic, a peculiar taste in the mouth, stomach cramps, black discoloration of the tongue, yellowing of the eyes and/or skin, loss of hair, changes in liver function, weight changes, excessive perspiration, flushing, frequent urination, drowsiness, dizziness, weakness, headache, and feelings of ill health.

Drug Interactions

• Interaction with monoamine oxidase (MAO) inhibitors can cause high fevers, convulsions, and occasionally death. Don't take MAO inhibitors until at least 2 weeks after Amitriptyline has been discontinued. Those who must take both an MAO inhibitor and Amitriptyline require close medical observation.

• Amitriptyline interacts with Guanethidine and Clonidine. Be sure to tell your doctor if you are taking any high-blood-pressure medicine.

• Amitriptyline increases the effects of barbiturates, tranquilizers and other sedative drugs, and alcohol. Also, barbiturates may decrease the effectiveness of Amitriptyline.

• Taking Amitriptyline and thyroid medicine together will enhance the effects of both medicines, possibly causing abnormal heart rhythms. The combination of Amitriptyline and Reserpine may cause overstimulation.

• Oral contraceptives can reduce the effect of Amitriptyline, as can smoking. Charcoal tablets can prevent antidepressant absorption into the blood. Estrogens can increase or decrease the effect of Amitriptyline.

• Drugs such as Bicarbonate of Soda, Acetazolamide, Quinidine, and Procainamide will increase the effect of Amitriptyline. Cimetidine, Methylphenidate, and Phenothiazine drugs (like Thorazine and Compazine) block the breakdown of Amitriptyline in the liver, causing it to stay in the body longer, which can cause severe drug side effects.

Food Interactions

You may take this drug with food if it upsets your stomach.

Usual Dose

Adult: 25 mg 3 times per day, increased to 150 mg per day if necessary. Dosage must be tailored to your specific needs.

Adolescent and Senior: lower doses are recommended, generally 30 to 50 mg per day.

Overdosage

Symptoms of overdose include confusion, inability to concentrate, hallucinations, drowsiness, lowered body temperature, abnormal heart rate, heart failure, enlarged pupils of the eyes, convulsions, severely lowered blood pressure, stupor, and coma. The overdose victim should be taken to an emergency room immediately. ALWAYS bring the medicine bottle.

Special Information

Avoid alcohol and other depressants while taking this drug. Do not stop taking this medicine unless your doctor specifically tells you to do so. Abruptly stopping this medicine may cause nausea, headache, and a sickly feeling.

This medicine can cause drowsiness, dizziness, and blurred vision. Be careful when driving or operating hazardous machinery. Avoid prolonged exposure to the sun or sunlamps.

Call your doctor immediately if you develop seizures, difficult or rapid breathing, fever and sweating, blood-pressure changes, muscle stiffness, loss of bladder control, or unusual tiredness or weakness. Dry mouth may lead to an increase in dental cavities and gum bleeding and disease. You should pay special attention to dental hygiene if you are taking Amitriptyline.

If you forget a dose of Amitriptyline, skip the dose and go back to your regular schedule. Do not take a double dose.

Special Populations

Pregnancy/Breast-feeding

Amitriptyline, like other antidepressants, crosses into the fetal circulation. Birth defects (heart, breathing, and urinary problems) have been reported if the drug is taken during the first 3 months of pregnancy. Avoid taking Amitriptyline while pregnant.

Small amounts of tricyclic antidepressants pass into breast milk and can sedate your baby. Nursing mothers taking Amitriptyline should bottle-feed their infants.

Seniors

Older adults are more sensitive to the effects of this drug, especially abnormal heart rhythms and other heart side effects, and often require a lower dose than younger adults to achieve the same results. Follow your doctor's directions and report any side effects at once.

Generic Name

Amlodipine

Brand Names

Norvasc

(Also available in generic form)

Type of Drug

Calcium channel blocker.

Prescribed for

Angina pectoris; Prinzmetal's angina; high blood pressure. Amlodipine has been studied for heart failure.

General Information

Amlodipine is one of a growing number of calcium channel blockers to be marketed in the United States. Calcium channel blockers work by blocking the passage of calcium into heart and smooth muscle. Since calcium is an essential factor in muscle contraction, any drug that affects calcium in this way will interfere with the contraction of these muscles. When this happens, the amount of oxygen used by the muscles is also reduced. Therefore, Amlodipine can be used in the treatment of angina, a type of heart pain related to poor oxygen supply to the heart muscles. Also, Amlodipine dilates (opens) the vessels that supply blood to the heart muscles and prevents spasm of these arteries. Amlodipine affects the movement of calcium only into muscle cells; it does not have any effect on calcium in the blood.

Cautions and Warnings

Amlodipine may, rarely, cause unwanted **low blood pressure** in some people taking it for reasons other than hypertension. This is more of a problem with other calcium channel blockers.

Amlodipine may worsen **heart failure** in some people and should be used with caution if heart failure is present.

Calcium channel blockers, alone and with Aspirin, have

caused bruises, black-and-blue marks, and bleeding due to an anticoagulant effect. This is mostly a problem with Nifedipine but should be considered for all members of the group.

Amlodipine may cause **angina pain** when treatment is first started, when dosage is increased, or if the drug is rapidly withdrawn. This can be avoided by gradual dosage reduction.

Studies have shown that people taking calcium channel blockers (usually those taken several times a day, not those taken only once daily) have a greater chance of having a **heart attack** than people taking beta blockers or other medicines for the same purposes. Discuss this with your doctor to be sure you are receiving the best possible treatment.

Do not take this drug if you have had an **allergic** reaction to it in the past.

People with severe **liver disease** break down Amlodipine much more slowly than people with less severe disease or normal livers. Your doctor should take this into account when determining your Amlodipine dosage.

Possible Side Effects

▼ Most common: headache, dizziness or light-headedness, anxiety, nausea, swelling in the arms or legs, heart palpitations, and flushing.

▼ Less common: sleepiness, muscle weakness, cramps or abdominal discomfort, itching, rash, sexual difficulties, wheezing or shortness of breath, muscle cramps, pain and inflammation.

▼ Rare: nervousness, psychiatric disturbances (depression, memory loss, paranoia, psychosis, hallucination), tingling in the hands or feet, sleeplessness, unusual dreams, anxiety, feelings of ill health, ringing or buzzing in the ears, hand or other muscle tremors, diarrhea, constipation, vomiting, dry mouth, excessive thirst, stomach gas, low blood pressure, slow heartbeat, abnormal heart rhythms, hair loss, bruising, black-and-blue marks, bleeding, stuffed nose, sinus inflammation, chest congestion, frequent or painful urination, joint stiffness or pain, weight gain, nosebleeds, cough, and appetite loss.

▼ Other: chest pain, blue discoloration of fingers or toes, difficulty swallowing, double vision, eye pain, ab-

Possible Side Effects *(continued)*

normal vision, conjunctivitis, heart failure, irregular pulse pulse, apathy, agitation, dry skin, skin discoloration, twitching, migraines, cold and clammy skin, loose stools, and taste changes.

Drug Interactions

• Amlodipine may interact with beta-blocking drugs to cause heart failure, very low blood pressure, or an increased incidence of angina pain.

• Amlodipine may cause unexpected blood-pressure reduction through interaction with other antihypertensive drugs in patients already taking medicine to control their high blood pressure, although this interaction is more likely with other calcium channel blockers.

• The combination of Quinidine (for abnormal heart rhythm) and Amlodipine must be used with caution because it can produce low blood pressure, very slow heart rate, abnormal heart rhythms, and swelling in the arms or legs.

• Amlodipine can increase the effects of Theophylline products (for asthma and other respiratory problems).

• Patients taking Amlodipine who are given Fentanyl as a short-term surgical anesthetic may experience very low blood pressure.

Food Interactions

Amlodipine can be taken without regard to food or meals.

Usual Dose

5 to 10 mg once a day.

Do not stop taking Amlodipine abruptly. The dosage should be gradually reduced over a period of time.

Overdosage

Overdose of Amlodipine can cause nausea, weakness, dizziness, confusion, and slurred speech. Take overdose victims to a hospital emergency room, or call your local Poison Center for directions. You may be asked to make the patient vomit to remove the medicine from his or her stomach. If you go to the hospital, ALWAYS bring the medicine bottle.

Special Information

Call your doctor if you develop constipation, nausea, weakness or dizziness, swelling in the hands or feet, difficulty breathing, or increased heart pains, or if other side effects are particularly bothersome or persistent.

If you are taking Amlodipine for high blood pressure, be sure to continue taking your medicine and follow any instructions for diet restriction or other treatments. High blood pressure is a condition with few recognizable symptoms; it may seem to you that you are taking medicine for no good reason. Call your doctor or pharmacist if you have any questions.

It is important to maintain good dental hygiene while taking Amlodipine and to use extra care when using your toothbrush or dental floss because of the chance that the drug will make you more susceptible to some infections.

If you forget a dose of Amlodipine, take it as soon as you remember. If it is almost time for your next regularly scheduled dose, skip the forgotten dose and continue with your regular schedule. Do not take a double dose.

Special Populations

Pregnancy/Breast-feeding

Animal studies with Amlodipine show that it may damage a developing fetus. Other calcium channel blockers can be used to treat severe high blood pressure associated with pregnancy, so there is no reason for pregnant women or those who might become pregnant to take Amlodipine.

It is not known if Amlodipine may pass into breast milk. Consider the possible effect of this medicine on the nursing infant.

Seniors

Older adults, especially those with liver disease, are more sensitive to the effects of this drug because it takes longer to pass out of their bodies. They should be given somewhat lower doses to start with. Follow your doctor's directions and report any side effects at once.

Generic Name

Amoxapine

Brand Name

Asendin Tablets

(Also available in generic form)

Type of Drug

Tricyclic antidepressant.

Prescribed for

Depression.

General Information

Amoxapine and other tricyclic antidepressants block the movement of certain stimulant chemicals (norepinephrine or serotonin) in and out of nerve endings, have a sedative effect, and counteract the effects of a hormone called *acetylcholine* (making them anticholinergic drugs). Amoxapine also works similarly to many of the antipsychotic medicines, including Chlorpromazine and Haloperidol, by blocking dopamine receptors in the brain. This is important because Amoxapine carries some of the same negatives as those drugs (neuroleptic malignant syndrome and tardive dyskinesia). One widely accepted theory says that people with depression have a chemical imbalance in their brains and that drugs such as Amoxapine work to reestablish a proper balance. It takes 2 to 4 weeks for Amoxapine's antidepressant effect to come into play. If symptoms are not affected after 6 to 8 weeks, contact your doctor. Tricyclics can also elevate mood, increase physical activity and mental alertness, and improve appetite and sleep patterns in a depressed patient. These drugs are mild sedatives and therefore useful in treating mild forms of depression associated with anxiety. Tricyclic antidepressants have been used in treating nighttime bed-wetting in young children, but they do not produce long-lasting relief. They are broken down in the liver.

Cautions and Warnings

Do not take Amoxapine if you are **allergic** or **sensitive** to this or other members of this class of drug. These drugs should not be used if you are recovering from a **heart attack**.

Amoxapine may be taken with caution if you have a history of **epilepsy** or other **convulsive disorders**, difficulty in **urination, glaucoma, heart disease, liver disease,** or **hyperthyroidism.** The condition of people who are **schizophrenic** or **paranoid** may worsen if they are given a tricyclic antidepressant. **Manic-depressive** people may switch phase: This can also happen if they are changing or stopping antidepressants. **Suicide** is always a possibility in severely depressed people, who should be allowed to have only minimal quantities of medication in their possession at any one time.

Amoxapine may cause **very high fevers, muscle rigidity, altered mental status, irregular pulse or blood pressure, sweating, abnormal heart rhythms,** and **rapid heartbeat.** This group of symptoms is called *neuroleptic malignant syndrome* and can be fatal. If it develops, stop your medicine at once and call your doctor, who may prescribe another antidepressant.

Amoxapine may also be associated with potentially irreversible **involuntary muscle movements** called *tardive dyskinesia* (symptoms include lip-smacking or puckering, puffing the cheeks, rapid or wormlike tongue movements, uncontrolled chewing motions, and uncontrolled arm and leg movements). This condition is more common among the elderly, especially elderly women. Call your doctor if this develops.

Possible Side Effects

▼ Most common: sedation and anticholinergic effects (blurred vision, disorientation, confusion, hallucinations, muscle spasms or tremors, seizures and/or convulsions, dry mouth, constipation [especially in older adults], difficult urination, worsening glaucoma, and sensitivity to bright light or sunlight).

▼ Less common: blood-pressure changes, abnormal heart rates, heart attack, anxiety, restlessness, excitement, numbness and tingling in the extremities, poor coordination, rash, itching, retention of fluids, fever, allergy, changes in composition of blood, nausea, vomiting, loss of appetite, stomach upset, diarrhea, enlargement of the breasts in males and females, changes in sex drive, and blood-sugar changes.

Possible Side Effects *(continued)*

▼ Rare: agitation, inability to sleep, nightmares, feeling of panic, a peculiar taste in the mouth, stomach cramps, black coloration of the tongue, yellowing eyes and/or skin, hair loss, changes in liver function, weight changes, excessive perspiration, flushing, frequent urination, drowsiness, dizziness, weakness, headache, nausea, and not feeling well. Neuroleptic malignant syndrome or tardive dyskinesia may also develop (see *Cautions and Warnings*).

Drug Interactions

• Interaction with monoamine oxidase (MAO) inhibitors can cause high fevers, convulsions, and occasionally death. Don't take MAO inhibitors until at least 2 weeks after Amoxapine has been stopped. Patients who must take both an MAO inhibitor and Amoxapine require close medical observation.

• Amoxapine interacts with Guanethidine and Clonidine. Be sure to tell your doctor if you are taking **any** high-blood-pressure medicine.

• Amoxapine increases the effects of alcohol, barbiturates, tranquilizers, and other sedative drugs. Also, barbiturates may decrease the effectiveness of Amoxapine.

• Taking Amoxapine and thyroid medicine together will enhance the effects of both medicines, possibly causing abnormal heart rhythms. The combination of Amoxapine and Reserpine may cause overstimulation.

• Oral contraceptives can reduce the effect of Amoxapine, as can smoking. Charcoal tablets can prevent Amoxapine's absorption into the blood. Estrogens can increase or decrease the effect of Amoxapine.

• Drugs such as Bicarbonate of Soda, Acetazolamide, Quinidine, and Procainamide will increase the effect of Amoxapine. Cimetidine, Methylphenidate, and Phenothiazine drugs (like Thorazine and Compazine) block the liver metabolism of Amoxapine, causing it to stay in the body longer, which can cause severe drug side effects.

Food Interactions

You may take Amoxapine with food if it upsets your stomach.

Usual Dose

Adult (age 17 years and older): 100 to 400 mg per day. Hospitalized patients may need up to 600 mg per day. Your dose must be tailored to your specific needs.

Senior: lower doses are recommended. For people over 60 years of age, usually 50 to 300 mg per day.

Child (16 years and under): do not use.

Overdosage

Symptoms include confusion, inability to concentrate, hallucinations, drowsiness, lowered body temperature, abnormal heart rate, heart failure, enlarged pupils, convulsions, severely lowered blood pressure, stupor, and coma. The overdose victim should be taken to a hospital emergency room immediately. ALWAYS bring the medicine bottle.

Special Information

Avoid alcohol and other depressants while taking Amoxapine. Do not stop taking this medicine unless your doctor specifically tells you to do so. Abruptly stopping this medicine may cause nausea, headache, and a sickly feeling.

This medicine can cause drowsiness, dizziness, and blurred vision. Be careful when driving or operating hazardous machinery. Avoid prolonged exposure to the sun or sunlamps.

Call your doctor at once if you develop seizures, difficult or rapid breathing, fever and sweating, blood-pressure changes, muscle stiffness, loss of bladder control, or unusual tiredness or weakness. Dry mouth may lead to an increase in dental cavities, gum bleeding, and disease; pay special attention to dental hygiene.

If you forget to take a dose of Amoxapine, skip it and go back to your regular schedule. Do not take a double dose.

Special Populations

Pregnancy/Breast-feeding

Amoxapine, like other antidepressants, crosses into your developing baby's circulation, and birth defects have been reported if it is taken during the first 3 months of pregnancy. Avoid taking Amoxapine while pregnant.

Tricyclic antidepressants pass into breast milk in low concentrations and sedate the baby. Nursing mothers taking Amoxapine should bottle-feed their babies.

Seniors
Older adults are more sensitive to the effects of this drug, especially abnormal rhythms and other heart side effects, and often require a lower dose than younger adults to achieve the same results. Follow your doctor's directions and report any side effects at once.

Amoxicillin

see ***Penicillin Antibiotics***, page 868

Amoxil

see ***Penicillin Antibiotics***, page 868

Type of Drug
Antacids

Brand Names

Ingredient: Aluminum

AlternaGEL	Amphojel
Aluminum Hydroxide Gel	Basaljel
Alu-Cap	Nephrox
Alu-Tab	

Ingredient: Calcium

Alkets	Equilet
Alka-Mints	Genelac
Amitone	Glycate
Calcium Carbonate	Mylanta Lozenges
Chooz	Maalox Antacid Caplets
Dicarbosil	Mallamint

Pama   Tums
Titracid   Tums Extra Strength
Titralac   [$]   Tums Ultra
Titralac Extra Strength   [$]

Ingredient: Magnesium

Magnesium Carbonate   Milk of Magnesia
Magnesium Oxide   Par-Mag
Magnesium Trisilicate   Phillips Chewable
Mag-Ox 400   Uro-Mag
Maox

Ingredient: Sodium Bicarbonate

Bell/ans   Sodium Bicarbonate

Ingredients: Aluminum + Magnesium

Alamag   Maalox Concentrate
Alenic Alka   Maalox Heartburn Relief
Alenic Alka, Extra Strength   Liquid
Algemol   Magnox
Algenic Alka   Magmalin
Algicon   Magnagel
Aludrox   Magnalox
Alumid   Magnatril
Creamalin   Mintox
Delcid   Neutrocomp
Escot   Noralac
Estomul-M   Remegel Squares
Gaviscon Liquid   Riopan
Genaton Liquid   RuLox
Kolantyl   TC Suspension
Kudrox   Tralmag
Lowsium   WinGel
Maalox

Ingredients: Aluminum + Magnesium + Sodium

Gaviscon 2 Tablets, Double Strength Genaton Tablets

Ingredients: Aluminum + Magnesium + Sodium + Calcium

Alenic Alka Tablets   Gaviscon Extra Strength
Foamicon Tablets   Relief Formula Tablets
Gaviscon Tablets   Genaton Tablets, Extra
                                  Strength

Ingredients: Aluminum + Calcium + Magnesium

Camalox   Duracid

Ingredients: Aluminum + Magnesium + Simethicone (an antigas ingredient)

Almacone
Almacone II
Alma-Mag
Aludrox
Alumid Plus
Anta Gel
Di-Gel
Gaviscon Extra Strength
Gelusil
Gelusil II
Gelusil-M
Iosopan Plus Liquid
Kudrox
Lostron Plus Liquid
Lowsium Plus
Maalox Plus
Maalox Extra Strength
Maalox Extra Strength Plus
Magaldrate Plus
  Suspension
Mi-Acid

Miacid II
Mintox Extra Strength
Mintox Plus
Mygel
Mylanta
Mylanta II
Mylanta Double Strength
  Tablets, Liquid
Mylagen II
Mygel Suspension
Mygel II Suspension
Riopan Plus
Riopan Plus Double
  Strength Tablets,
  Suspension
RuLox Plus Tablets,
  Suspension
Silain Gel
Simaal
Simeco

Ingredients: Aluminum + Magnesium + Calcium + Simethicone

Tempo

Ingredients: Calcium + Magnesium

Alkets
Bisodol
Lo-Sol
Marblen
Mi-Acid Gelcaps

Mylagen Gelcaps
Mylanta Gelcaps
Ratio
Spastoced

Ingredients: Calcium + Simethicone

Titralac Plus Tablets

Ingredients: Calcium + Magnesium + Simethicone

Advanced Formula Di-Gel

Effervescent Powder or Tablet

Alka-Seltzer	Bromo Seltzer
Alka-Seltzer	Citrocarbonate
with Aspirin	ENO
Bisodol Powder	Flavored Alka-Seltzer

(Also available in generic form)

Prescribed for

Relief of heartburn, acid indigestion, sour stomach, gastro-esophageal reflux disease (GERD), and other conditions related to stomach upset and excess acidity. These drugs are also prescribed for excess acid in the stomach or intestine associated with ulcer, gastritis, esophagitis, and hiatal hernia. Antacid therapy will help these conditions to heal more quickly.

Aluminum antacids are prescribed for kidney failure patients to prevent phosphate from being absorbed into the body. Only Aluminum Hydroxide (all brands) and Basaljel have been shown to be useful as phosphate binders.

General Information

In spite of the large number of antacid products available, there are basically only a few different kinds. All antacids work against stomach acid by neutralizing the acid through a chemical reaction. The choice of an antacid is based upon its "neutralizing capacity," that is, how much acid is neutralized by a given amount of antacid. Sodium and calcium have the greatest neutralizing capacity, but should not be used for long-term or ulcer therapy because of the other effects large amounts of sodium and calcium can have on your body. Of the other products, Magnesium Hydroxide has the greatest neutralizing capacity, followed by mixtures of magnesium and aluminum compounds, Magnesium Trisilicate, Aluminum Hydroxide, and Aluminum Phosphates. The neutralizing capacity of an antacid product also depends upon how it is formulated, how much antacid is put in the mixture, and what the form of the mixture is. Antacid suspensions have greater neutralizing capacity than either powders or tablets.

Calcium antacids have been recommended as a source of extra calcium to prevent osteoporosis. Four to six tablets per day are needed to provide the proper amount of calcium. Although Tums has been widely recommended, any product listed under Calcium Antacids will do the job. Magnesium antacids can be used to treat magnesium deficiency.

Cautions and Warnings

People with **high blood pressure** or **heart failure** and those on **low-sodium diets** must avoid antacids with a high sodium content. Many antacids are considered to be low in sodium (Riopan is the lowest). Your pharmacist can advise you which of these drugs are considered low-sodium antacids.

Aluminum antacids should be used with caution by people who have just had **severe bleeding** in the **stomach** or **intestines**. Excessive amounts of aluminum antacids can lead to low blood-phosphate levels.

Sodium Bicarbonate is easily absorbed and may result in a condition called *systemic alkalosis* (a condition where the blood becomes less acidic, affecting the kidney, blood, and salt balance) if it is taken for a long period of time. Magnesium antacids must be used with caution by patients with kidney disease.

Calcium Carbonate and Sodium Bicarbonate may have a **rebound effect;** that is, after you stop taking an antacid, your problem returns worse than it was when you first took it. They and other antacids can also cause *milk-alkali syndrome* (headache, nausea, irritability, and weakness). Over the longer term, milk-alkali syndrome can cause kidney disease and failure, high blood-calcium levels, and alkalosis.

Possible Side Effects

▼ Most common: diarrhea (magnesium products) and constipation (aluminum and calcium products). Aluminum/magnesium combinations are usually used to avoid affecting the bowel.

People with kidney failure who take magnesium antacids may develop magnesium toxicity.

Possible Side Effects *(continued)*

Calcium and sodium antacids may cause a rebound effect, with more acid produced after the antacid is stopped than before it was started.

Magnesium Trisilicate antacids used over long periods may result in the development of silicate renal stones.

Drug Interactions

• Antacids can interfere with the absorption of most drugs into the body by interfering with the disintegration of tablets in your stomach and then preventing them from being absorbed; and by changing the acid balance in your kidneys, thus affecting how drugs are released from the body. In a few cases, antacids can actually increase the drug's effect. Separate your antacid from other oral medicines by 1 or 2 hours.

• Aluminum antacids interfere with Allopurinol, Chloroquine, Corticosteroids, Diflunisal, Digoxin, Ethambutol, histamine H_2 antagonists, Iron salts, Isoniazid, Penicillamine, Phenothiazine drugs, Tetracycline antibiotics, thyroid hormones, and Ticlopidine. Aluminum antacids **increase** the absorption of benzodiazepine tranquilizers into the blood.

• Calcium antacids interfere with fluoroquinolone antibacterial drugs, hydantoin antiseizure medicines, Iron, Aspirin and other salicylates, and Tetracycline antibiotics. Calcium antacids can **increase** the amount of Quinidine absorbed into the blood.

• Magnesium antacids interfere with benzodiazepine tranquilizers, Chloroquine, corticosteroid drugs, Digoxin, histamine H_2 antagonists, hydantoin antiseizure drugs, Nitrofurantoin, Penicillamine, phenothiazine drugs, Tetracycline antibiotics, and Ticlopidine. Magnesium antacids **increase** the absorption of Dicumarol (a blood-thinner), Quinidine, and sulfonylurea antidiabetes medicines.

• Magnesium-aluminum antacid combinations interfere with benzodiazepine tranquilizer drugs, Captopril, corticosteroids, fluoroquinolone antibacterials, histamine H_2 antagonists, hydantoin antiseizure drugs, Iron salts, Ketoconazole, Penicillamine, phenothiazine drugs, Aspirin and other salicylates, Tetracycline antibiotics, and Ticlopidine. Magnesium aluminum combinations **increase** the absorption of Levodopa, Quinidine, sulfonylurea antidiabetes drugs, and Valproic Acid. Magnesium-aluminum antacids can lead to kidney failure and alkalosis when taken with sodium polystyrene sulfonate (for high blood cholesterol).

• Sodium bicarbonate interferes with benzodiazepine tranquilizers, Iron salts, Ketoconazole, Lithium, Methenamine, Methotrexate, Aspirin and other salicylates, sulfonylurea antidiabetes drugs, and Tetracycline antibiotics. Sodium bicarbonate **increases** the absorption of amphetamines, Flecainide, Quinidine, and sympathomimetic drugs (stimulants and decongestants).

Food Interactions

Antacids are best taken on an empty stomach but may be taken with food.

Usual Dose

The dose of antacids must be individualized to your specific needs. For ulcers, antacids are given every hour for the first 2 weeks (during waking hours), and 1 to 3 hours after meals and at bedtime thereafter. For GERD, the usual dose is 1 tablespoonful ½ hour after meals and at bedtime.

Overdosage

Symptoms of overdosage include stomach gas, nausea, and vomiting. Call your doctor or hospital emergency room for more information. Treatment is rarely needed unless large numbers of tablets have been swallowed.

Special Information

Be sure to chew antacid tablets completely. Swallow with milk or water. Effervescent antacid tablets must be allowed to completely dissolve in water before you drink the bubbly solution.

Aluminum antacids may cause speckling or add a whitish discoloration to the stool and can cause constipation.

Magnesium antacids may have a laxative effect by drawing water into the large intestines and can cause diarrhea.

Severe stomach or abdominal pain, cramps, and nausea may be signs of appendicitis, which cannot be treated with antacids.

Call your doctor if you do not get relief from your antacid or if your stool becomes black and tarry or takes on the characteristics of "coffee grounds," which indicates bleeding in the intestines or stomach.

Children under age 6 should not take antacids unless directed by their doctor.

Special Populations

Pregnancy/Breast-feeding

Antacids can be safely taken in low doses for short periods of time during pregnancy. Be sure your doctor knows you are taking antacids.

Antacids may be taken during breast-feeding.

Seniors

Seniors can safely use most antacids without special restriction. However, do not use more than the usual dose of antacid unless so directed by your doctor, and avoid those that contain aluminum.

Type of Drug

Antidiabetes Drugs (Oral Sulfonylureas)

Generic Name	Brand Name
Acetohexamide	Dymelor*
Chlorpropamide	Diabinese*
Glimepiride	Amaryl
Glipizide	Glucotrol
	Glucotrol XL
Glyburide	DiaBeta*
	Glynase PresTab
	Micronase*
Tolazamide	Tolinase*
Tolbutamide	Orinase*

(*Also available in generic form)

Prescribed for

Diabetes mellitus (sugar in the urine). Chlorpropamide (200 to 500 mg per day) may also be used to treat diabetes insipidus (a hormonal condition unrelated to body sugar).

General Information

Oral sulfonylurea antidiabetes drugs work by stimulating the production and release of insulin from the pancreas. These drugs differ from each other in how long they take to start working, the duration of their effectiveness, and the amount of each required to produce a roughly equivalent antidiabetic effect. (See table for details.) These drugs do not lower blood sugar directly; they require some working pancreas cells. The 'second-generation' antidiabetes drugs, Glipizide and Glyburide, belong to the same chemical class as the older "first-generation" ones, but lower doses of the second-generation agents are required to accomplish the same effect. Other minor differences between the two groups are considered clinically unimportant, and the second-generation drugs offer no advantage over the first-generation agents.

Drug	Equivalent Dose (mg)	Hours to Start Working	Hours of Effectiveness
Acetohexamide	500	1	12 to 24
Chlorpropamide	250	1	up to 60
Glimepiride	4	1	24
Glipizide	10	1 to 1½	10 to 16
Glyburide (DiaBeta, Micronase)	5	2 to 4	24
Glyburide (Glynase Prestab)	3	1	12 to 24
Tolazamide	250	4 to 6	12 to 24
Tolbutamide	1000	1	6 to 12

Cautions and Warnings

Mild stress (such as infection, minor surgery, or emotional upset) reduces the effectiveness of oral sulfonylurea antidiabetes drugs. Remember that while you are taking these drugs you must be **under your doctor's continuous care.**

Oral sulfonylurea antidiabetics drugs are not oral Insulin, nor are they a substitute for Insulin. They do not lower blood sugar by themselves. Studies have found that people taking an oral sulfonylurea antidiabetic drug are more likely to have **fatal heart trouble** than those who can control their diabetes with diet alone or diet plus Insulin.

The treatment of diabetes is your responsibility. **Follow your doctor's instructions** about diet, body weight, exercise, personal hygiene, and all measures to avoid infection.

Oral sulfonylurea antidiabetics are broken down in the liver. They generally should be used with caution if you have **serious liver, kidney, or endocrine disease;** you should monitor your blood sugar very closely.

Possible Side Effects

▼ Most common: loss of appetite, nausea, vomiting, and stomach upset. At times you may experience weakness or tingling in the hands and feet. To eliminate these effects, ask your doctor to reduce your daily dosage or, if necessary, switch you to another oral sulfonylurea antidiabetes drug.

▼ Less common: oral sulfonylurea antidiabetics may produce abnormally low blood-sugar levels when too much is taken for your immediate requirements. (Other factors that may cause lowering of blood sugar are liver or kidney disease, diseases of the glands, malnutrition, old age, and drinking alcohol.)

▼ Other: these drugs may cause a yellowing of the eyes or skin, itching, or rash. Usually these reactions will disappear in time. If they persist, you should contact your doctor.

Drug Interactions

• The following drugs may increase your need for your oral

sulfonylurea antidiabetes drug: beta blockers, Cholestyramine, Diazoxide, Phenytoin and other Hydantoin drugs, Rifampin, thiazide diuretics, charcoal tablets, and anything that makes your urine less acidic.

• The following drugs may decrease your need for your oral sulfonylurea antidiabetes drug: androgens (male hormones), sulfa drugs, Aspirin and other salicylates, Chloramphenicol, Clofibrate, Fenfluramine, Gemfibrozil, Cimetidine, Ranitidine, Famotidine, Nizatidine, Oxyphenbutazone, Magnesium, Methyldopa, Phenylbutazone, Probenecid, Dicumarol, Bishydroxycoumarin, Warfarin, Phenyramidol, Sulfinpyrazone, tricyclic antidepressants, vitamin C (in large doses), citrus fruits and other foods that make your urine more acidic, and monoamine oxidase (MAO) inhibitor drugs. These drugs tend to prolong and enhance the action of oral sulfonylurea antidiabetes drugs. Insulin may be used with an oral sulfonylurea antidiabetes drug, but only under the strict control of a physician. If used indiscriminately, this combination can cause severely low blood sugar.

• Interaction with alcoholic beverages causes flushing of the face and body, as well as breathlessness. Other possible adverse effects are throbbing pain in the head and neck, breathing difficulty, nausea, vomiting, increased sweating, excessive thirst, chest pains, palpitations, lowered blood pressure, weakness, dizziness, blurred vision, and confusion. If you experience any of these reactions, contact your doctor immediately.

• Oral sulfonylurea antidiabetics may increase blood levels of the Digitalis drugs, increasing their effects on your body.

• Because of the stimulant ingredients found in many nonprescription cough, cold, and allergy remedies, avoid them unless your doctor advises otherwise.

Food Interactions

All oral sulfonylurea antidiabetes drugs (except Glipizide) may be taken with food. Glipizide should be taken 30 minutes before a meal for best results.

Dietary management is an important part of controlling your diabetes. Be sure to follow your doctor's directions about which foods you should avoid.

Usual Dose

Acetohexamide
250 to 1500 mg per day.

Chlorpropamide
Begin with 1 to 2 grams per day; your doctor will then increase or decrease your dosage according to your response. Maintenance dose: 250 mg to 2 (or, rarely, 3) grams per day.

Glimepiride
4 to 8 mg once per day.

Glipizide
5 mg once per day. Seniors may be started on 2.5 mg per day. Doses up to 40 mg per day divided into two daily doses may be needed to control more severe diabetes. Single daily doses should not be greater than 15 mg.

Glyburide
DiaBeta/Micronase: 2.5 to 20 mg once per day, usually with breakfast or the first main meal. Seniors may be started with 1.25 mg per day.

Glynase: 1.5 to 12 mg per day, usually with breakfast or the first main meal. Seniors may be started with 0.75 mg per day.

Note: The micronized form of Glyburide, Glynase, is not equivalent to DiaBeta or Micronase and may not be substituted for either of them. DiaBeta and Micronase are interchangeable.

Tolazamide
Moderate diabetes: 100 to 250 mg daily.
Severe diabetes: 500 to 1000 mg daily.

Tolbutamide
Begin with 1 to 2 grams per day; your doctor will then increase or decrease your dosage based on your response. Maintenance dose: 250 mg to 2 (or, rarely, 3) grams per day.

Overdosage

A mild overdose lowers blood sugar, which can be treated by consuming sugar in such forms as candy, orange juice, or glucose tablets. Low-blood-sugar symptoms include tingling of the lips and tongue, nausea, lethargy, yawning, confusion, agitation, nervousness, rapid heartbeat, increased sweating, tremors, and hunger. Ultimately, low blood sugar can lead to convulsions, stupor, and coma. Call your doctor, local poison control center, or hospital emergency room to find out if the overdose victim should be taken to a hospital emergency room for treatment. ALWAYS bring the medicine bottle.

Special Information

Diet remains of primary importance in the treatment of your diabetes. Follow the diet plan your doctor has prescribed and avoid alcoholic beverages.

Call your doctor if you develop low blood sugar (see *Overdosage* for symptoms) or high blood sugar (excessive thirst or urination, sugar, or ketones in the urine), if you are not feeling well, or if you have symptoms such as itching, rash, yellowing of the skin or eyes, abnormally light-colored stools, a low-grade fever, sore throat, diarrhea, or unusual bruising or bleeding.

Do not stop taking these medicines, except under your doctor's supervision. If you forget a dose of an oral sulfonylurea antidiabetes drug, take it as soon as you remember. If it is almost time for your next dose, skip the one you forgot and continue with your regular schedule. Do not take a double dose.

Special Populations

Pregnancy/Breast-feeding

Animal studies have shown that all oral sulfonylurea antidiabetes drugs (except Glyburide) cause birth defects or interfere with fetal development. Check with your doctor before taking an oral sulfonylurea antidiabetes drug if you are, or might be, pregnant. Blood-sugar control is essential in pregnant diabetics because high blood sugar is also associated with more birth defects. Pregnant women are best treated with Insulin, because oral sulfonylurea antidiabetes drugs generally won't control their blood sugar. Birth defects and other problems are 3 to 4 times more common in diabetic mothers than in nondiabetics.

If you take oral sulfonylurea antidiabetics while nursing, the baby's blood-sugar level may be reduced; nursing mothers taking one of these drugs should bottle-feed their babies.

Seniors

Older adults, especially those with reduced kidney function, are very sensitive to the blood-sugar-lowering effects and side effects of these medicines because they don't eliminate them from the body as efficiently as younger people. Low blood sugar, the major sign of drug overdose, may be more difficult to identify in seniors. Also, low blood sugar is more likely to cause nervous-system side effects in seniors.

Older adults taking oral sulfonylurea antidiabetes drugs must keep in close contact with their doctors and follow their directions.

Type of Drug

Antihistamine–Decongestant Combination Products

Brand Names

Ingredients: Acrivastine + Pseudoephedrine

Semprex-D Capsules

Ingredients: Azatadine + Pseudoephedrine

Trinalin Repetabs

Ingredients: Brompheniramine + Phenylpropanolamine

Bromaline Elixir	Dimetapp	E.N.T.
Bromanate Elixir S A	Dimetapp Cold and Allergy Chewable	Genatap Elixir S A
Bromatapp Cold and Allergy Elixir S A	Dimetapp Elixir A	Vicks DayQuil Allergy Relief 12 Hour Tablets
Dimaphen	Dimetapp Extentabs	Vicks DayQuil Allergy Relief
Dimaphen Elixir	Dimetapp 4-Hour Liqui-Gel	4 Hour Tablets
Dimaphen Release Tablets		

Ingredients: Brompheniramine + Phenylephrine directions.

Dimetane Decongestant Caplets and Elixir

Ingredients: Brompheniramine + Phenylephrine + Phenylpropanolamine

Bromophen T.D. Tablets   Tamine S.R. Tablets

Ingredients: Brompheniramine + Pseudoephedrine

12-Hour Cold
  Tablets
Allent
Bromfed Tablets
  and Syrup
Bromfed-PD
Bromfed-DM
Cheracol Sinus

Dallergy-JR
Disobrom
Dexaphen-SA
Disophrol
Disophrol
  Chronotabs
Drixoral Cold and
  Allergy

Drixoral Syrup 🅐
Endafed
Lodrane LD
Respahist
Touro A & H
ULTRAbrom
ULTRAbrom-PD

Ingredients: Carbinoxamine + Pseudoephedrine

Carbiset
Carbiset-TR
Carbodec Tablets
  and Syrup

Carbodec TR
Cardec-S Syrup
Rondec

Rondec Syrup and
  Drops 🅢 🅐
Rondec-TR

Ingredients: Chlorpheniramine + Pseudoephedrine

Allerest Maximum
  Strength 12 Hour
Anamine
  Syrup 🅢 🅐
Anamine TD
Anaplex
  Liquid 🅢 🅐
Atrohist Pediatric
Brexin LA
Chlorafed HS
  Timecelles
Chlorafed
  Timecelles
Chlorafed
  Liquid 🅢 🅐
Chlordrine SR
Chlorfedrine SR
ChlorTrimeton
  4 Hour Relief
  Tablets
ChlorTrimeton
  12 Hour Relief
  Tablets
Codimal LA

Codimal LA Half
  Capsules
Colfed-A
Cophene No.2
CoPyronil 2
Deconamine
Deconamine SR
Deconamine
  Syrup 🅐
Deconomed SR
Dorcol Children's
  Cold Formula
  Liquid 🅐
Duralex
Dura-Tap /PD
  Capsules
Fedahist
Fedahist Gyrocaps
Fedahist Timecaps
Hayfebrol
  Liquid 🅢 🅐
Histalet Syrup 🅐
Klerist
Klerist-D

Kronofed A
Kronofed-A Jr.
  Capsules
ND Clear
Novafed A
Pedia-Care
  Cold-Allergy
  Chewables
Pseudo-Chlor
Pseudo-Gest Plus
Rescon ED
Rescon Jr
Rhinosyn Liquid
Rhinosyn-PD
  Liquid
Rinade B.I.D.
Ryna Liquid 🅢 🅐
Sudafed Plus
  Tablets
Sudafed Plus
  Liquid
Tanafed
Time-Hist

Ingredients: Chlorpheniramine + Phenylephrine

Dallergy-D Syrup Ⓐ
Ed A-Hist
Histatab Plus

Histor-D Syrup
Novahistine Elixir Ⓢ
Prehist

Rolatuss Plain Liquid
Ru-Tuss Liquid

Ingredients: Chlorpheniramine + Phenylpropanolamine

A.R.M. Caplets
12 Hour Cold Capsules
Allerest Maximum Strength 12 Hour
Allerest Children's Tablets
Chlor-Rest
Cold-Gest Cold Capsules
Contac 12 Hour
Contac Maximum Strength 12 Hour
Demazin Tablets and Syrup
Drize

Dura/Vent A Capsules
Genamin Cold Syrup
Gencold
Ornade Spansules
Resaid
Rescon Liquid Ⓢ Ⓐ
Rhinolar-EX
Rhinolar-EX 12
Silaminic Cold Syrup
Teldrin 12-Hour Allergy Relief Capsules

Temazin Cold Syrup
Thera-Hist Syrup Ⓐ
Triaminic
Triaminic Chewable
Triaminic Syrup Ⓐ
Triaminic Allergy Tablets
Triaminic-12
Tri-Nefrin Extra Strength
Tri-Phenyl Syrup

Ingredients: Chlorpheniramine + Phenylephrine + Phenylpropanolamine

Hista-Vadrin Decongestant Tablets

Ingredients: Chlorpheniramine + Phenindamine + Phenylpropanolamine

Nolamine Tablets

Ingredients: Chlorpheniramine + Phenyltoloxamine + Phenylephrine

Comhist Tablets
Comhist LA Capsules

Ingredients: Chlorpheniramine + Phenyltoloxamine + Phenylephrine + Phenylpropanolamine

Naldecon Tablets	Nalgest	Tri-Phen-Chlor
Naldecon Syrup	Syrup 🆂 🅰	Pediatric
Naldecon	Nalgest Pediatric	Syrup 🆂
Pediatric Drops	Drops	Tri-Phen-Mine
Naldecon	Nalgest Pediatric	Pediatric Drops
Pediatric Syrup	Syrup	Tri-Phen-Mine
Naldelate Syrup	Tri-Phen-Chlor	Pediatric
Naldelate	Tablets	Syrup 🆂 🅰
Pediatric Syrup	Tri-Phen-Chlor	Uni-Decon
Naldelate	Syrup	
Pediatric Drops		

Ingredients: Chlorpheniramine + Pyrilamine + Phenylephrine

Atrohist Pediatric	R-Tannamine	Tanoral
Suspension	Pediatric	Triotann
Rhinatate	Suspension	Tritan
R-Tannate Tablets	Rynatan Pediatric	Tri-Tannate
R-Tannate	Suspension	Tablets
Suspension	Rynatan-S	Tri-Tannate
R-Tannamine	Pediatric	Pediatric
Tablets	Suspension	Suspension

Ingredients: Chlorpheniramine + Pyrilamine + Phenylephrine + Phenylpropanolamine

Histalet Forte Tablets
Vanex Forte Caplets

Ingredients: Clemastine + Phenylpropanolamine

Tavist-D Tablets

Ingredients: Diphenhydramine + Pseudoephedrine

Actifed Allergy Tablets: Night
Banophen
Benadryl Allergy Decongestant Liquid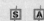

Ingredients: Loratadine + Pseudoephedrine

Claritin-D

Ingredients: Pheniramine + Pyrilamine + Phenylpropanolamine

Triaminic Oral Infant Drops & TR Tablets

Ingredients: Pheniramine + Phenyltoloxamine + Pyrilamine + Phenylpropanolamine

Liqui-Histine-D Elixir
Poly-Histine-D

Ingredients: Promethazine + Phenylephrine

Phenergan VC Syrup
Promethazine VC Syrup
Prometh VC Plain Liquid

Ingredients: Terfenadine + Pseudoephedrine

Seldane-D Tablets

Ingredients: Triprolidine + Pseudoephedrine

Actagen Tablets	Allerfrim Tablets	Genac
Actagen Syrup	Allerfrim Syrup	Silafed Syrup
Actifed Tablets	Aprodine Tablets	Triofed Syrup
Actifed Syrup	Aprodine Syrup	Triposed Tablets
Allercon	Cenafed	Triposed Syrup
Allerfed Syrup		

Prescribed for

Relieving common cold symptoms, allergies, or other upper respiratory conditions, including sneezing, watery eyes, runny nose, itchy or scratchy throat, and nasal congestion.

General Information

The antihistamine-decongestant combinations listed above are among the hundreds of different prescription-only and nonprescription cold and allergy remedies. The basic formula that appears in each of these is always the same: an antihistamine to relieve allergy symptoms and a decongestant to treat the symptoms of either a cold or allergy.

Most of these products are taken several times a day, while others are long-acting and are taken once or twice a day. Since nothing can cure a cold or allergy, the best you can hope to achieve from this or any other cold and allergy remedy is simply symptom relief.

Cautions and Warnings

The antihistamines in these products can cause **drowsiness**. Clemastine, the antihistamine ingredient in Tavist-D, and Terfenadine, the antihistamine ingredient in Seldane-D, cause less drowsiness than other products. Decongestants can cause you to become overly **anxious** and **nervous** and may **interfere with sleep**.

People who are **allergic** to antihistamine or decongestant products should use these medicines with caution. Check with your doctor or pharmacist for further information.

People with **narrow-angle glaucoma, prostate disease, certain stomach ulcers,** and **bladder obstruction** should not take these medicines. Also, people having an **asthma attack** and those taking a **monoamine oxidase (MAO) inhibitor-type antidepressant** should not take these medications. People with serious **liver disease** and those taking **Erythromycin, Ketoconazole,** or **Itraconazole** should not take Terfenadine.

Possible Side Effects

▼ Most common: restlessness, nervousness, sleeplessness, drowsiness, sedation, excitation, dizziness, poor coordination, and upset stomach. Terfenadine has been associated with some abnormal heart rhythms, especially when taken by people with liver disease or when taken together with Erythromycin, Ketoconazole, or Itraconazole.

▼ Less common: low blood pressure, heart palpitations, rapid heartbeat and abnormal heart rhythm, chest pain, anemia, fatigue, confusion, tremors, headache, irritability, euphoria (feeling "high"), tingling or heaviness in the hands, tingling in the feet or legs, blurred or double vision, convulsions, hysterical reactions, ringing or buzzing in the ears, fainting, changes in appetite (increase or decrease), nausea, vomiting, diarrhea or constipation, frequent urination, difficulty urinating, early menstrual periods, loss of sex drive, difficulty breathing, wheezing with chest tightness, stuffed nose, itching, rashes, unusual

> **Possible Side Effects** (continued)
>
> sensitivity to the sun, chills, excessive perspiration, and dry mouth, nose, or throat.

Drug Interactions

• Interaction with alcoholic beverages, antianxiety drugs, tranquilizers, and narcotic-type pain relievers may lead to excessive drowsiness or difficulty concentrating.

• These products should be avoided if you are taking an MAO inhibitor for depression or high blood pressure, because the MAO inhibitor may cause a very rapid rise in blood pressure or increase some side effects (dry mouth and nose, blurred vision, abnormal heart rhythms).

• Terfenadine should not be taken with Erythromycin, Ketoconazole, or Itraconazole because of the rare possibility of developing serious abnormal heart rhythms.

• The decongestant portion of these products may interfere with the normal effects of blood-pressure-lowering medicines and can aggravate diabetes, heart disease, hyperthyroid disease, high blood pressure, prostate disease, stomach ulcers, and urinary blockage.

• If your doctor has prescribed one of these products, do not self-medicate with an additional over-the-counter drug for the relief of cold symptoms. This combination may aggravate high blood pressure, heart disease, diabetes, or thyroid disease.

Food Interactions

These drugs are best taken on an empty stomach, but may be taken with food if they upset your stomach.

Usual Dose

Follow package directions for the specific dosage of the product you are taking. Generally, these medicines are taken every 4 to 12 hours.

Overdosage

The main symptoms of overdose are drowsiness, chills, dry mouth, fever, nausea, nervousness, irritability, rapid or irregular heartbeat, heart pains, and urinary difficulty. Most cases are not severe, but should be treated by inducing vomiting as soon as possible with Syrup of Ipecac (available in any pharmacy). Then call your local poison control center for more information and/or take the victim to a hospital emergency room. ALWAYS bring the medicine container with you.

Special Information

Since the antihistamine component in most of these medicines can slow your central nervous system, you must take extra caution while doing anything that requires concentration, such as driving a car or operating hazardous machinery.

Call your doctor if your side effects are severe or gradually become intolerable. There are so many different cold and allergy products available that one is sure to be the right combination for you.

If you forget to take a dose of your medicine, take it as soon as you remember. If it is almost time for your next dose, skip the one you forgot and go back to your regular schedule. Do not take a double dose.

Special Populations

Pregnancy/Breast-feeding

The ingredients in these products have not been proven to cause birth defects or other problems in pregnant women, although studies in animals have shown that some antihistamines, used mainly against nausea and vomiting, may cause birth defects. Do not take any of these products without your doctor's knowledge.

Small amounts of antihistamine or decongestant medicines pass into breast milk and may affect a nursing infant. Nursing mothers should either not take this medicine or use alternative feeding methods while taking it.

Seniors

Seniors are more sensitive to the side effects of these medications. Confusion, difficult or painful urination, dizziness, drowsiness, a faint feeling, dry mouth, nose, or throat, nightmares or excitement, nervousness, restlessness, or irritability are more likely to occur among older adults.

Generic Name

Apraclonidine Hydrochloride

Brand Name
Iopidine

Type of Drug
Sympathomimetic.

Prescribed for
Post-surgical increases in eye pressure. Apraclonidine is also prescribed as additional short-term treatment in people who are using other glaucoma medicines.

General Information
Apraclonidine reduces both elevated and normal fluid pressure inside the eye and selectively blocks certain nerve endings without acting as a local anesthetic. The exact way it works is not known, but Apraclonidine, like other drugs that reduce eye pressure, may work by decreasing the production of eye fluid. Because permanent damage to the eye nerve can be caused by sharp increases in eye pressure, this agent can be used after laser eye surgery to prevent this from happening. Apraclonidine has a minimal effect on the heart and blood vessels. The drug starts to work within an hour after it is put into the eye and reaches its maximum effect in 3 to 5 hours.

Cautions and Warnings
Do not use Apraclonidine if you are **allergic** to it or to Clonidine. This drug can cause an allergic-like reaction, including **red eye, swelling of the lid and white of the eye, itching, burning,** and the **feeling of something in your eye.** If this happens, stop using the drug and call your doctor. Taking this drug together with a **monoamine oxidase (MAO) inhibitor drug** can result in severe side effects; do not mix them.

Using this medicine with other eye-pressure-lowering drugs may not provide additional benefit because other drugs work in the same way and no further effect may be possible.

The ability of Apraclonidine to lower eye pressure decreases over time. Most people continuously **benefit** for **less than 1 month.**

People with **kidney or liver disease** should be monitored by their doctors while taking this medicine.

Possible Side Effects

▼ Most common: eye redness, itching, tearing, eye discomfort, lid swelling, dry mouth, feeling of something in your eye, headache, and weakness.

▼ Less common: blanching of the eye, upper lid elevation, dilated pupils, blurred vision and other eye disorders, allergic reactions, lid crusting, abnormal vision, eye pain, abdominal pain, diarrhea, stomach discomfort, vomiting, dry mouth or nose, nasal burning, runny nose, sore throat, worsening asthma, constipation and nausea, slow heartbeat, heart palpitations, abnormal heart rhythms, chest pain, fainting, swelling, difficulty sleeping, irritability, reduced sex drive, pain, numbness, or tingling in the hands or feet, clammy or sweaty palms, taste changes, a feeling of having a head cold, and skin rash.

Drug Interactions

• Apraclonidine can reduce pulse and blood pressure. If you are also taking drugs to treat high blood pressure or other cardiovascular drugs, check your pulse and blood pressure.

• MAO·inhibitor drugs can slow the breakdown of Apraclonidine and increase the chance of drug side effects. This combination should be avoided.

Food Interactions

None.

Usual Dose

Adult: 1 or 2 drops in the affected eye 3 times a day.

Overdosage

Exaggerated side effects, especially those that affect the nervous system, are symptoms of overdose. Call your local poison control center for more information. ALWAYS take the medicine bottle with you if you go to the hospital for treatment.

Special Information

This drug can cause dizziness and tiredness. Be careful doing anything that requires concentration, coordination, or alertness while taking this medicine.

To administer eyedrops, lie down or tilt your head backward and look at the ceiling. Hold the dropper above your eye, hold out your lower lid to make a small pouch, and drop the medicine inside while looking up. Release the lower lid and keep your eye open. Don't blink for about 30 seconds. Press gently on the bridge of your nose at the inside corner of your eye for about a minute to help circulate the medicine around your eye. To prevent infection, don't touch the dropper tip to your finger or eyelid. Wait 5 minutes before using any other eyedrop or ointment.

If you forget a dose of Apraclonidine, take it as soon as you remember. If it is almost time for your next dose, take one dose as soon as you remember and then go back to your regular schedule. Do not take a double dose.

Special Populations

Pregnancy/Breast-feeding

In animal studies, Apraclonidine was toxic to developing embryos when given by mouth. There are no studies of this drug in pregnant women, and it should be used with caution during pregnancy.

It is not known if this drug passes into breast milk, but nursing mothers should bottle-feed their babies while using this medicine.

Seniors

Seniors may use this medicine without special precautions.

Generic Names

Aspirin, Buffered Aspirin

Brand Names

A.S.A.	Ascriptin Extra Strength
Alka-Seltzer with Aspirin	Aspergum
Arthritis Pain Formula	Bayer
Ascriptin A/D	Bayer, 8-Hour

Bufferin
Bufferin Arthritis Strength
Bufferin, Extra Strength
Cama Arthritis Pain Reliever
Ecotrin
Ecotrin Maximum Strength

Empirin
Maximum Bayer
Measurin
Norwich Extra-Strength
ZORprin

(Also available in generic form)

Type of Drug

Analgesic; anti-inflammatory agent.

Prescribed for

Mild to moderate pain; fever; arthritis or inflammation of bones, joints, or other body tissues. Men who have had a stroke or TIA (oxygen shortage to the brain) because of a problem with blood coagulation may be prescribed Aspirin to reduce the risk of having another such attack. Aspirin may also be prescribed as an anticoagulant (blood-thinning) drug in people with unstable angina, and to protect against heart attack. The long-term effect of Aspirin in preventing cataracts is now being studied.

General Information

Aspirin may be the closest thing we have to a wonder drug. It has been used for more than a century for pain and fever relief, and is now used for its effect on the blood as well.

Aspirin is the standard against which all other drugs are compared for pain relief and for reduction of inflammation. Chemically, Aspirin is a member of the group of drugs called *salicylates*. Other salicylates include Sodium Salicylate, Sodium Thiosalicylate, Choline Salicylate, and Magnesium Salicylate (Trilisate). These drugs are no more effective than regular Aspirin, although two of them (Choline Salicylate and Magnesium Salicylate) may be a little less irritating to the stomach. They are all more expensive than Aspirin.

Aspirin reduces fever by causing the blood vessels in the skin to open, allowing heat to leave the body more rapidly. Its effects on pain and inflammation are thought to be related to its ability to prevent the manufacture of complex body hormones called prostaglandins. Of all the salicylates, Aspirin has the greatest effect on prostaglandin production.

Many people find that they can take Buffered Aspirin but not regular Aspirin. The addition of antacids to Aspirin can be important to patients who must take large doses of Aspirin for chronic arthritis or other conditions. In many cases, Aspirin is the only effective drug and can be tolerated only with the antacids present.

Cautions and Warnings

People with **liver damage** should avoid Aspirin. People who are **allergic to Aspirin** may also be allergic to drugs such as Indomethacin, Sulindac, Ibuprofen, Fenoprofen, Naproxen, Tolmetin, and Meclofenamate Sodium or to products containing *tartrazine* (a commonly used orange dye and food coloring). People with asthma and/or nasal polyps are more likely to be allergic to Aspirin.

Alcoholic beverages can aggravate the stomach irritation caused by Aspirin. The risk of Aspirin-related ulcers is increased by alcohol.

Do not use Aspirin if you develop dizziness, hearing loss, or ringing or buzzing in your ears.

Reye's syndrome is a life-threatening condition characterized by vomiting and stupor or dullness and may develop in children with influenza (flu) or chickenpox if treated with Aspirin or other salicylates. Up to 30 percent of people who develop Reye's syndrome can die, and permanent brain damage is possible in those who survive. Because of this, the U.S. Surgeon General, the Centers for Disease Control and Prevention, and pediatric physicians' associations advise against the use of Aspirin or other salicylates in children under age 17, especially those with chickenpox or the flu. Products with Acetaminophen are suggested instead.

Aspirin can interfere with normal blood coagulation and should be avoided for 1 week before surgery for this reason. It would be wise to ask your surgeon or dentist their recommendation before taking Aspirin for pain after surgery.

Possible Side Effects

▼ Most common: nausea, upset stomach, heartburn, loss of appetite, and loss of small amounts of blood in the stool.

Possible Side Effects *(continued)*

▼ Other: hives, rashes, liver damage, fever, thirst, and difficulties with vision. Aspirin may contribute to the formation of stomach ulcers and bleeding. People who are allergic to Aspirin and those with a history of nasal polyps, asthma, or rhinitis may experience breathing difficulty and a stuffed nose.

Drug Interactions

• People taking anticoagulants (blood-thinning drugs) should avoid Aspirin. The effect of the anticoagulant will be increased.

• Aspirin may increase the possibility of stomach ulcer when taken together with adrenal corticosteroids, Phenylbutazone, or alcoholic beverages.

• Aspirin will counteract the uric-acid-eliminating effect of Probenecid and Sulfinpyrazone. Aspirin may counteract the blood-pressure-lowering effect of ACE Inhibitor and betablocking drugs. Aspirin may also counteract the effects of some diuretics in people with severe liver disease.

• Aspirin may increase blood levels of Methotrexate and of Valproic Acid when taken with either of these drugs, leading to increased chances of drug toxicity. Aspirin and Nitroglycerin tablets may lead to an unexpected drop in blood pressure.

• Do not take Aspirin with a nonsteroidal anti-inflammatory drug (NSAID). There is no benefit to the combination, and the chance of side effects, especially stomach irritation, is vastly increased.

• Large Aspirin doses (2000 mg per day or more) can lower blood sugar. This can be a problem in diabetics who take Insulin or oral antidiabetes drugs to control their condition.

Food Interactions

Because Aspirin can cause upset stomach or bleeding, take each dose with food, milk, or a glass of water.

Usual Dose

Adult: for aches, pains, and fever, 325 to 650 mg every 4

hours; for arthritis and rheumatic conditions, up to 5200 mg (16 325-mg tablets) per day; for rheumatic fever, up to 7800 mg (24 325-mg tablets) per day; to prevent heart attack, stroke, or TIA in men, 325 mg every 2 days or 160 mg per day.

Child (age 16 and under): not recommended because of the risk of Reye's syndrome (see *Cautions and Warnings*).

Overdosage

The approximate lethal dose of Aspirin is 30 to 90 regular-strength (325-mg) tablets (20 to 40 maximum-strength [500-mg] tablets) for adults and 12 regular-strength tablets (8 maximum-strength tablets) for children.

Symptoms of mild overdosage are rapid and deep breathing, nausea, vomiting, dizziness, ringing or buzzing in the ears, flushing, sweating, thirst, headache, drowsiness, diarrhea, and rapid heartbeat.

Severe overdosage may cause fever, excitement, confusion, convulsions, liver or kidney failure, coma, or bleeding.

The initial treatment of Aspirin overdose involves making the patient vomit to remove any Aspirin remaining in the stomach. Further treatment depends on how the situation develops and what must be done to maintain the patient. **Do not induce vomiting until you have spoken with your doctor or poison control center.** If in doubt, go to a hospital emergency room.

Special Information

Contact your doctor if you develop continuous stomach pain or ringing or buzzing in the ears.

Do not use an Aspirin product if it has a strong odor of vinegar. This is an indication that the product has started to break down in the bottle.

If you forget to take a dose of Aspirin, take it as soon as you remember. If it is almost time for your next dose, skip the forgotten dose and continue with your regular schedule. Do not take a double dose.

Special Populations

Pregnancy/Breast-feeding

Check with your doctor before taking any Aspirin-containing

product during pregnancy. Aspirin can cause bleeding problems in the developing fetus during the last 2 weeks of pregnancy. Taking Aspirin during the last 3 months of pregnancy may lead to a low-birth-weight infant, prolong labor, and extend the length of pregnancy; it can also cause bleeding in the mother before, during, or after delivery.

Aspirin has not caused any problems among nursing mothers or their infants.

Seniors

Aspirin, especially in the larger doses that an older adult may take to treat arthritis and rheumatic conditions, may be irritating to the stomach. Older adults with liver disease should not use Aspirin.

Generic Name

Astemizole

Brand Name

Hismanal

Type of Drug

Antihistamine.

Prescribed for

Seasonal allergy, stuffed and runny nose, itchy eyes, scratchy throat caused by allergies, and other symptoms of allergy (such as rash, itching, or hives).

General Information

Astemizole is a nonsedating antihistamine available only by prescription. It may be used by people who find other antihistamines unacceptable because of the drowsiness and tiredness they cause.

Cautions and Warnings

Astemizole should not be taken by people who have had an allergic reaction to it in the past. People with **asthma** or **other**

deep-breathing problems, glaucoma (pressure in the eye), or **stomach ulcer** or **other stomach problems** should avoid Astemizole because it may aggravate these problems.

In high doses (20 or 30 mg per day) or cases of drug overdose, Astemizole may cause serious **abnormal heart rhythms** or other, possibly fatal **cardiac effects**. It should not be taken by people with **serious liver disease** or by those **taking Erythromycin, Ketoconazole, or Itraconazole**.

Possible Side Effects

The most important side effects of Astemizole are the rare cardiac consequences that most often occur in people with liver disease and those taking Erythromycin, Ketoconazole, or Itraconazole. Dizziness or fainting may be the first sign of a cardiac problem with Astemizole.

▼ Most common: headache; nervousness; weakness; upset stomach; nausea; vomiting; dry mouth, nose, or throat; cough; stuffed nose; change in bowel habits; sore throat; and nosebleeds. In scientific studies, Astemizole was found to cause the same amount of drowsiness as a placebo (inactive pill). Ironically, about half of the other antihistamines sold in the United States also cause a similar degree of drowsiness. Most commonly used antihistamines cause more sedation than Astemizole. Astemizole may also cause increased appetite or weight gain.

▼ Less common: hair loss, allergic reactions, depression, sleeplessness, muscle aches, menstrual irregularities, increased sweating, tingling in the hands or feet, frequent urination, and visual disturbances. A few people taking this drug have developed liver damage.

Drug Interactions

• Antihistamines may decrease the effects of oral anticoagulant (blood-thinning) drugs.

• People taking Erythromycin, Ketoconazole, or Itraconazole have been reported to develop serious and possibly fatal cardiac side effects, though this is rare. Do not take any of these medicines with Astemizole.

Food Interactions

Take Astemizole 1 hour before or 2 hours after meals.

Usual Dose

Adult and Adolescent (age 12 and older): 10 mg once a day.
Child (under age 12): not recommended.

Overdosage

Astemizole overdose is likely to cause serious cardiac effects or exaggerated side effects. Overdose victims should be given Syrup of Ipecac to make them vomit; they should then be taken to a hospital emergency room. ALWAYS bring the prescription bottle.

Special Information

Dizziness or fainting may be the first sign of serious drug side effects; call your doctor at once if you experience these or any other unusual side effects while taking Astemizole.

If you forget to take a dose of Astemizole, take it as soon as you remember. If it is almost time for your next dose, skip the forgotten dose and continue with your regular schedule. Do not take a double dose.

Special Populations

Pregnancy/Breast-feeding

Astemizole has been studied in pregnant lab animals, and no damage to developing fetuses was found. Nevertheless, this drug should be used by pregnant women only if it is absolutely necessary.

It is not known if this drug passes into breast milk. Nursing mothers should avoid using this drug. If you must use Astemizole, you should bottle-feed your baby.

Seniors

Older adults may be more sensitive to the side effects of Astemizole, and should be treated with the minimum effective dose, 10 mg per day.

Generic Name

Atenolol

Brand Name

Tenormin*

Combination Product

Atenolol + Chlorthalidone

Tenoretic*

(*Also available in generic form)

Type of Drug

Beta-adrenergic-blocking agent.

Prescribed for

High blood pressure, abnormal heart rhythms, angina pectoris, preventing second heart attack, preventing migraine headaches, alcohol withdrawal, stage fright and other anxieties, and bleeding from the esophagus.

General Information

Atenolol, a beta-adrenergic blocker, interferes with the action of a specific part of the nervous system. Beta receptors are found all over the body and affect many body functions, which accounts for the usefulness of beta blockers against many conditions. The first member of this group, *Propranolol*, was found to affect the entire beta-adrenergic portion of the nervous system. Newer beta blockers, like Atenolol, have been refined to affect only a portion of that system, making them more useful in treating cardiovascular disorders and less so for other purposes. Other beta blockers are mild stimulants to the heart or have other characteristics.

Cautions and Warnings

People with **angina** who take Atenolol for high blood pressure should have their drug dosage reduced gradually over 1 to 2 weeks rather than suddenly discontinued to avoid possible aggravation of the angina.

Atenolol should be used with caution if you have **liver or kidney disease,** because your ability to eliminate this drug from your body may be impaired.

Atenolol reduces the amount of blood the heart pumps. This reduction in blood flow can worsen the condition of people with **poor circulation** or **circulatory disease**.

If you are undergoing **major surgery,** your doctor may want you to stop taking Atenolol at least 2 days before to permit the heart to respond more quickly to things that happen during the procedure. This is still controversial and may not hold true for all people preparing for surgery.

Possible Side Effects

Side effects are usually mild and relatively uncommon, develop early in the course of treatment, and are rarely a reason to stop taking Atenolol.

▼ Most common: male impotence.

▼ Other: unusual tiredness or weakness, slow heartbeat, heart failure (swelling of the legs, ankles, or feet), dizziness, breathing difficulty, bronchospasm, mental depression, confusion, anxiety, nervousness, sleeplessness, disorientation, short-term memory loss, emotional instability, cold hands and feet, constipation, diarrhea, nausea, vomiting, upset stomach, increased sweating, urinary difficulty, cramps, blurred vision, skin rash, hair loss, stuffy nose, facial swelling, aggravation of lupus erythematosus (a disease of the body's connective tissues), itching, chest pains, back or joint pains, colitis, drug allergy (fever, sore throat), and liver toxicity.

Drug Interactions

• Atenolol may interact with surgical anesthetics to increase the risk of heart problems during surgery. Some anesthesiologists recommend gradually stopping your medicine 2 days before surgery.

• Atenolol may interfere with the normal signs of low blood sugar and can interfere with oral antidiabetic drugs.

• Atenolol enhances the blood-pressure-lowering effects of other such agents (e.g., Clonidine, Guanabenz, Reserpine) and calcium channel blockers (e.g., Nifedipine).

• Aspirin-containing drugs, Indomethacin, Sulfinpyrazone, and estrogen drugs can interfere with the blood-pressure-lowering effect of Atenolol.

• Cocaine may reduce the effects of all beta-blocking drugs.

• Atenolol may worsen the condition of cold hands and feet associated with taking ergot alkaloids (for migraine headaches). Gangrene is a possibility in people taking an ergot and Atenolol.

• Atenolol will counteract the effects of thyroid hormone replacement medicines.

• Calcium channel blockers, Flecainide, Hydralazine, oral contraceptives, Propafenone, Haloperidol, phenothiazine tranquilizers (Molindone and others), quinolone antibacterials, and Quinidine may increase the amount of Atenolol in the bloodstream and its effect on the body.

• Atenolol should not be taken within 2 weeks of taking a monoamine oxidase (MAO) inhibitor antidepressant drug.

• Cimetidine increases the amount of Atenolol absorbed into the bloodstream from oral tablets.

• Atenolol may interfere with the effectiveness of Theophylline, Aminophylline, and some antiasthma drugs (especially Ephedrine and Isoproterenol).

• The combination of Atenolol and Phenytoin or Digitalis drugs can result in excessive slowing of the heart, possibly causing heart block.

• If you stop smoking while taking Atenolol, your dose may have to be reduced because your liver will break down the drug more slowly after you stop.

Food Interactions

Atenolol may be taken without regard to food or meals.

Usual Dose

Adult: starting dose, 50 mg per day, taken all at once. The daily dose may be gradually increased up to 200 mg. The maintenance dose is 50 to 200 mg once a day. People with kidney disease may need only 50 mg every other day.

Senior: older adults may need lower doses and should be treated more cautiously.

Overdosage

Symptoms are changes in heartbeat (unusually slow, unusually fast, or irregular), severe dizziness or fainting, difficulty breathing, bluish-colored fingernails or palms, and seizures. The victim should be taken to a hospital emergency room. ALWAYS bring the medicine bottle.

Special Information

Atenolol is meant to be taken continuously. Do not stop taking it unless directed to do so by your doctor; abrupt withdrawal may cause chest pain, difficulty breathing, increased sweating, and unusually fast or irregular heartbeat. The dose should be lowered gradually over a period of about 2 weeks.

Call your doctor at once if any of these symptoms develop: back or joint pains, difficulty breathing, cold hands or feet, depression, skin rash, or changes in heartbeat. Atenolol may produce an undesirable lowering of blood pressure, leading to dizziness or fainting. Call your doctor if this happens. Call your doctor about the following side effects only if they persist or are bothersome: anxiety, diarrhea, constipation, impotence, headache, itching, nausea or vomiting, nightmares or vivid dreams, upset stomach, insomnia, stuffed nose, frequent urination, unusual tiredness, or weakness.

Atenolol can cause drowsiness, light-headedness, dizziness, or blurred vision. Be careful when driving or performing complex tasks.

It is best to take your medicine at the same time each day. If you forget a dose, take it as soon as you remember. If you take it once a day and it is within 8 hours of your next dose, skip the forgotten tablet and continue with your regular schedule. If you take Atenolol twice a day, and it is within 4 hours of your next dose, skip the forgotten dose and continue with your regular schedule. Do not take a double dose.

Special Populations

Pregnancy/Breast-feeding

Infants born to women who took a beta blocker while pregnant weighed less at birth and had low blood pressure and reduced heart rate. Atenolol should be avoided by pregnant women and those who might become pregnant while taking it. When the drug is considered essential by your doctor, its potential benefits must be carefully weighed against its risks.

Atenolol passes into breast milk in concentrations greater than those found in the bloodstream. Nursing mothers should avoid taking Atenolol.

Seniors

Older adults may absorb and retain more Atenolol, thus requiring less medicine to achieve the same results. Your doctor will need to adjust your dosage to meet your individual needs. Seniors taking this medicine may be more likely to suffer from cold hands and feet, reduced body temperature, chest pains, general feelings of ill health, sudden breathing difficulty, increased sweating, or changes in heartbeat.

Generic Name

Atovaquone

Brand Name

Mepron Suspension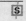

Type of Drug

Anti-infective.

Prescribed for

Pneumocystis carinii pneumonia (PCP) in people who cannot take Trimethoprim-Sulfamethoxazole (TMP-SMZ).

General Information

Atovaquone is an anti-infective with specific activity against PCP pneumonia, an infection commonly associated with AIDS. In studies comparing Atovaquone with TMP-SMZ, the two drugs provided a roughly similar improvement for people with PCP (about 60 percent improved); *however, more people died on Atovaquone of PCP and other infections*. Of those who died, most had less Atovaquone in their bloodstream. In studies comparing oral Atovaquone with intravenous Pentamidine for PCP in people with AIDS, both drugs were equally effective (14 percent), but there was a direct correlation between the amount of Atovaquone in the blood and survival. Sixty percent of people with less than 5 micrograms of drug per milliliter of blood died, while only 9 percent of those with 5 or more micrograms of drug per milliliter of blood died. In clinical trials of Atovaquone for PCP using doses of 750 mg three times a day, average blood levels were almost 14 micrograms per milliliter of blood, well above the threshold level of 5. The drug stays in the body for several days and is eliminated via breakdown in the liver.

Cautions and Warnings

Do not take Atovaquone if you are or may be **allergic** to any of this product's components.

This drug has not been studied for **PCP prevention** or **severe PCP** or in those who are failing on TMP-SMZ.

Atovaquone does not work against anything except PCP. People with PCP who have bacterial, viral, fungal, or other infections of the lung may continue to worsen despite Atovaquone therapy. If this happens, it may be a sign that another kind of infecting organism is the cause. Your doctor will have to **prescribe additional medicine.**

Since Atovaquone **absorption** is so **strongly influenced by food,** people who cannot eat sufficiently may not be able to absorb enough drug, and may have to take alternative intravenous PCP treatments while taking Atovaquone.

Possible Side Effects

It is often difficult to detect Atovaquone-related side effects because they often resemble the underlying medical condition of people who generally take this medicine. Overall, only 4 to 7 percent of people stopped taking the drug because of side effects, much less than those on other PCP treatments. This drug has not been associated with any life-threatening or fatal side effects.

▼ Most common: rash, nausea, diarrhea, headache, vomiting, fever, sleeplessness, weakness, itching, oral fungal infections, abdominal pain, upset stomach, appetite loss, constipation, cough, dizziness, pains, increased sweating, anxiety, sinus inflammation, and runny nose.

▼ Less common: taste changes, low blood sugar, and low blood pressure.

Drug Interactions

• Atovaquone may increase levels of Warfarin, oral antidiabetes drugs, Digoxin, and other drugs that strongly bind to blood proteins.

• Rifampin and Rifabutin may reduce blood levels of Atovaquone, possibly reducing its effectiveness.

• Taking Atovaquone together with TMP-SMZ has resulted in reduced blood levels of TMP-SMZ. This should not affect the ability of TMP-SMZ to do its job.

• Taking Atovaquone with Zidovudine causes the body to drastically reduce the rate at which Zidovudine is eliminated from the body. For most people, this is not a problem.

Food Interactions

Atovaquone is highly fat-soluble. Its absorption into the blood is highly affected by food, especially a high-fat meal, which can increase the amount absorbed by **300 percent!** Take Atovaquone with food or meals to improve drug absorption.

Usual Dose

750 mg 2 times per day for 3 weeks, taken with food.

Overdosage

There is little experience with Atovaquone overdose; symptoms are likely to be exaggerated drug side effects. If the overdose is taken without food in the stomach, the amount absorbed may not be enough to be harmful. Call your local poison control center or hospital emergency room for more information. If you go to the hospital, ALWAYS bring the medicine bottle.

Special Information

Taking Atovaquone regularly and with food is essential to the drug's effectiveness. If you cannot eat 2 meals a day, your doctor may have to prescribe another PCP treatment.

Call your doctor if you develop any persistent or bothersome side effects.

If you forget a dose, take it as soon as you remember. If it is almost time for your next dose, space your remaining doses equally throughout the rest of the day so that you can still take a total daily dose of 1500 mg (two teaspoonfuls).

Special Populations

Pregnancy/Breast-feeding

In animal studies, Atovaquone has affected fetal development in doses that are roughly equal to human doses. This drug should be used only if the potential risks and benefits have been weighed by you and your doctor. If you are not pregnant, use effective contraception while taking Atovaquone.

It is not known if Atovaquone passes into breast milk or if the drug affects a nursing infant. In animal studies, Atovaquone was found in breast milk at levels equal to 1/3 of those in the blood. Nursing mothers should bottle-feed their babies while taking Atovaquone.

Seniors

This drug has not been systematically tested in people over age 65. Older adults, especially those with kidney, heart, or liver disease, may be more sensitive to Atovaquone side effects. Report any unusual side effects to your doctor.

Atrovent

see *Ipratropium Bromide*, page 542

Augmentin

see *Penicillin Antibiotics*, page 868

Brand Name

Auralgan Otic Solution

Ingredients

Antipyrine
Benzocaine
Glycerin

Other Brand Names

Allergen Ear Drops
Auroto Otic Solution
Otocalm Ear

(Also available in generic form)

Type of Drug

Analgesic.

Prescribed for

Earache.

General Information

This drug is a combination product containing Benzocaine, a local anesthetic (to deaden nerves inside the ear that transmit painful impulses); Antipyrine, an analgesic (to provide additional pain relief); and Glycerin (to remove any water present in the ear). This drug is often used to treat painful conditions caused by water in the ear canal, such as "swimmer's ear." This drug does not contain antibiotics and should not be used to treat any infection or condition other than the one for which it is prescribed.

Cautions and Warnings

Do not use if you are **allergic** to any of the ingredients.

Possible Side Effects

▼ Most common: local irritation.

Drug Interactions

• Do not apply any other medicines at the same time as Auralgan.

Food Interactions

None known.

Usual Dose

Place drops of Auralgan in the ear canal until the canal is filled. Saturate a piece of cotton with Auralgan, and put it in the ear canal to keep the drug from leaking out. Leave the drug in the ear for several minutes. Repeat 3 to 4 times per day.

Overdose

Auralgan overdose is not likely to cause serious effects. Call your local poison control center for more information.

Special Information

Before using, warm the medicine bottle to body temperature by holding it in your hand for several minutes. Do not warm the bottle to a temperature above normal body temperature. Protect the bottle from light.

Call your doctor if you develop a burning or itching feeling or if the pain does not go away after 2 to 4 days of treatment.

If you forget a dose of Auralgan, take it as soon as you remember. If it is almost time for your next dose, skip the forgotten dose and continue with your regular schedule.

Special Populations

Pregnancy/Breast-feeding

Pregnant and breast-feeding women may use this product without special restrictions.

Seniors

Older adults may use this product without restriction.

Axid

see **Nizatidine**, page 815

Generic Name

Azithromycin

Brand Name

Zithromax

Type of Drug

Macrolide antibiotic.

Prescribed for

Infections of virtually any part of the body. It is prescribed for upper and lower respiratory tract infections, skin infections, and some sexually transmitted diseases.

General Information

Azithromycin is a member of the *azalide* group of antibiotics, a subgroup of the *macrolide* antibiotics. The macrolides (which also include Erythromycin and Clarithromycin) are either bactericidal (they kill the bacteria directly) or bacteriostatic (they slow the bacteria's growth so that the body's natural protective mechanisms can kill them). Whether these drugs are bacteriostatic or bactericidal depends on the organism in question and the amount of antibiotic present in the blood or other body fluid.

Azithromycin is rapidly absorbed from the gastrointestinal tract and distributed to all parts of the body. Because the action of this antibiotic depends on its concentration within the invading bacteria, it is imperative that you follow your doctor's directions regarding the spacing of the doses as well as the number of days you should continue taking the medication. The effectiveness of this antibiotic can be severely reduced if these instructions are not followed.

Cautions and Warnings

Do not take Azithromycin if you are **allergic** to it or any of the macrolide antibiotics.

Azithromycin is excreted primarily through the liver. People with **liver disease or damage** should exercise caution by watching for possible drug side effects. Those on long-term therapy with this drug should have periodic blood tests.

A form of **colitis** (bowel inflammation) has been associated with all antibiotics, including Azithromycin. Diarrhea may be an indication of this problem.

Abnormal heart rhythms have been associated with other macrolide antibiotics and should be considered as possible side effects of Azithromycin treatment, even though they have yet to be seen with this drug.

Azithromycin is considered appropriate only for the treatment of more **mild forms of pneumonia in nonhospitalized patients.** Other people, including those with other underlying conditions, those who are immunocompromised, and those who contracted their pneumonia while in a hospital or other institutional setting, probably should be treated with other antibiotics.

Possible Side Effects

Most side effects are mild and will go away once you stop taking Azithromycin.

▼ Most common: nausea, vomiting, stomach cramps, stomach gas, and diarrhea. Colitis may develop after taking Azithromycin.

▼ Less common: heart palpitations, chest pain, hairy tongue, vaginal irritation, kidney inflammation, dizziness, headache, fainting, fatigue, tiredness, unusual sensitivity to the sun, skin rash, and swelling.

Drug Interactions

• Azithromycin may increase Warfarin's anticoagulant (blood-thinning) effects in people who take it regularly, especially seniors. People taking anticoagulants who must also take Azithromycin may need their anticoagulant dose adjusted.

• Azithromycin may interfere with the elimination of Theophylline from the body, in a manner similar to Erythromycin. People taking this combination should be carefully monitored by their doctors for changes in blood-Theophylline levels.

• Antacid products containing Aluminum or Magnesium

may delay the absorption of Azithromycin into the blood.
Separate your antacid dose from your Azithromycin dose by
at least 1 hour.

Food Interactions

Food in the stomach will cut the amount of Azithromycin
absorbed into the blood in half. Take it on an empty stomach
or 1 hour before or 2 hours after meals.

Usual Dose

Adult and Adolescent (age 16 and older): 500 mg as a single
dose on the first day of treatment, then 250 mg once a day for
4 more days. For some sexually transmitted diseases, 1000
mg is taken as a single dose.

Child (6 months to 15 years): 2.25 to 5.5 mg per pound (up
to 500 mg) daily for 5 days.

Child (under 6 months): not recommended.

Overdosage

Azithromycin overdose may result in exaggerated side effects, especially nausea, vomiting, stomach cramps, and
diarrhea. Call your local poison control center or hospital
emergency room for more information.

Special Information

Call your doctor if you develop nausea, vomiting, diarrhea,
stomach cramps, or severe abdominal pain, or any unusual
side effects.

Since Azithromycin is taken only once a day, take it at the
same time each day to help you remember your medicine. If
you forget a dose of Azithromycin, take it as soon as you
remember. If it is almost time for your next dose, skip the
missed dose and go back to your regular schedule. Remember to complete the full course of therapy prescribed by your
doctor, even if you feel perfectly well after only 1 or 2 days of
taking the antibiotic.

Special Populations

Pregnancy/Breast-feeding

It is not known if Azithromycin passes into the circulation of the developing fetus. This medication should be taken by pregnant women only if it is clearly needed.

It is not known if Azithromycin passes into breast milk. Nursing mothers should discuss the risks and possible benefits of taking this medicine with their doctor.

Seniors

Older adults, except those with liver disease, may generally use this product without restriction or dose adjustment. Older adults who have pneumonia or who are especially sickly or debilitated probably should be treated with another medication.

Azmacort

see **Corticosteroid Inhalers**, page 280

Brand Name

Azo Gantrisin

Ingredients

Phenazopyridine
Sulfisoxazole

Other Brand Names

Azo-Sulfisoxazole

(Also available in generic form)

Type of Drug

Urinary anti-infective.

Prescribed for

Urinary tract infections.

General Information

Azo Gantrisin is one of many combination products used to

treat urinary tract infections. The primary active ingredient is the sulfa drug *Sulfisoxazole*. The other ingredient, *Phenazopyridine*, is added to relieve urinary tract pain.

Cautions and Warnings

Do not take Azo Gantrisin if you know you are **allergic** to it (or other sulfa drugs), **salicylates,** or similar agents, or if you have a condition called *porphyria.* Azo Gantrisin should not be used by people with **advanced kidney disease.**

Possible Side Effects

▼ Most common: headache, itching, rash, sensitivity to bright lights (particularly sunlight), nausea, vomiting, abdominal pains, feelings of tiredness or fatigue, hallucinations, dizziness, ringing in the ears, chills, and feelings of ill health.

▼ Less common: reduced white-blood-cell counts and platelet counts, changes in other blood components, itchy eyes, arthritis-type pain, diarrhea, loss of appetite, stomach cramps or pains, hearing loss, drowsiness, fever, hair loss, yellowing of the skin and/or eyes, and reduction of sperm count.

Drug Interactions

• When Azo Gantrisin is taken with an anticoagulant (blood-thinning) drug, any diabetes drug, Methotrexate, Phenylbutazone, salicylates (Aspirin-like drugs), Phenytoin, or Probenecid, it will cause unusually large amounts of these drugs to be released into the bloodstream, possibly producing symptoms of overdosage. If you must take Azo Gantrisin for an extended period, your physician should reduce the dosage of these interactive drugs. Also, avoid large doses of vitamin C.

Food Interactions

Sulfa drugs should be taken with a full glass of water on an empty stomach, but they can be taken with food if they upset your stomach.

Usual Dose

First dose, 4 to 6 tablets, then 2 tablets every 4 hours. Take each dose with a full glass of water.

Overdosage

Give the overdose victim Syrup of Ipecac (available in any pharmacy) to induce vomiting as soon as possible. Follow package directions. Take the victim to a hospital emergency room. ALWAYS bring the medicine bottle.

Special Information

Azo Gantrisin can cause photosensitivity (a severe reaction to strong sunlight): Avoid prolonged sun exposure.

Sore throat, fever, unusual bleeding or bruising, rash, and feeling tired are early signs of serious blood disorders and should be reported to your doctor immediately.

The Phenazopyridine ingredient in Azo Gantrisin is an orange-red dye and will discolor the urine. This is a normal effect of the drug, but if you are diabetic, the dye may interfere with testing your urine for sugar. This dye may also appear in your sweat and tears. Note that this dye may discolor certain types of contact lenses.

If you miss a dose of Azo Gantrisin, take it as soon as possible. If it is almost time for your next dose, skip the missed dose and continue with your regular schedule. Do not take a double dose.

Special Populations

Pregnancy/Breast-feeding

This drug may cause birth defects or interfere with fetal development. Check with your doctor before taking it if you are, or might be, pregnant.

The sulfa ingredient in this combination may pass into breast milk and can cause problems in infants suffering from G6PD deficiency, a rare genetic disorder. Other infants are usually not affected by this drug.

Seniors

Older adults may take this drug without special restriction.

Beconase AQ

see **Corticosteroids, Nasal,** page 284

Generic Name

Benazepril Hydrochloride

Brand Name

Lotensin

Type of Drug

Angiotensin-converting-enzyme (ACE) inhibitor.

Prescribed for

High blood pressure.

General Information

Benazepril Hydrochloride belongs to the class of drugs known as angiotensin-converting-enzyme (ACE) inhibitors. ACE inhibitors prevent the conversion of a hormone called *angiotensin I* to another hormone called *angiotensin II*, a potent blood-vessel constrictor. Preventing this conversion relaxes (dilates) blood vessels and helps to reduce blood pressure and relieve the symptoms of heart failure by making it easier for a failing heart to pump blood through the body. The production of other hormones and enzymes that participate in the regulation of blood-vessel dilation is also affected by Benazepril and probably plays a role in its effectiveness. Benazepril starts working in 1 hour and continues for about 24 hours.

Some people, especially heart-failure patients, who start taking Benazepril after they are already on a diuretic (water pill) experience a rapid blood-pressure drop after their first dose or when their dose is increased. To prevent this from happening, your doctor may tell you to stop taking your diuretic 2 or 3 days before starting Benazepril or increase your salt intake during that time. The diuretic may then be restarted gradually.

Cautions and Warnings

Do not take Benazepril Hydrochloride if you have had an **allergic** reaction to it in the past. It can (rarely) cause **very low blood pressure** and **affect kidney function**. Your doctor should check your urine for protein content during the first few months of treatment.

Because this drug is generally eliminated from the body via the kidneys, dosage adjustment of Benazepril is necessary if you have **reduced kidney function**.

Benazepril can affect **white-blood-cell counts**, possibly increasing your susceptibility to infection. Your doctor should monitor your blood counts periodically.

Possible Side Effects

▼ Most common: dizziness, tiredness, headache, and chronic cough. The cough usually goes away a few days after you stop taking the medicine. Nausea can also occur.

▼ Rare: low blood pressure, chest pains, dizziness when rising from a sitting or lying position, fainting, heart palpitations, sleeping difficulty, tingling in the hands or feet, vomiting, constipation, abdominal pain, blood in the stool, itching, rash, flushing, anxiety, nervousness, reduced sex drive, impotence, muscle and joint aches, arthritis, asthma, bronchitis, breathing difficulty, weakness, increased sweating, urinary tract infection, and swelling of the arms, legs, lips, tongue, face, and throat.

Drug Interactions

• The blood-pressure-lowering effect of Benazepril is additive with diuretics and beta blockers. Any other drug that causes a rapid blood-pressure drop should be used with caution if you are taking Benazepril.

• Benazepril may increase blood-potassium levels, especially if taken with Dyazide or other potassium-sparing diuretics.

• Benazepril may increase the effect of Lithium; this combination should be used with caution.

• Antacids may reduce the amount of Benazepril absorbed

into the blood. Separate doses of these 2 medicines by at least 2 hours.

• Capsaicin may cause or aggravate the cough associated with Benazepril therapy.

• Indomethacin may reduce the blood-pressure-lowering effects of Benazepril.

• Phenothiazine tranquilizers and antivomiting drugs may increase the effects of Benazepril.

• Combining Allopurinol and Benazepril increases the risk of adverse drug reactions. Avoid this combination.

• Benazepril increases blood levels of Digoxin, possibly increasing the chance of Digoxin-related side effects.

Food Interactions

Benazepril may be taken without regard to food. You may take it with food if it upsets your stomach.

Usual Dose

10 to 40 mg once or twice a day. People with poor kidney function may need less medicine to lower blood pressure.

Overdosage

The principal effect of Benazepril overdose is a rapid drop in blood pressure, as evidenced by dizziness or fainting. Take the overdose victim to a hospital emergency room immediately. ALWAYS bring the medicine bottle.

Special Information

Benazepril Hydrochloride can cause swelling of the face, lips, hands, and feet. This swelling can also affect the larynx (throat) and tongue, and interfere with breathing. If this happens, go to a hospital at once. Call your doctor if you develop a sore throat, mouth sores, abnormal heartbeat, sudden difficulty breathing, chest pain, a persistent rash, or loss of taste perception.

You may get dizzy if you rise to your feet too quickly from a sitting or lying position. Avoid strenuous exercise and/or very hot weather because heavy sweating or dehydration can cause a rapid blood-pressure drop.

Avoid nonprescription diet pills, decongestants, and stimulants that can raise blood pressure while taking Benazepril.

If you take Benazepril once a day and forget to take a dose, take it as soon as you remember. If it is within 8 hours of your next dose, skip the one you forgot and continue with your regular schedule.

If you take it twice a day and miss a dose, take it right away. If it is within 4 hours of your next dose, take one dose then and another in 5 or 6 hours, and then go back to your regular schedule. Do not take a double dose.

Special Populations

Pregnancy/Breast-feeding

ACE inhibitors have caused low blood pressure, kidney failure, slow formation of the skull, and death in developing fetuses when taken during the last 6 months of pregnancy. Women who are, or may become, pregnant should not take any ACE inhibitor drugs. Sexually active women who must take Benazepril must use an effective contraceptive method, or use a different medicine. If you become pregnant, stop taking the medicine, and call your doctor immediately.

Relatively small amounts of Benazepril pass into breast milk, and the effect on a nursing infant is likely to be small. However, nursing mothers who must take this drug should consider bottle-feeding with formula because infants, especially newborns, are more susceptible to this medicine's effects than adults.

Seniors

Older adults may be more sensitive to the effects of this drug because of normal age-related declines in kidney or liver function. Dosage must be tailored to suit your needs.

Generic Name

Benztropine Mesylate

Brand Name

Cogentin*

Note: The information in this profile also applies to:

Generic Name: Biperiden

Akineton

Generic Name: Ethopropazine

Parsidol

Generic Name: Procyclidine

Kemadrin

Generic Name: Trihexiphenidyl Hydrochloride

Artane Tablets,* Elixir
Artane Sequels
Trihexy-2
Trihexy-5

(*Also available in generic form)

Type of Drug

Anticholinergic.

Prescribed for

Treatment of all forms of Parkinson's disease. Also used to prevent or manage uncontrolled muscle spasms caused by the phenothiazines and other drugs.

General Information

Benztropine Mesylate has an action on the body similar to that of Atropine Sulfate, but its side effects are less frequent and less severe. This drug, an anticholinergic, counteracts the effects of *acetylcholine*, one of the body's major nerve impulse transmitters. It has the ability to reduce muscle spasms by about 20 percent, and also reduces other symptoms of Parkinson's disease, like drooling. This property makes the drug useful in treating Parkinson's disease and other diseases associated with spasms of skeletal muscles.

Cautions and Warnings

Benztropine Mesylate should be used with caution if you have **narrow-angle glaucoma, stomach ulcers, heart disease, obstructions in the gastrointestinal tract, prostatitis,** or **myasthenia gravis.**

　　When **taken in hot weather,** especially by seniors, chronically ill people, alcoholics, those with nervous-system disease, or those who work in hot environments, Benztropine Mesylate will reduce **your ability to perspire**, interfering with your body's heat-control mechanisms, thus making you more likely to develop heat exhaustion or heat stroke. In severe instances, this can be fatal.

Possible Side Effects

▼ Most common: difficulty or hesitancy in urination, painful urination, constipation, blurred vision, and increased sensitivity to bright light.

▼ Less common: rash, disorientation, confusion, memory loss, hallucinations, psychosis, agitation, nervousness, delusions, delirium, paranoid feelings, listlessness, depression, drowsiness, euphoria (feeling "high"), excitement, light-headedness, dizziness, headache, weakness, giddiness, heaviness or tingling in the hands or feet, rapid heartbeat, palpitations, mild reduction in heart rate, low blood pressure, dizziness when rising quickly from a sitting or lying position, dry mouth (possibly extreme), swollen glands, nausea, vomiting, upset stomach, interference with normal bowel function, duodenal ulcer, double vision, dilated pupils, glaucoma, muscle weakness or cramping, high temperature, flushing, decreased sweating, heat stroke, and, in men, difficulty in achieving and keeping an erection.

Drug Interactions

• Side effects may increase if Benztropine Mesylate is taken with antihistamines, phenothiazines, antidepressants, or other anticholinergic drugs. This drug should be used with caution by people taking barbiturates. Avoid alcoholic beverages.

• Benztropine may reduce the absorption and effect of some drugs, including Levodopa, Haloperidol, and phenothiazines, leading to reduced drug effects.

• Amantadine plus Benztropine may result in excessive drug side effects.

Food Interactions

This medicine (except Procyclidine) is best taken on an empty stomach, but it may be taken with food if it upsets your stomach.

Usual Dose

Benztropine: 0.5 to 6 mg per day.
Biperiden: 2 to 8 mg a day.
Ethopropazine: 50 to 600 mg daily.
Procyclidine: 2.5 to 5 mg 3 times a day after meals.
Trihexiphenidyl: 1 or 2 mg to start, increased gradually to 6 to 10 mg daily. Sequels are a more convenient way to take a high daily dosage.

Overdosage

Signs of drug overdose include the following: clumsiness or unsteadiness; severe drowsiness; severely dry mouth, nose, or throat; hallucinations; mood changes; difficulty breathing; rapid heartbeat; and unusually warm and dry skin. Overdose victims should be taken to a hospital emergency room at once. ALWAYS bring the medicine bottle.

Special Information

Dry mouth, nose, and throat can be easily relieved with candy or gum. These side effects can lead to tooth and gum disease. Maintain good oral hygiene to prevent cavities and gum disease while taking Benztropine.

A stool softener, like Docusate, will usually relieve constipation. Sunglasses will reduce the irritation brought on by bright lights.

Benztropine can interfere with driving or other tasks that require concentration and reliable vision. Be cautious while taking this medicine, and avoid alcohol and nervous-system depressants.

Call your doctor if you develop confusion, rash, eye pain, or a pounding heartbeat.

This medicine will make you less tolerant of hot weather because it makes you sweat less. Avoid exposure to hot weather because of the chance of developing heat stroke.

If you forget to take a dose of your medicine and you take it several times a day, take it as soon as you remember. If it is within 2 hours of your next regular dose, go back to the regular schedule and skip the missed dose. Do not take a

double dose. If you take your medicine twice a day and forget
a dose, take it as soon as you remember. If it is within 4 hours
of your next dose, take your medicine and then take the next
two doses 8 hours apart. Then, continue with your regular
schedule.

Special Populations

Pregnancy/Breast-feeding

Drugs of this type have not been proven to be a cause of birth
defects or of other problems in pregnant women. However,
women who are, or may become, pregnant while taking this
medication should discuss the possibility of birth defects
and/or changing medication with their doctor.

This medication may reduce the amount of breast milk
produced by a nursing mother. Infants are also particularly
sensitive to Benztropine; nursing mothers who must take it
should bottle-feed their babies.

Seniors

Seniors taking this medication on a regular basis may be
more sensitive to drug side effects, including a predisposition
to developing glaucoma, confusion, disorientation, agitation,
and hallucinations.

Generic Name

Bepridil Hydrochloride

Brand Name

Vascor

Type of Drug

Calcium channel blocker.

Prescribed for

Prevention of angina-type heart pains.

General Information

Bepridil is one of many calcium channel blockers available in
the United States. These drugs work by blocking the passage

of calcium into heart and smooth muscle. Since calcium is an essential factor in muscle contraction, any drug that affects calcium in this way will interfere with the contraction of these muscles. When this happens, the amount of oxygen used by the muscles is also reduced. Therefore, Bepridil is used to treat angina, a type of heart pain related to poor oxygen supply to the heart muscles. Bepridil affects the movement of calcium only into muscle cells. It does not have any effect on calcium in the blood. Other calcium channel blockers are used for high blood pressure, abnormal heart rhythms, diseases involving blood vessel spasm (migraine headache, Raynaud's syndrome), heart failure, and cardiomyopathy.

Cautions and Warnings

Do not take this drug if you have had an **allergic** reaction to it. It should be used with extreme caution if you have a history of **problems related to heart rhythm.**

Bepridil has caused serious **derangement of heart rhythm** and has affected **white-blood-cell counts;** therefore, it is usually reserved only for people who do not respond to other treatments.

Low blood pressure may occur, especially in people also taking a beta blocker.

Use Bepridil with caution if you have **heart failure,** since the drug can worsen the condition. Bepridil may cause **angina pain** when treatment is first started, when dosage is increased, or if the drug is rapidly withdrawn. This can be avoided by gradual dosage reduction.

Studies have shown that people taking calcium channel blockers (usually those taken several times a day, not those taken only once daily) have a greater chance of having a **heart attack** than people taking beta blockers or other medicines for the same purposes. Discuss this with your doctor to be sure you are receiving the best possible treatment.

Calcium channel blockers can affect **blood platelets,** leading to possible **bruising, black-and-blue marks,** and **bleeding.**

People with **serious liver disorders** should use this product with care because it is primarily eliminated from the body by breakdown in the liver. Drug dosage should be reduced.

People with **kidney problems** need to have their Bepridil dosage adjusted because the drug's breakdown products pass out of the body through the kidneys.

Possible Side Effects

Calcium channel blocker side effects are generally mild and rarely cause people to stop taking them.

▼ Most common: diarrhea, nausea, and light-headedness.

▼ Less common: abnormal heart rhythms, very slow or very rapid heartbeat, breathing difficulty, coughing or wheezing (possible signs of lung congestion or heart failure), constipation, headache, and unusual tiredness or weakness.

▼ Rare: low blood pressure, fainting, and swelling in the ankles, feet, or legs. Other rare side effects can affect a wide variety of body systems. Call your doctor if something unusual develops.

Drug Interactions

• Bepridil may interact with the beta-blocking drugs to cause heart failure, very low blood pressure, or an increased incidence of angina pain. However, in many cases these drugs have been taken together with no problem.

• Bepridil may, in rare instances, increase the effects of anticoagulant (blood-thinning) drugs.

• Some calcium channel blockers may increase the amount of Digoxin in the blood, but this interaction does not occur with Bepridil.

• Additional drug interactions occur with other members of this class but have not been seen with Bepridil.

Food Interactions

Taking Bepridil with food has a minor effect on the absorption of the drug. You may take it with food if it upsets your stomach.

Usual Dose

200 to 400 mg per day in 2 doses. Do not stop taking this drug abruptly. The dosage should be gradually reduced over a period of time.

Overdosage

Overdose of Bepridil can cause nausea, dizziness, weakness, drowsiness, confusion, slurred speech, very low blood pressure, reduced heart efficiency, and unusual heart rhythms. Victims of a Bepridil overdose should be taken to a hospital emergency room for treatment. ALWAYS bring the medicine bottle.

Special Information

Call your doctor if you develop swelling in the arms or legs, difficulty breathing, abnormal heartbeat, increased heart pains, dizziness, constipation, nausea, light-headedness, or very low blood pressure.

If you forget to take a dose of Bepridil, take it as soon as you remember. If it is almost time for your next regularly scheduled dose, skip the forgotten dose and continue with your regular schedule. Do not take a double dose.

Special Populations

Pregnancy/Breast-feeding

Very high doses of Bepridil have been found to affect the development of animal fetuses in laboratory studies. Bepridil has not caused human birth defects, but pregnant women, or those who might become pregnant while taking this drug, should take it only with their doctor's approval. When the drug is considered essential by your doctor, the potential risk of taking the medicine must be carefully weighed against the benefit it might produce.

Bepridil passes into breast milk. This drug has caused no problems among breast-fed infants. However, if you must take Bepridil, you should consider the potential effect on your infant before nursing.

Seniors

No problems have been reported in older adults. However, older adults are likely to have age-related reduction in kidney or liver function. This factor should be taken into account by your doctor when determining the dosage of this medication. Follow your doctor's directions and report any side effects at once. Older adults require more frequent monitoring by their doctors after treatment has started.

Generic Name

Betaxolol

Brand Names

Betoptic Ophthalmic Solution
Betoptic S Ophthalmic Suspension
Kerlone Tablets

Type of Drug

Beta-adrenergic-blocking agent.

Prescribed for

High blood pressure and glaucoma.

General Information

Betaxolol is one of 14 beta-adrenergic-blocking drugs that interfere with the action of a specific part of the nervous system. Beta receptors are found all over the body and affect many body functions. This accounts for the usefulness of beta blockers in a wide variety of conditions. The original member of this group, *Propranolol*, affects the entire beta-adrenergic section of the nervous system. Newer beta blockers have been refined to affect only a portion of that system, making them more useful in the treatment of cardiovascular disorders and less useful for other purposes. Other beta blockers are mild stimulants to the heart or have other characteristics that make them more useful for a specific purpose or better for certain people.

When applied to the eye, Betaxolol reduces pressure by slowing the production of eye fluids and slightly increasing the rate at which they flow through and leave the eye. Beta blockers produce a greater drop in eye pressure than either Pilocarpine or Epinephrine (other glaucoma drugs) and may be combined with these or other drugs to produce a more pronounced drop in eye pressure.

Betaxolol eyedrops differ from Timolol eyedrops in that they do not strongly affect lung function or heart rate; thus, Betaxolol may be used by some people who cannot use Timolol or Levobunolol.

Cautions and Warnings

You should be **cautious about taking Betaxolol** if you have **asthma, severe heart failure, a very slow heart rate,** or **heart block** because the drug may aggravate these conditions. Compared with the other beta blockers, Betaxolol has less of an effect on your pulse and bronchial muscles (asthma), and less of a rebound effect when discontinued; it also produces less tiredness, depression, and intolerance to exercise than other beta-blocking drugs.

People with **angina** who take Betaxolol for high blood pressure should have their **drug dosage reduced gradually** over 1 to 2 weeks rather than suddenly discontinued to avoid possible aggravation of the angina.

Liver or kidney problems can reduce your ability to eliminate Betaxolol from your body.

Betaxolol reduces the amount of blood your heart pumps with each beat. This reduction in blood flow can aggravate or worsen the condition of people with **poor circulation** or **circulatory disease**.

If you are undergoing **major surgery,** your doctor may want you to stop taking Betaxolol at least 2 days before surgery to permit the heart to respond more acutely to things that happen during the surgery. This is still controversial and may not hold for all surgical patients.

Betaxolol eyedrops should not be used by people who cannot take oral beta-blocking drugs (such as Propranolol).

Possible Side Effects

Side effects are usually mild, are relatively uncommon, develop early in the course of treatment, and are rarely a reason to stop taking Betaxolol.

▼ Most common: male impotence.

▼ Infrequent: unusual tiredness or weakness, slow heartbeat, heart failure (swelling of the legs, ankles, or feet), dizziness, breathing difficulty, bronchospasm, mental depression, confusion, anxiety, nervousness, sleeplessness, disorientation, short-term memory loss, emotional instability, cold hands and feet, constipation, diarrhea, nausea, vomiting, upset stomach, increased sweating, urinary difficulty, cramps, blurred vision, skin rash, hair loss,

Possible Side Effects *(continued)*

stuffy nose, facial swelling, aggravation of lupus erythematosus (a disease of the body's connective tissues), itching, chest pains, back or joint pains, colitis, drug allergy (fever, sore throat), and liver toxicity.

Drug Interactions

• Betaxolol may interact with surgical anesthetics to increase the risk of heart problems during surgery. Some anesthesiologists recommend gradually stopping your medicine 2 days before surgery.

• Betaxolol may interfere with the normal signs of low blood sugar and can interfere with the action of oral antidiabetes medicines.

• Betaxolol enhances the blood-pressure-lowering effects of other blood-pressure-reducing agents (including Clonidine, Guanabenz, and Reserpine) and calcium-channel-blocking drugs (such as Nifedipine).

• Aspirin-containing drugs, Indomethacin, Sulfinpyrazone, and estrogen drugs can interfere with the blood-pressure-lowering effect of Betaxolol.

• Cocaine may reduce the effects of all beta-blocking drugs.

• Betaxolol may increase the cold hands and feet associated with taking ergot alkaloids (for migraine headaches). Gangrene is a possibility in people taking an ergot and Betaxolol.

• Betaxolol will counteract the effects of thyroid-hormone-replacement medicines.

• Calcium channel blockers, Flecainide, Hydralazine, oral contraceptives, Propafenone, Haloperidol, phenothiazine tranquilizers (Molindone and others), quinolone antibacterials, and Quinidine may increase the amount of Betaxolol in the bloodstream and the effect of that drug on the body.

• Betaxolol should not be taken within 2 weeks of taking a monoamine oxidase (MAO) inhibitor antidepressant drug.

• Cimetidine increases the amount of Betaxolol absorbed into the bloodstream from oral tablets.

• Betaxolol may lessen the effectiveness of Theophylline,

Aminophylline, and some antiasthma drugs (especially Ephedrine and Isoproterenol).

• The combination of Betaxolol and Phenytoin or Digitalis drugs can result in excessive slowing of the heart, possibly causing heart block.

• If you stop smoking while taking Betaxolol, your dose may have to be reduced because your liver will break down the drug more slowly after you stop.

• If you take other glaucoma eye medicines, separate them to avoid physically mixing them. Small amounts of Betaxolol are absorbed into the general circulation and may interact with some of the same drugs as beta blockers taken by mouth, but this is unlikely.

Food Interactions

Betaxolol tablets may be taken without regard to food.

Usual Dose

Tablets

5 to 20 mg once a day. People with kidney failure should take 5 mg to start, and then 5 to 20 mg once every 2 weeks.

Eyedrops

1 drop in the affected eye twice a day.

Overdosage

Symptoms of overdosage are changes in heartbeat (unusually slow, unusually fast, or irregular), severe dizziness or fainting, difficulty breathing, bluish-colored fingernails or palms, and seizures. The overdose victim should be taken to a hospital emergency room where proper therapy can be given. ALWAYS bring the medicine bottle.

Special Information

Betaxolol is meant to be taken continuously. Do not stop taking it unless directed to do so by your doctor; abrupt withdrawal may cause chest pain, difficulty breathing, increased sweating, and unusually fast or irregular heartbeat. The dose should be lowered gradually over a period of about 2 weeks.

Call your doctor at once if any of the following symptoms develop: back or joint pains, difficulty breathing, cold hands or feet, depression, skin rash, or changes in heartbeat. This drug may produce an undesirable lowering of blood pressure, leading to dizziness or fainting. Call your doctor if this happens to you. Call your doctor about the following side effects only if they persist or are bothersome: anxiety, diarrhea, constipation, sexual impotence, headache, itching, nausea or vomiting, nightmares or vivid dreams, upset stomach, trouble sleeping, stuffy nose, frequent urination, unusual tiredness, or weakness.

Betaxolol can cause drowsiness, light-headedness, dizziness, or blurred vision. Be careful when driving or performing complex tasks.

It is best to take your medicine at the same time each day. If you forget a dose of Betaxolol, take it as soon as you remember. If you take your medicine once a day and it is within 8 hours of your next dose, skip the forgotten tablet and continue with your regular schedule. If you take Betaxolol twice a day and it is within 4 hours of your next dose, skip the forgotten dose and continue with your regular schedule. Do not double the dose.

To administer eyedrops, lie down or tilt your head backward and look at the ceiling. Hold the dropper above your eye and drop the medicine inside your lower lid while looking up. To prevent infection, keep the dropper from touching your fingers, eyelids, or any surface. Release the lower lid and keep your eye open. Don't blink for about 30 seconds. Press gently on the bridge of your nose at the inside corner of your eye for about 1 minute. This will help circulate the medicine around your eye. Wait at least 5 minutes before using any other eyedrops.

If you forget to take a dose of Betaxolol eyedrops, take it as soon as you remember. If it is almost time for your next dose, skip the one you forgot and continue with your regular schedule. Do not take a double dose.

Special Populations

Pregnancy/Breast-feeding

Infants born to women who took a beta blocker weighed less at birth, and had low blood pressure and reduced heart rate. Betaxolol should be avoided by pregnant women and those who might become pregnant while taking it. When the drug is considered essential by your doctor, its potential benefits must be carefully weighed against its risks.

Beta blockers pass into breast milk in varying concentrations, but problems are rare. Still, nursing mothers taking Betaxolol should bottle-feed their babies.

Seniors

Older adults may absorb and retain more Betaxolol, thus requiring less medicine to achieve the same results. Your doctor will need to adjust your dosage to meet your individual needs. Seniors taking this medicine may be more likely to suffer from cold hands and feet, reduced body temperature, chest pains, general feelings of ill health, sudden breathing difficulty, increased sweating, or changes in heartbeat.

Biaxin

see Clarithromycin, page 219

Generic Name

Bicalutamide

Brand Name

Casodex

Type of Drug

Antiandrogen.

Prescribed for

Advanced prostate cancer.

General Information

Bicalutamide is a nonsteroidal antiandrogenic hormone that inhibits the action of androgen. Prostate cancer is androgen-sensitive and responds to any treatment that counteracts the effects of androgen or removes the source of androgen. When Bicalutamide is given by itself, levels of other hormones, testosterone and estradiol, rise. To prevent this, Bicalutamide is combined with a second drug (Goserelin or Leuprolide).

Cautions and Warnings

Do not take this drug if you are **sensitive** or **allergic** to it. Bicalutamide should be used with caution if you have moderate to severe **liver disease.** Bicalutamide may reduce sperm production.

Possible Side Effects

▼ Most common: hot flashes, breast swelling and pain, generalized pain, and infection.

▼ Common: back pain, weakness, pain in the pelvic area, abdominal pain, constipation, nausea, diarrhea, liver irritation, swelling in the arms or legs, dizziness, tingling in the hands or feet, sleeplessness, sweating, rash, nighttime urination, blood in the urine, urinary infection, impotence, anemia, and breathing difficulty.

▼ Less common: flu, high blood pressure, high blood sugar, vomiting, weight loss, loss of urinary control, bone pain, headache, swelling, fever, neck pain, chills, blood infection, cancers, angina pains, heart failure, upset stomach, rectal bleeding, dry mouth, blood in the stool, diabetes, weight gain, dehydration, gout, muscle aches or weakness, arthritis, broken bones, anxiety, depression, reduced sex drive, confusion, muscle stiffness or spasms, confusion, sleepiness, nervousness, nerve damage, cough, sore throat, bronchitis, pneumonia, stuffy or runny nose, lung disease, itching, dry skin, hair loss, frequent urination, pain or difficulty on urination, and perceived need to urinate.

Drug Interactions

• Bicalutamide increases the effects of oral anticoagulant (blood-thinning) drugs. If you are taking an anticoagulant and start on Bicalutamide, your dosage will have to be adjusted.

Food Interactions

This drug may be taken without regard to food or meals.

Usual Dose

Adult: 50 mg once a day.
Child: not recommended.

Overdosage

Studies have been carried out with people taking 200 mg a day of Bicalutamide. Exact dosage levels at which Bicalutamide would be an overdose have not been established. Call your local poison center for more information. Overdose victims should be taken to a hospital emergency room for treatment. ALWAYS bring the medicine bottle with you.

Special Information

Take this drug at the same time each day. You should be taking Bicalutamide together with a luteinizing hormone-releasing hormone (LH-RH) drug such as Goserelin or Leuprolide. These drugs should be taken together and stopped only on the advice of your doctor.

If you forget a dose of Bicalutamide, take it as soon as you remember. If it is almost time for your next dose, skip the forgotten dose and continue with your regular schedule. Call your doctor if you miss a dose.

Special Populations

Pregnancy/Breast-feeding

Bicalutamide can harm a developing fetus and should never be taken by a pregnant woman. It is meant for use only by men.

It is not known if this drug passes into breast milk.

Seniors

Bicalutamide can be taken without special precaution by older adults.

Generic Name

Bisoprolol Fumarate

Brand Name

Zebeta

Combination Product

Bisoprolol + Hydrochlorothiazide

Ziac

Type of Drug

Beta-adrenergic-blocking agent.

Prescribed for

High blood pressure, angina pectoris, and abnormal heart rhythms. The combination of Bisoprolol and Hydrochlorothiazide is prescribed only for high blood pressure.

General Information

Bisoprolol is one of 14 beta-adrenergic-blocking drugs that interfere with the action of a specific part of the nervous system. Beta receptors are found all over the body and affect many body functions. This accounts for the usefulness of beta blockers against a wide variety of conditions. The first member of this group, *Propranolol*, was found to affect the entire beta-adrenergic portion of the nervous system. Newer beta blockers have been refined to affect only a portion of that system, making them more useful in the treatment of cardiovascular disorders and less useful for other purposes. Other beta blockers are mild stimulants to the heart or have other characteristics that make them more useful for a specific purpose or better for certain people. Bisoprolol is available in a single-tablet combination with Hydrochlorothiazide, a diuretic that also lowers blood pressure.

Cautions and Warnings

People with **angina** who take Bisoprolol for high blood pressure should have their drug dosage reduced gradually over 1 to 2 weeks rather than suddenly discontinued to avoid possible aggravation of the angina.

Bisoprolol should be used with caution if you have **liver or kidney disease,** because your ability to eliminate this drug from your body may be impaired.

Bisoprolol reduces the amount of blood pumped by the heart with each beat. This reduction in blood flow can aggravate or worsen the condition of people with **poor circulation or circulatory disease.**

If you are undergoing **major surgery,** your doctor may want you to stop taking Bisoprolol at least 2 days before surgery to permit the heart to respond more acutely to things that happen during the surgery. This is still controversial and may not hold true for all people preparing for surgery.

Possible Side Effects

Side effects are usually mild, relatively uncommon, develop early in the course of treatment, and are rarely a reason to stop taking Bisoprolol.

▼ Most common: male impotence.

▼ Other: unusual tiredness or weakness, slow heartbeat, heart failure (swelling of the legs, ankles, or feet), dizziness, breathing difficulty, bronchospasm, mental depression, confusion, anxiety, nervousness, sleeplessness, disorientation, short-term memory loss, emotional instability, cold hands and feet, constipation, diarrhea, nausea, vomiting, upset stomach, increased sweating, urinary difficulty, cramps, blurred vision, skin rash, hair loss, stuffy nose, facial swelling, aggravation of lupus erythematosus (a disease of the body's connective tissues), itching, chest pains, back or joint pains, colitis, drug allergy (fever, sore throat), and liver toxicity.

Drug Interactions

• Bisoprolol may interact with surgical anesthetics to increase the risk of heart problems during surgery. Some anesthesiologists recommend gradually stopping your medicine 2 days before surgery.

• Bisoprolol may interfere with the normal signs of low

blood sugar and can interfere with the action of oral antidiabetes medicines.

• Bisoprolol enhances the blood-pressure-lowering effects of other blood-pressure-reducing agents (including Clonidine, Guanabenz, and Reserpine) and calcium-channel-blocking drugs (such as Nifedipine).

• Aspirin-containing drugs, Indomethacin, Sulfinpyrazone, and estrogen drugs can interfere with the blood-pressure-lowering effect of Bisoprolol.

• Cocaine may reduce the effects of all beta-blocking drugs.

• Bisoprolol may worsen the condition of cold hands and feet associated with taking ergot alkaloids (for migraine headaches). Gangrene is a possibility in people taking an ergot and Bisoprolol.

• Bisopropol will counteract the effects of thyroid hormone replacement medicines.

• Calcium channel blockers, Flecainide, Hydralazine, oral contraceptives, Propafenone, Haloperidol, phenothiazine tranquilizers (Molindone and others), quinolone antibacterials, and Quinidine may increase the amount of Bisoprolol in the bloodstream and the effect of that drug on the body.

• Bisoprolol should not be taken within 2 weeks of taking a monoamine oxidase (MAO) inhibitor antidepressant drug.

• Cimetidine increases the amount of Bisoprolol absorbed into the bloodstream from oral tablets.

• Bisoprolol may lessen the effectiveness of Theophylline, Aminophylline, and some antiasthma drugs (especially Ephedrine and Isoproterenol).

• The combination of Bisoprolol and Phenytoin or Digitalis drugs can result in excessive slowing of the heart, possibly causing heart block.

• If you stop smoking while taking Bisoprolol, your dose may have to be reduced because your liver will break down the drug more slowly after you stop.

Food Interactions

Bisoprolol may be taken without regard to food or meals.

Usual Dose

Adult: Starting dose: 5 mg once daily. The daily dose may be gradually increased up to 20 mg. Maintenance dose: 5 to 10 mg once daily.

Senior: may respond to lower doses and should be treated more cautiously.

People with kidney or liver disease may need only 2.5 mg a day to start.

Overdosage

Symptoms of overdosage are changes in heartbeat (unusually slow, unusually fast, or irregular), severe dizziness or fainting, difficulty breathing, bluish-colored fingernails or palms, and seizures. The overdose victim should be taken to a hospital emergency room, where proper therapy can be given. ALWAYS bring the medicine bottle.

Special Information

Bisoprolol is meant to be taken continuously. Do not stop taking it unless directed to do so by your doctor, because abrupt withdrawal may cause chest pain, difficulty breathing, increased sweating, and unusually fast or irregular heartbeat. The dose should be lowered gradually over a period of about 2 weeks.

Call your doctor at once if any of the following symptoms develop: back or joint pains, difficulty breathing, cold hands or feet, depression, skin rash, or changes in heartbeat. Bisoprolol may produce an undesirable lowering of blood pressure, leading to dizziness or fainting. Call your doctor if this happens to you. Call your doctor about the following side effects only if they persist or are bothersome: anxiety, diarrhea, constipation, sexual impotence, headache, itching, nausea or vomiting, nightmares or vivid dreams, upset stomach, trouble sleeping, stuffed nose, frequent urination, unusual tiredness, or weakness.

Bisoprolol can cause drowsiness, dizziness, blurred vision, or light-headedness. Be careful when driving or performing complex tasks. It is best to take your medicine at the same time every day.

If you forget a dose of Bisoprolol, take it as soon as you remember. If it is within 8 hours of your next dose, skip the forgotten tablet and continue with your regular schedule. Do not take a double dose.

Special Populations

Pregnancy/Breast-feeding

Infants born to women who took a beta blocker weighed less

at birth, and had low blood pressure and reduced heart rate. Bisoprolol should be avoided by pregnant women and those who might become pregnant while taking it. When the drug is considered essential by your doctor, its potential benefits must be carefully weighed against its risks.

It is not known if Bisoprolol pases into breast milk. Still, nursing mothers taking this medication should bottle-feed their babies.

Seniors

Older adults may absorb and retain more Bisoprolol in their bodies, thus requiring less medicine to achieve the same results. Your doctor will need to adjust your dosage to meet your individual needs. Seniors taking this medicine may be more likely to suffer from cold hands and feet, reduced body temperature, chest pains, general feelings of ill health, sudden breathing difficulty, increased sweating, or changes in heartbeat.

Generic Name

Bitolterol Mesylate

Brand Name

Tornalate

Type of Drug

Bronchodilator.

Prescribed for

Asthma and bronchospasm.

General Information

Bitolterol is currently available only as an inhalant. It may be taken in combination with other medicines to control your asthma. The drug starts working 3 to 4 minutes after it is taken and continues to work for 5 to 8 hours. It can be used only when needed to treat an asthmatic attack or on a regular basis to prevent an attack. Each dose of Bitolterol Mesylate inhalant delivers 0.37 mg of medication.

Cautions and Warnings

Bitolterol should be used with caution if you have had **angina** (chest tightness/pain), **heart disease, high blood pressure,** a **history of stroke or seizures, diabetes, prostate disease,** or **glaucoma.**

Using **excessive amounts** of Bitolterol can lead to **increased difficulty breathing,** instead of providing breathing relief. In the most extreme cases, people have had heart attacks after using excessive amounts of inhalant.

Possible Side Effects

Bitolterol's side effects are similar to those associated with other bronchodilator drugs.

▼ Most common: tremors, cough, and dry or sore throat.

▼ Common: restlessness, weakness, anxiety, shakiness and nervousness, tension, sleeplessness, dizziness and fainting, headache, pallor, sweating, nausea, vomiting, and muscle cramps.

▼ Less common: light-headedness, angina, abnormal heart rhythms, heart palpitations, breathing difficulty or bronchospasm, and flushing.

▼ Other: Bitolterol has been associated with abnormalities in blood tests for the liver and white-blood-cell counts, and in tests for urine protein, but the importance of these reactions is not known.

Drug Interactions

• Bitolterol's effects may be enhanced by monoamine oxidase (MAO) inhibitor drugs, antidepressants, thyroid drugs, other bronchodilators, and some antihistamines. It is antagonized by beta-blocking drugs (Propranolol and others).

• Bitolterol may antagonize the effects of blood-pressure-lowering drugs, especially Reserpine, Methyldopa, and Guanethidine.

• The chances of cardiotoxicity may be increased in people taking Bitolterol and Theophylline.

Food Interactions

Bitolterol does not interact with food because it is taken only by inhalation into the lungs.

Usual Dose

Adult and Adolescent (age 12 and older): To treat an attack: 2 inhalations at an interval of at least 1 to 3 minutes, followed by a third inhalation, if needed. To prevent an attack: 2 inhalations every 8 hours.

Do not take more than 3 puffs in 6 hours or 2 every 4 hours.

Overdosage

Bitolterol overdosage can result in exaggerated side effects, including heart pains and high blood pressure, although the pressure can drop to a low level after a short period of elevation. People who inhale too much Bitolterol should see a doctor or go to a hospital emergency room, where they will probably be given a beta-blocking drug like Atenolol or Metoprolol to counter the bronchodilator's effects.

Special Information

The drug should be inhaled during the second half of your breath. This allows the medicine to reach more deeply into your lungs.

Be sure to follow your doctor's directions for the use of Bitolterol. Using more than is prescribed can lead to drug tolerance and actually cause your condition to worsen. If your condition worsens instead of improves after taking your dose, stop taking it and call your doctor at once.

Call your doctor at once if you develop chest pains, rapid heartbeat, palpitations, muscle tremors, dizziness, headache, or facial flushing, or if you still have trouble breathing after using the medicine.

If a dose of Bitolterol is forgotten, take it as soon as you remember. If it is almost time for your next dose, skip the forgotten one and continue with your regular schedule. Do not take a double dose.

Special Populations

Pregnancy/Breast-feeding

Bitolterol should be used by a pregnant or breast-feeding

woman only when it is absolutely necessary. The potential benefit of using this medicine must be weighed against the potential, but unknown, hazard it can pose to your baby.

It is not known if Bitolterol passes into breast milk. Nursing mothers must look for any possible drug effect on their infants while taking this medication. You may want to consider bottle-feeding your infant.

Seniors

Older adults are more sensitive to the effects of this drug. They should closely follow their doctor's directions and report any side effects at once.

Generic Name

Bupropion Hydrochloride

Brand Name

Wellbutrin

Type of Drug

Antidepressant.

Prescribed for

Depression.

General Information

Bupropion is generally not prescribed for the treatment of severe or major depression until after other drugs have been tried, because of the higher-than-usual chance of developing seizures while taking it. Bupropion is chemically different from other antidepressants, but it is similar to Diethylpropion, an appetite suppressant.

Bupropion is not likely to work until you have taken it for 3 to 4 weeks. The drug takes about 2 weeks to clear from your system after you have stopped taking it.

Cautions and Warnings

People with **seizure disorders,** people who have had **a seizure in the past,** and people with **eating disorders** should be very careful about taking Bupropion because of the greatly increased chance of having a seizure while taking it. In doses up to 450 mg a day, about 4 of every 1000 people taking Bupropion will develop a seizure. This is about 4 times the seizure rate associated with other antidepressants. The chance of developing a seizure increases by about 10 times when the dosage is between 450 and 600 mg per day. About half of all people who developed a seizure on Bupropion had a risk factor such as a history of head injury, a previous seizure, or a nervous system tumor, or were taking another medicine associated with increased seizure risk.

People with **unstable heart disease** or a **recent heart attack** should take this drug with caution because of possible side effects. Many people taking Bupropion experience some **restlessness, agitation, anxiety,** and **sleeplessness,** especially soon after they start taking the drug. Some even require sleeping pills to counter this effect, and others find the stimulation so severe that they have to stop taking Bupropion.

People taking Bupropion may experience **hallucinations, delusions,** and **psychotic episodes**. Dosage reduction or drug withdrawal is usually necessary to minimize these reactions. One-quarter of the people who take Bupropion lose their appetites and 5 or more pounds of body weight. Most other antidepressants cause weight gain. People who have **lost weight** because of their depression should be cautious about taking Bupropion.

People switching from Bupropion to a monoamine oxidase (MAO) inhibitor antidepressant, or vice versa, should allow at least **2 weeks to pass before switching.** In animal studies, Bupropion has caused **liver damage** and tumors, but these effects have not been seen in people.

People with **kidney or liver disease** require less medication at the beginning of treatment. Dosage should be increased cautiously.

People with a **history of drug abuse** should probably be treated with a different antidepressant because they experience mild stimulation while taking Bupropion and may require a larger-than-usual dose. However, they are still susceptible to seizures at the higher doses. Severely depressed individuals are more likely to attempt suicide; therefore, they should not be given a large number of Bupropion tablets at one time.

Possible Side Effects

▼ Most common: dry mouth, dizziness, rapid heart-beat, headaches (including migraines), excessive sweating, nausea, vomiting, constipation, loss of appetite, weight changes, sedation, agitation, sleeplessness, and tremors.

▼ Less common: upset stomach, diarrhea, increased appetite, menstrual complaints, impotence, urinary difficulties, slowing of movements, salivation, muscle spasms, warmth, uncontrolled muscle movements, feeling compelled to move around or change positions often, abnormal heart rhythms, blood-pressure changes, heart palpitations, fainting, itching, redness and rash, confusion, hostility, loss of concentration, reduced sex drive, anxiety, delusions, euphoria (feeling "high"), fatigue, joint pains, fever or chills, respiratory infections, and visual, taste, and hearing disturbances.

Many other side effects have been reported with Bupropion, but their link to the drug is not well established. About 1 in 10 people who take this drug have to stop it because of intolerable side effects.

Drug Interactions

• Bupropion may increase the rate at which the body breaks down Carbamazepine, Cimetidine, Phenobarbital, or Phenytoin. Dosage adjustments may be needed if the combination continues to be used.

• People taking both Bupropion and Levodopa experience more side effects than other people. Levodopa users should have their Bupropion dosages increased more slowly and gradually than others.

• Phenelzine, an MAO inhibitor antidepressant, increases the toxic effects of Bupropion. Allow at least 2 weeks to pass between stopping an MAO inhibitor and starting Bupropion.

• The combination of Bupropion and other drugs that increase the chance of seizures (including tricyclic antidepressants, Haloperidol, Lithium, Loxapine, Molindone, phenothiazine tranquilizers, or thioxanthene tranquilizers) should be avoided.

Food Interactions

Bupropion may be taken with food if it upsets your stomach.

Usual Dose

200 to 450 mg a day, divided into 3 or 4 daily doses. The usual dose is 300 mg.

Overdosage

Overdose symptoms are likely to be exaggerated drug side effects. Most people who take a Bupropion overdose recover without a serious problem, but overdose victims may experience seizures, hallucinations, loss of consciousness, and rapid heartbeat. Death has occurred rarely in people taking massive overdoses of this drug. Overdose victims should be taken to an emergency room at once. ALWAYS bring the medicine bottle.

Special Information

Do not stop taking Bupropion without your doctor's approval. Suddenly stopping the medicine may precipitate a drug-withdrawal reaction and drug side effects.

Call your doctor if you have any of the following symptoms: agitation or excitement, restlessness, or confusion; trouble sleeping; a fast or abnormal heart rhythm; severe headache; seizure; skin rash; or fainting; or if symptoms are unusually persistent or severe.

To reduce the risk of a seizure, take this medication in 3 or 4 equal doses each day. The total daily dose should not be more than 450 mg, and single doses should not be greater than 150 mg.

Bupropion can make you tired, dizzy, or light-headed. Be careful when performing tasks requiring concentration and coordination (such as driving).

Alcohol, tranquilizers, or other nervous-system depressants will increase the depressant effects of this drug. Alcohol also increases the chance of a seizure.

If you forget a dose of Bupropion, take it as soon as you remember. If it is almost time for your next dose, take 1 dose as soon as you remember and another in 3 or 4 hours, then go back to your regular schedule. Do not take a double dose.

Special Populations

Pregnancy/Breast-feeding

Pregnant women should take Bupropion only if it is absolutely necessary.

Nursing mothers who must use Bupropion should bottle-feed their babies because of the severe side effects caused by this medicine.

Seniors

No special problems have been reported in older adults. However, older adults are likely to have age-related reduction in kidney and/or liver function. This factor should be taken into account by your doctor when determining the dosage of this drug.

BuSpar

see Buspirone, page 142

Generic Name

Buspirone

Brand Name

BuSpar

Type of Drug

Minor tranquilizer; antianxiety drug.

Prescribed for

Anxiety. Buspirone may also be prescribed for the aches, pains, fatigue, and cramps of premenstrual syndrome (PMS).

General Information

This drug is chemically distinct from the benzodiazepines, the most widely prescribed antianxiety drugs in America, but Buspirone has a potent antianxiety effect. Although it is approved by the United States Food and Drug Administration

(FDA) for short-term relief of anxiety, it appears that Buspirone can be safely used for longer periods of time (more than 4 weeks). The exact way that Buspirone works is not known, but it seems to lack the addiction dangers associated with other antianxiety drugs, including the benzodiazepines. It does not severely depress the nervous system or act as an anticonvulsant or muscle relaxant, as other antianxiety drugs do. Minor improvement will be apparent after only 7 to 10 days of drug treatment, but the maximum effect does not occur until 3 to 4 weeks after starting treatment.

Cautions and Warnings

Do not take Buspirone if you are **allergic** to it.

Buspirone should be used cautiously by people with **liver or kidney disease**.

Buspirone does not have any antipsychotic effect and should **not be taken for symptoms of psychosis**.

Although Buspirone has not shown a potential for drug abuse, you should be aware of this possibility.

Possible Side Effects

▼ Most common: dizziness, nausea, headache, fatigue, nervousness, light-headedness, and excitement.

▼ Common: heart palpitations, muscle aches and pains, tremors, skin rash, sweating, and clamminess.

▼ Less common: sleeplessness, chest pain, rapid heartbeat, low blood pressure, fainting, stroke, heart attack, heart failure, dream disturbances, difficulty concentrating, euphoria (feeling "high"), anger or hostility, depression, depersonalization or disassociation, fearfulness, loss of interest, hallucinations, suicidal tendencies, claustrophobia, stupor, slurred speech, intolerance to noise, and intolerance to cold temperatures.

▼ Infrequent: ringing or buzzing in the ears, a "roaring" sensation in the head, sore throat, red and itchy eyes, changes in taste and smell, inner ear problems, eye pain, intolerance to bright light, dry mouth, stomach or intestinal upset or cramps, diarrhea, constipation, stomach gas, changes in appetite, excess salivation, urinary difficulty, menstrual irregularity, pelvic inflammatory disease,

Possible Side Effects *(continued)*

muscle cramps and spasms, numbness, tingling in the
hands or feet, bed-wetting, poor coordination, involuntary movements, slowed reaction time, rapid breathing,
shortness of breath, chest congestion, changes in sex
drive, itching, facial swelling or flushing, easy bruising,
hair loss, dry skin, blisters, fever, feelings of ill health,
unusual bleeding or bruising, and voice loss.

▼ Rare: very slow heartbeat, high blood pressure,
seizures and psychotic reactions, blurred vision, stuffy
nose, pressure on the eyes, thyroid abnormalities, irritable colon, bleeding from the rectum, burning of the
tongue, periodic spotting, painful urination, muscle weakness, nosebleeds, delayed ejaculation and impotence
(men), thinning of the nails, and hiccups.

Drug Interactions

• The combination of Buspirone with monoamine oxidase
(MAO) inhibitor drugs may produce very high blood pressure
and can be dangerous.

• The effects of Buspirone together with other drugs that
work in the central nervous system are not known. Do not
take other tranquilizers or antianxiety or psychoactive drugs
with Buspirone unless prescribed by a doctor who knows
your complete medication history.

• The combination of Buspirone and Haloperidol results in
high blood levels of Haloperidol, increasing the chances of
Haloperidol side effects.

• Studies show that Buspirone is not affected by alcohol,
but this combination should still be used with caution because Buspirone causes drowsiness and dizziness.

• The combination of Buspirone and Trazodone may cause
liver inflammation.

Food Interactions

Food tends to double the amount of drug absorbed into the
bloodstream, although it decreases the rate at which the drug
is absorbed. This drug can be taken either with or without
food, but for the most consistent results, always take your

dose at the same time of day in the same way (that is, with or without food).

Usual Dose

15 mg per day in 3 divided doses to start. Dosage may be increased gradually to 60 mg per day.

Overdosage

Symptoms of overdose are nausea, vomiting, dizziness, drowsiness, pinpointed pupils, and upset stomach. To date, no deaths have been caused by Buspirone overdose. There is no specific antidote for Buspirone overdose. Go to a hospital emergency room. ALWAYS bring the medicine bottle with you.

Special Information

Buspirone can cause nervous-system depression, drowsiness, and dizziness. Be careful while driving or operating hazardous equipment. Avoid other central-nervous-system drugs and alcoholic beverages because they will enhance Buspirone's effects.

Contact your doctor if you become restless, or develop uncontrolled or repeated movements of the head, face, or neck, or have any intolerable side effects. About 1 out of 10 people who were included in drug studies had to stop taking Buspirone because of drug side effects.

If you miss a dose of Buspirone, take it as soon as you remember. If it is almost time for your next dose, skip the missed dose and go back to your regular dose schedule. Do not take a double dose.

Special Populations

Pregnancy/Breast-feeding

Make sure your doctor knows if you are or are planning to become pregnant, or if you will be breast-feeding while taking this medicine.

Buspirone has not been found to cause birth defects. When the drug is considered essential by your doctor, its potential benefits must be carefully weighed against its risks.

It is not known how much Buspirone passes into breast milk. Consider the chance of drug side effects on a nursing infant.

Seniors

Several hundred older adults participated in drug evaluation studies without any unusual problems. However, the effect of this drug in older adults is not well known, and special problems may surface in older adults, particularly in those with kidney or liver disease.

Generic Name

Butoconazole

Brand Name

Femstat

Type of Drug

Antifungal.

Prescribed for

Treatment of fungal infections in the vagina.

General Information

Butoconazole is used as a vaginal cream. About 5 percent of each dose is absorbed into the bloodstream. It may also be applied to the skin to treat common fungal infections. It is effective against common fungal infections, but the exact mechanism of action is not known.

Cautions and Warnings

Do not use Butoconazole if you know you are **allergic** to it. **Proper diagnosis** is essential for effective treatment. Do not use this product without first consulting your doctor.

Possible Side Effects

▼ Most common: vaginal burning, itching, or irritation.

▼ Other: vaginal discharge, swelling of the vulva, soreness, and itchy fingers.

Drug and Food Interactions

None known.

Usual Dose

One applicatorful into the vagina at bedtime for 3 to 6 days. Pregnant women who use Butoconazole cream should use it for 6 days and only during the last 6 months of pregnancy.

Special Information

When using the vaginal cream, insert the whole applicatorful of cream high into the vagina. Be sure to complete the full course of treatment as prescribed. Call your doctor if you develop burning or itching.

Refrain from sexual intercourse or use a condom while using this product to avoid reinfection. Sanitary napkins may prevent staining of your clothing by Butoconazole.

If you forget to take a dose of Butoconazole, take it as soon as you remember. If it is almost time for your next dose, skip the missed dose and continue with your regular schedule. Do not take a double dose.

Special Populations

Pregnancy/Breast-feeding

Pregnant women should avoid using this product during pregnancy because the use of a vaginal applicator may cause problems. If it is to be used, it must be avoided during the first 3 months of pregnancy. The effect of Butoconazole on the developing fetus is not known.

It is not known if Butoconazole passes into breast milk. Nursing mothers using this product should watch their infants for possible drug side effects.

Seniors

Older adults may take this medication without special restriction. Follow your doctor's directions and report any side effects at once.

Calan SR

see **Verapamil**, page 1169

Generic Name

Calcitonin

Brand Name

Micalcin Nasal Spray

Type of Drug

Peptide hormone.

Prescribed for

Osteoporosis (bone calcium depletion) in women who have gone through menopause. Calcitonin is also used for Paget's disease of bone.

General Information

Calcitonin is a naturally occuring hormone, produced within the thyroid gland, that has a role in helping to regulate calcium and bone production and maintenance in the body. It also directly affects calcium in the body by working on the kidneys and gastrointestinal (GI) tract. The Calcitonin used in this product comes from salmon; although it is essentially identical to human calcitonin, it is much more potent. Calcitonin helps to drive calcium into bone, strengthening it, and slows the natural process in which bone is naturally broken down (resorption). People with osteoporosis have low bone mass and a deteriorated bone structure, causing bone to be brittle and easily broken. People with osteoporosis also experience fractures of their vertebrae (back bones) that are associated with back pain and a loss of height. Calcitonin helps reverse these situations. Calcitonin has been available for some years as an injection, but the nasal spray makes it easier to use and more accessible for the average person.

Cautions and Warnings

This drug should not be used if you are **sensitive** or **allergic** to salmon Calcitonin. Because Calcitonin is a naturally derived hormone, allergic reactions are possible, but none have been experienced to date with the nasal spray. Serious allergic reactions were reported with the injectable form of salmon Calcitonin.

Changes in the lining of your nose are possible with extended use of this product. Periodic **nasal examinations** are recommended.

Possible Side Effects

▼ Most common: stuffy and runny nose and other nasal symptoms, and back pain.

▼ Less common: flulike symptoms, fatigue, red rash, muscle aches, joint problems, sinus irritation, upper respiratory infection, bronchial spasm, high blood pressure, angina pain, upset stomach, constipation, abdominal pains, nausea, diarrhea, cystitis, dizziness, tingling in the hands or feet, eye tearing, red eyes, swollen lymph glands, infections, and depression.

▼ Rare: swelling around the eyes, fever, skin ulcers, eczema, baldness, itching, sweating, arthritis, stiffness, sore throat, bronchitis, pneumonia, coughing, breathing difficulty, taste and smell changes (including phantom smells), rapid heartbeat, heart palpitation, heart attack, vomiting, stomach gas, increased appetite, gastric irritation, dry mouth, hepatitis, thirst, gallstones, weight gain, goiter, overactive thyroid, blood in the urine, urinary infection, fainting, migraines, nerve pain, urine, urinary infection, fainting, migraines, nerve pain, agitation, hearing loss, ringing or buzzing in the ears, earache, blurred vision, particles floating (floaters) in eye fluid, flushing, stroke, vein irritation, anemia, sleeplessness, anxiety, appetite loss.

Drug Interactions

• No drug interactions have been found with the ingredients in this nasal spray.

Food Interactions

None known.

Usual Dose

Adult: one puff (200 I.U.) per day.
Child: not recommended.

Overdosage

No cases of Calcitonin nasal spray overdose have been reported, and no adverse effects have been reported after high doses. Call your local poison center for more information. Overdose victims should be taken to a hospital emergency room for treatment. ALWAYS bring the medicine bottle with you.

Special Information

Alternate nostrils every day when using this nasal spray.

Before you take the first dose of this product, you must activate the pump. Hold the bottle upright and press the 2 white arms toward the bottle 6 times until a faint spray is emitted. Once you have seen the spray, the pump is activated and can be used. It is not necessary to reactivate the pump every day.

If you forget a dose of Calcitonin nasal spray, take it as soon as you remember. If it is almost time for the next dose, skip the forgotten dose and continue with your regular schedule.

Call your doctor if you forget your medicine for 2 or more days or if you develop a severe nose irritation or any other unusual or intolerable symptom.

Special Populations

Pregnancy/Breast-feeding

Animal studies have associated injectable salmon Calcitonin with low birth weight, but Calcitonin does not cross into the baby's blood circulation. This product is not recommended for use during pregnancy. It should be used only if the possible benefits of taking it outweigh the risks.

Animal studies have shown that Calcitonin reduces the amount of milk produced, but it is not known if Calcitonin passes into breast milk. Nursing mothers who must use Calcitonin should discuss it with their doctor.

Seniors
Studies of salmon Calcitonin have included people up to age 77. Seniors may use this product without special restriction.

Capoten

see **Captopril**, page 153

Generic Name

Capsaicin

Brand Name
Zostrix

Type of Drug
Local pain reliever.

Prescribed for
Temporary relief of pain associated with rheumatoid arthritis, osteoarthritis, and neuralgias (nerve pain), such as shingles. It may also be prescribed for pain associated with psoriasis, vitiligo, untreatable itching, phantom-limb syndrome, and vulvar irritations.

General Information
Capsaicin is a natural substance that seems to work by depleting and preventing the body from rebuilding stores of a chemical called *substance P* in nerve endings that sense pain. Substance P is thought to be a principal participant in the transmission of painful impulses from the skin to the brain.

Cautions and Warnings
Capsaicin is highly **irritating**. It must only be applied to the skin. **Do not apply it to the eye** or allow it to get into your eye

after application to your skin. You may want to use an applicator or wear gloves while applying Capsaicin cream.

Do not use for more than 28 days. Call your doctor if your condition gets worse or fails to improve after that time.

Possible Side Effects

▼ Most common: burning, stinging, swelling, cough, and respiratory irritation.

Drug Interactions

• Capsaicin may worsen or initiate the cough normally experienced by people taking angiotensin-converting-enzyme (ACE) inhibitors for hypertension.

Food Interactions

None known.

Usual Dose

Apply to affected areas no more than 3 or 4 times per day.

Overdosage

Overdose will cause skin irritation and burning. If Capsaicin cream gets into your eyes, call your local poison control center as soon as possible.

Special Information

Do not tightly bandage areas to which Capsaicin cream has been applied. Use gloves or an applicator to avoid getting this cream in your eyes. Wash your hands thoroughly after each application.

This drug is less sedating than most other antihistamines, but it still may cause some sedation and should not be mixed with alcohol or other nervous-system depressants.

If you forget to apply a dose of Capsaicin, apply it as soon as you remember. If it is almost time for your next regularly scheduled dose, skip the one you forgot and continue with your regular schedule. Do not apply a double dose.

Special Populations

Pregnancy/Breast-feeding

There is no known effect of this product on pregnant women or nursing mothers. Exercise caution with all medicines.

Seniors

Seniors may use this medicine without special restriction.

Generic Name

Captopril

Brand Name

Capoten

(Also available in generic form)

Combination Product

Captopril + Hydrochlorothiazide

Capozide

(This combination of Captopril with the diuretic Hydrochlorothiazide is used for the treatment of high blood pressure.)

Type of Drug

Antihypertensive; angiotensin-converting-enzyme (ACE) inhibitor.

Prescribed for

High blood pressure and congestive heart failure. Low doses may be used to treat mild to moderate high blood pressure. It is also used for the treatment of diabetic kidney disease, as well as high blood pressure associated with some other medical conditions (scleroderma and Takayasu's disease). Captopril also has been studied as a treatment for rheumatoid arthritis, diagnosis of certain kidney diseases and of primary aldosteronism, swelling and fluid accumulation, Bartter's syndrome (corrects low blood potassium), relief of Raynaud's disease, and post-heart-attack treatment when the function of the left ventricle is affected.

General Information

Captopril belongs to the class of drugs known as *angiotensin-converting-enzyme (ACE) inhibitors.* ACE inhibitors work by preventing the conversion of a hormone called *angiotensin I* to another hormone called *angiotensin II,* a potent blood-vessel constrictor. Preventing this conversion relaxes blood vessels and helps to reduce blood pressure and relieve the symptoms of heart failure by making it easier for a failing heart to pump blood through the body. The production of other hormones and enzymes that participate in the regulation of blood-vessel dilation is also affected by Captopril and probably plays a role in the effectiveness of this medicine. Captopril usually begins working about 1 hour after taking it.

Some people who start taking Captopril after they are already on a diuretic (water pill) experience a rapid blood-pressure drop after their first dose or when their dose is increased. To prevent this from happening, your doctor may tell you to stop taking your diuretic 2 or 3 days before starting Captopril or increase your salt intake during that time. The diuretic may then be restarted gradually. Heart-failure patients generally have been on Digoxin and a diuretic before beginning Captopril treatment.

Cautions and Warnings

Do not take Captopril if you are **allergic** to it. It can (rarely) cause very **low blood pressure.** It may also affect your **kidneys,** especially if you have **congestive heart failure.** Your doctor should **check your urine** for protein content during the first few months of treatment.

Captopril may cause a decline in **kidney function.** Dosage adjustment of Captopril is necessary if you have reduced kidney function because it is generally eliminated from the body via the kidneys.

Captopril can affect **white-blood-cell counts,** possibly increasing your susceptibility to infection. Your doctor should monitor your blood counts periodically.

Possible Side Effects

▼ Most common: rash, itching, and cough; the cough usually goes away a few days after you stop taking the drug.

▼ Less common: dizziness, tiredness, sleep disturbances, headache, tingling in hands or feet, chest pain, heart palpitations, feeling ill, abdominal pains, nausea, vomiting, diarrhea, constipation, loss of appetite, dry mouth, breathing difficulty, and hair loss.

▼ Other: fever, angina (chest tightness/pain), heart attack, stroke, abdominal pain, low blood pressure, dizziness when rising from a sitting or lying position, abnormal heart rhythms, sleeping difficulty, hepatitis and jaundice, blood in the stool, unusual skin sensitivity to the sun, flushing, nervousness, reduced sex drive, muscle cramps or weakness, muscle aches, arthritis, bronchitis or other respiratory infections, sinus irritation, weakness, confusion, depression, increased sweating, kidney problems, urinary infection, blurred vision, and swelling of the arms, legs, lips, tongue, face, and throat.

Drug Interactions

• The blood-pressure-lowering effect of Captopril is additive with diuretic drugs and beta blockers. Any other drug that causes a rapid blood-pressure drop should be used with caution if you are taking Captopril.

• Captopril may increase blood-potassium levels, especially when taken with Dyazide or other potassium-sparing diuretics.

• Captopril may increase the effects of Lithium; this combination should be used with caution.

• Antacids may reduce the amount of Captopril absorbed into the blood. Separate doses of these 2 medicines by at least 2 hours.

• Capsaicin may cause or aggravate the cough associated with Captopril therapy.

• Indomethacin may reduce the blood-pressure-lowering effect of Captopril.

• Phenothiazine tranquilizers and antivomiting agents may increase the effects of Captopril.

- Probenecid increases blood levels of Captopril, thus increasing the drug's effect as well as the chance of side effects.
- The combination of Allopurinol and Captopril increases the chance of an adverse drug reaction.
- Captopril can increase blood levels of Digoxin, which possibly increases the chance of Digoxin-related side effects.

Food Interactions

Captopril is affected by food in the stomach and should be taken on an empty stomach or at least 1 hour before or 2 hours after a meal.

Usual Dose

Adult: 75 mg per day to start. Dose may be increased up to 450 mg per day in divided doses, if needed. The dose of this medicine must be tailored to your needs. People with poor kidney function must take less medicine.

Child: about 0.15 mg per pound of body weight 3 times a day.

Overdosage

The principal effect of Captopril overdose is a rapid drop in blood pressure, which can lead to dizziness or fainting. Take the overdose victim to a hospital emergency room immediately. ALWAYS bring the medicine bottle.

Special Information

Captopril can cause swelling of the face, lips, hands, and feet. This swelling can also affect the larynx (throat) and tongue, and interfere with breathing. If this happens, go to a hospital emergency room at once. Call your doctor if you develop a sore throat, mouth sores, abnormal heartbeat, chest pain, a persistent rash, or loss of taste perception.

You may get dizzy if you rise to your feet too quickly from a sitting or lying position. Avoid strenuous exercise and/or very hot weather because heavy sweating or dehydration can cause a rapid blood-pressure drop.

Avoid nonprescription diet pills, decongestants, and stimulants that can raise blood pressure while taking Captopril.

If you forget to take a dose of Captopril, take it as soon as you remember. If it is within 4 hours of your next dose, take 1 dose and then another in 5 or 6 hours, then go back to your regular schedule. Do not take a double dose.

Special Populations

Pregnancy/Breast-feeding

ACE inhibitors have caused low blood pressure, kidney failure, slow skull formation, and death in developing fetuses when taken during the last 6 months of pregnancy. Women who are, or may become, pregnant should not take any ACE inhibitors. Sexually active women taking Captopril must use an effective contraceptive method to prevent pregnancy, or use an alternative medicine. If you become pregnant, stop taking the medicine, and call your doctor immediately.

Relatively small amounts of Captopril pass into breast milk, and the effect on a nursing infant has not been determined. Mothers who must take this drug should consider bottle-feeding with formula because infants, especially newborns, are more susceptible to this medicine's effects than adults.

Seniors

Older adults may be more sensitive to the effects of Captopril because of normal age-related declines in kidney or liver function. The dosage must be tailored to individual needs.

Generic Name

Carbamazepine

Brand Name

Tegretol

(Also available in generic form)

Type of Drug

Anticonvulsant.

Prescribed for

Seizure disorders and trigeminal neuralgia. Carbamazepine is also prescribed for diabetes insipidus (a hormonal disease leading to severe water retention), some forms of severe pain, some psychiatric disorders (including bipolar disorder in people who cannot tolerate Lithium or antipsychotic drugs alone), psychotic disorders, and alcohol withdrawal.

General Information

Carbamazepine was first approved for the relief of the severe pain of trigeminal neuralgia. Over the years, though, it has gained much greater acceptance for seizure control, especially for people whose seizures are not controlled by Phenytoin, Phenobarbital, or Primidone, or who have suffered severe side effects from these medicines.

This drug is not a simple pain reliever and should not be taken for everyday aches and pains. It has some potentially fatal side effects.

Cautions and Warnings

This drug should not be used if you have a history of **bone marrow depression** or if you are sensitive or **allergic** to this drug or to the **tricyclic antidepressants. Monoamine oxidase (MAO) inhibitors** should be discontinued 2 weeks before Carbamazepine treatment is begun.

Carbamazepine can cause severe, possibly life-threatening **blood reactions**. Your doctor should have a complete blood count done before you start taking this medicine and repeat that examination weekly during the first 3 months of treatment and then every month for the next 2 or 3 years.

Carbamazepine may aggravate **glaucoma** and should be used with caution by people with this condition. This drug may activate underlying **psychosis, confusion,** or **agitation,** especially in older adults.

Possible Side Effects

▼ Most common: dizziness, drowsiness, unsteadiness, nausea, and vomiting. Other common side effects are blurred or double vision, confusion, hostility, headache, and severe water retention.

Possible Side Effects *(continued)*

▼ Less common: mood and behavior changes (especially in children). Hives, itching or skin rash, and other allergic reactions may also occur.

▼ Rare: chest pain, fainting, trouble breathing, continuous back-and-forth eye movements, slurred speech, depression, restlessness, nervousness, muscle rigidity, ringing or buzzing in the ears, trembling, uncontrolled body movement, hallucinations, darkening of the stool or urine, yellow eyes or skin, mouth sores, unusual bleeding or bruising, unusual tiredness or weakness, changes in urination patterns (more frequent, or a sudden decrease in urine production), swelling of the feet or lower legs, numbness, tingling, pain or weakness in the hands or feet, pain, tenderness, a bluish discoloration of the legs or feet, and swollen glands.

Drug Interactions

• The level of Carbamazepine in the blood may be increased by taking Cimetidine, Danazol, Diltiazem, Isoniazid, Propoxyphene, Erythromycin, Mexiletine, Nicotinamide, Troleandomycin, or Verapamil, leading to possible Carbamazepine toxicity. Consult your doctor.

• Women taking oral contraceptives may experience breakthrough bleeding with Carbamazepine.

• Charcoal tablets or powder, Phenobarbital, Phenytoin, or Primidone may decrease the amount of Carbamazepine absorbed into the bloodstream.

• Carbamazepine decreases the effect of Acetaminophen, Warfarin, an anticoagulant (blood-thinning) drug, and Theophylline (for asthma). People taking these combinations may need more medicine to retain the desired effects. Other drugs counteracted by Carbamazepine are Cyclosporine, Dacarbazine, Digitalis drugs, Disopyramide, Doxycycline, Haloperidol, Levothyroxine, and Quinidine.

• When taking Carbamazepine with other seizure-control medicines, including the Hydantoins, Succinimides, and Valproic Acid, the outcome is difficult to predict because the action of these drugs can be affected in different ways.

Combination treatments to control seizures must be customized to each patient.

• If Carbamazepine is taken together with Lithium, increased nervous-system toxicity can occur.

Food Interactions

Take Carbamazepine with food if it causes stomach upset.

Usual Dose

Adult and Adolescent (age 13 and older): 400 to 1200 mg per day, depending on the condition being treated. The usual maintenance dose is 400 to 800 mg per day in 2 divided doses.

Child (age 6 to 12): 200 to 1000 mg per day, or 10 to 15 mg per pound of body weight per day, divided into 3 or 4 equal doses.

Overdosage

Carbamazepine is a potentially lethal drug. The lowest known single lethal dose is 60 grams. Adults have survived single doses of 30 grams and children have survived single doses of 5 to 10 grams.

Overdose symptoms appear 1 to 3 hours after the drug is taken. The most prominent effects are irregularity or difficulty in breathing, rapid heartbeat, changes in blood pressure, shock, loss of consciousness or coma, convulsions, muscle twitching, restlessness, uncontrolled body movements, drooping eyelids, psychotic mood changes, nausea, vomiting, and reduced urination.

Successful treatment depends on prompt elimination of the drug from the body: Give the victim Syrup of Ipecac (available at any pharmacy) to make him or her vomit. The overdose victim then must be taken to a hospital emergency room for treatment immediately. ALWAYS bring the medicine bottle with you.

Special Information

Carbamazepine can cause dizziness and drowsiness. Take care while driving or operating hazardous equipment.

Call your doctor at once if you develop a yellow discoloration of the eyes or skin, unusual bleeding or bruising, abdominal pain, pale stools, dark urine, impotence (men), mood changes, nervous-system symptoms, swelling, fever, chills, sore throat, or mouth sores. These may be signs of a potentially fatal drug side effect.

Do not abruptly stop taking Carbamazepine without your physician's advice. If you forget to take a dose, however, skip the missed dose and go back to your regular dose schedule. If you miss more than 1 dose in a day, check with your doctor before continuing with your medication schedule.

Special Populations

Pregnancy/Breast-feeding

Carbamazepine has been shown to cause birth defects in animal studies. However, women taking this drug for a seizure problem should continue taking it because of the possibility that stopping the drug will cause a seizure, which could be just as dangerous for the unborn child. If possible, anticonvulsant drugs should be stopped before the pregnancy begins.

Carbamazepine passes into breast milk in concentrations of about 60 percent of the concentration in the mother's bloodstream and can affect a nursing infant. Nursing mothers who must take Carbamazepine should bottle-feed their babies.

Seniors

Older adults are more likely to develop Carbamazepine-induced heart problems, psychosis, confusion, or agitation.

Cardizem CD

see *Diltiazem Hydrochloride, page 342*

see *Diltiazem Hydrochloride, page 342*

Generic Name

Carteolol

Brand Names

Cartrol
Ocupress Eye Drops

Type of Drug

Beta-adrenergic-blocking agent.

Prescribed for

High blood pressure; angina pectoris; glaucoma (eyedrops).

General Information

Carteolol is one of 14 beta-adrenergic-blocking drugs that interfere with the action of a specific part of the nervous system. Beta receptors are found all over the body and affect many body functions. This accounts for the usefulness of beta blockers against a wide variety of conditions. The first member of this group, *Propranolol*, was found to affect the entire beta-adrenergic portion of the nervous system. Newer beta blockers have been refined to affect only a portion of that system, making them more useful in the treatment of cardio-vascular disorders and less useful for other purposes. Other beta blockers are mild stimulants to the heart or have other characteristics that make them more useful for a specific purpose or better for certain people.

When applied to the eye, Carteolol reduces fluid pressure inside the eye by reducing the production of eye fluids and slightly increasing the rate at which fluids flow through and leave the eye. Carteolol produces a greater drop in eye pressure than either Pilocarpine or Epinephrine (other glau-coma drugs), but may be combined with these or other drugs to produce a more pronounced drop in eye pressure.

Cautions and Warnings

You should be **cautious about taking Carteolol** if you have **asthma, severe heart failure, a very slow heart rate,** or **heart block** because the drug may aggravate these conditions. Compared with many other beta blockers, Carteolol has less of an effect on your pulse and bronchial muscles (asthma), has less of a rebound effect when discontinued, and produces less tiredness, depression, and intolerance to exercise.

People with **angina** who take Carteolol for high blood pressure should have their **drug dosage reduced gradually** over 1 to 2 weeks rather than suddenly discontinued to avoid possible aggravation of the angina.

Carteolol should be used with caution if you have **liver or kidney disease** because the ability to eliminate this drug from your body may be impaired.

Carteolol reduces the amount of blood pumped by the heart with each beat. This reduction in blood flow can aggravate or worsen the condition of people with **poor circulation** or **circulatory disease.**

If you are undergoing **major surgery,** your doctor may want you to stop taking Carteolol at least 2 days before surgery to permit the heart to respond more acutely to things that happen during the surgery. This is still controversial and may not hold true for all people preparing for surgery.

Carteolol eyedrops should not be used by people who cannot take oral beta-blocking drugs, such as Propranolol.

Possible Side Effects

Side effects are usually mild, are relatively uncommon, develop early in the course of treatment, and are rarely a reason to stop taking Carteolol.

▼ Most common: impotence.

▼ Other: unusual tiredness or weakness, slow heart-beat, heart failure (swelling of the legs, ankles, or feet), dizziness, breathing difficulty, bronchospasm, mental depression, anxiety, nervousness, sleeplessness, disorientation, short-term memory loss, emotional instability, cold hands and feet, constipation, diarrhea, nausea, vomiting, upset stomach, increased sweating, urinary difficulty, cramps, blurred vision, skin rash, hair loss, stuffy nose, facial swelling, aggravation of lupus erythematosus (a disease of the body's connective tissues), itching, chest pains, back or joint pains, colitis, and drug allergy (fever, sore throat).

Drug Interactions

• Carteolol may interact with surgical anesthetics to increase the risk of heart problems during surgery. Some anesthesiologists recommend gradually stopping your medicine 2 days before surgery.

• Carteolol may interfere with the normal signs of low

blood sugar and can interfere with the action of oral antidiabetes medicines.

• Carteolol enhances the blood-pressure-lowering effects
of other blood-pressure-reducing agents (including Clonidine,
Guanabenz, and Reserpine) and calcium-channel-blocking
drugs (such as Nifedipine).

• Aspirin-containing drugs, Indomethacin, Sulfinpyrazone,
and estrogen drugs can interfere with the blood-pressure-
lowering effect of Carteolol.

• Cocaine may reduce the effects of all beta-blocking drugs.

• Carteolol may increase the cold hands and feet associ-
ated with taking ergot alkaloids (for migraine headaches).
Gangrene is a possibility in people taking an ergot and
Carteolol.

• Carteolol will counteract the effects of thyroid-hormone-
replacement medicines.

• Calcium channel blockers, Flecainide, Hydralazine, oral
contraceptives, Propafenone, Haloperidol, phenothiazine tranquilizers (Molindone and others), quinolone antibacterials,
and Quinidine may increase the amount of Carteolol in the
bloodstream and the effect of that drug on the body.

• Carteolol should not be taken within 2 weeks of taking a
monoamine oxidase (MAO) inhibitor antidepressant drug.

• Cimetidine increases the amount of Carteolol absorbed
into the bloodstream from oral tablets.

• Carteolol may reduce the effect of Theophylline, Aminophylline, and some antiasthma drugs (especially Ephedrine
and Isoproterenol).

• The combination of Carteolol and Phenytoin or Digitalis
drugs can result in excessive slowing of the heart, possibly
causing heart block.

• If you stop smoking while taking Carteolol, your dose
may have to be reduced because your liver will break down
the drug more slowly after you stop.

• If you take other glaucoma eye medicines, separate them
from Carteolol to avoid physically mixing them. Small amounts
of Carteolol are absorbed into the general circulation and
may interact with some of the same drugs as other beta
blockers, but this is unlikely.

Food Interactions

Carteolol may be taken without regard to food or meals.

Usual Dose

Tablets

2.5 to 10 mg once a day. Taking more than 10 mg per day is not likely to improve the drug's effect. Those with poor kidney function may take their medication dosage as infrequently as once every 72 hours.

Eyedrops

One drop in the affected eye 1 or 2 times per day.

Overdosage

Symptoms of overdosage are changes in heartbeat (unusually slow, unusually fast, or irregular), severe dizziness or fainting, difficulty breathing, bluish-colored fingernails or palms, and seizures. The overdose victim should be taken to a hospital emergency room where proper therapy can be given. ALWAYS bring the medicine bottle with you.

Special Information

Carteolol should be taken continuously. Do not stop taking it unless directed to do so by your doctor; abrupt withdrawal may cause chest pain, difficulty breathing, increased sweating, and unusually fast or irregular heartbeat. The dose should be lowered gradually over a period of about 2 weeks.

Call your doctor at once if any of the following symptoms develop: back or joint pains, difficulty breathing, cold hands or feet, depression, skin rash, or changes in heartbeat. This drug may produce an undesirable lowering of blood pressure, leading to dizziness or fainting. Call your doctor if this happens to you. Call your doctor about the following side effects only if they persist or are bothersome: anxiety, diarrhea, constipation, sexual impotence, headache, itching, nausea or vomiting, nightmares or vivid dreams, upset stomach, trouble sleeping, stuffy nose, frequent urination, unusual tiredness, or weakness.

Carteolol can cause drowsiness, light-headedness, dizziness, or blurred vision. Be careful when driving or performing complex tasks.

It is best to take your medicine at the same time each day. If you forget a dose of Carteolol tablets, take it as soon as you remember. If you take your medicine once a day and it is within 8 hours of your next dose, skip the forgotten tablet and continue with your regular schedule. If you take your medicine twice a day and it is within 4 hours of your next dose, skip the forgotten dose and continue with your regular schedule. Do not double the dose.

To administer the eyedrops, lie down or tilt your head backward and look at the ceiling. Hold the dropper above your eye and drop the medicine inside your lower lid while looking up. To prevent possible infection, don't allow the dropper to touch your fingers, eyelids, or any surface. Release the lower lid and keep your eye open. Don't blink for about 30 seconds. Press gently on the bridge of your nose at the inside corner of your eye for about 1 minute. This will help circulate the medicine around your eye. Wait at least 5 minutes before using any other eyedrops.

If you forget to take a dose of Carteolol eyedrops, take it as soon as you remember. If it is almost time for your next dose, skip the one you forgot and continue with your regular schedule. Do not take a double dose.

Special Populations

Pregnancy/Breast-feeding

Infants born to women who took a beta blocker weighed less at birth, and had low blood pressure and reduced heart rate. Carteolol should be avoided by pregnant women and those who might become pregnant while taking it. When the drug is considered essential by your doctor, its potential benefits must be carefully weighed against its risks.

It is not known if Carteolol passes into breast milk. Nursing mothers taking this medicine should bottle-feed their babies.

Seniors

Older adults may absorb and retain more Carteolol, thus requiring less medicine to achieve the same results. Your doctor will need to adjust your dosage to meet your individual needs. Seniors taking this medicine may be more likely to suffer from cold hands and feet, reduced body temperature, chest pains, general feelings of ill health, sudden breathing difficulty, increased sweating, or changes in heartbeat.

Generic Name

Carvedilol

Brand Name

Coreg

Type of Drug

Alpha-beta-adrenergic blocker.

Prescribed for

High blood pressure. Also used for congestive heart failure, angina pains, and cardiomyopathy.

General Information

Carvedilol blocks both the alpha- and beta-adrenergic portions of the nervous system. This unique combination of actions produces the following effects on the body: It reduces the amount of blood pumped with each heartbeat and also decreases the responsiveness of the heart to various kinds of stimulation that normally cause tachycardia, or very rapid heartbeat. Its beta-blocking effects begin within an hour of taking the first dose of Carvedilol, and maximum blood pressure lowering happens after 1 or 2 weeks. The drug also causes blood vessels to widen, and makes it easier for the heart to pump blood more efficiently. People with heart failure have traditionally been warned against taking beta-blocking drugs, but a study reported late in 1995 showed that Carvedilol provided an important benefit for people with heart failure.

Because Carvedilol blocks the alpha-nervous-system receptors, it lowers blood pressure more when you are standing than when you are lying down. This effect leads to a greater chance of dizziness when rising quickly from a sitting or lying position than with other drugs.

Cautions and Warnings

Carvedilol may injure the liver in about 1 of every 100 people who take it. Those who already have **severe liver disease** should not take this medicine. Call your doctor at once if you develop **signs of liver damage** (severe itching, dark urine, unexplained flu, loss of appetite, yellowing of the eyeballs or skin). Check with your doctor about continuing Carvedilol if you are having **general anesthesia.** Heart function depressed by anesthetics can be made worse if you are also taking Carvedilol.

Carvedilol can mask the signs of low blood sugar and may **increase the effects of Insulin or oral antidiabetes drugs,** making it more difficult to recover from low blood sugar.

Carvedilol can also **mask the symptoms of an overactive thyroid gland.** Abruptly stopping Carvedilol can bring on an attack of hyperthyroidism.

Possible Side Effects

Most Carvedilol side effects are considered mild or moderate.

▼ Most common: dizziness, sleepiness or sleeplessness, diarrhea, abdominal pain, slow heartbeat, dizziness when rising from a sitting or lying position, swelling of the hands or feet, sore throat, breathing difficulty, fatigue, back pain, urinary infection, viral infections, high blood-triglyceride levels, low blood platelet counts.

▼ Less common: extra heartbeats, palpitation, blood pressure changes, fainting, reduced blood supply to the arms and legs (aches, cramps, pain or tiredness on walking, or in the foot, thigh, hip, or buttocks), tingling in the hands or feet, reduced feeling, fainting, depression, nervousness, constipation, stomach gas, liver irritation, cough, male impotence and reduced sex drive, itching, rash, visual difficulties, ringing or buzzing in the ears, high blood cholesterol, sugar or uric acid, anemia, weakness, hot flushes, leg cramps, dry mouth, feelings of ill health, sweating, muscle aches.

▼ Rare: angina pain, abnormal heart rhythms, heart failure, migraines, neuralgia, confusion, forgetfulness, slight paralysis, asthma, allergy, bronchial spasm, blood in the urine, frequent urination, hair loss, hearing loss, weight gain and sugar in the urine, kidney function loss, potassium level changes.

Drug Interactions

- Carvedilol increases the effects of Insulin and oral antidiabetes drugs. People who must take this combination must monitor their blood sugar regularly. Call your doctor if there is any change from your normal pattern.

- Carvedilol increases the effects of Verapamil, Diltiazem, or similar calcium-channel-blocking drugs.

- Carvedilol increases the blood-pressure-lowering effect of Clonidine. People taking this combination may need less medicine to control their pressure.

- Carvedilol increases the amount of Digoxin in the blood by about 15 percent when the drugs are taken together. Digoxin doses may have to be adjusted when you are starting, taking, or stopping Carvedilol.

- Cimetidine increases the amount of Carvedilol absorbed into the blood by about 30 percent, but it may not affect you.

- Rifampin increases the breakdown of Carvedilol and reduces the amount of Carvedilol in the blood by about 70 percent. Dosage adjustment is necessary if you must mix these medicines.

Food Interactions

Food slows the rate at which Carvedilol is absorbed into the blood. Take each dose of Carvedilol with food to reduce the risk of dizziness or fainting.

Usual Dose

Adult: 6.25 mg twice a day to start, increased up to 25 mg twice a day if needed.

Child: not recommended.

Overdosage

Carvedilol overdose may cause very low blood pressure (dizziness, fainting), slow heartbeat, and other heart problems, including shock and heart attack. Breathing problems, bronchial spasm, vomiting, periods of unconsciousness, and seizures may also develop. Three cases of overdose are known (including a 2-year-old); all victims all fully recovered. Overdose victims must be taken to a hospital emergency room for treatment. ALWAYS bring the medicine bottle with you.

Special Information

Carvedilol is meant to be taken continuously. Do not stop taking it unless directed to do so by your doctor; abrupt withdrawal may cause chest pain, difficulty breathing, increased sweating, and unusually fast or irregular heartbeat. The dose should be gradually reduced over a period of about 2 weeks.

People taking Carvedilol may become dizzy and even faint on standing. If this happens to you, sit or lie down until you feel better. Carvedilol can also cause drowsiness, light-headedness, or blurred vision. Be careful when driving or performing complex tasks.

Contact lens wearers are more likely to experience dry eyes if taking Carvedilol.

It is best to take your medicine at the same time each day. If you forget a dose, take it as soon as you remember. If it is within 4 hours of your next dose, skip the missed dose and continue with your regular schedule. Do not take a double dose of Carvedilol.

Special Populations

Pregnancy/Breast-feeding

Animal studies indicate that Carvedilol passes into the fetal bloodstream and can interfere with a normal pregnancy, but there is no human information available. This drug should be taken during pregnancy only if its possible benefits outweigh its risks.

It is not known if Carvedilol passes into human breast milk, though it passes into rat breast milk. Beta-blocking drugs may affect babies' hearts. Nursing mothers who must take this drug should bottle-feed their babies.

Seniors

Seniors break down Carvedilol less efficiently than younger adults and may have 50 percent more drug in their blood than younger people. Older adults may be more likely to develop drug side effects, especially dizziness.

Ceclor

see *Cephalosporin Antibiotics*, page 171

Cefaclor

see *Cephalosporin Antibiotics*, page 171

Ceftin

see *Cephalosporin Antibiotics*, page 171

Cefzil

see *Cephalosporin Antibiotics*, page 171

Cephalexin

see *Cephalosporin Antibiotics*, page 171

Type of Drug

Cephalosporin Antibiotics

Generic Name	Brand Name
Cefaclor	Ceclor*
Cefadroxil	Duricef*
	Ultracef*
Cefixime	Suprax
Cefpodoxime Proxetil	Vantin
Cefprozil	Cefzil

Ceftibuten	Cedax
Cefuroxime Axetil	Ceftin
Cephalexin	Keflet*
	Keflex*
Cephalexin Hydrochloride	Keftab
Cephradine	Anspor*
	Velosef*
Loracarbef	Lorabid

(*Also available in generic form)

Prescribed for

Bacterial infections.

General Information

These antibiotics are all related to *Cephalosporin A*, which was isolated from a micro-organism discovered in the sea near Sardinia in 1948. Over the years, researchers have manipulated the Cephalosporin A molecule, which is similar to Penicillin, to produce more than 20 different antibiotic drugs. The cephalosporin antibiotics included in *The Pill Book* can be taken orally as a liquid, tablet, or capsule. Injectable cephalosporins are not included.

Cautions and Warnings

A small number of people (about 5 percent) with an **allergy to Penicillin** may also be allergic to cephalosporin. Be sure your doctor knows about any Penicillin allergies. The most common allergic reaction to a cephalosporin is a hivelike condition with redness over large areas of the body. Other sensitivity reactions to cephalosporin antibiotics can include skin rashes or other reactions, fever, or joint aches or pains. When this happens, the reactions generally occur after a few days of taking the antibiotic and resolve within a few days after the antibiotic is stopped.

Prolonged or repeated use of a cephalosporin antibiotic can lead to the **overgrowth** of a fungus or bacteria that are not susceptible to the antibiotic, causing a secondary infection.

Occasionally, people taking a cephalosporin may develop **drug-related colitis.** Call your doctor if you develop diarrhea while taking one of these medicines.

People with **kidney disease** who receive high doses of a cephalosporin antibiotic may develop seizure in rare instances. Call your doctor if this happens.

The dosage of some cephalosporins must be adjusted for people with **poor kidney function.**

Possible Side Effects

Most cephalosporin side effects are quite mild.

▼ Most common: abdominal pains and gas, upset stomach, nausea, vomiting, diarrhea, itching, and rashes.

▼ Less common: headache, dizziness, tiredness, tingling in the hands or feet, seizures, confusion, drug allergy, fever, joint pains, chest tightness, redness, muscle aches and swelling, loss of appetite, and changes in taste perception. Colitis may develop during treatment because of changes in the normal micro-organisms found in the gastrointestinal tract.

Cefaclor may cause serum sickness (a combination of fever, joint pains, and rash).

Cephalosporins may cause changes in some blood cells, but this problem is not generally seen with those drugs that can be taken orally. Some cephalosporins have caused kidney problems, liver inflammation, and jaundice, but these are also rarely a problem with oral cephalosporins.

Drug Interactions

• The cephalosporins should not be taken with Erythromycin or Tetracycline, because of conflicting antibacterial action.

• Some cephalosporin antibiotics may increase the blood-thinning effects of anticoagulant drugs.

• Probenecid may increase blood levels of the cephalosporins by preventing their elimination through the kidneys.

• Cephalosporins may cause a false-positive test for sugar in the urine with Clinitest tablets or similar products. Enzyme-based tests like Tes-Tape and Clinistix are not affected.

• Cefuroxime may cause a false-positive test for blood sugar.

Food Interactions

Generally, the cephalosporins may be taken with food or milk if they upset your stomach.

Food interferes with the absorption of Cephalexin and Cefaclor into the blood. They should be taken on an empty stomach, 1 hour before or 2 hours after meals.

Cefpodoxime and Cefuroxime should be taken with food to increase the amount of drug absorbed into the blood.

Cefadroxil, Cefixime, Cefprozil, Cephradine, and Loracarbef may be taken without regard to food or meals.

Usual Dose

Cefaclor
Adult: 250 to 500 mg every 8 hours.
Child: 3 to 6 mg per pound of body weight every 8 hours.

Cefadroxil
Adult: 1 to 2 grams per day in 1 or 2 doses.
Child: 13 mg per pound of body weight per day in 1 or 2 doses.

Cefixime
Adult: 400 mg per day in 1 or 2 doses.
Child: 3.5 mg per pound of body weight per day in 1 or 2 doses.

Cefpodoxime Proxetil
Adult: 200 to 400 mg per day in 1 or 2 doses.
Child (age 6 months to 12 years): 2.5 to 5 mg per pound of body weight up to 400 mg per day.

Cefprozil
Adult: 250 to 1000 mg per day.
Child (age 6 months to 12 years): 13 mg per pound of body weight every 12 hours.

Ceftibuten
Adult: 400 mg once a day.
Child: 4 mg per pound of body weight once a day, up to 400 mg.

Cefuroxime
Adult and Child (age 12 and older): 125 to 500 mg every 12 hours.
Child and Infant (under age 12): 125 to 250 mg every 12 hours.

Cephalexin

Adult: 250 to 1000 mg every 6 hours. Some urinary infections may be treated with 500 mg every 12 hours.

Child: 11 to 23 mg per pound of body weight per day. The dose may be increased to 46 mg per pound of body weight to treat middle-ear infections.

Cephradine

Adult: 250 to 500 mg every 6 to 12 hours.

Child (9 months and older): 11 to 45 mg per pound of body weight per day in 2 or 4 doses.

Loracarbef

Adult and Child (age 13 and older): 200 to 400 mg every 12 hours.

Child (age 6 months to 12 years): 6.5 to 13 mg per pound of body weight per day.

Overdosage

The most common symptoms of a cephalosporin overdose are nausea, vomiting, and upset stomach. These symptoms can be treated with milk or an antacid. Cephalosporin overdoses are generally not serious, but you may want to contact a hospital emergency room or local poison control center for more information.

Special Information

Proper diagnosis is key to the effective use of any antibiotic. Don't take any of these medicines without first consulting your doctor. The cephalosporins, like all antibiotics, will make you feel better within 2 or 3 days. However, to obtain the maximum benefit from any antibiotic, you must take the full prescribed dose for 7 to 14 days.

If you miss a dose of a cephalosporin that you take once a day and it is almost time for your next dose, take the dose you forgot right away and your next one 10 to 12 hours later. Then go back to your regular schedule.

If you take the medicine 2 times a day, take the dose you forgot right away and the next dose 5 to 6 hours later. Then go back to your regular schedule.

If you take the medicine 3 or more times a day, take the

dose you missed right away and your next dose 2 to 4 hours later. Then go back to your regular schedule.

Most cephalosporin liquids must be kept in the refrigerator to maintain their strength. Only Cefixime liquid does not require refrigeration. All of the liquid cephalosporins have a very limited shelf life. Do not keep any of these liquids beyond the 10 days to 2 weeks specified on the label. Check with your pharmacist if you're not sure about how long you can keep the antibiotic.

The cephalosporins may interfere with the Clinitest tablets used to test for sugar in the urine. They do not interfere with enzyme-based tests like Tes-Tape and Clinistix.

Special Populations

Pregnancy/Breast-feeding
These drugs are considered to be relatively safe during pregnancy. However, they should be taken only if the potential benefit outweighs any harm they could cause.

Small amounts of cephalosporin antibiotic pass into breast milk. Nursing mothers who must take a cephalosporin antibiotic should bottle-feed their babies to avoid possible problems.

Seniors
Seniors with reduced kidney function should be regularly monitored for possible antibiotic side effects. Otherwise, seniors may take oral cephalosporin antibiotics without special restriction. Be sure to report any unusual side effects to your doctor.

Generic Name

Cetirizine

Brand Name
Zyrtec

Type of Drug
Antihistamine.

Prescribed for

Seasonal allergy, stuffy and runny nose, itching of the eyes, scratchy throat caused by allergies, and other allergic symptoms, such as rash, itching, or hives. Cetirizine may be prescribed for the treatment of asthma in people whose disease is triggered by allergies.

General Information

Cetirizine causes less sedation than most other antihistamines available in the United States. It has been widely used and accepted by people who find other antihistamines unacceptable because of the drowsiness and tiredness they cause. Cetirizine appears to work in exactly the same way as Chlorpheniramine and other widely used antihistamines.

Cautions and Warnings

Do not take Cetirizine if you are **allergic** to it.

People with **kidney disease** should receive a lower than normal dosage of Cetirizine because they are unable to clear the drug as rapidly from their bodies as others.

Possible Side Effects

▼ Rare: headache, nervousness, weakness, upset stomach, nausea, vomiting, sore throat, nosebleeds, cough, stuffy nose, changes in bowel habits, and dry mouth, nose, or throat.

Drug Interactions

• Cetirizine is less likely to interact than other antihistamines.

Food Interactions

Cetirizine should be taken on an empty stomach, 1 hour before or 2 hours after food or meals, although it may be taken with food or milk if it upsets your stomach.

Usual Dose

Adult and Adolescent (age 12 and older): 5 to 20 mg once a day. Reduce dosage in people with kidney disease.

Child (age 6–11): 10 mg a day.
Child (age 2–5): 5 mg a day.

Overdosage

Cetirizine overdose is likely to cause exaggerated side effects. Overdose victims should be given Syrup of Ipecac to make them vomit and then should be taken to a hospital emergency room. ALWAYS bring the prescription bottle with you.

Special Information

Report sore throat, unusual bleeding, bruising, tiredness, or weakness or any other unusual side effects to your doctor. This drug is less sedating than most other antihistamines, yet it still may cause some drowsiness and should not be mixed with alcohol or other nervous-system depressants.

If you forget to take a dose of Cetirizine, take it as soon as you remember. If it is almost time for your next regularly scheduled dose, skip the one you forgot and continue with your regular schedule. Do not take a double dose.

Special Populations

Pregnancy/Breast-feeding

Do not take any antihistamine without your doctor's knowledge. Animal studies of Cetirizine have shown that doses several times larger than the human dose lower the baby's weight and increase the risk of the baby's death.

Small amounts of antihistamine medicines pass into breast milk and may affect a nursing infant. Nursing mothers should avoid antihistamines or use alternative feeding methods while taking the medicine.

Seniors

Seniors are unlikely to experience nervous-system effects with this antihistamine.

Generic Name

Chlordiazepoxide

Brand Names

Libritabs
Librium
Lipoxide

(Also available in generic form)

Type of Drug

Benzodiazepine tranquilizer.

Prescribed for

Relief of symptoms of anxiety, tension, fatigue, and agitation. Also used for irritable bowel syndrome and panic attacks.

General Information

Chlordiazepoxide is a member of the group of drugs known as *benzodiazepines*. These drugs have some activity as either antianxiety agents, anticonvulsants, or sedatives. Some are more suited to a specific role because of differences in their chemical makeup that give them greater activity in a certain area or characteristics that make them more desirable for a certain function. Often, individual drugs are limited by the applications for which their research has been sponsored. Benzodiazepines work by a direct effect on the brain. In doing so, they can relax you and make you either more tranquil or sleepier, or can slow nervous-system transmissions in such a way as to act as an anticonvulsant, depending on which drug you use and how much you take. Many doctors prefer the benzodiazepines to other drugs that can be used for similar effects because they tend to be safer, have fewer side effects, and are usually as, if not more, effective.

Cautions and Warnings

Do not take Chlordiazepoxide if you know you are **sensitive** or **allergic** to it or another member of the group, including Clonazepam.

Chlordiazepoxide can aggravate **narrow-angle glaucoma,** but if you have open-angle glaucoma, you may take it. Check with your doctor.

Other conditions in which Chlordiazepoxide should be avoided are severe depression, severe lung disease, sleep apnea (intermittent breathing during sleep), liver disease, drunkenness, and kidney disease. In these conditions, the depressive effects of Chlordiazepoxide may be enhanced and/or could be detrimental to your overall situation.

Chlordiazepoxide should **not be taken by psychotic people,** because it doesn't work for them and can cause unusual excitement, stimulation, and rage.

Chlordiazepoxide is **not intended for more than 3 to 4 months of continuous use.** Your condition should be reassessed before continuing Chlordiazepoxide beyond that time.

Chlordiazepoxide may be **addictive,** and you can experience drug withdrawal symptoms if you suddenly stop taking your medicine after as little as 4 to 6 weeks of treatment. Withdrawal generally begins with increased feelings of anxiety and continues with tingling in the extremities, sensitivity to bright lights or the sun, long periods of sleep or sleeplessness, a metallic taste, flulike illness, fatigue, difficulty concentrating, restlessness, loss of appetite, nausea, irritability, headache, dizziness, sweating, muscle tension or cramps, tremors, and feeling uncomfortable or ill at ease. Other major withdrawal symptoms include confusion, abnormal perception of movement, depersonalization, paranoid delusions, hallucinations, psychotic reactions, muscle twitching, seizures, and memory loss.

Possible Side Effects

Weakness and confusion may occur, especially in seniors and those who are more sickly.

▼ Most common: mild drowsiness during the first few days of therapy.

▼ Less common: depression, lethargy, disorientation, headache, inactivity, slurred speech, stupor, dizziness, tremor, constipation, dry mouth, nausea, inability to control urination, sexual difficulties, irregular menstrual cycle, changes in heart rhythm, lowered blood pressure, fluid

Possible Side Effects *(continued)*

retention, blurred or double vision, itching, rash, hiccups, nervousness, inability to fall asleep, and occasional liver dysfunction. If you experience any of these symptoms, stop taking the medicine and contact your doctor immediately.

▼ Infrequent: diarrhea, coated tongue, sore gums, vomiting, appetite changes, swallowing difficulty, increased salivation, upset stomach, incontinence, changes in heart rate, blood pressure changes, palpitations, swelling, stuffy nose, hearing difficulty, hair loss, hairiness, increased sweating, fever, tingling in the hands or feet, breast pain, muscle disturbances, breathing difficulty, changes in the components of your blood, and joint pain.

Drug Interactions

• Chlordiazepoxide is a central-nervous-system depressant. Avoid alcohol, other tranquilizers, narcotics, barbiturates, monoamine oxidase (MAO) inhibitors, antihistamines, and antidepressants. Taking Chlordiazepoxide with these drugs may result in excessive depression, tiredness, sleepiness, difficulty breathing, or similar symptoms.

• Smoking may reduce the effectiveness of Chlordiazepoxide by increasing the rate at which it is broken down by the body.

• The effects of Chlordiazepoxide may be prolonged when it is taken with Cimetidine, oral contraceptives, Disulfiram, Fluoxetine, Isoniazid, Ketoconazole, Metoprolol, Probenecid, Propoxyphene, Propranolol, Rifampin, or Valproic Acid.

• Theophylline may reduce Chlordiazepoxide's sedative effects.

• If you take antacids, separate them by at least 1 hour from your Chlordiazepoxide dose to prevent them from interfering with the passage of Chlordiazepoxide into the bloodstream.

• Chlordiazepoxide may increase blood levels of Digoxin and the chances for Digoxin toxicity.

• Levodopa's effectiveness may be reduced by Chlordiazepoxide.

• Phenytoin blood concentrations may be increased when

taken with Chlordiazepoxide, resulting in possible Phenytoin toxicity.

Food Interactions

Chlordiazepoxide is best taken on an empty stomach but may be taken with food if it upsets your stomach.

Usual Dose

Adult: 5 to 100 mg per day. This tremendous range in dosage is due to individual response related to age, weight, disease severity, and other characteristics.

Child (age 6 and older): this drug may be given if deemed appropriate by a doctor. Initially, the lowest available dose (5 mg 2 to 4 times per day) is used. The dose may be increased in some children to 30 to 40 mg per day but must be individualized to obtain maximum benefit.

Overdosage

Symptoms of overdosage are confusion, sleepiness, poor coordination, lack of response to pain such as a pin stick, loss of reflexes, shallow breathing, low blood pressure, and coma. The victim should be taken to a hospital emergency room for treatment. ALWAYS bring the medicine bottle with you.

Special Information

Chlordiazepoxide can cause tiredness, drowsiness, inability to concentrate, or similar symptoms. Be careful if you are driving, operating machinery, or performing other activities that require concentration.

If you forget a dose of Chlordiazepoxide, take it as soon as you remember. If it is almost time for your next dose, skip the forgotten pill and continue with your regular schedule. Do not take a double dose.

Special Populations
Pregnancy/Breast-feeding

Chlordiazepoxide may cross into the developing fetal circulation and may cause birth defects if taken during the first 3 months of pregnancy. Avoid Chlordiazepoxide while pregnant.

Chlordiazepoxide may pass into breast milk. Because infants break the drug down more slowly than adults, it is possible for the medicine to accumulate and have an undesired effect on the baby. Tell your doctor if you become pregnant or are nursing an infant.

Seniors

Older adults, especially those with liver or kidney disease, are more sensitive to the effects of Chlordiazepoxide and generally require smaller doses to achieve the same effect. Follow your doctor's directions, and report any side effects at once.

Generic Name

Chlorhexidine Gluconate

Brand Name

Peridex Oral Rinse
PerioGard

Type of Drug

Oral disinfectant.

Prescribed for

Swelling and redness of the gums. Chlorhexidine is also prescribed for severe gum disease as part of an overall treatment program. It may be used to treat or prevent mouth irritation or infection after periodontal surgery and in cancer or bone marrow transplant patients, to reduce dental plaque, and to treat minor ulcers inside the mouth. Chlorhexidine may also be prescribed for gum irritations caused by ill-fitting dentures.

General Information

Chlorhexidine Gluconate kills bacteria that contribute to gum redness, swelling, and bleeding. It is absorbed by the tissues it comes into contact with and is slowly released over a 24-hour period after rinsing with it, providing a continuous antibacterial effect. Studies have shown that the bacterial content of dental plaque is reduced by up to 97 percent after using Chlorhexidine rinse for 6 months. Chlorhexidine is also used in surgical scrub products and other topical disinfectants.

Cautions and Warnings

People who have had an **allergic reaction** to Chlorhexidine skin disinfectants should avoid this product, though generalized allergic reactions to this product are rare. Its use is **not recommended** for **children under 18 years of age.**

Chlorhexidine may permanently **discolor your teeth** or **tooth-filling** edges. People with front-tooth fillings should be careful about using this product because it can create the need for cosmetic treatment of the front teeth.

Your **taste perception** may change while using this product but will return to normal after you stop using it.

Possible Side Effects

▼ Most common: tooth staining, increased tooth calculus formation, and temporary changes in the sense of taste.

▼ Other: minor mouth irritation and tissue loss (especially in children) and occasional irritation of glands in your mouth or throat.

Drug Interactions

• Do not mix Chlorhexidine with any other oral drug product.

Food Interactions

Do not dilute Chlorhexidine rinse with any food or liquid. To get the maximum benefit from each treatment, do not eat or drink for several hours after using Chlorhexidine rinse.

Usual Dose

Adult (age 18 years and older): rinse with 1 tablespoonful of Chlorhexidine (marked in product cap) for 30 seconds twice a day after flossing and brushing your teeth.

Denture irritation: soak your dentures twice a day for 1 to 2 minutes. Rinse your mouth for 30 seconds twice a day. Or you may be asked to brush your dentures and gums with Chlorhexidine rinse 2 times a day.

Overdosage

Small children swallowing 1 or 2 ounces of Chlorhexidine rinse may develop upset stomachs or signs of alcohol intoxication (the product is 11.6% alcohol). If a small child (22 pounds or less) swallows 4 ounces or more, or if signs of drunkenness develop, take the victim to a hospital emergency room. ALWAYS bring the medicine bottle.

Special Information

Do not use Chlorhexidine except under the supervision of a dentist, who will remove tooth deposits before Chlorhexidine use. People using Chlorhexidine rinse may develop more solid deposits on tooth surfaces (called calculus) while using it. See your dentist every 6 months to have these removed.

Chlorhexidine rinse should be used after flossing and brushing your teeth. Rinse your mouth completely before using Chlorhexidine rinse. Swish the rinse in your mouth for 30 seconds and spit it out. Do not swallow the rinse. Do not rinse with water immediately after a Chlorhexidine rinse, because this will increase the product's bitter taste.

If you forget a dose of Chlorhexidine, take it as soon as you remember. If it is almost time for your next dose, skip the dose you forgot and continue with your regular schedule. Do not take a double dose.

Special Populations

Pregnancy/Breast-feeding

There are no reports of adverse effects of Chlorhexidine on developing fetuses. Also, animal studies have revealed no problems with the drug. Pregnant women and those who might become pregnant should use this mouthwash only after weighing its possible risks versus its benefits.

It is not known if Chlorhexidine passes into breast milk. No problems have been found in nursing infants or in laboratory animal studies. Use caution if you nurse while using this product.

Seniors

Older adults may use this product without special restriction.

Generic Name

Chlorpheniramine Maleate

Brand Names

Aller-Chlor	Chlor-Trimeton	Phenetron
Chlo-Amine	Chlor-Trimeton	Telachlor
Chlorate	Repetabs	Teldrin
Chlortab	Pfeiffer's Allergy	

(Also available in generic form)

Note: The information in this profile also applies to:

Generic Name: Azatadine Maleate

Optimine

Generic Name: Brompheniramine Maleate

Bromphen	Dimetane	Veltane
Diamine T.D.	Dimetane	
	Extentabs	

Generic Name: Cyproheptadine Hydrochloride

Periactin

Generic Name: Dexchlorpheniramine Maleate

Dexchlor	Polaramine	Polargen
Poladex		

Generic Name: Tripelennamine Hydrochloride

PBZ/PBZ-SR (long-acting)
Pelamine

(All of these brand-name products are also available in generic form *except* Optimine.)

Type of Drug

Antihistamine.

Prescribed for

Seasonal allergy, stuffed and runny nose, itchy eyes, scratchy throat caused by allergy, and other allergic symptoms (such as skin rash, itching, or hives).

General Information

Antihistamines usually act by blocking the release of histamine from the cell at the H_1 histamine receptor site. Antihistamines dry up the secretions of the nose, throat, and eyes.

Cautions and Warnings

Antihistamines should not be used if you are **allergic** to them. Use these drugs with care if you have a history of **thyroid disease, heart disease, high blood pressure**, or **diabetes**. These drugs should be avoided or used with extreme care if you have **narrow-angle glaucoma** (pressure in the eye), **stomach ulcer** or **other stomach problems, enlarged prostate**, or **problems passing urine**. They should not be used by people who have deep-breathing problems, such as **asthma**.

Possible Side Effects

▼ Less common: skin rash or itching, sensitivity to bright light, increased perspiration, chills, lowered blood pressure, headache, rapid heartbeat, sleeplessness, dizziness, disturbed coordination, confusion, restlessness, nervousness, irritability, euphoria (feeling "high"), tingling in the hands or feet, blurred or double vision, ringing in the ears, stomach upset, loss of appetite, nausea, vomiting, constipation, diarrhea, difficulty in urination, tightness of the chest, wheezing, nasal stuffiness, and dryness of the mouth, nose, or throat. Young children can also develop nervousness, irritability, tension, and anxiety.

Drug Interactions

• Anthihistamines should not be taken with monoamine oxidase (MAO) inhibitors, because of possibly severe reactions.

• Interaction with tranquilizers, benzodiazepines, sedatives, and sleeping medications will increase the effect of these drugs; it is extremely important that your doctor knows if you are taking any other medicines together with an antihistamine so that doses of those drugs can be properly adjusted. Be extremely cautious when drinking alcoholic beverages while taking Chlorpheniramine, which will enhance the intoxicating and sedating effects of alcohol.

Food Interactions

You may take this drug with food if it upsets your stomach.

Usual Dose

Azatadine
1 to 2 mg twice per day.

Brompheniramine
Adult and Adolescent (age 13 and older): 4 mg 3 to 4 times per day.

Child (age 6 to 12): 2 to 4 mg 3 to 4 times per day, not more than 12 mg per day.

Child (under age 6): 1/4 mg per pound per day in divided doses.

Chlorpheniramine
Adult and Adolescent (age 13 and older): 4-mg tablet every 4 to 6 hours; not more than 24 mg per day.

Child (age 6 to 12): 2-mg tablet every 4 to 6 hours; not more than 8 mg per day.

Child (age 2 to 5): 1 mg every 4 to 6 hours; not more than 4 mg per day.

Timed-release Chlorpheniramine (capsule or tablet)
Adult and Adolescent (age 13 and older): 8 to 12 mg at bedtime or every 8 to 12 hours during the day.

Child (age 6 to 12): 8 mg during the day or at bedtime.

Child (under age 6): do not use.

Cyproheptadine
Adult: 4 to 20 mg daily (maximum dose: 32 mg).

Child (age 7 to 14): 4 mg, 2 to 3 times per day (maximum dose: 16 mg).

Child (age 2 to 6): 2 mg, 2 to 3 times per day (maximum dose: 12 mg).

Dexchlorpheniramine

Adult and Adolescent (age 12 and older): 2 mg every 4 to 6 hours. *Timed-release tablets:* 4 to 6 mg every 8 to 10 hours and at bedtime.

Child (age 6 to 11): 1 mg every 4 to 6 hours. *Timed-release tablets:* 4 mg once a day and at bedtime.

Child (age 2 to 5): 0.5 mg every 4 to 6 hours. *Timed-release tablets:* do not use.

Tripelennamine

Adult and Adolescent (age 12 and older): 25 to 50 mg every 4 to 6 hours. Up to 600 mg per day may be used. Adult patients may take up to 3 of the 100-mg long-acting (PBZ-SR) tablets per day, although this much is not usually needed.

Infant and Child: 2 mg per pound of body weight per day in divided doses. No more than 300 mg should be given per day. Older children may take up to 3 of the extended-release (long-acting) tablets per day, if needed.

Overdosage

Symptoms of overdosage are depression or stimulation (especially in children), dry mouth, fixed or dilated pupils, flushing of the skin, and stomach upset. Overdose victims should be made to vomit as soon as possible with Syrup of Ipecac (available at any pharmacy) to remove excess drug from the stomach. Follow directions on the package label and be sure to prevent the victim from inhaling his or her own vomit. Take the victim to a hospital emergency room immediately if the victim is unconscious or if you cannot make him or her vomit. ALWAYS bring the medicine bottle.

Special Information

Antihistamines can make you feel tired or lose your concentration: Be extremely cautious when driving or doing anything that requires close attention.

If you forget a dose of Chlorpheniramine Maleate, take it as soon as you remember. If it is almost time for your next dose, skip the one you forgot and continue with your regular schedule. Do not take a double dose.

Special Populations

Pregnancy/Breast-feeding

Antihistamines have not generally been proven to cause birth defects or other problems in pregnant women, although studies in animals have shown that some antihistamines (Meclizine and Cyclizine, used mainly against nausea and vomiting) may cause birth defects. Do not take any antihistamine without your doctor's knowledge, especially during the last 3 months of pregnancy, because newborns and premature infants may have severe reactions to antihistamines.

Small amounts of some antihistamines pass into breast milk, and others have not been proven safe for use in infants or young children. If you must take an antihistamine, you should bottle-feed your baby.

Seniors

Seniors are more sensitive to antihistamine side effects, particularly confusion; difficult or painful urination; dizziness; drowsiness; feelings of faintness; nightmares; excitement; nervousness; restlessness; irritability; and dry mouth, nose, and throat.

Generic Name

Chlorpromazine

Brand Name

Thorazine Tablets, Suppositories, Concentrate   [S]
Thorazine Syrup*   [A]

The information contained in this drug profile also applies to the following:

Generic Name	Brand Name	
Fluphenazine Hydrochloride	Permitil Tablets and Concentrate	[S]
	Prolixin Tablets, Elixir and Concentrate	
Mesoridazine	Serentil Tablets and Concentrate	[S]
Thioridazine Hydrochloride	Mellaril Tablets and Concentrate*	
	Mellaril-S Suspension*	
Trifluoperazine	Stelazine Tablets and Concentrate*	

(*Also available in generic form)

Type of Drug

Phenothiazine antipsychotic.

Prescribed for

Psychotic disorders, moderate to severe depression with anxiety, control of agitation or aggressiveness in disturbed children, alcohol withdrawal symptoms, intractable pain, and senility. Chlorpromazine may also be used to relieve nausea, vomiting, hiccups, restlessness, and apprehension before surgery or other special therapy.

General Information

Chlorpromazine and the other medicines listed above are members of the *phenothiazine* group of drugs, which act upon a portion of the brain called the *hypothalamus*. They affect parts of the hypothalamus that control metabolism, body temperature, alertness, muscle tone, hormone balance, and vomiting and may be used to treat problems related to any of these functions. This drug is available in suppositories and liquid forms for those who have trouble swallowing tablets.

Cautions and Warnings

Chlorpromazine can **depress the cough (gag) reflex**. Some people who have taken it have accidentally **choked to death** because the cough reflex failed to protect them. Because of its effect in reducing vomiting, Chlorpromazine can obscure signs of toxicity due to overdose of other drugs or symptoms of disease.

Do not take Chlorpromazine if you are allergic to it or any of the other phenothiazine drugs. Do not take it if you have very low blood pressure, Parkinson's disease, or any blood, liver, kidney, or heart disease.

If you have glaucoma, epilepsy, ulcers, or difficulty passing urine, Chlorpromazine should be used with caution and under your doctor's strict supervision.

Avoid exposure to extreme heat, because this drug can upset your body's normal temperature control mechanism.

Possible Side Effects

▼ Most common: drowsiness, especially during the first or second week of therapy. If the drowsiness becomes troublesome, contact your doctor. Do not allow the liquid forms of this medicine to come in contact with your skin, because they are highly irritating.

▼ Less common: changes in blood components including anemias, raised or lowered blood pressure, abnormal heart rates, heart attack, and faintness or dizziness.

▼ Other: Chlorpromazine can cause jaundice (yellowing of the eyes or skin), usually within the first 2 to 4 weeks. The jaundice usually goes away when the drug is discontinued, but there have been cases when it did not. If you notice this effect, or if you develop symptoms such as fever and general feelings of ill health, contact your doctor immediately.

Phenothiazines can produce extrapyramidal effects, such as spasm of the neck muscles, rolling back of the eyes, convulsions, difficulty in swallowing, and symptoms associated with Parkinson's disease. These effects seem very serious but usually disappear after the drug has been withdrawn; however, symptoms affecting the face, tongue, or jaw may persist for as long as several years, especially in older adults with a history of brain damage. If you experience extrapyramidal effects, contact your doctor immediately.

Chlorpromazine may cause an unusual increase in psychotic symptoms or may cause paranoid reactions, tiredness, lethargy, restlessness, hyperactivity, confusion at night, bizarre dreams, inability to sleep, depression, and euphoria (feeling "high"). Other reactions are itching, swelling, unusual sensitivity to bright light, red skin or rash, stuffy nose, headache, nausea, vomiting, loss of appetite, change in body temperature, loss of facial color, excessive salivation or perspiration, constipation, diarrhea, changes in urine and bowel habits, worsening of glaucoma, blurred vision, weakening of eyelid muscles, spasms in bronchial or other muscles, increased appetite, excessive thirst, and changes in the coloration of skin,

Possible Side Effects *(continued)*

particularly in areas exposed to the sun. There have been cases of breast enlargement, false-positive pregnancy tests, and changes in menstrual flow in females, and impotence and changes in sex drive in males.

Drug Interactions

• Be cautious about taking Chlorpromazine with barbiturates, sleeping pills, narcotics or other tranquilizers, or any other medication that may produce a depressive effect; avoid alcoholic beverages for the same reason.

• Aluminum antacids may interfere with the absorption of phenothiazine drugs into the bloodstream, reducing their effectiveness.

• Chlorpromazine can reduce the effects of Bromocriptine and appetite suppressants.

• Anticholinergic drugs can reduce the effectiveness of Chlorpromazine and increase the chance of drug side effects.

• The blood-pressure-lowering effect of Guanethidine may be counteracted by phenothiazine drugs.

• Taking Lithium together with a phenothiazine drug may lead to disorientation, loss of consciousness, or uncontrolled muscle movements.

• Mixing Propranolol and a phenothiazine drug may lead to unusually low blood pressure.

• Blood concentrations of tricyclic antidepressant drugs may increase if they are taken together with a phenothiazine drug. This can lead to antidepressant side effects.

Food Interactions

Take liquid Chlorpromazine with fruit juice or other liquids. You may also take it with food if it upsets your stomach.

Usual Dose

Adult: 30 to 1000 mg or more per day, individualized according to your disease and response.

Child (age 6 months and older): 0.25 mg per pound of body weight every 4 to 6 hours, up to 200 mg or more per day (by various routes, including rectal suppositories), depending on disease, age, and response to therapy.

Overdosage

Symptoms of overdosage are depression, extreme weakness, tiredness, lowered blood pressure, agitation, restlessness, uncontrolled muscle spasms, convulsions, fever, dry mouth, abnormal heart rhythms, and coma. The victim should be taken to a hospital emergency room immediately. ALWAYS bring the medicine bottle.

Special Information

Call your doctor at once if you develop sore throat, fever, rash, weakness, visual problems, tremors, muscle movements or twitching, yellowing of the skin or whites of the eyes, or urine darkening.

This medication may cause drowsiness. Use caution when driving or operating hazardous equipment, and avoid alcoholic beverages while taking the medicine.

Chlorpromazine and other medicines listed above may also cause unusual sensitivity to the sun and can turn your urine reddish-brown to pink.

If dizziness occurs, avoid rising quickly from a sitting or lying position and avoid climbing stairs. Use caution in hot weather, because this medicine may make you more prone to heat stroke.

If you are using sustained-release capsules, do not chew them or break them: Swallow them whole. Liquid forms of Chlorpromazine and the other medicines listed above must be protected from light. Don't take them out of the opaque bottle in which they are dispensed from the pharmacy.

If you forget to take a dose of Chlorpromazine, take it as soon as you remember. If you are taking just 1 dose per day and miss a dose, skip the forgotten dose and continue your regular dose schedule the next day. If you take more than 1 dose per day, skip the missed dose and continue with your regular schedule. Do not take a double dose.

Special Populations

Pregnancy/Breast-feeding

Infants born to women taking this medication have experienced drug side effects (liver jaundice, nervous-system effects) immediately after birth. Check with your doctor about taking this medicine if you are, or might become, pregnant.

This drug may pass into breast milk and affect a nursing infant. Consider alternative feeding methods if you must take Chlorpromazine.

Seniors

Older adults are more sensitive to the effects of this medication and usually require a lower dosage to achieve the desired results. Also, seniors are more likely to develop drug side effects, and some experts feel that they should be treated with ½ to ¼ the usual adult dose.

Generic Name

Chlorzoxazone

Brand Names

Paraflex
Parafon Forte DSC
Remular-S

(Also available in generic form)

Combination Products

Chlorzoxazone + Acetaminophen

Flexaphen
Mus-Lax

(Also available in generic form)

Type of Drug

Skeletal muscle relaxant.

Prescribed for

Relief of pain and spasm of muscular conditions (including strains, sprains, lower back pain, or muscle bruises).

General Information

Chlorzoxazone is one of several drugs used to treat pain associated with muscle aches, strains, or a bad back. It gives only temporary relief, and is not a substitute for other types of therapy (such as rest, surgery, or physical therapy).

Chlorzoxazone acts primarily at the spinal cord level and on areas of the brain, acting as a mild sedative. This results in fewer muscle spasms, less pain, and greater mobility. It does not directly relax tense muscles.

Cautions and Warnings

Do not take Chlorzoxazone if you are **allergic** to it or if you have a condition known as *porphyria* (a hereditary condition characterized by abdominal pain, psychoses, and nervous-system disorders).

People with **poor liver or kidney function** should take this medicine with caution because it is broken down by the liver and passes out of the body in the urine.

Chlorzoxazone may worsen depression or interact with other drugs that cause nervous system depression (see *Drug Interactions*).

On rare occasions, people have abused this drug. People with a history of substance abuse should take it with caution.

Possible Side Effects

▼ Most common: dizziness, drowsiness, and light-headedness.

▼ Less common: headache, stimulation, stomach cramps or pain, diarrhea, constipation, heartburn, nausea, and vomiting.

▼ Rare: stomach or intestinal bleeding (black or tarry stools, vomiting blood or a "coffee-ground"-like material); a rapid drop in white-blood-cell count (fever with or without chills, sores, ulcers, or white spots on the lips or mouth, sore throat); unusual tiredness or weakness; liver inflammation (yellow discoloration of the skin or eyes); allergic reactions (changes in facial color, skin rash, hives, itching, rapid or irregular breathing, difficulty breathing, chest tightness, or wheezing); large hive-like swellings on the face, eyelids, mouth, or tongue; and skin rash.

Drug Interactions

• The depressive effects of Chlorzoxazone may be enhanced by taking it with alcohol, tranquilizers, sleeping pills,
or other nervous-system depressants. Avoid these combinations.

Food Interactions

Take this drug with food if it upsets your stomach. Chlorzoxazone tablets may be crushed and mixed with food.

Usual Dose

Adult: 250 to 750 mg 3 to 4 times per day.
Child: 125 to 500 mg 3 to 4 times per day.
Do not take more medication than is prescribed.

Overdosage

Possible early overdose signs are nausea, vomiting, diarrhea,
drowsiness, dizziness, light-headedness, or headache. Victims may also feel sluggish or sickly and lose the ability to
move their muscles. Breathing may become slow or irregular,
and blood pressure may drop. Contact your doctor immediately or go to a hospital emergency room for treatment.
ALWAYS bring the medicine bottle.

Special Information

Chlorzoxazone can make you drowsy or reduce your concentration, so be extremely careful while driving or operating
hazardous equipment; avoid alcoholic beverages.

A breakdown product of Chlorzoxazone can turn your urine
orange to purple-red: This is not dangerous.

Call your doctor if you develop drowsiness, weakness, an
allergic reaction, breathing difficulty, black or tarry stools,
vomiting of "coffee-ground"-like material, liver problems, or
other severe or bothersome side effects.

If you miss a dose of Chlorzoxazone by more than an hour,
skip the forgotten dose and continue with your regular
schedule. Do not take a double dose.

Special Populations

Pregnancy/Breast-feeding

This drug has not been found to cause birth defects. Nevertheless, pregnant women and those who might become pregnant should not take it without their doctor's approval.

It is not known if Chlorzoxazone passes into breast milk, but it has not caused problems among breast-fed infants. Consider the potential effect on your nursing infant if breast-feeding while taking this medicine.

Seniors

Older adults, especially those with severe liver disease, are more sensitive to the effects of this drug because they retain it in their bodies longer than younger people. Follow your doctor's directions and report any side effects at once.

Generic Name

Cholestyramine Resin

Brand Names

Questran
Questran Light

The information in this drug profile also applies to:

Generic Name: Colestipol

Colestid Granules/Tablets

Type of Drug

Antihyperlipidemic (blood-fat reducer).

Prescribed for

High blood cholesterol, generalized itching associated with bile-duct obstruction (Cholestyramine only), some forms of colitis, Digitalis overdose, and pesticide poisoning.

General Information

This medication reduces blood cholesterol by removing bile acids from the biliary system. Since cholesterol is used by the body to make bile acids, which are necessary for the digestion of dietary fats, the only way the body can continue to digest fats is to make more bile acids from cholesterol, resulting in a lowering of blood-cholesterol levels. These medicines work entirely within the bowel and are never absorbed into the bloodstream. They begin to lower blood-cholesterol levels in 4 to 7 days. Though usually given 3 to 4 times a day, there appears to be no advantage to taking this medicine more often than 2 times a day. The cholesterol-lowering effect of Cholestyramine may be addictive when taken with one of the HMG-CoA inhibitors or Nicotinic Acid.

In some kinds of hyperlipidemia, Colestipol may be more effective in lowering total blood cholesterol than Clofibrate another antihyperlipidemic drug. There are 6 different types of hyperlipidemia. Check with your doctor as to the kind you have and the proper drug treatment for your condition.

Cautions and Warnings

Do not use these medicines if you are **sensitive** to them or if your **bile duct is blocked**. The **powder** form **should not be taken dry.** Doing so can expose you to inhaling some of the powder into your lungs or to clogging the esophagus.

Possible Side Effects

▼ Most common: constipation, which may be severe and result in bowel impaction. Hemorrhoids may be worsened.

▼ Less common: abdominal pain and bloating, bleeding disorders, or black-and-blue marks due to interference with the absorption of vitamin K, a necessary factor in the clotting process. One person developed night-blindness because the medicine interfered with vitamin A absorption into the blood.

▼ Other: belching, gas, nausea, vomiting, diarrhea, heartburn, appetite loss, rashes, irritation of the tongue and anus, osteoporosis, black stools (your stool may have an unusual appearance because of a high fat level), stomach ulcers, dental bleeding, hiccups, a sour taste, pancreas inflammation, ulcer attack, gallbladder attack, itching and rash, backache, muscle and joint pains, arthritis, headache, anxiety, dizziness, fatigue, ringing or buzzing in the ears, fainting, tingling in the hands or feet,

---

Possible Side Effects *(continued)*

blood in the urine, frequent or painful urination, an unusual urine odor, swollen glands, swelling of the arms or legs, and shortness of breath.

Drug Interactions

• These medications interfere with the absorption of virtually all other oral medicines; this effect has been proven for Acetaminophen, Amiodarone, Cephalexin, Chenodiol, Clindamycin, corticosteroids, Iron, Digitalis drugs, Gemfibrozil, Glipizide, Penicillins, Phenobarbital, Phenylbutazone, Piroxicam, Tetracycline, Thiazide diuretics, thyroid drugs, Trimethoprim, Warfarin and other anticoagulant (blood-thinning) medicines, and vitamins A, D, E, and K. Take other medicines at least 1 hour before or 4 to 6 hours after taking Cholestyramine or Colestipol.

Food Interactions

Take these medications before meals. They may be mixed with soda, water, juice, cereal, or pulpy fruits (such as applesauce or crushed pineapple). Cholestyramine bars should be thoroughly chewed and taken with plenty of fluids.

Usual Dose

Cholestyramine Resin
4 grams (1 packet) taken 1 to 6 times per day.

Colestipol
5 to 30 grams (1 to 6 packets) per day in 2 to 4 divided doses.

Overdosage

The most severe effect of overdosage with either of these medicines is bowel impaction. Take the overdose victim to a hospital emergency room for evaluation and treatment. ALWAYS bring the medicine container with you.

Special Information

Do not swallow the granules or powder in their dry form.

Prepare each packet of powder by mixing it with a soup, cereal, or pulpy fruit. Alternatively, the powder may be added to a glass of 6 ounces or more of a liquid, such as a carbonated beverage. Some of the drug may stick to the sides of the glass; this should be rinsed with liquid and drunk.

Constipation, stomach gas, nausea, and heartburn may occur and then disappear with continued use of this medication. Call your doctor if these side effects continue or if you develop unusual problems, such as bleeding from the gums or rectum.

If you miss a dose, skip it and continue on your regular schedule. Do not take a double dose.

Special Populations

Pregnancy/Breast-feeding

Cholestyramine and Colestipol are not absorbed into the blood and will not directly affect a developing fetus. However, they can prevent the absorption of some vitamins and other nutrients essential to fetal development, even when you take a prenatal vitamin supplement.

Because these medicines are not absorbed into the blood, they will not affect a nursing infant. However, they reduce the amounts of some vitamins and other nutrients absorbed, making your milk less nutritious. Nursing mothers who must take these medicines should bottle-feed their babies.

Seniors

Older adults are more likely to suffer side effects from these medications, especially those relating to the bowel.

Generic Name

Ciclopirox Olamine

Brand Name

Loprox Cream/Lotion

Type of Drug

Antifungal.

Prescribed for

Fungal and yeast infections of the skin, including athlete's foot and candidiasis.

General Information

Ciclopirox slows the growth of a wide variety of fungus organisms and yeasts, and kills many others. The drug penetrates the skin very well and is present in levels sufficient to kill or inhibit most fungus organisms. In addition, it penetrates the hair, hair follicles, and skin sweat glands.

Cautions and Warnings

Do not use this product if you are **allergic** to it.

Possible Side Effects

▼ Common: burning, itching, and stinging at the application site.

Usual Dose

Apply enough of the cream or lotion to cover affected areas and massage it into the skin twice a day.

Overdosage

If this drug is accidentally swallowed, the victim may be nauseated and have an upset stomach. Little is known about Ciclopirox overdose; you should call your local poison control center or hospital for more information.

Drug and Food Interactions

None known.

Special Information

Clean the affected areas before applying Ciclopirox, unless otherwise directed by your doctor.

This product is quite effective and can be expected to relieve symptoms within the first week of use. Follow your doctor's directions for the complete 2- to 4-week course of treatment to gain maximum benefit from this product. Stopping it too soon may not completely eliminate the fungus and can lead to a relapse.

Call your doctor if the affected area burns, stings, or becomes red after you use this product. Also, notify your doctor if your symptoms don't clear up after 4 weeks of treatment, because it is unlikely that after that length of treatment the cream will be effective at all.

If you forget a dose of Ciclopirox, apply it as soon as you remember. Do not apply more than prescribed to make up for the missed dose.

Special Populations

Pregnancy/Breast-feeding
Ciclopirox may pass into the developing fetus in very small amounts. However, there is no proof that it causes damage to the fetus. When the drug was given by mouth to animals in doses 10 times the amount normally applied to the skin, it was found to be nontoxic to the fetuses.

Ciclopirox is not known to pass into breast milk. As with all drugs, caution should be exercised when using Ciclopirox during pregnancy and while breast-feeding.

Seniors
Older adults may use this drug without special restriction.

Generic Name
Cimetidine

Brand Name
Tagamet
Tagamet HB (nonprescription form)

(Also available in generic form)

Type of Drug
Histamine H_2 antagonist.

Prescribed for
Ulcers of the stomach and upper intestine (duodenum). It is

also prescribed for upset stomach, gastroesophageal reflux disease (GERD), benign stomach ulcers, bleeding in the stomach and upper intestines, colorectal cancer, prevention of stress ulcers, hyperparathyroidism, fungal infections of the hair and scalp, herpes virus infection, excessive hairiness in women, chronic itching of unknown cause, skin reactions, warts, Acetaminophen overdose, and other conditions characterized by the production of large amounts of gastric fluids. Surgeons may prescribe Cimetidine for a surgical procedure when it is desirable for the production of stomach acid to be stopped completely.

The nonprescription version of Cimetidine is sold for heartburn, indigestion, and upset stomach.

General Information

Cimetidine, approved in 1977, was the first histamine H_2 antagonist in the United States. It works against ulcers and other gastrointestinal conditions by actually turning off the system that produces stomach acid and other secretions.

Cimetidine is effective in treating the symptoms of ulcer and preventing complications of the disease. However, since all of the histamine H_2 antagonists work in the exact same way, it is doubtful that an ulcer that does not respond to one will be effectively treated by another. Histamine H_2 antagonists differ only in their potency. Cimetidine is the least potent, with 1000 mg roughly equal to 300 mg of Nizatidine and Ranitidine or 40 mg of Famotidine. The ulcer healing rates of all of these drugs are roughly equivalent, as is the chance of drug side effects with each.

Cautions and Warnings

Do not take Cimetidine if you have had an **allergic** reaction to it or to another histamine H_2 antagonist. Cimetidine has a mild antiandrogen effect. This is probably the reason why some people experience **painful, swollen breasts** after taking this medicine for a month or more.

Caution must be exercised by people with **kidney or liver disease** because Cimetidine is broken down in the liver and passes out of the body through the kidneys.

A positive response to this medicine **does not preclude the chance of stomach cancer,** which can have similar symptoms. Make sure your doctor screens for possible malignancy.

Confusion, agitation, psychosis, hallucinations, depression, anxiety, and **disorientation** can occur, mostly in very ill people. If this happens, it usually does so within 2 or 3 days after starting on Cimetidine and stops 3 to 4 days after stopping the medicine. Call your doctor if this happens.

Possible Side Effects

Most people taking Cimetidine do not experience serious drug side effects.

▼ Most common: mild diarrhea, dizziness, skin rash, painful breast swelling, nausea and vomiting, headache, confusion, drowsiness, hallucinations, and male impotence.

▼ Less common: liver inflammation, a peeling or a red and swollen rash, difficulty breathing, tingling in the hands or feet, delirious feelings, and oozing fluid from the nipples.

▼ Rare: Cimetidine can affect white blood cells or blood platelets. Some symptoms of these effects are unusual bleeding or bruising, unusual tiredness, and weakness. Other rare side effects are inflammation of the pancreas, hair loss (reversible), abnormal heart rhythms, heart attacks, muscle or joint pains (reversible), and reversible drug reactions.

Drug Interactions

• The effects of Cimetidine may be reduced if it is taken with an antacid. This minor interaction may be avoided by separating Cimetidine from antacid doses by about 3 hours. Other drugs that can reduce the absorption of Cimetidine are anticholinergic drugs (drugs that counteract the effect of acetycholine, including Trihexyphenidyl Hydrochloride, Oxybutynin, and Benztropine Mesylate) and Metoclopramide.

• Cigarette smoking has also been shown to reverse the ulcer healing effect of Cimetidine.

• Cimetidine may increase the effects of a variety of drugs by preventing their breakdown or elimination from the body, possibly leading to drug toxicity. These drugs include alcohol, Aminophylline, oral antidiabetes drugs, benzodiazepine tranquilizers and sleeping pills (except Lorazepam, Oxazepam, and Temazepam), caffeine, calcium-channel-blocking drugs, Carbamazepine, Carmustine, Chloroquine, Flecainide, Fluorouracil, Labetalol, Lidocaine, Metoprolol, Metronidazole, Moricizine, Mexiletine, narcotic pain-relieving drugs, Ondansetron, Pentoxifylline, Phenytoin, Procainamide, Propafenone, Propranolol, Quinine, Quinidine, Tacrine, Theophylline drugs (except Dyphylline), Triamterene, tricyclic antidepressants, Valproic Acid, and Warfarin (a blood-thinning drug).

• Drugs whose absorption may be decreased by Cimetidine are Iron, Indomethacin, Fluconazole, Ketoconazole, and the Tetracycline antibiotics.

• Enteric-coated tablets should not be taken with Cimetidine. The change in stomach acidity will cause the tablets to disintegrate prematurely in the stomach.

• The effects of Digoxin and Tocainide may decrease while you are taking Cimetidine.

Food Interactions

Cimetidine may be taken without regard to food or meals.

Usual Dose

Adult: 400 to 800 mg at bedtime; 300 mg 4 times per day with meals and at bedtime; or 400 mg twice a day. For GERD, the usual dose is 400 mg 4 times per day. Do not exceed 2400 mg per day.

Seniors and those with impaired kidney function: smaller doses may be as effective for seniors or patients with impaired kidney function.

Nonprescription dose: 2 tablets (100 mg each) with water; no more than 8 pills a day.

Overdosage

Cimetidine overdose victims usually show exaggerated side-effect symptoms, but little else is known. Two deaths were reported in people who supposedly took 40,000 mg (40 grams) of Cimetidine at once. Your local poison control center may advise giving the victim Syrup of Ipecac (available at any pharmacy) to cause vomiting, which will hopefully remove any remaining drug from the stomach. Victims who have definite symptoms should be taken to a hospital emergency room for observation and possible treatment. ALWAYS bring the prescription bottle.

Special Information

You must take this medicine exactly as directed, and follow your doctor's instructions for diet and other treatments in order to get the maximum benefit from it.

Cigarettes are known to be associated with stomach ulcers and will reverse the effect of Cimetidine on stomach acid.

Call your doctor at once if any unusual side effects develop, especially unusual bleeding or bruising, unusual tiredness, diarrhea, dizziness, rash, or hallucinations. Black, tarry stools or vomiting "coffee-ground"-like material may indicate your ulcer is bleeding.

If you miss a dose of Cimetidine, take it as soon as possible. If it is almost time for your next dose, skip the missed dose and go back to your usual dose schedule. Do not take a double dose.

Special Populations

Pregnancy/Breast-feeding

Studies with laboratory animals have revealed no fetal damage, though Cimetidine does pass into the fetal blood. Cimetidine's potential risk must be carefully weighed against any benefit it might produce.

Large amounts of Cimetidine pass into breast milk. Nursing mothers who must take it should bottle-feed their babies.

Seniors

Seniors respond well to Cimetidine, but may need less medication to achieve the desired response, since the drug is eliminated through the kidneys and kidney function tends to decline with age. Older adults may be more susceptible to some side effects of this drug, especially confusion and other nervous system effects (see *Cautions and Warnings*).

Generic Name

Cinoxacin

Brand Name

Cinobac

(Also available in generic form)

Type of Drug

Urinary anti-infective.

Prescribed for

Urinary tract infections in adults caused by susceptible microorganisms.

General Information

Cinoxacin treats urinary infections by interfering with DNA reproduction in those bacteria.

Cautions and Warnings

Do not take Cinoxacin if you have had an **allergic** reaction to it or another quinolone in the past, or if you have had a reaction to related medications like Nalidixic Acid. **Severe, possibly fatal, allergic reactions** can occur **even after the very first dose,** including cardiovascular collapse, loss of consciousness, tingling, swelling of the face or throat, breathing difficulty, itching, or rash. Stop taking the drug if any of these happen and seek medical help at once.

This drug should **not be used by infants or children,** because of the possibility that it could produce joint and/or cartilage erosion, affecting their development.

Cinoxacin should be used with caution by anyone who has had **seizures or another nervous system problem** that leads to seizures. A few people taking anti-infectives similar to Cinoxacin have experienced convulsions, stimulation, tremors, restlessness, confusion, or hallucinations. Report anything unusual to your doctor.

Possible Side Effects

▼ Most common: nausea, headache, dizziness, rash, itching, and redness.

▼ Less common: vomiting, appetite loss, abdominal cramps, diarrhea, altered taste sensations, burning in the area surrounding the rectum, sleeplessness, confusion, drowsiness, tingling sensations, blurred vision, ringing or buzzing in the ears, sensitivity to the sun or bright light, and drug reactions. Cinoxacin may also affect some laboratory tests that reflect liver and kidney function.

Drug Interactions

• Probenecid blocks the excretion of Cinoxacin through the kidneys, causing the drug to accumulate in the body.

Food Interactions

Food slows the rate at which Cinoxacin is absorbed into the bloodstream, but does not affect the total amount absorbed. Cinoxacin may be taken without regard to food or meals.

Usual Dose

1000 mg a day, divided into 2 or 4 doses, for 1 or 2 weeks. For preventive treatment: 250 mg at bedtime. People with reduced kidney function take lower dosages.

Overdosage

Symptoms are appetite loss, nausea, vomiting, stomach upset, and diarrhea. Stomach upset and diarrhea worsen with increased dose. Headache, dizziness, sensitivity to bright light, ringing or buzzing in the ears, and a tingling sensation have also occurred. Other symptoms may be related to another condition or be due to a drug reaction, not an overdose. Take the victim to a hospital emergency room for treatment. ALWAYS bring the prescription bottle.

Special Information

Take each dose with a full glass of water, and drink a total of 8 glasses a day while you are taking this medicine.

Call your doctor if you become dizzy while taking Cinoxacin. This dizziness can interfere with driving or any other activity that requires concentration. Your eyes may be more sensitive to bright light, which is a normal side effect of Cinoxacin use. Wearing sunglasses will help you tolerate bright light.

If you take Cinoxacin twice per day and forget a dose, take it as soon as you remember. If it is almost time for your next dose, take one dose as soon as you remember and another in 5 or 6 hours, then go back to your regular schedule.

If you take Cinoxacin 3 or 4 times per day and forget a dose, take it as soon as you remember. If it is almost time for your next dose, take one dose right away and another in 3 or 4 hours, then go back to your regular schedule.

Special Populations

Pregnancy/Breast-feeding

Cinoxacin should not be used by pregnant women, or women who might become pregnant, because of the possibility that it could affect joint and cartilage development in the fetus.

It is not known if Cinoxacin passes into breast milk. Nursing mothers should bottle-feed because this drug may cause joint and connective tissue changes in the nursing infant.

Seniors

Seniors are likely to require a reduced dose of Cinoxacin due to their normal tendency toward reduced kidney function.

Cipro

see *Ciprofloxacin*, page 210

Generic Name

Ciprofloxacin

Brand Names

Ciloxan Eyedrops
Cipro Tablets*

(*Also available in generic form)

Type of Drug

Fluoroquinolone anti-infective.

Prescribed for

Lower respiratory infections, skin infections, bone and joint infections, treating and preventing urinary tract infections, infectious diarrhea, lung infections in people with cystic fibrosis, bronchitis, pneumonia, prostate infection, and traveler's diarrhea. Ciprofloxacin does not work against the common cold, flu, or other viral infections.

General Information

The fluoroquinolone antibacterials are widely used and work against many organisms that traditional antibiotic treatments have trouble killing. These medications are chemically related to an older antibacterial called *Nalidixic Acid* but work better than that drug against urinary tract infections. Ciprofloxacin, the first of the fluoroquinolones, is used to treat a wide variety of infections all over the body. It is also available as eyedrops to treat ocular infections.

Cautions and Warnings

Do not take Ciprofloxacin if you have had an **allergic** reaction to it or another fluoroquinolone in the past, or if you have had a reaction to related medications, like Nalidixic Acid. **Severe,** possibly fatal, **allergic reactions** can occur **even after the very first dose.** Reactions include cardiovascular collapse, loss of consciousness, tingling, swelling of the face or throat, breathing difficulty, itching, or rash. Stop taking the drug if any of these happen, and seek medical help at once.

Dosage must be adjusted in the presence of **kidney failure.**

Ciprofloxacin may cause **increased pressure** on parts of the brain, leading to **convulsions** and **psychotic reactions.** Other possible adverse effects include **tremors, restlessness, light-headedness, confusion,** and **hallucinations.** Ciprofloxacin should be used with caution in people with **seizure disorders** or other conditions of the nervous system.

People taking fluoroquinolone medicines can be **unusually sensitive to direct or indirect sunlight** (photosensitivity). Avoid the sun while taking this drug and for several days following therapy, *even if you are using a sunscreen!*

As with any other anti-infective, people taking Ciprofloxacin may develop **colitis** that could range from mild to very serious. See your doctor if you develop diarrhea or cramps while taking this drug.

Prolonged use of Ciprofloxacin can lead to **fungal overgrowth**. Follow your doctor's directions exactly.

Possible Side Effects

▼ Most common: nausea, vomiting, and diarrhea.

▼ Common: abdominal pain, headache, and liver inflammation.

▼ Rare: dry mouth, mouth pain, swallowing difficulty, upset stomach, constipation, gas, colitis, stomach bleeding, yellowing of the skin or whites of the eyes, fatigue, feelings of ill health, depression, sleeplessness, seizures, confusion, restlessness, psychotic reactions, tingling in the hands or feet, irritability, tremors, weakness, worsening of myasthenia gravis, appetite loss, flushing, hallucinations, nightmares, sensitivity to the sun, skin peeling, drug reactions, visual disturbances, eye pain, ringing or buzzing in the ears, uncontrolled rolling of the eyes, hearing loss, vaginal infection, high blood pressure, heart palpitations, angina pains, heart attack, blood clots in the lung or brain, general dizziness or dizziness when rising from a sitting or lying position, fainting, chills, fever, kidney damage, bronchial spasms, breathing difficulty, nosebleeds, vomiting blood, hiccups, swelling of the throat, fluid in the lungs, bad taste in the mouth, oral infections, and swelling in the ankles, legs, or arms.

Drug Interactions

• Antacids, Didanosine, Iron supplements, Sucralfate, and Zinc will decrease the amount of Ciprofloxacin absorbed into the bloodstream. If you must take any of these products, separate them from your Ciprofloxacin dosage by at least 2 hours.

• Probenecid cuts the amount of Ciprofloxacin released through your kidneys by half, and may increase the chance of drug side effects. Cimetidine may also increase blood levels of Ciprofloxacin.

• Ciprofloxacin may increase the effect of oral anticoagulant drugs. Your anticoagulant dose may have to be reduced.

• Ciprofloxacin may increase the toxic effects of Cyclosporine (for organ transplants) on your kidneys.

• Ciprofloxacin may reduce the rate at which Theophylline is released from your body, increasing Theophylline blood levels and the chance for Theophylline-related side effects.

• Azlocillin may decrease the amount of Ciprofloxacin released through your kidneys, and may increase the chance of drug side effects.

• Ciprofloxacin decreases the total body clearance of caffeine, possibly increasing its effect on your system.

• Anticancer drugs may decrease the amount of Ciprofloxacin in your blood.

• Nitrofurantoin may antagonize Ciprofloxacin's antibacterial effects. Do not take these drugs together.

• Ciprofloxacin may reduce blood levels of Phenytoin (for seizures), requiring alteration of your daily dose.

Food Interactions

Food slows the rate at which Ciprofloxacin is absorbed into the bloodstream but does not affect the total amount absorbed. Dairy products interfere with the absorption of Ciprofloxacin and should be avoided. Take this drug at least 1 hour before or 2 hours after meals.

Usual Dose

Tablets
500 to 1500 mg a day. Dosage is adjusted in the presence of kidney failure.

Eyedrops
1 or 2 drops in the affected eye several times per day as prescribed.

Overdosage

One person experienced kidney failure when he took an overdose of Ciprofloxacin. Generally, the symptoms of Ciprofloxacin overdose are the same as those found under *Possible Side Effects*. Consult the local poison control center or hospital emergency room for specific instructions. You may be asked to induce vomiting with Syrup of Ipecac (available at any pharmacy) to remove excess medication from the victim's stomach. Overdose victims should be taken to a hospital emergency room for treatment. ALWAYS bring the medicine bottle with you.

Special Information

Take each dose with a full glass of water. Be sure to drink at least 8 glasses of water a day while taking this medicine to promote removal of the drug from your system and to help avoid side effects.

If you are taking an Antacid, Didanosine, Sucralfate, or an Iron or Zinc supplement while taking Ciprofloxacin, be sure to separate the doses by at least 2 hours to avoid a drug interaction.

Drug sensitivity reactions can develop even after only one dose of this medicine! Stop taking it and get immediate medical attention if you faint or if you develop itching, rash, facial swelling, difficulty breathing, convulsions, depression, visual disturbances, dizziness, headache, light-headedness, or any sign of a drug reaction.

Colitis can be caused by any anti-infective medication. If diarrhea develops after taking Ciprofloxacin, call your doctor at once.

Avoid excessive sunlight or exposure to a sunlamp while taking Ciprofloxacin. Call your doctor if you become unusually sensitive to the sun.

Follow your doctor's directions exactly. Do not stop taking it even if you begin to feel better after a few days, unless directed to do so by your doctor.

Since Ciprofloxacin can cause visual changes, dizziness, drowsiness, or light-headedness, it can affect your ability to drive a car or do other things requiring full concentration.

If you forget to take a dose of Ciprofloxacin (including the eyedrops), take it as soon as you remember. If it is almost time for your next dose, skip the missed dose and continue with your regular schedule. Do not take a double dose.

To administer eyedrops, lie down or tilt your head back. Hold the dropper above your eye, gently squeeze your lower lid to make a small pouch, and drop the medicine inside while looking up. Release the lower lid and keep your eye open. Don't blink for about 40 seconds. Press gently on the bridge of your nose at the inside corner of your eye for about a minute to help circulate the medicine around your eye. To avoid infection, don't touch the dropper tip to your finger or eyelid. Wait 5 minutes before using another eyedrop or ointment.

Call your doctor at once if your eyes sting, itch, burn, swell, or become red or irritated, if pain gets worse, or if you have trouble seeing.

Special Populations

Pregnancy/Breast-feeding

Pregnant women should not take Ciprofloxacin unless its benefits clearly outweigh its risks. Animal studies have shown that Ciprofloxacin may reduce your chances for a successful pregnancy or damage a developing fetus.

Nursing infants swallow small amounts of Ciprofloxacin through breast milk. Nursing mothers who must take Ciprofloxacin should bottle-feed their babies. Be sure your doctor knows if you are breast-feeding.

Seniors

Studies in healthy seniors showed that Ciprofloxacin is released from their bodies more slowly because of natural decreases in kidney function. Dosage reductions may be made according to kidney function.

Older adults may use Ciprofloxacin eyedrops without special restriction. Some seniors may have weaker eyelid muscles; this creates a small reservoir for the eyedrops, which may actually increase the drug's effect by keeping it in contact with their eyes for a longer period. Your dosage may need to be adjusted.

Generic Name

Cisapride

Brand Name

Propulsid Tablets/Suspension

Type of Drug

Gastrointestinal stimulant.

Prescribed for

Nighttime heartburn caused by gastroesophageal reflux disease (GERD).

General Information

Cisapride restores the normal ability of the stomach and intestines to move food through the gastrointestinal (GI) tract. It does this by stimulating the release of the hormone *acetylcholine* at key nerve endings throughout the GI tract. By stimulating movement of the GI tract, it increases pressure in the lower esophagus and helps to pull through any stomach contents that might have refluxed (come back up into the lower esophagus without vomiting). People with GERD have about half the normal lower esophageal pressure; Cisapride restores that pressure to normal levels. Cisapride increases the rate of speed at which food moves through the stomach. This is helpful in treating nighttime heartburn caused by GERD. Cisapride has no consistent effect on daytime heartburn, regurgitation (food from the stomach coming back up to the mouth without vomiting), or changes in the esophagus, and it does not work as an antacid. Cisapride is related to Metoclopramide, but is more specific and targeted in its effects.

Cautions and Warnings

Cisapride should not be taken by people with **stomach or intestinal bleeding, bowel obstruction or perforation,** or other conditions where increasing GI tract activity could be harmful.

Rare cases of serious **abnormal heart rhythms** have occurred in people taking this medicine.

Animal studies indicate that high doses of Cisapride may **interfere with female fertility.**

Possible Side Effects

▼ Most common: headache, diarrhea, abdominal pain, nausea, constipation, and runny nose.

▼ Less common: stomach upset, stomach gas, sinus inflammation, upper respiratory infections, coughing,

---

Possible Side Effects *(continued)*

pains, fever, urinary infections, frequent urination, sleep-lessness, anxiety, nervousness, rash, itching, viral infections, joint pains, vision changes, and vaginal irritation.

▼ Rare: dizziness, vomiting, sore throat, chest pain, back pain, depression, dehydration, muscle aches, dry mouth, tiredness, heart palpitations, migraines, tremors, swelling in the feet or legs, seizures, uncontrollable muscle movements, rapid heartbeat, liver inflammation, hepatitis, and reduced counts of white blood cells and blood platelets.

Drug Interactions

• Mixing Cisapride with Ketoconazole (an antifungal) results in high blood levels of Cisapride and serious cardiac abnormalities. Itraconazole, Miconazole (intravenous), and Troleandomycin may also do this.

• Cisapride's stimulating effect on the GI tract interferes with the absorption of most oral drug products into the bloodstream by moving them through the system before they can be adequately absorbed. Your doctor should check to be sure that any other medicines you are taking are not affected.

• When Cimetidine and Cisapride are taken together, the amount of both drugs absorbed into the blood is increased. Cisapride also increases the amount of Ranitidine absorbed.

• Cisapride may increase the effects of anticoagulant (blood-thinning) drugs. Your anticoagulant dose may need to be adjusted, or you may have to stop taking Cisapride.

• Anticholinergic drugs (including Atropine, Benztropine, Donnatal, Oxybutynin, and Trihexyphenidyl) interfere with the effects of Cisapride.

Food Interactions

Take this drug 15 minutes before meals and at bedtime.

Usual Dose

40 to 80 mg a day.

Overdosage

Symptoms of overdosage include stomach rumbling, stomach gas, and frequent stools and frequent urination. Other possible symptoms are droopy eyelids, tremors, convulsions, breathing difficulty, catatonic reactions, loss of muscle tone, and diarrhea. Doses as low as 80 mg per pound of body weight have been lethal in animal studies. Overdose victims should be taken to a hospital emergency room. ALWAYS bring the medicine bottle.

Special Information

Take Cisapride with care if you take a benzodiazepine tranquilizer or sleeping medicine; avoid alcoholic beverages.

Call your doctor if any side effects become intolerable, bothersome, or interfere with regular daily activities.

If you forget a dose of Cisapride, take it as soon as you remember, as long as it is before a meal. If it is almost time for the next dose, skip the missed dose and continue with your regular schedule. Do not take a double dose.

Special Populations

Pregnancy/Breast-feeding

Animal studies have indicated that Cisapride may be harmful to a developing fetus. There are no conclusive studies of this drug in people, but women who are or who might become pregnant should take Cisapride only after weighing its possible risks and benefits.

Cisapride passes into breast milk in 1/20 the concentration found in the blood. Nursing mothers taking it should observe their nursing infants for possible drug-related side effects.

Seniors

After taking the same dose as other adults, seniors, especially those with kidney or liver disease, have more Cisapride in the bloodstream. Nevertheless, dosage is usually not altered for seniors.

Generic Name

Clarithromycin

Brand Name

Biaxin Tablets/Suspension

Type of Drug

Macrolide antibiotic.

Prescribed for

Mild to moderate infections of the sinus, upper and lower respiratory tract infections and middle-ear infections in children. Clarithromycin is also prescribed in the treatment of some skin and other infections and in some infections associated with AIDS.

General Information

Clarithromycin is a member of the *macrolide* group of antibiotics. These medicines, which also include Erythromycin and Azithromycin, are either bactericidal (they kill the bacteria directly) or bacteriostatic (they slow the bacteria's growth so that the body's natural protective mechanisms can kill them). Whether these drugs are bacteriostatic or bactericidal depends on the organism in question and the amount of antibiotic present in the blood or other body fluid. They are effective against all varieties of organisms, with each of the macrolide antibiotics working against a somewhat different profile of bacteria.

Clarithromycin is rapidly absorbed into the blood and distributed through the bloodstream to all parts of the body. It is gentler on the digestive tract than Erythromycin.

Because the action of this antibiotic depends on its concentration within the invading bacteria, it is imperative that you follow your doctor's directions regarding the spacing of doses as well as the number of days you should continue taking the medication. The effectiveness of this antibiotic can be severely reduced if these instructions are not followed.

Cautions and Warnings

Do not take Clarithromycin if you're **allergic** to it or any of the macrolide antibiotics.

Clarithromycin is primarily eliminated from the body through the liver and kidneys. People with **severe kidney disease** may require dosage adjustments. Liver disease generally does not require dose adjustments.

All antibiotics, including Clarithromycin, have been associated with a particular form of **colitis** (bowel inflammation). **Diarrhea** that begins after you start taking this drug may be an indication of this problem.

Possible Side Effects
___

Most side effects are mild and will go away once you stop taking Clarithromycin.

▼ Most common: nausea, vomiting, upset stomach, taste distortions, stomach cramps, stomach gas, and headache. Colitis may develop after taking Clarithromycin.

Drug Interactions

• Clarithromycin may increase the anticoagulant (blood-thinning) effects of Warfarin in people who take it regularly, especially older adults.

• Clarithromycin may raise blood levels of Carbamazepine, in a manner similar to Erythromycin. People taking this combination should be carefully monitored by their doctors for changes in blood Carbamazepine levels.

• Clarithromycin may raise blood levels of Theophylline, possibly leading to a Theophylline overdose. It can also increase the effects of caffeine, which is chemically related to Theophylline.

• Clarithromycin may increase blood levels of Terfenadine, a nonsedating antihistamine broken down in the liver. This drug interaction may lead to serious cardiac toxicity and should be avoided.

• Clarithromycin may increase blood levels of Digoxin.

• Taking Clarithromycin with Zidovudine (AZT) can reduce the amount of Zidovudine in the blood.

Food Interactions

Clarithromycin can be taken without regard to food or meals.

Usual Dose

Adult: 250 to 500 mg every 12 hours. Dosage must be reduced in people with severe kidney disease.

Child: 3.4 mg per pound of body weight every 12 hours, up to 250 or 500 mg per dose, depending on the offending organism.

Overdosage

Clarithromycin overdose may result in exaggerated side effects, especially nausea, vomiting, stomach cramps, and diarrhea. Call your local poison center or hospital emergency room for more information.

Special Information

Call your doctor if you develop nausea, vomiting, diarrhea, stomach cramps, or severe abdominal pain.

Remember to complete the full course of treatment as prescribed by your doctor, even if you feel perfectly well after only a few days of Clarithromycin.

Because Clarithromycin is taken twice a day, you should take it at the same time each day to help you remember your medicine. But if you forget a dose of oral Clarithromycin, take it as soon as you remember. If it is within 4 hours of your next dose, skip the missing dose and go back to your regular schedule.

Special Populations

Pregnancy/Breast-feeding

Animal studies have shown that Clarithromycin can have an effect on a developing fetus. Pregnant women should take Clarithromycin only if there is no alternative.

Clarithromycin passes into the breast milk of pregnant animals. Other macrolides pass into human milk, but it is not known if this is true of Clarithromycin. Nursing mothers should be cautious about taking this medicine.

Seniors

Older adults should have their Clarithromycin dose adjusted with age-related changes in kidney function. Those with kidney disease should also take a reduced dose.

Claritin

see **Loratadine**, *page 625*

Claritin D

see **Antihistamine-Decongestant Combination Products**,
page 78

Generic Name

Clemastine

Brand Names

Tavist
Tavist-1

Type of Drug

Antihistamine.

Prescribed for

Seasonal allergy; stuffed and runny nose; itchy eyes; scratchy
throat caused by allergies; and other allergic symptoms, such
as rash, itching, or hives.

General Information

Clemastine is distinguished from many of the other antihistamines in that it is somewhat less sedating. It is not less
sedating than Astemizole, Loratadine, or Terfenadine (the
newest and least sedating of this group). Antihistamines,
including Clemastine, generally act by blocking the release of
histamine from the cell at the H_1 histamine receptor site.
Antihistamines work by drying up the secretions of the nose,
throat, and eyes.

Cautions and Warnings

Clemastine should not be taken if you have had an **allergic** reaction to it. People with **asthma** or other deep-breathing problems, **glaucoma** (pressure in the eye), **stomach ulcers,** or other stomach problems should avoid Clemastine because its side effects can aggravate these problems.

Possible Side Effects

▼ Most common: headache, weakness, nervousness, upset stomach, nausea, vomiting, cough, stuffed nose, changes in bowel habits, sore throat, nosebleeds, and dry mouth, nose, or throat.

▼ Less common: drowsiness, hair loss, allergic reactions (itching, rash, breathing difficulty), depression, sleeplessness, menstrual irregularities, muscle aches, sweating, tingling in the hands or feet, frequent urination, visual disturbances.

Drug Interactions

• Taking Clemastine with alcohol, tranquilizers, sleeping pills, or other nervous system depressants can increase the depressant effects of Clemastine. Do not mix these drugs.

• The effects of oral anticoagulant (blood-thinning) drugs may be decreased by Clemastine. Do not take this combination without your doctor's knowledge.

• Monoamine oxidase (MAO) inhibitor drugs (for depression or high blood pressure) may increase the drying and other effects of Clemastine. This combination can also increase urinary difficulty.

Food Interactions

Clemastine is best taken on an empty stomach or at least 1 hour before or 2 hours after food or meals, but may be taken with food if it upsets your stomach.

Usual Dose

Adult and Adolescent (age 12 and older): 1.34 mg 2 times

per day to 2.68 mg 3 times per day. Do not take more than 8.04 mg (7 tablets of Tavist-1 or 3 1/2 tablets of Tavist).

Child (under age 12): not recommended.

Overdosage

Clemastine overdose is likely to cause exaggerated side effects. Overdose victims should be given Syrup of Ipecac (available at any pharmacy) to induce vomiting, and then taken to a hospital emergency room for treatment. ALWAYS bring the medicine bottle with you.

Special Information

Clemastine can make it difficult for you to concentrate and perform complex tasks like driving a car. Be sure to report any unusual side effects to your doctor.

If you forget to take a dose of Clemastine, take it as soon as you remember. If it is almost time for your next dose, skip the forgotten one and continue with your regular schedule. Do not take a double dose.

Special Populations

Pregnancy/Breast-feeding

Antihistamines have not been proven to be a cause of birth defects. Regardless, if you are pregnant, do not take any antihistamine, including Clemastine, without your doctor's knowledge. This is especially important during the last 3 months of your pregnancy, since premature babies and newborns can have severe reactions to antihistamines.

Small amounts of this medicine pass into breast milk and can affect a nursing infant. Nursing mothers should not take Clemastine.

Seniors

Seniors are more sensitive to Clemastine side effects such as confusion; difficult or painful urination; dizziness; drowsiness; feeling faint; dry mouth, nose, or throat; nightmares or excitement; nervousness; restlessness; or irritability.

Generic Name

Clindamycin

Brand Names

Cleocin Hydrochloride Capsules*
Cleocin T Topical Gel/Lotion/Solution
Cleocin Vaginal Cream

(*Also available in generic form)

Type of Drug

Antibiotic.

Prescribed for

Bacterial infections that are found to be susceptible to this drug. Clindamycin vaginal cream is used to treat bacterial vaginosis. Topical Clindamycin is used to treat acne and rosacea, a skin condition.

General Information

Clindamycin is one of the few oral drugs that is effective against anaerobic organisms (bacteria that grow only in the absence of oxygen and are frequently found in infected wounds, lung abscesses, abdominal infections, and infections of the female genital tract). It is also effective against the organisms usually treated by Penicillin or Erythromycin.

Clindamycin may be useful for treating certain skin or soft tissue infections where susceptible organisms are present. It kills bacteria commonly found to be a cause of acne. Another topical antimicrobial, Azelaic Acid (Azelex Cream) works on these bacteria and also normalizes skin processes that can worsen acne.

Cautions and Warnings

Do not take Clindamycin if you are **allergic** to it or Lincomycin (another antibiotic).

Clindamycin can cause a severe intestinal irritation called *colitis*, **which can be fatal.** Signs of colitis are diarrhea, bloody diarrhea, and abdominal cramps. This can occur with **any form of this drug,** including products applied to the skin and the vaginal cream. Because of this, Clindamycin should be **reserved for serious infections** due to organisms known to be affected by it. It should not be used for treatment of the common cold or other moderate infections, or for infections that can be successfully treated with other drugs.

Clindamycin should be used with caution if you have **kidney or liver disease.**

Possible Side Effects

▼ Most common: stomach pain, nausea, vomiting, diarrhea (in up to 30 percent of people who take this drug) and pain when swallowing (oral); skin dryness, redness, burning, peeling, oiliness/oily skin, and itching (topical); cervicitis, vaginitis, and irritation (vaginal).

▼ Less common: itching, rash, or more serious signs of drug sensitivity (such as difficulty in breathing, yellowing of the skin or the eyes), colitis (severe and persistent—possibly bloody—diarrhea, severe abdominal cramps), occasional effects on components of the blood, and joint pain (oral); diarrhea, pains, colitis, and GI upset (topical); nausea, vomiting, diarrhea, constipation, abdominal pain, dizziness, headache, and fainting (vaginal).

Drug Interactions

• Clindamycin and Erythromycin may antagonize each other; these drugs should not be taken together.
• The absorption of Clindamycin capsules into the bloodstream is delayed by Kaolin-Pectin Suspension (for diarrhea).

Food Interactions

Take the oral medication with a full glass of water or food to prevent irritation of the stomach or intestine.

Usual Dose

Capsules
  Adult: 150 to 450 mg every 6 hours.
  Child: 4 to 11 mg per pound of body weight per day in divided doses. No child should be given less than 37.5 mg 3 times per day, regardless of weight.

Topical Lotion
Apply enough to cover the affected area(s) lightly twice a day.

Vaginal Cream
Insert one applicatorful at bedtime for 7 consecutive days.

Special Information

Unsupervised use of Clindamycin can lead to secondary infections from susceptible organisms such as fungi. As with any antibiotic treatment, take this drug for the full course of therapy as indicated by your physician.

If you develop severe diarrhea or abdominal pains, call your doctor at once.

Women using the vaginal cream should refrain from vaginal intercourse until the course of treatment is complete.

If you miss an oral dose of Clindamycin, take it as soon as possible. If it is almost time for your next dose, double that dose and go back to your regular dose schedule.

Special Populations

Pregnancy/Breast-feeding
This drug crosses into fetal blood circulation but has not been found to cause birth defects. When the drug is considered essential by your doctor, its potential benefits must be carefully weighed against its risks.

Clindamycin passes into breast milk but has caused no problems among breast-fed infants. You should consider bottle-feeding your baby if taking Clindamycin by mouth.

Seniors
Older adults with other illnesses may be unable to tolerate diarrhea and other Clindamycin side effects. Be sure to report any Clindamycin complications at once.

Generic Name

Clofibrate

Brand Name

Atromid-S

(Also available in generic form)

Type of Drug

Antihyperlipidemic (blood-fat reducer).

Prescribed for

Reduction of high blood levels of triglycerides. Clofibrate is also used to lower cholesterol and LDL cholesterol, but it is less predictable and effective than other cholesterol-lowering medicines. It is usually prescribed for people whose blood fats remain high despite changes in diet, weight control, and exercise. Clofibrate has also been used to treat a condition known as *diabetes insipidus*; however, this condition is usually treated with other medicines.

General Information

Although we don't know exactly how Clofibrate works, we do know that it works on both blood cholesterol and triglycerides by interfering with the natural systems that make those blood fats and by increasing the rate at which they are removed from the body. Clofibrate is generally much more effective in reducing blood triglycerides than cholesterol.

Lower blood-fat levels are considered beneficial in reducing the chances of developing heart disease. But people with high cholesterol and low triglycerides should not take Clofibrate because it is most effective in lowering triglycerides.

Clofibrate is only part of the therapy for high blood-fat levels. Diet and weight control are also very important. This medicine is not a substitute for exercise or dietary restrictions that have been prescribed by your doctor.

Cautions and Warnings

Clofibrate causes **liver cancer in rats.** It should be used with caution if you are **allergic** to the drug or if you have **cirrhosis of the liver, heart disease, gallstones** (Clofibrate users have twice the risk of developing gallstones as people who don't take this drug!), **liver disease, an underactive thyroid,** or **stomach ulcer.** People with **kidney disease** may take Clofibrate as long as their daily dosage is calibrated for their degree of kidney function loss.

Clofibrate does not reduce the number of **fatal heart attacks.** A 1978 study suggested that taking Clofibrate regularly for many years increases the chances of dying from noncardiac causes, but this has not been confirmed by more recent work. Another study showed an increase in certain side effects among people taking Clofibrate, including abnormal heart rhythms and intermittent leg pains due to blood-vessel spasm. Clofibrate should be used only by people whose other efforts to solve their triglyceride or cholesterol problems have not worked.

Possible Side Effects

▼ Most common: nausea.

▼ Less common: vomiting, nausea, loose stools, stomach upset, gas, abdominal pain, liver enlargement, gastric irritation, mouth sores, headache, dizziness, tiredness, cramped muscles, aching and weakness, rash, itching, brittle hair or hair loss, abnormal heart rhythms, blood clots in the lungs or veins, gallstones (especially in people who have taken Clofibrate for a long time), decreased sex drive, and sexual impotence.

If you suffer from angina pectoris (a specific type of chest pain), Clofibrate may increase or decrease this pain. It may cause you to produce smaller amounts of urine than usual, and it has been associated with blood in the urine, tiredness, weakness, drowsiness, and mildly increased appetite and weight gain. Some experts claim that Clofibrate causes stomach ulcers, stomach bleeding, arthritis-like symptoms, uncontrollable muscle spasms, increased perspiration, blurred vision, breast enlargement, and some effects on the blood.

Drug Interactions

• If you are taking an anticoagulant (blood-thinner) and get a new prescription for Clofibrate, your anticoagulant dose may have to be reduced by up to one-half. It is absolutely essential that your doctor knows you are taking both drugs so that the proper dose adjustments can be made.

• Taking Clofibrate with an anticholesterol drug like Lovastatin or Pravastatin can result in a reaction that leads to some skeletal muscle destruction.

• The effect of Chenodiol may be decreased when it is taken together with Clofibrate.

• Clofibrate may increase the effect of oral antidiabetics and can increase the effects of any drug used to treat diabetes insipidus, including Carbamazepine, Chlorpropamide, Desmopressin, some diuretics, and hormone replacement products.

• Contraceptive drugs can interfere with the effectiveness of Clofibrate.

• Probenecid can increase the effectiveness and side effects of Clofibrate.

• Rifampin can increase the rate at which Clofibrate is broken down in the liver, reducing its effectiveness.

• Clofibrate can interfere with a number of blood tests. Make sure your doctor knows you are taking the drug before any blood tests are done.

Food Interactions

Take this drug with food or milk to prevent stomach upset.

Usual Dose

2000 mg per day.

Overdosage

Overdose symptoms are most likely to be exaggerated drug side effects. Take the overdose victim to a hospital emergency room. ALWAYS bring the medicine bottle with you.

Special Information

Call your doctor if you develop chest pains, difficulty breathing, abnormal heart rates, severe stomach pains (with nausea and vomiting), fever and chills, sore throat, blood in the urine, swelling of the legs, weight gain, blood in the urine, or any change in urinary habits, or if other side effects become intolerable.

Follow your diet; limit your intake of alcoholic beverages.

Clofibrate should be stored at room temperature in a dry place (not in a bathroom medicine cabinet) to protect this drug's soft gelatin covering.

Regular visits to your doctor are necessary while taking Clofibrate to be sure the drug is still working and to be screened with blood counts and liver function tests, which may uncover possible drug side effects.

If you miss a dose, take it as soon as possible. If it is almost time for your next dose, skip the missed dose and go back to your regular dose schedule. Do not take a double dose.

Special Populations

Pregnancy/Breast-feeding

Pregnant women should not take Clofibrate because large amounts of this drug pass into the developing fetus, which cannot break it down. If you are planning to become pregnant, stop taking Clofibrate several months before trying to conceive.

Clofibrate passes into breast milk and should not be taken by nursing mothers. Bottle-feed your baby if you must take this drug.

Seniors

Older adults generally take Clofibrate without special restriction. Normal age-related losses of kidney function may require your doctor to adjust your daily dosage.

Generic Name

Clomipramine

Brand Name

Anafranil

Type of Drug

Tricyclic antidepressant.

Prescribed for

Obsessive-compulsive disorder (with or without depression). Clomipramine is also prescribed for narcolepsy and pain from migraines, tension headaches, diabetic disease, tic douloureux, cancer, herpes lesions, arthritis, and other sources.

General Information

Clomipramine belongs to a group of drugs called *tricyclic antidepressants*. These drugs block the movement of certain stimulant chemicals in and out of nerve endings, have a sedative effect, and counteract the effects of a hormone called *acetylcholine* (they are anticholinergic). They prevent the reuptake of important neurohormones (norepinephrine or serotonin) at the nerve ending. One widely accepted theory says that people with depression have a chemical imbalance in their brains and that drugs such as Clomipramine work to reestablish a proper balance. Although Clomipramine and similar medications immediately block neurohormones, it takes 2 to 4 weeks for their clinical antidepressant effect to come into play. They can also elevate mood, increase physical activity and mental alertness, and improve appetite and sleep patterns in depressed individuals. If symptoms are not affected after 6 to 8 weeks, contact your doctor. Occasionally Clomipramine and other tricyclic antidepressants have been used in treating nighttime bed-wetting in young children, but they do not produce long-lasting relief. Tricyclic antidepressants are broken down in the liver.

Cautions and Warnings

Do not take Clomipramine if you are **allergic or sensitive to it** or **other tricyclic drugs** such as Imipramine, Doxepin, Nortriptyline, Trimipramine, Amitriptyline, Desipramine, Protriptyline, and Amoxapine. None of these drugs should be used if you are recovering from a heart attack.

If you have a history of **epilepsy or other convulsive disorders, difficulty in urination, glaucoma, heart disease, liver disease,** or **hyperthyroidism,** Clomipramine may be taken with caution. People who are **schizophrenic or paranoid** may get worse if given a tricyclic antidepressant, and **manic-depressive people** may switch phase. This can also happen if they are changing or stopping antidepressants.

Possible Side Effects

▼ Most common: sedation and anticholinergic effects (blurred vision, disorientation, confusion, hallucinations, muscle spasms or tremors, seizures and/or convulsions, dry mouth, constipation [especially in older adults], difficult urination, worsening glaucoma, and sensitivity to bright light or the sun). Men taking Clomipramine have a good chance of sexual function problems.

Possible Side Effects *(continued)*

▼ Less common: blood-pressure changes, abnormal heart rates, heart attack, anxiety, restlessness, excitement, numbness and tingling in the extremities, poor coordination, rash, itching, retention of fluids, fever, allergy, changes in composition of blood, nausea, vomiting, loss of appetite, stomach upset, diarrhea, enlargement of the breasts in males and females, and blood-sugar changes.

▼ Rare: agitation, inability to sleep, nightmares, feeling of panic, a peculiar taste in the mouth, stomach cramps, black discoloration of the tongue, yellowing of the eyes and/or skin, changes in liver function, increased or decreased weight, excessive perspiration, flushing, frequent urination, drowsiness, dizziness, weakness, headache, loss of hair, and not feeling well.

Drug Interactions

• Taking Clomipramine with monoamine oxidase (MAO) inhibitors can cause high fevers, convulsions, and occasionally death. Don't take MAO inhibitors until at least 2 weeks after Clomipramine has been discontinued. Patients who must take both Clomipramine and an MAO inhibitor require close medical observation.

• Clomipramine interacts with Guanethidine and Clonidine. Be sure to tell your doctor if you are taking **any** high-blood-pressure medicine.

• Clomipramine increases the effects of barbiturates, tranquilizers, other sedative drugs, and alcohol. Also, barbiturates may decrease the effectiveness of Clomipramine.

• Taking Clomipramine and thyroid medicine together will enhance the effects of both medicines, possibly causing abnormal heart rhythms. The combination of Clomipramine and Reserpine may cause overstimulation.

• Oral contraceptives can reduce the effect of Clomipramine, as can smoking. Charcoal tablets can prevent Clomipramine's absorption into the bloodstream. Estrogens can either increase or decrease the effect of Clomipramine.

• Drugs such as Bicarbonate of Soda, Acetazolamide, Quinidine, or Procainamide will increase the effect of Clomipramine. Cimetidine, Methylphenidate and phenothiazine drugs (like Thorazine and Compazine) block the liver metabolism of Clomipramine, causing it to stay in the body longer, which can cause severe drug side effects.

Food Interactions

Take Clomipramine with food if it upsets your stomach.

Usual Dose

Adult: 25 to 250 mg per day.
Child: 25 to 100 mg per day.
After the most effective dose has been determined, the total daily dose may be taken at bedtime to minimize daytime sedation.

Overdosage

Symptoms of overdosage are confusion, inability to concentrate, hallucinations, drowsiness, lowered body temperature, abnormal heart rate, heart failure, enlarged pupils of the eyes, convulsions, severely lowered blood pressure, stupor, and coma. Agitation, stiffening of body muscles, vomiting, and high fever may also develop. The overdose victim should be taken to a hospital emergency room immediately. ALWAYS bring the medicine bottle with you.

Special Information

Avoid alcohol and other depressants while taking Clomipramine. Do not stop taking this medicine unless your doctor specifically tells you to do so. Abruptly stopping this medicine may cause nausea, headache, and a sickly feeling. Avoid exposure to the sun or sunlamps.

This drug can cause drowsiness, dizziness, and blurred vision. Be careful driving or operating hazardous machinery.

Call your doctor at once if you develop seizures, difficult or rapid breathing, fever and sweating, blood-pressure changes, muscle stiffness, loss of bladder control, or unusual tiredness or weakness. Dry mouth may lead to an increase in dental cavities, gum bleeding, and gum disease. People taking Clomipramine should pay special attention to dental hygiene.

If you forget a dose of Clomipramine, skip the one you forgot and go back to your regular schedule. Do not take a double dose.

Special Populations

Pregnancy/Breast-feeding
Clomipramine, like other antidepressants, crosses into your developing baby's circulation, and birth defects have been reported if taken during the first 3 months of pregnancy. There have been reports of newborn infants suffering from heart, breathing, and urinary problems after their mothers had taken an antidepressant of this type immediately before delivery. Avoid taking this medication while pregnant.

Tricyclic antidepressants pass into breast milk in low concentrations and sedate the baby. Nursing mothers should consider alternate feeding methods if taking Clomipramine.

Seniors
Older adults are more sensitive to the effects of Clomipramine, especially abnormal rhythms and other heart side effects, and often require a lower dose to have the same effect. Follow your doctor's directions and report any side effects at once.

Generic Name

Clonazepam

Brand Name
Klonopin

Type of Drug
Anticonvulsant.

Prescribed for
Petit mal and other seizures. Clonazepam has also been used to treat panic attacks, periodic leg movements during sleep, speaking difficulty associated with Parkinson's disease, acute manic episodes, nerve pain, and schizophrenia.

General Information

Clonazepam is a member of the family of drugs known as *benzodiazepines*, including Diazepam, Chlordiazepoxide, Flurazepam, and Triazolam. Unlike the other benzodiazepine drugs, Clonazepam is not used as a sedative or hypnotic. It is used only to control petit mal seizures in people who have not responded to other drug treatments, such as Ethosuximide. Clonazepam is generally considered safe and effective for such seizures and shares many of the same side effects, precautions, and interactions as its benzodiazepine cousins.

Unfortunately, people commonly become tolerant to the effects of Clonazepam within about 3 months of starting on it. This happens because of the body's natural tendency to be more efficient in breaking the drug down and eliminating it from the circulation. Your doctor may have to raise your Clonazepam dosage to maintain the drug's effect.

Cautions and Warnings

Do not take Clonazepam if you are **sensitive or allergic** to it or another benzodiazepine.

When stopping Clonazepam treatments, it is essential that the drug be **discontinued gradually** over a period of time to allow for safe withdrawal. Abrupt discontinuance of any benzodiazepine, including Clonazepam, may lead to drug withdrawal symptoms. In the case of Clonazepam, the withdrawal symptoms can include severe seizures. Other symptoms include tremors, abdominal cramps, muscle cramps, vomiting, and increased sweating.

Clonazepam should be used with caution if you have a **chronic respiratory illness,** since the drug tends to increase salivation and other respiratory secretions, and can make breathing more labored. Other conditions where benzodiazepines should be avoided are **severe depression, severe lung disease, sleep apnea** (intermittent breathing while sleeping), **liver disease, drunkenness,** and **kidney disease.** In all of these conditions, the depressive effects of benzodiazepines may be enhanced and/or could be detrimental to your overall condition.

Clonazepam can aggravate **narrow-angle glaucoma,** but if you have open-angle glaucoma, you may take it. Check with your doctor.

Possible Side Effects

▼ Most common: drowsiness, poor muscle control, and behavior changes.

▼ Infrequent: abnormal eye movements, loss of voice and/or the ability to express a thought, double vision, coma, a glassy-eyed appearance, headache, temporary paralysis, labored breathing, shortness of breath, slurred speech, tremors, dizziness, fainting, confusion, depression, forgetfulness, hallucination, increased sex drive, hysteria, sleeplessness, psychosis, suicidal acts, chest congestion, stuffy nose, heart palpitations, hair loss or gain, rash, swelling of the face or ankles, increase or decrease in appetite or body weight, coated tongue, constipation, diarrhea, involuntary passing of feces, dry mouth, stomach irritation, nausea, sore gums, difficulty urinating, pain upon urination, bed-wetting, nighttime urination, muscle weakness or pain, reduced red- and white-blood-cell and platelet levels, enlarged liver, liver inflammation, dehydration, a deterioration in general health, fever, and swollen lymph glands.

Drug Interactions

• The depressant effects of Clonazepam are increased by tranquilizers, sleeping pills, narcotic pain relievers, antihistamines, alcohol, monoamine oxidase (MAO) inhibitors, tricyclic antidepressants, and other anticonvulsants.

• The combination of Valproic Acid and Clonazepam may produce severe petit mal seizures.

• Phenobarbital or Phenytoin may reduce Clonazepam's effectiveness by increasing the rate at which it is eliminated from the body.

• Smoking may reduce Clonazepam's effectiveness.

• Clonazepam treatment may increase the requirement for other anticonvulsant drugs because of its effects on people who suffer from multiple types of seizures.

• The effects of Clonazepam may be prolonged when it is taken with Cimetidine, oral contraceptives, Disulfiram, Fluoxetine, Isoniazid, Ketoconazole, Metoprolol, Probenecid, Propoxyphene, Propranolol, Rifampin, or Valproic Acid.

- Theophylline may reduce the drug's sedative effects.
- If you take antacids, separate them from your Clonazepam dose by at least 1 hour to prevent them from interfering with the passage of Clonazepam into the bloodstream.
- Clonazepam may increase blood levels of Digoxin and the chances for Digoxin toxicity.
- The effect of Levodopa may be decreased if it is taken with Clonazepam.

Food Interactions

Clonazepam is best taken on an empty stomach but may be taken with food if it upsets your stomach.

Usual Dose

Adult and Child (age 10 and older): 0.5 mg 3 times per day to start. The dose is increased in increments of 0.5 to 1 mg every 3 days until seizures are controlled or side effects develop. The maximum daily dose is 20 mg. Other uses for Clonazepam involve doses from 0.5 to 16 mg per day, depending on the condition being treated and its severity.

Infant and Child (up to age 9, or 66 pounds): 0.004 to 0.013 mg per pound of body weight per day to start. The dosage can be gradually increased to a maximum of 0.045 to 0.09 mg per pound of body weight.

The dosage of Clonazepam must be reduced in people with impaired kidney function because this drug is primarily released from the body via the kidneys.

Overdosage

Clonazepam overdosage may cause confusion, coma, poor reflexes, sleepiness, low blood pressure, labored breathing, and other depressive effects. If the overdose is discovered within a few minutes, and the victim is still conscious, it may be helpful to make him or her vomit with Syrup of Ipecac (available at any pharmacy) to remove any remaining medicine from the stomach. All victims of Clonazepam overdose must be taken to a hospital emergency room. ALWAYS bring the medicine bottle with you.

Special Information

Clonazepam may interfere with your ability to drive a car or perform other complex tasks because it can cause drowsiness and difficulty concentrating.

Your doctor should perform periodic blood counts and liver function tests while you are taking this drug to check for possible drug side effects.

Do not suddenly stop taking the medicine, because doing so could result in severe seizures. The dosage must be discontinued gradually by your doctor.

If you miss a dose, and it is within an hour of that dose time, take it right away. Otherwise skip the missed dose and go back to your regular dose schedule. Do not take a double dose.

Carry identification or wear a bracelet indicating that you have a seizure disorder for which you take Clonazepam.

Special Populations

Pregnancy/Breast-feeding
Clonazepam crosses into the fetal circulation and can affect the developing infant. Clonazepam should be avoided by women who are or might become pregnant. In those situations where the drug is deemed essential, its potential benefits must be carefully weighed against its risks.

Some reports suggest a strong link between anticonvulsant drugs and birth defects, though most of the information pertains to Phenytoin and Phenobarbital, not Clonazepam. It is also possible that the epileptic condition itself or genetic factors common to people with seizure disorders may also figure in the higher incidence of birth defects.

Mothers taking Clonazepam should bottle-feed their babies because of the chance that the drug will pass into their breast milk and affect the baby.

Seniors
Older adults, especially those with liver or kidney disease, are more sensitive to the effects of this drug (especially dizziness and drowsiness) and may require smaller doses. Follow your doctor's directions, and report any side effects at once.

Generic Name

Clonidine

Brand Names

Catapres Tablets*
Catapres-TTS Transdermal Patch

(*Also available in generic form)

Type of Drug

Antihypertensive.

Prescribed for

High blood pressure. Clonidine has also been used to treat hypertensive emergencies (where diastolic blood pressure is over 120). Other uses are childhood growth delay, Tourette's syndrome, migraine headaches, ulcerative colitis, painful or difficult menstruation, flushing related to menopause, diagnosis of an unusual tumor called *pheochromocytoma*, diabetic diarrhea, nicotine dependence, Methadone/opiate detoxification, withdrawal from alcohol and benzodiazepines (e.g., Valium), nerve pain following herpes attacks, and reduction of some allergic reactions in people with asthma triggered from external sources. Clonidine (by epidural injection) has been used to treat cancer pain in people who are intolerant to the effects of epidural narcotic analgesics.

General Information

Clonidine acts in the brain to stimulate a set of nerve endings called *alpha-adrenergic receptors.* At first, this causes a minor increase in blood pressure. But once the drug starts producing its major effect on brain receptors, it produces the opening, or dilation, of certain blood vessels, decreasing blood pressure. The drug produces its effect very quickly, causing a decline in blood pressure within 1 hour. The other effects of Clonidine may be traced to its stimulating effects on alpha receptors throughout the body.

Cautions and Warnings

Do not take Clonidine if you are **allergic** to it or to any other product that has Clonidine as one of its ingredients. People who have had a **recent heart attack, chronic kidney failure, cardiac insufficiency,** or **disease of blood vessels in the brain** should avoid Clonidine.

Some people **develop a tolerance to their usual dose** of Clonidine. If this happens to you, your blood pressure may increase, and you will require a change in your Clonidine dose.

If you **abruptly stop taking Clonidine,** you may experience an **unusual increase in blood pressure** with symptoms of **agitation, headache,** and **nervousness.** These effects can be reversed by simply resuming therapy or by taking another drug to lower the blood pressure. Under no circumstances should you stop taking Clonidine without your doctor's knowledge. Abruptly stopping this medication may cause severe reactions and possibly even death. Be sure you always have an adequate supply on hand.

Animal studies of Clonidine have shown a tendency toward degeneration of the retina. People taking this drug on a regular basis should have their **eyes examined** periodically.

If you are going to have **surgery,** your doctor will continue your Clonidine until about 4 hours before surgery and then continue it as soon as possible afterward.

People who develop **skin sensitivity** (rash, itching, or swelling) to **Catapres-TTS,** the Clonidine skin patch, may find that oral Clonidine also produces the same reactions.

Possible Side Effects

▼ Most common: dry mouth, drowsiness, and sedation (tablets); dry mouth and drowsiness (skin patches).

▼ Common: constipation, dizziness, headache, and fatigue (tablets). These tend to diminish within 4 to 6 weeks.

▼ Less common: loss of appetite, swelling or pain of glands in the throat, nausea, vomiting, weight gain, blood-sugar elevation, breast pain or enlargement, worsening of congestive heart failure, heart palpitations, rapid heartbeat, dizziness when rising quickly from a sitting or lying position, painful blood-vessel spasm, abnormal heart rhythms, electrocardiogram changes, feelings of ill

Possible Side Effects (continued)

health, changes in dream patterns, nightmares, difficulty sleeping, hallucinations, feelings of delirium, anxiety, depression, nervousness, restlessness, headache, rash, hives, thinning or loss of scalp hair, difficult or painful urination, nighttime urination, retaining urine, decreased or loss of sex drive, weakness, muscle or joint pain, leg cramps, increased alcohol sensitivity, dryness and burning of the eyes, dry nose, loss of color, and fever (tablets); constipation, nausea, changes in taste perception, dry throat, fatigue, headache, lethargy, changes in sleep patterns, nervousness, dizziness, impotence, sexual difficulties, and mild skin reactions, including itching, swelling, contact dermatitis, skin discoloration, burning, skin peeling, throbbing, white patches on the skin, and a generalized rash (skin patches). Rashes of the face and tongue have also occurred but cannot be specifically tied to the Clonidine skin patch.

Drug Interactions

• Clonidine has a depressive effect and will increase the depressive effects of alcohol, barbiturates, sedatives, and tranquilizers: Avoid them. Antidepressants, Fenfluramine and other appetite suppressants, estrogens, stimulants, Indocin, and other nonsteroidal anti-inflammatory drugs (NSAIDs) may counteract the effects of Clonidine.

• Taking Clonidine together with a beta blocker can cause a much more severe drug-withdrawal reaction and rebound high blood pressure. Also, this combination has actually caused blood pressure to rise in some people.

Food Interactions

Clonidine tablets are best taken on an empty stomach but may be taken with food if they upset your stomach.

Usual Dose

Tablets

Adult: The starting dose of 0.1 mg twice per day may be raised by 0.1 to 0.2 mg per day until maximum control is achieved. The dose must be tailored to your individual needs. It is recommended that no one take more than 2.4 mg per day.

Opiate Detoxification

Up to 0.008 mg per pound of body weight in divided doses.

Senior: Start with a lower dose and increase more slowly.

Child: 5 to 25 micrograms for every 2.2 pounds each day, divided into 4 doses given every 6 hours.

Transdermal Patch

Adult: 0.1-mg patch applied every 7 days. Two 0.3-mg patches have not been shown to increase effectiveness.

Child: not recommended.

Overdosage

Symptoms are slow heartbeat, nervous-system depression, very slow breathing or no breathing at all, low body temperature, pinpoint pupils, seizures, lethargy, agitation, irritability, nausea, vomiting, abnormal heart rhythms, mild increases in blood pressure followed by a rapid drop in blood pressure, dizziness, weakness, loss of reflexes, and vomiting. The overdose victim should be taken to a hospital emergency room immediately. ALWAYS bring the medicine bottle with you.

Special Information

Clonidine causes drowsiness in about one third of those who take it: Be extremely careful while driving or operating any potentially hazardous appliance or machinery. This effect is prominent during the first few weeks of therapy, then tends to decrease.

Avoid taking nonprescription cough and cold medicines unless so directed by your doctor.

Call your doctor if you become depressed or have vivid dreams or nightmares while taking Clonidine, develop swelling in your feet and/or legs, develop paleness or coldness in your fingertips or toes, or develop other side effects that are persistent or bothersome.

Apply the patch to a hairless area of skin like the upper arm or torso. Use a different skin site each time. If the patch becomes loose during the 7 days, apply the specially supplied adhesive directly over the patch. If the patch falls off, apply a new one. The patch should not be removed for bathing.

If you miss a dose of the oral medication, take it as soon as possible and go back to your regular dose schedule. If you miss 2 or more doses in a row, consult your doctor; missing doses can cause your blood pressure to go up and severe adverse effects to occur. Do not take a double dose.

Special Populations

Pregnancy/Breast-feeding
Animal studies have shown this drug to be able to damage a developing fetus in doses as low as one third the maximum human dose. Pregnant women and those who might become pregnant should avoid this drug.

Clonidine passes into breast milk, but no effects on nursing infants have been noted. Nursing mothers should avoid this drug or bottle-feed their babies.

Seniors
Older adults are more susceptible to the effects of this drug and should be treated with lower than normal doses.

Generic Name

Clorazepate Dipotassium

Brand Names

Tranxene-SD Tablets
Tranxene T Tablets

(Also available in generic form)

Type of Drug

Benzodiazepine tranquilizer.

Prescribed for

Relief of symptoms of anxiety, tension, fatigue, and agitation. Also used for irritable bowel syndrome and panic attacks.

General Information

Clorazepate Dipotassium is a member of a group of drugs known as *benzodiazepines*, used as either antianxiety agents, anticonvulsants, or sedatives. Some are more suited to a specific role because of differences in their chemical makeup that give them greater activity in certain areas or characteristics that make them more desirable for a certain function. Often, individual drugs are limited by the applications for which their research has been sponsored. Benzodiazepines all directly affect the brain. In doing so, they can relax you and make you more tranquil or sleepier, or can slow nervous-system transmissions in such a way as to act as an anticonvulsant, depending on which drug you use and how much you take. Many doctors prefer the benzodiazepines to other drugs that can be used for similar effects because they tend to be safer, have fewer side effects, and are usually as, if not more, effective.

Cautions and Warnings

Do not take Clorazepate if you know you are **sensitive** or **allergic** to it or another benzodiazepine drug, including Clonazepam.

Clorazepate can aggravate **narrow-angle glaucoma**. However, if you have open-angle glaucoma, you may take it. Check with your doctor.

Other **conditions where Clorazepate should be avoided** are severe depression, severe lung disease, sleep apnea (intermittent breathing while sleeping), liver disease, drunkenness, and kidney disease. In all of these conditions, the depressive effects of Clorazepate may be enhanced and/or could be detrimental to your overall condition.

Clorazepate should **not be taken by psychotic patients**, because it doesn't work for those people and can cause unusual excitement, stimulation, and rage in them.

Clorazepate is **not intended to be used for more than 3 to 4 months at a time.** Your doctor should reassess your condition before continuing your prescription beyond that time.

Clorazepate may be **addictive.** You can experience drug withdrawal symptoms if you suddenly stop taking it after as little as 4 to 6 weeks of treatment. Withdrawal generally begins with increased feelings of anxiety and continues with tingling in the extremities, sensitivity to bright lights or the sun, long periods of sleep or sleeplessness, a metallic taste, flulike illness, fatigue, difficulty concentrating, restlessness, loss of appetite, nausea, irritability, headache, dizziness, sweating, muscle tension or cramps, tremors, and feeling uncomfortable or ill at ease. Other major withdrawal symptoms include confusion, abnormal perception of movement, depersonalization, paranoid delusions, hallucinations, psychotic reactions, muscle twitching, seizures, and memory loss.

Possible Side Effects

Weakness and confusion may occur, especially in seniors and those who are more sickly.

▼ Most common: mild drowsiness during the first few days of therapy.

▼ Less common: confusion, depression, lethargy, disorientation, headache, inactivity, slurred speech, stupor, dizziness, tremors, constipation, dry mouth, nausea, inability to control urination, sexual difficulties, irregular menstrual cycle, changes in heart rhythm, lowered blood pressure, fluid retention, blurred or double vision, itching, rash, hiccups, nervousness, inability to fall asleep, and occasional liver dysfunction. If you have any of these symptoms, stop taking the medicine, and contact your doctor at once.

▼ Other: diarrhea, coated tongue, sore gums, vomiting, appetite changes, swallowing difficulty, increased salivation, upset stomach, changes in sex drive, urinary difficulties, changes in heart rate, palpitations, swelling, stuffy nose, hearing difficulty, hair loss or gain, sweating, fever, tingling in the hands or feet, breast pain, muscle disturbances, breathing difficulty, changes in the components of your blood, and joint pain.

Drug Interactions

• Clorazepate is a central-nervous-system depressant. Avoid alcohol, other tranquilizers, narcotics, barbiturates, monoamine oxidase (MAO) inhibitors, antihistamines, and antidepressants.

Taking Clorazepate with these drugs may result in excessive depression, tiredness, sleepiness, difficulty breathing, or similar symptoms.

• Smoking may reduce the effectiveness of Clorazepate by increasing the speed at which it is broken down by the body.

• The effects of Clorazepate may be prolonged when it is taken together with Cimetidine, oral contraceptives, Disulfiram, Fluoxetine, Isoniazid, Ketoconazole, Metoprolol, Probenecid, Propoxyphene, Propranolol, Rifampin, or Valproic Acid.

• Theophylline may reduce Clorazepate's sedative effects.

• If you take antacids, separate them from your Clorazepate dose by at least 1 hour to prevent them from interfering with the absorption of Clorazepate into the bloodstream.

• Clorazepate may increase blood levels of Digoxin and the chances for Digoxin toxicity.

• The effect of Levodopa may be decreased if it is taken together with Clorazepate.

• Phenytoin blood concentrations may be increased if taken with Clorazepate, resulting in possible Phenytoin toxicity.

Food Interactions

Clorazepate is best taken on an empty stomach, but it may be taken with food if it upsets your stomach.

Usual Dose

Tranxene-T

Adult and Child (age 9 and older): 15 to 60 mg daily; average dose, 30 mg in divided quantities. The dose must be adjusted to individual response for maximum effect.

Child (under age 9): not recommended.

Tranxene-SD

Adult: Tranxene-SD, a long-acting form of Clorazepate, may be given as a single dose, either 11.25 or 22.5 mg, once every 24 hours.

Child: not recommended.

Overdosage

Symptoms of overdosage are confusion, sleepiness, poor coordination, lack of response to pain (such as a pin stick), loss of reflexes, shallow breathing, low blood pressure, and coma. The victim should be taken to a hospital emergency room. ALWAYS bring the medicine bottle with you.

Special Information

Clorazepate can cause tiredness, drowsiness, inability to concentrate, or similar symptoms. Be careful if you are driving, operating machinery, or performing other activities that require concentration.

People taking Clorazepate for more than 3 or 4 months at a time may develop drug-withdrawal reactions if the medication is stopped suddenly (see *Cautions and Warnings*).

If you forget a dose of Clorazepate, take it as soon as you remember. If it is almost time for your next dose, skip the forgotten pill and continue with your regular schedule. Do not take a double dose.

Special Populations

Pregnancy/Breast-feeding

Clorazepate may cross into the developing fetal circulation and may cause birth defects if taken during the first 3 months of pregnancy. Avoid this drug if you are or think you might be pregnant.

Clorazepate may pass into breast milk. Since infants break the drug down more slowly than adults, it is possible for the medicine to accumulate and have an undesired effect on the baby. Nursing mothers who must take Clorazepate should bottle-feed their babies.

Seniors

Older adults, especially those with liver or kidney disease, are more sensitive to the effects of Clorazepate and generally require smaller doses to achieve the same effect. Follow your doctor's directions, and report any side effects at once.

Generic Name

Clotrimazole

Brand Names

Femcare Vaginal Cream
Gyne-Lotrimin Vaginal
    Cream/Tablets/
    Combination Pak
Lotrimin Cream/Lotion/
    Solution

Mycelex-7 Cream/Troches
Mycelex Twin Pack
Mycelex-G Vaginal Cream/
    Tablets

(Also available in generic form)

Type of Drug

Antifungal.

Prescribed for

Fungal infections of the mouth, skin, and vaginal tract.

General Information

Clotrimazole is one of a group of antifungal drugs available without a prescription in the United States. It is useful against a wide variety of fungus organisms that other drugs do not affect. The exact way in which Clotrimazole produces its effect is not known.

Cautions and Warnings

If Clotrimazole causes **local itching and/or irritation,** stop using it. Do **not** use Clotrimazole **in your eyes. Proper diagnosis is essential** for effective treatment. Do not use this product without first consulting your doctor.

Possible Side Effects

Side effects do not occur very often and are usually mild.
    ▼ Most common: redness, stinging, blistering, peeling, itching, and swelling of local areas (cream or solution); mild burning, skin rash, mild cramps, frequent

---

Possible Side Effects *(continued)*

urination, and burning or itching in a sexual partner
(vaginal tablets); stomach cramps or pain, diarrhea, nausea, and vomiting (oral tablets).

Drug Interactions

None known.

Food Interactions

The oral form of Clotrimazole is best taken on an empty
stomach, at least 1 hour before or 2 hours after meals.
However, you may take it with food as long as you allow the
tablet to dissolve in your mouth like a lozenge.

Usual Dose

Topical Cream and Solution
Apply to affected areas, morning and night.

Vaginal Cream
One applicatorful at bedtime for 7 to 14 days.

Vaginal Tablet
1 tablet inserted into the vagina at bedtime for 7 days, or 2
tablets per day for 3 days.

Lozenge
1 lozenge 5 times per day for 2 weeks or more.

Overdosage

This drug is not well absorbed into the blood. Call your local
poison control center for information.

Special Information

If treating a vaginal infection, you should refrain from sexual
activity or be sure that your partner wears a condom until the
treatment is finished. Call your doctor if burning or itching
develops or if the condition does not show improvement
within 7 days.

If you are using the vaginal cream, you may want to wear a sanitary napkin to avoid staining your clothing.

Dissolve the lozenge slowly in the mouth.

This medicine must be taken on consecutive days. If you forget to take a dose of oral Clotrimazole, take it as soon as you remember. Do not double any doses.

Special Populations

Pregnancy/Breast-feeding

No problems have been found in children of women who used Clotrimazole during their pregnancy. Pregnant women, or women who might become pregnant while using this drug, should talk to their doctor about the risks associated with this medicine versus the benefits it can provide. Women who are in the first 3 months of pregnancy should use this drug only if directed to do so by their doctors. If you are pregnant, your doctor may want you to insert vaginal tablets by hand rather than use a vaginal applicator.

This drug is poorly absorbed into the bloodstream and is not likely to pass into breast milk. Nursing mothers need not worry about adverse effects on their infants while taking Clotrimazole.

Seniors

Seniors may use this medication without special restriction.

Generic Name

Clozapine

Brand Name

Clozaril

Type of Drug

Antipsychotic.

Prescribed for

Severely ill schizophrenics who do not respond to other medicines.

General Information

Clozapine is a unique antipsychotic that has the capacity to treat people who either do not respond to other drugs or suffer from severe side effects of those drugs. Chemically, it is a distant cousin of the benzodiazepine tranquilizers and anticonvulsants, but it works by a mechanism that differs from those of other antipsychotic drugs.

A very small number of people who take Clozapine develop a rapid drop in their white-blood-cell count, a condition called *agranulocytosis.* This effect usually reverses itself when the drug is stopped, but the drug must be stopped **AS SOON AS IT IS DISCOVERED.** An unusually large number of people who have developed Clozapine agranulocytosis in the United States are of Eastern European Jewish descent, but the association is not very strong. Most cases of agranulocytosis occur between week 4 and week 10 of treatment. It is essential that blood samples be taken every week or so to watch for this effect and for 4 weeks after the drug is stopped. Also, because of the possibility of agranulocytosis, no one should start taking Clozapine until he or she has tried at least 2 other antipsychotic medicines to make sure that nothing else will work.

Some people taking antipsychotic drugs develop a group of potentially irreversible, uncontrollable movements. The fact that this has not been reported with Clozapine is seen as a major advantage of the drug over other antipsychotic medicines. However, there is still a possibility that this set of symptoms could occur with Clozapine.

Cautions and Warnings

Women, seniors, people with **serious illnesses,** those who are **emaciated,** those with a **history of diseases affecting the white blood cells,** or those who are **taking other medicines that could affect white blood cells** may be more susceptible to Clozapine agranulocytosis. There is no easy way to know who is likely to develop Clozapine agranulocytosis.

About 5 percent of people taking the drug experience a **seizure** in the first year of treatment. Seizure is most likely to occur at higher drug doses.

People with **heart disease** should be carefully monitored while on Clozapine because of possible cardiac risks.

A more serious set of side effects, known as *neuroleptic malignant syndrome* (NMS), includes **a high fever** and has been associated with Clozapine when it is used together with

Lithium or other drugs. The other symptoms that make up NMS include **muscle rigidity, mental changes, irregular pulse or blood pressure, increased sweating,** and **abnormal heart rhythms.** NMS is potentially fatal and requires immediate medical attention.

Use this drug with caution if you have **glaucoma, prostate problems,** or **liver, kidney, or heart disease.**

Clozapine may interfere with **mental or physical abilities** because of the sedation it usually causes in the first few weeks of treatment.

Possible Side Effects

▼ Most common: rapid heartbeat, low blood pressure, dizziness, fainting, drowsiness or sedation, salivation, and constipation.

▼ Less common: headache, tremor, sleep disturbances, restlessness, slow muscle motions, absence of movement, agitation, convulsions, rigidity, restlessness, confusion, sweating, dry mouth, visual disturbances, high blood pressure, nausea, vomiting, heartburn or abdominal discomfort, fever, and weight gain.

▼ Rare: agranulocytosis (reduced white-blood-cell count) and other changes in blood components, electrocardiogram changes, fatigue, sleeplessness, rapid movements, general weakness, muscle weakness, lethargy, slurred speech, tremors, depression, seizures, tardive dyskinesia (characterized by lip smacking or puckering, puffing of the cheeks, rapid tongue movement, and uncontrolled chewing motions), neuroleptic malignant syndrome (characterized by convulsions, difficulty breathing, pains in the back, neck, or legs), muscle spasms, angina pains, electrocardiogram changes, diarrhea, abnormal liver function, appetite loss, loss of bladder control, abnormal ejaculation, frequent or infrequent urination, the feeling of having to urinate, breathing difficulty, sore throat, stuffed nose, and numbness or soreness of the tongue.

Drug Interactions

• Clozapine's anticholinergic effects (blurred vision, dry

mouth, and confusion) may be enhanced by other anticholinergics (e.g., the tricyclic antidepressants, including Amitriptyline).

• Drugs that reduce blood pressure may enhance the blood-pressure-lowering effects of Clozapine.

• Alcohol and other nervous-system depressants, including benzodiazepines and other antianxiety drugs, may enhance Clozapine's sedative actions. There is at least one known case of a patient dying while taking a combination of Diazepam and Clozapine.

• Clozapine may increase blood levels of Digoxin, Warfarin, Heparin, or Phenytoin.

• The combination of Lithium and Clozapine may cause seizures, confusion, and NMS (see *Cautions and Warnings*).

• Cigarette smoking may increase the rate at which the liver breaks down Clozapine, altering dosage requirements. This is usually a problem only if a person changes his or her smoking habits while taking the drug.

Food Interactions

Clozapine may be taken without regard to food or meals.

Usual Dose

25 mg twice a day to start, with gradual dosage increases to a daily maximum of 900 mg, although no more than 300 to 450 mg daily is usually required.

Overdosage

Usual symptoms of overdose are delirium, drowsiness, changes in heart rhythm, unusual excitement, nervousness, restlessness, hallucinations, excessive salivation, dizziness or fainting, slow or irregular breathing, and coma. Overdose victims must be taken to a hospital emergency room immediately. ALWAYS take the medicine bottle with you.

Special Information

Clozapine may cause a fever during the first few weeks of treatment. Generally, the fever is not important, but it may occasionally be necessary to stop treatment due to persistent fever. This decision is made by the supervising doctor.

Regular blood tests are necessary to monitor blood composition for any changes that might be caused by Clozapine. Call your doctor at once if you develop lethargy or weakness, a flu-like infection, sore throat, a sickly feeling, sweating, muscle rigidity, mental changes, irregular pulse or blood pressure, mouth ulcers, or dry mouth that lasts for more than 2 weeks. Dry mouth, a common side effect of Clozapine, may be countered by using gum, candy, ice, or a saliva substitute (such as Orex or Moi-Stir).

Do not stop taking Clozapine without your doctor's knowledge and approval, because a gradual dosage reduction may be necessary to prevent side effects.

Avoid alcohol or any other nervous-system depressant while taking Clozapine.

Some of the side effects of Clozapine (drowsiness, blurred vision, or seizures) may interfere with the performance of complex tasks like driving or operating hazardous equipment.

While taking Clozapine, rapidly rising from a sitting or lying position may cause you to become dizzy or faint.

If you take Clozapine twice a day and forget a dose, take it as soon as you remember. If it is almost time for your next dose, take one dose as soon as you remember and another in 5 or 6 hours, then go back to your regular schedule. Do not take a double dose.

If you take Clozapine 3 times a day and forget a dose, take it as soon as you remember. If it is almost time for your next dose, take one dose as soon as you remember and another in 3 or 4 hours, then go back to your regular schedule. Do not take a double dose.

Special Populations

Pregnancy/Breast-feeding
This drug should be used during pregnancy only if your doctor determines that it is absolutely necessary.

Clozapine may pass into breast milk. Nursing mothers who must take this drug should bottle-feed their babies.

Seniors
Older adults may be more sensitive to the side effects of Clozapine (such as dizziness on rapidly rising from a sitting or lying position, confusion, and excitement) than younger adults. Older men are also more likely to have prostate problems, a cause for caution with Clozapine.

Generic Name

Codeine

(Available only in generic form)

Type of Drug

Narcotic pain reliever; cough suppressant.

Prescribed for

Relief of moderate pain and cough suppression.

General Information

Codeine is a narcotic drug with some pain-relieving and cough-suppressing activity. As an analgesic it is useful for mild to moderate pain. The pain-relieving effect of 30 to 60 mg of Codeine is approximately equal to that of 2 Aspirin tablets (650 mg). Codeine may be less active than Aspirin for types of pain associated with inflammation, because Aspirin reduces inflammation and Codeine does not. Codeine suppresses the cough reflex but does not cure the underlying cause of the cough. In fact, sometimes it may not be desirable to overly suppress a cough, because cough suppression reduces your ability to naturally eliminate excess mucus produced during a cold or allergy attack. Other narcotic cough suppressants are stronger than Codeine, but Codeine remains the best cough medicine available today.

Cautions and Warnings

Do not take Codeine if you know you are **allergic or sensitive** to it. Use this drug with extreme caution if you suffer from **asthma** or other breathing problems. Long-term use of Codeine may cause drug **dependence or addiction.** Narcotics may make it difficult to monitor the progress of people who have suffered head injuries and should be used with caution in these patients.

Possible Side Effects

▼ Most common: light-headedness, dizziness, sleepiness, nausea, vomiting, loss of appetite, and sweating. If these occur, ask your doctor about lowering your Codeine dose. Most of these side effects disappear if you simply lie down.

▼ Less common: euphoria (feeling "high"), sleepiness, headache, agitation, uncoordinated muscle movement, minor hallucinations, disorientation and visual disturbances, dry mouth, loss of appetite, constipation, flushing of the face, rapid heartbeat, palpitations, faintness, urinary difficulties or hesitancy, reduced sex drive and/or impotency, itching, rashes, anemia, lowered blood sugar, and yellowing of the skin and/or whites of the eyes. Narcotic analgesics may aggravate convulsions in those who have had convulsions in the past.

More serious side effects of Codeine are shallow breathing or difficulty in breathing.

Drug Interactions

• Because of Codeine's depressant effect and potential effect on breathing, avoid combining it with alcohol, sleeping medicine, tranquilizers, or other depressant drugs.

• Combining Cimetidine with a narcotic pain reliever such as Codeine can cause confusion, disorientation, breathing difficulty, and seizures.

Food Interactions

Codeine may be taken with food to reduce stomach upset.

Usual Dose

Adult: 15 to 60 mg 4 times per day for relief of pain; 10 to 20 mg every few hours as needed to suppress cough.

Child: 1 to 2 mg per pound of body weight in divided doses for relief of pain; 0.5 to 0.75 mg per pound of body weight in divided doses to suppress cough.

Overdosage

Symptoms of overdosage are depression of respiration (breathing), extreme tiredness progressing to stupor and then coma, pinpointed pupils of the eyes, no response to pain stimulation (such as a pin stick), cold and clammy skin, slowing down of the heartbeat, lowering of blood pressure, convulsions, and cardiac arrest. The victim should be taken to a hospital emergency room immediately. ALWAYS bring the medicine bottle with you.

Special Information

Codeine is a respiratory depressant and affects the central nervous system, producing sleepiness, tiredness, and/or inability to concentrate. Be careful if you are driving, operating hazardous machinery, or performing other functions requiring concentration. Avoid alcohol while taking Codeine because it enhances these effects.

Call your doctor if you develop breathing difficulty, constipation, dry mouth, or any other side effect that is prominent or persistent.

If you forget a dose of Codeine, take it as soon as you remember. If it is almost time for your next dose, skip the one you forgot and continue with your regular schedule. Do not take a double dose.

Special Populations

Pregnancy/Breast-feeding

No studies of this medication have been done in women and no reports of human birth defects exist, but animal studies show that large quantities of the drug can cause problems in a developing fetus. Pregnant women and those who might become pregnant should talk to their doctors about the risks of taking Codeine versus its possible benefits.

This drug passes into breast milk, but no problems in nursing infants have been seen. However, breast-feeding women should bottle-feed their babies to avoid possible adverse effects on their nursing infants.

Too much (large amounts taken for a long time) of any narcotic, including Codeine, taken during pregnancy and/or breast-feeding may cause the baby to become dependent on the narcotic. Narcotics may also cause breathing problems in the infant during delivery.

Seniors

Seniors are more likely to be sensitive to side effects of this drug and should be treated with the smallest effective dose.

Generic Name

Colchicine

(Available only in generic form)

Type of Drug

Antigout drug.

Prescribed for

Treatment and prevention of gouty arthritis. May also be prescribed for Mediterranean fever, cirrhosis of the liver, biliary cirrhosis, Behçet's disease, pseudogout (caused by calcium deposits), amyloidosis, skin reactions (scleroderma, psoriasis, and other skin conditions), and nerve problems associated with chronic progressive multiple sclerosis.

General Information

While no one knows exactly how Colchicine works, it appears to help people with gout by reducing their inflammatory response to uric acid crystals that form inside joints and by interfering with the body's mechanism for making uric acid. Unlike drugs that affect uric-acid levels, Colchicine does not block the progression of gout to chronic gouty arthritis; it will, however, relieve the pain of acute attacks and lessen the frequency and severity of attacks. It has no effect on other kinds of pain.

Cautions and Warnings

Do not use Colchicine if you suffer from any serious **blood, kidney, liver, stomach,** or **cardiac conditions**.

Vomiting, abdominal pain, diarrhea, nausea, kidney damage, and **blood in the urine** can occur with Colchicine, especially at maximal doses. This can **worsen existing gastrointestinal or other conditions**. Stop taking the medication if you develop one of these symptoms and call your doctor.

The **weakness** that people develop while taking Colchicine is frequently related to high levels of Colchicine in the blood caused by **poor kidney function** and will resolve without treatment 3 to 4 weeks after you stop taking the drug. This reaction is often mistaken for other conditions.

Periodic **blood counts** should be done if you are taking Colchicine for long periods of time.

Colchicine may affect the process of **sperm generation** in men.

The safety and effectiveness for use by **children** have not been established.

Possible Side Effects

▼ Common: vomiting, diarrhea, and abdominal pain may occur if you take maximal doses of Colchicine for an acute gout attack. You may also experience severe diarrhea, kidney and blood-vessel damage, blood in the urine, and reduced urination.

▼ Less common: hair loss, skin rash, appetite loss, muscle and nerve weakness.

▼ Other: (with long-term Colchicine therapy) reduced white-blood-cell and platelet counts, nerve inflammation, blood-clotting problems, hair loss, skin rash, and other drug reactions. Colchicine may interfere with sperm formation.

Drug Interactions

- Colchicine interferes with the absorption of vitamin B_{12}.
- Colchicine may increase sensitivity to central-nervous-system depressants, such as tranquilizers and alcohol.
- The following drugs can reduce Colchicine's effectiveness: anticancer drugs, Bumetanide, Diazoxide, Thiazide diuretics, Ethacrynic Acid, Furosemide, Mecamylamine, Pyrazinamide, and Triamterene.
- Taking Phenylbutazone together with Colchicine increases the chance of drug side effects.

Food Interactions

This drug may be taken without regard to food or meals.

Usual Dose

Acute Gout Attack

1 mg to 1.2 mg. This dose may be followed by 0.5 mg to 1.2

mg every 1 to 2 hours until pain is relieved or nausea, vomiting, or diarrhea occurs. The total dose needed to control pain and inflammation during an attack varies from 4 to 8 mg.

Gout-Attack Prevention
0.5 mg to 1.8 mg daily. In mild cases, 0.5 mg or 0.6 mg may be taken only 3 or 4 days a week.

Overdosage

Usually 1 to 3 days pass between the time that an overdose is taken and symptoms begin. The lethal dose is estimated at 65 mg, though people have died after taking as little as 7 mg at once. Overdose symptoms start with nausea, vomiting, stomach pain, diarrhea (which may be severe and bloody), and burning sensations in the throat or stomach or on the skin. If you think you are experiencing overdose symptoms, contact your doctor immediately, or go to a hospital emergency room. ALWAYS bring the medicine bottle with you.

Special Information

Call your doctor if you develop skin rash, sore throat, fever, unusual bleeding or bruising, tiredness, or numbness or tingling. Older adults are more likely to develop drug side effects and should use this drug with caution.

Stop taking maximum doses of Colchicine as soon as gout pain is relieved, and reduce your dose to a maintenance level if your doctor has prescribed it for gout prevention. Also, stop taking the drug at the first sign of nausea, vomiting, stomach pain, or diarrhea, and contact your doctor.

If you forget a dose of Colchicine, take it as soon as possible. If it is almost time for your next dose, skip the forgotten dose and continue with your regular schedule. Do not take a double dose.

Special Populations

Pregnancy/Breast-feeding
Colchicine can harm the fetus. Pregnant women should not take it unless the benefits clearly outweigh the potential risk of harming the fetus.

It is not known if Colchicine passes into breast milk. No problems with nursing infants are known, but you should consider bottle-feeding your baby if you must take Colchicine.

Seniors
Older adults and sick people are more likely to develop drug side effects and should use this drug with caution.

Generic Name
Contraceptives

Brand Names

Low-Dose Estrogen/Low-Dose Progestin Single-Phase Combinations

Brevicon	Loestrin Fe 1/20	Norethin 1/50 M
Genora 0.5/35	Modicon	Norinyl 1+35
Genora 1/35	N.E.E. 1/35 E	Norinyl 1+50
Genora 1/50	Nelova 0.5/35 E	Ortho-Novum 1/35
Loestrin 21 1.5/30	Nelova 1/35 E	Ortho-Novum 1/50
Loestrin 21 1/20	Nelova 1/50 M	Ovcon-35
Loestrin Fe 1.5/30		

Low-Dose Estrogen/Intermediate-Dose Progestin Single-Phase Combinations

Demulen 1/35	Lo/Ovral	Ortho-Cept
Desogen	Nordette	Ortho-Cyclen
Levlen		

Intermediate-Dose Estrogen/Low-Dose Progestin Single-Phase Combinations

Ovcon-50

Intermediate-Dose Estrogen/Intermediate-Dose Progestin Single-Phase Combinations

Demulen 1/50

Intermediate-Dose Estrogen/High-Dose Progestin Single-Phase Combination

Ovral

Low-Dose Estrogen/Low-Dose Progestin 2-Phase Combinations

Nelova 10/11
Ortho-Novum 10/11

Low-Dose Estrogen/Low-Dose Progestin 3-Phase Combinations

Ortho-Novum 7/7/7	Tri-Norinyl
Tri-Levlen	Triphasil

Low-Dose Progestin Mini-Pill

Ovrette

High-Dose Progestin Mini-Pills

Micronor
Nor-Q.D.

Implant Systems

Levonorgestrel Implant (Norplant System)
Progesterone Intrauterine Insert (Progestasert)

Type of Drug

Contraceptive.

Prescribed for

Prevention of pregnancy; postcoital (morning-after) pill; endometriosis; excessive menstruation; cyclic withdrawal bleeding.

General Information

Oral contraceptives ("the Pill") are synthetic hormones containing either a Progestin hormone alone or a Progestin hormone combined with an Estrogen hormone. These hormones are similar to naturally occurring female hormones that control the menstrual cycle and prepare a woman's body to accept a fertilized egg. Natural hormones cannot be used as contraceptives, because very large doses would be needed. Synthetic hormones are much more potent and can be given in much smaller doses.

Once an egg has been fertilized and is accepted (implanted)

in the womb, no more eggs may be released from the ovaries until the pregnancy is over. Oral contraceptives interfere with these natural processes; they may not allow sperm to reach the unfertilized egg, not allow the acceptance of a fertilized egg, and/or not allow ovulation (the release of an unfertilized egg).

Oral contraceptives provide a very high rate of protection from pregnancy. They are from 97 to 99 percent effective, depending upon which product is used and how closely you follow your doctor's directions. With no contraceptive at all, the normal pregnancy rate is 60 to 80 percent.

The many different kinds of combination products available contain different amounts of Estrogen and Progestin and different hormone products. Products with the smallest amount of Estrogen may be less effective in some women than others. In general, the product that contains the lowest amount of hormones but is effective and keeps side effects to a minimum is preferred.

The mini-pill, a Progestin-only product, may cause irregular menstrual cycles and may be less effective than combination products. Mini-pills may be used in older women or women who should avoid Estrogens (see *Cautions and Warnings*).

Single-phase products provide a fixed amount of Estrogen and Progestin throughout the entire pill cycle.

In the 2-phase combination, the amount of Progestin first increases and then decreases. This is supposed to allow normal changes to take place in the uterus. The amount of Estrogen remains at a steady low level throughout the cycle. The newest combination products are triple-phase in design. Throughout the cycle, the Estrogen portion remains the same, but the Progestin changes to create a wave pattern in 3 parts. The 3-phase products are supposed to act most like normal hormone cycles and reduce breakthrough bleeding. Breakthrough bleeding may be seen with the older combination products beginning with the 8th through 16th days. The amount of Estrogen in these new products is considered to be in the low category.

Levonorgestrel implants provide effective contraception for up to 5 years after implantation in the skin of your upper arm by your doctor. They can be removed at any time, reversing the contraceptive effect, but should be replaced by your doctor at least once every 5 years. The intrauterine insert provides a continuous flow of Progestin, and effective contraception, for about 1 year. The medicines contained in both of these systems are of the same type as the Progestin-only mini-pills and can be associated with many of the same side effects and precautions as the oral pills.

Every woman taking or thinking of using a contraceptive, whether it is a pill or an implantable device, should be fully aware of the problems associated with this type of contraception. The highest risk is in women over 35 who smoke and have high blood pressure.

Cautions and Warnings

You should not use oral contraceptives if you are or might be **pregnant** or if you have or have had **blood clots of the veins or arteries, stroke, any disease affecting blood coagulation, known or suspected cancer of the breast or sex organs, liver cancer,** or **irregular or scanty menstrual periods.** Oral contraceptives can cause some **eye problems.** Call your doctor at once if you develop **visual difficulties** of any kind.

Your doctor should carefully consider the risks of contraceptive products if you are **physically immobile** or if you have **asthma, cardiac insufficiency, epilepsy, migraine headaches, kidney problems,** a **strong family history of breast cancer, benign breast disease, diabetes, endometriosis, gallbladder disease** or **gallstones, liver problems** (including jaundice), **high blood cholesterol, high blood pressure, Estrogen** or **Progestin intolerance, depression, tuberculosis,** or **varicose veins.**

There is an increased risk of **heart attack** in women who take oral contraceptives for more than 10 years or who are between age 40 and 49 and have other coronary risk factors (cigarettes, obesity, high blood pressure, diabetes, high blood cholesterol); this risk remains even after the medication is stopped. **Smokers** who use oral contraceptives have a 5 times greater chance of having a heart attack as nonsmoking Pill users and a 10 to 12 times greater chance of heart attack than nonsmoking, non-Pill users.

Women who should avoid Estrogen-containing products are those with a history of **headaches, high blood pressure,** and **varicose veins. Older women** and women who have experienced **side effects** from Estrogen also should not take Estrogen products.

Oral contraceptives can mask the **onset of menopause.**

Progestin-only products carry an increased risk of blood-clotting problems, but the exact risk is not well understood.

Possible Side Effects

The ideal oral contraceptive will have virtually no side effects. Your doctor will choose a product suited to you but may have to change products from time to time depending on the side effects you develop. If you are taking too much Estrogen, for example, you may experience nausea, bloating, high blood pressure, migraines, or breast tenderness. If you have too little Estrogen, you may develop early or mid-cycle breakthrough bleeding, spotting, or reduced periodic flow. Too much Progestin is associated with weight gain and increased appetite, tiredness or weakness, low periodic flow, acne, depression, breast regression, and oily scalp. Too little Progestin is associated with late breakthrough bleeding, excessive periodic bleeding, or no period at all.

▼ Other: abdominal cramps, possible infertility after coming off the Pill, breast tenderness, weight change, headaches, rash, vaginal itching and burning, general vaginal infection, nervousness, dizziness, depression, formation of eye cataract, changes in sex drive, loss of hair, and unusual sensitivity to the sun.

▼ Rare: women who take oral contraceptives are more likely to develop several serious conditions, including the formation of blood clots in the deep veins, stroke, heart attack, liver cancer, gallbladder disease, and high blood pressure. Women who smoke cigarettes are much more likely to develop some of these adverse effects.

Drug Interactions

• Interaction with Rifampin decreases the effectiveness of oral contraceptives. The same may be true of barbiturates, Phenylbutazone, Phenytoin, Ampicillin, Neomycin, Penicillin, Tetracycline, Chloramphenicol, sulfa drugs, Griseofulvin, Nitrofurantoin, tranquilizers, and antimigraine medication.

• Oral contraceptives can reduce the breakdown of certain Benzodiazepine tranquilizers and sleeping pills, Caffeine, Metoprolol, Corticosteroids, Theophylline drugs, and tricyclic antidepressants, increasing the amount of drug in the blood and the chances for drug side effects and toxicities.

• Oral contraceptives may increase the toxic effect of Acetaminophen on your liver. Also, Acetaminophen effectiveness may be reduced by your oral contraceptive. Another interaction may reduce the effect of anticoagulant (blood-thinning) drugs, but an increased effect has also been reported. Discuss this with your doctor.

• Oral contraceptives may decrease the effects of salicylate pain relievers (including Aspirin), Clofibrate, Lorazepam, Oxazepam, and Temazepam by increasing the rate at which they are broken down by the liver.

• The Pill can increase blood-cholesterol (fat) levels, and can interfere with blood tests for thyroid function and blood sugar.

Food Interactions

These drugs may be taken without regard to food or meals.

Usual Dose

The first day of bleeding is the first day of the menstrual cycle. At the start, 1 tablet, beginning on the 5th day of the menstrual cycle, is taken every day for 20 to 21 days according to the number of contraceptive tablets supplied by the manufacturer. If menstrual flow has not begun 7 days after taking the last tablet, begin the next month's cycle of pills.

Manufacturers of some Pills recommend starting them on a Sunday to make it easy to remember to take them. If yours is one of these, start on the first Sunday after your period begins. If menstruation begins on a Sunday, take the first tablet on that day.

Progestin-only mini-pills are taken every day, 365 days a year.

Overdosage

Overdosage may cause nausea and withdrawal bleeding in adult females. Accidental overdosage in children who take their mothers' pills has not caused serious adverse effects; however, overdose victims should be taken to a hospital emergency room for evaluation and treatment. ALWAYS bring the medicine package with you.

Special Information

Use an alternative method of birth control during the first 3 weeks you are taking the Pill to be sure to prevent an accidental pregnancy at this time.

Take your Pill at the same time each day to establish a routine and ensure maximum contraceptive protection.

Call your doctor immediately if you develop sudden, severe abnominal pains; severe or sudden headaches; pains in the chest, groin, or leg (especially the calf); sudden slurring of your speech; changes in vision; weakness, numbness, or unexplained pains in an arm or leg; or if you start coughing up blood; lose coordination; or become suddenly short of breath.

Other problems that may develop and require medical attention are bulging eyes; changes in vaginal bleeding patterns; fainting; frequent or painful urination; a gradual increase in blood pressure; breast lumps or secretions; mental depression; yellow eyes or skin; skin rash; redness or irritation; upper abdominal swelling, pain, or tenderness; an unusual or dark-colored mole; thick, white vaginal discharge; or vaginal itching or tenderness. Other symptoms that may develop while taking contraceptive products require medical attention only if they are unusually bothersome or persistent.

See your doctor every 6 to 12 months to check on your progress.

Some manufacturers include 7 blank or 7 iron pills in their packages, to be taken on days when the Pill is not taken. These pills have the number 28 as part of the brand name, and a pill should be taken every day.

For the single or 2-phase pills: If you forget to take the Pill for 1 day, take 2 pills the following day. If you miss 2 consecutive days, take 2 pills for the next 2 days. Then continue to take 1 pill daily. If you miss 3 consecutive days, don't take any Pills for the next 7 days and use another form of contraception; then start a new cycle.

For the 3-phase pills: If you forget to take the Pill for 1 day, take 2 pills the following day and then continue with your regular dose. If you miss 2 consecutive days, take 2 pills for the next 2 days. Then continue to take 1 pill daily. If you forget to take the Pill for 3 days in a row, stop taking the medicine and use an alternate means of contraception until your period comes. ALWAYS use a backup contraceptive method for the remainder of your cycle if you forget even one 3-phase pill.

Forgetting to take the Pill reduces your protection: If you keep forgetting to take it, you should use another means of birth control.

If you must take any medication listed in the *Drug Interactions* section, use a backup contraceptive method during that cycle to prevent accidental pregnancy.

It is important to maintain good dental hygiene while taking this drug and to use extra care when using your toothbrush or dental floss because of the chance that the drug will make you more susceptible to some infections. See your dentist regularly while taking a contraceptive product. Check with your dentist if you notice swelling or bleeding of your gums.

You may be more sensitive to the sun while taking oral contraceptives.

You may become intolerant to contact lenses because of minor changes in the shape of your eyes.

All oral contraceptive prescriptions must come with a "patient package insert" for you to read. It gives detailed information about the drug and is required by federal law.

Special Population

Pregnancy/Breast-feeding

Oral contraceptives cause birth defects or can interfere with your baby's development. They are not safe for use during pregnancy.

Oral contraceptives reduce the amount of breast milk you make and can affect its quality. Some of the hormone passes into breast milk, but the effect on a nursing infant is not known. Do not breast-feed while you are taking oral contraceptives.

Type of Drug

Corticosteroids

Brand Names

Generic Name: Betamethasone

Celestone Tablet/Syrup

Generic Name: Cortisone Acetate*

Cortone

Generic Name: Dexamethasone*

Decadron Tablet/Elixir	Hexadrol Tablets/Elixir
Dexameth Tablet	Maxidex Tablets
Dexone Tablets	

Generic Name: Hydrocortisone*

Cortef Tablet/Suspension
Cortenema
Hydrocortone

Generic Name: Methylprednisolone*

Medrol

Generic Name: Prednisolone*

Delta-Cortef
Prelone

Generic Name: Prednisone*

Deltasone	Panasol-S	Sterapred
Liquid Pred	Prednicen-M	Sterapred DS
Meticorten	Prednisone	
Orasone	Intensol	

Generic Name: Triamcinolone*

Aristocort   Kenacort

(*Also available in generic form)

Prescribed for

Corticosteroids are prescribed for a wide variety of disorders, from skin rash to cancer. They may be used to treat adrenal gland disease because one of the hormones produced by the adrenal gland is very similar to these synthetic corticosteroid drugs. If patients are not producing enough adrenal hormones, corticosteroids may be used as replacement therapy. They may also be prescribed to treat the following: bursitis; arthritis; severe skin reactions (such as psoriasis or other rashes); severe or disabling allergies; asthma; drug or serum sickness; severe respiratory diseases (including pneumonitis); blood disorders; gastrointestinal diseases (including ulcerative colitis); and inflammation of the nerves, heart, or other organs.

Dexamethasone is also used to treat "mountain sickness," vomiting, bronchial disease in premature babies, the diagnosis of depression (controversial), and excessive hairiness, and to reduce hearing loss associated with bacterial meningitis.

General Information

The major differences among the corticosteroids are potency of medication and variation in some secondary effects. Choosing one corticosteroid for a specific disease is usually a matter of doctor preference and past experience. Taking 5 mg of Prednisone as the basic drug for comparison purposes, equivalent doses of other corticosteroids are: Betamethasone (0.6 mg to 0.75 mg), Cortisone (25 mg), Dexamethasone (0.75 mg), Hydrocortisone (20 mg), Methylprednisolone (4 mg), Prednisolone (5 mg), and Triamcinolone (4 mg).

Cautions and Warnings

If you are **allergic** to one corticosteroid, chances are you are allergic to all; you should avoid using corticosteroids.

Corticosteroids can **mask the symptoms** of a current infection, and **new infections** may appear during their use because your immune system is compromised by these drugs. Should this happen, a relatively minor infection that would respond to ordinary treatments can turn into a major problem. Corticosteroids may impair the immune response to **hepatitis B**, prolonging recovery. They can **reactivate** dormant **amebiasis**, an infection usually acquired in the tropics. Corticosteroids should not be taken if you have a **fungus blood infection**, because they could actually make it easier for the infection to spread. They should be used with caution by people with **tuberculosis**.

Long-term use of any corticosteroid drug can increase your chances of developing **cataracts**, **glaucoma**, or **eye infections** (viral or fungal, especially).

Because of the effect of corticosteroids on your adrenal glands, it is essential that when it is time for you to stop taking the drug, the dose be **gradually reduced by your doctor** over a period of time. If you stop taking this medication suddenly or without the advice of your doctor, you could experience adrenal gland failure, which can have extremely serious consequences.

If you are taking large corticosteroid doses, you should not be **vaccinated** with any **live virus vaccines,** because corticosteroids will interfere with the body's normal reaction to the vaccine. Discuss this with your doctor before you receive any vaccine.

Hydrocortisone and Cortisone can lead to **high blood pressure** because of their effect on blood sodium and other electrolytes. This is less of a problem with other corticosteroids.

Corticosteroids should be used with caution if you have **severe kidney disease**.

High-dose or long-term corticosteroid therapy may aggravate or worsen **stomach ulcers**. For Prednisone, this may not happen until the total dose reaches 1000 mg. For other corticosteroids, the dose required to have this effect depends on the drug: Betamethasone and Dexamethasone (150 mg), Cortisone (5000 mg), Hydrocortisone (4000 mg), Prednisolone (1000 mg), Triamcinolone and Methylprednisolone (800 mg).

People who have recently stopped taking a corticosteroid and who are going through **stressful situations** may need small doses of a rapid-acting corticosteroid (Hydrocortisone) to get them through the period of stress. Call your doctor if you think this is happening to you.

Use corticosteroids with care if you have had a recent **heart attack,** or if you have **ulcerative colitis, heart failure, high blood pressure, blood-clotting tendencies, thrombophlebitis, osteoporosis, antibiotic-resistant infections, Cushing's disease, myasthenia gravis, metastatic cancer, diabetes, underactive thyroid disease, cirrhosis of the liver,** or **seizure disorders**.

Corticosteroid **psychosis** (euphoria or feeling "high," delirium, sleeplessness, mood swings, personality changes, and severe depression) may develop in people taking large doses of Prednisone or Prednisolone (more than 40 mg a day). These symptoms can develop with other corticosteroids taken in equivalent doses (see *General Information* for drug equivalencies). Symptoms usually develop within 15 to 30 days of taking the drug; these symptoms may also be linked to other factors, including a **family history of psychosis** and **female gender**.

Corticosteroids may be used for speeding the recovery from attacks of **multiple sclerosis,** but they don't fight the underlying disease or slow its progression.

Corticosteroid products often contain **tartrazine dyes** (to add color) and **sulfites** (preservatives), two chemicals to which many people are **allergic** (wheezing, rashes, etc). Check with your pharmacist to determine if the product you are using contains tartrazine dyes or sulfites.

Possible Side Effects

▼ Most common: stomach upset, which may, in some cases, lead to stomach or duodenal ulcers.

▼ Common: water retention, heart failure, potassium loss, muscle weakness, loss of muscle mass, slow wound healing, black-and-blue marks on the skin, increased sweating, allergic skin rash, itching, convulsions, dizziness, and headache. Corticosteroids may also cause a loss of calcium, which may result in bone fractures and a condition known as *aseptic necrosis* of the femoral and humoral heads (the ends of the large bones in the hip degenerate from loss of calcium).

▼ Less common: irregular menstrual cycles, slow growth in children (particularly after the medication has been taken for long periods of time), adrenal and/or pituitary gland suppression, developing diabetes, drug sensitivity or allergic reactions, blood clots, insomnia, weight gain, increased appetite, nausea, and feelings of ill health. Psychological derangements may appear, which range from euphoria (feeling "high") to mood swings, personality changes, and severe depression. Prednisone may also aggravate existing emotional instability.

Drug Interactions

• Tell your doctor if you are taking any oral anticoagulant (blood-thinning) drugs if a corticosteroid is being considered; the anticoagulant dose may have to be changed.

• Interaction with diuretics (such as Hydrochlorothiazide) may cause the loss of blood potassium. Signs of low blood-potassium levels include weakness, muscle cramps, and tiredness; report any of these symptoms to your physician. Eat high-potassium foods such as bananas, citrus fruits, melons, and tomatoes. Digitalis drug side effects may be increased because of low blood potassium.

• Oral contraceptives, Estrogens, Erythromycin, Azithromycin, Clarithromycin, and Ketoconazole may increase the effects of corticosteroid drugs, increasing the chance of corticosteroid side effects.

• Barbiturates, Aminoglutethimide, Phenytoin and other hydantoin anticonvulsants, Rifampin, Ephedrine, Colestipol, and Cholestyramine may reduce corticosteroid effectiveness.

• Corticosteroids may decrease the effects of Aspirin (and other salicylate drugs), growth hormones, and Isoniazid.

• Corticosteroids and Theophylline drugs may interact to alter the requirements of either or both drugs. Your doctor will have to determine the proper dosage levels of each.

• Corticosteroids can interfere with laboratory tests. Tell your doctor if you are taking any of these drugs so that the tests can be properly analyzed.

Food Interactions

Take these medications with food or a small amount of antacid to avoid stomach upset. If stomach upset continues, notify your doctor.

Usual Dose

Betamethasone

Initial dose: 0.6 to 7.2 mg a day. *Maintenance dose:* 0.6 to 7.2 mg a day, depending on response.

Cortisone

Initial dose: 25 to 300 mg a day. *Maintenance dose:* 25 to 300 mg a day, depending on response.

Dexamethasone

Initial dose: 0.75 to 9 (or more) mg a day. *Maintenance dose:* 0.75 to 9 mg a day, depending on response and disease being treated. The lowest effective dose is desirable. Stressful situations may cause a need for a temporary increase in your Dexamethasone dose. Dexamethasone may also be given in "alternate-day" therapy (twice the usual daily dose is given every other day).

Hydrocortisone

Initial dose: 20 to 240 mg a day. *Maintenance dose:* 20 to 240 mg a day, depending on individual response.

Methylprednisolone

Initial dose: 4 to 48 (or more) mg a day. *Maintenance dosage:* varies according to your response and the disease being treated. The lowest effective dose is desirable. Stressful situations may cause a need for a temporary increase in your Methylprednisolone dose. It may be given in "alternate-day" therapy (twice the usual daily dose is given every other day).

Prednisone and Prednisolone

Initial dose: 5 to 60 (or more) mg a day. *Maintenance dose:* 5 to 60 mg a day, depending on your response and the disease being treated. The lowest effective dose is desirable. Stressful situations may cause a need for a temporary increase in your Prednisone or Prednisolone dose. Prednisone and Prednisolone may be given in "alternate-day" therapy (twice the usual daily dose is given every other day).

Overdosage

Symptoms of corticosteroid overdosage are anxiety, depression and/or stimulation, stomach bleeding, increased blood sugar, high blood pressure, and water retention. The victim should be taken to a hospital emergency room immediately, where stomach pumping, oxygen, intravenous fluids, and other supportive treatments are available. ALWAYS bring the medicine bottle with you.

Special Information

Do not stop taking this medicine on your own. Suddenly stopping any corticosteroid drug can have severe consequences; the dosage must be gradually reduced by your doctor.

Call your doctor if you develop unusual weight gain, black or tarry stools, swelling of the feet or legs, muscle weakness, vomiting of blood, menstrual irregularity, prolonged sore throat, fever, cold or infection, appetite loss, nausea and vomiting, diarrhea, weight loss, weakness, dizziness, or low blood sugar.

If you miss a corticosteroid dose and you take several doses a day, take the missed dose as soon as you can. If it is almost time for your next dose, skip the missed dose and double the next dose.

If you take one dose a day and you do not remember the

missed dose until the next day, skip the missed dose and take your usual dose. Do not take a double dose.

If you take a corticosteroid every other day, take the missed dose if you remember it that morning. If it is much later in the day, skip the missed dose and take it the following morning, then go back to your usual dose schedule. Do not take a double dose.

Special Populations

Pregnancy/Breast-feeding

Studies have shown that taking large doses of corticosteroids over long periods can cause birth defects. Chronic use during the first 3 months of pregnancy can lead to birth defects. Pregnant women should not take a corticosteroid unless the risks have been considered.

Corticosteroid drugs taken by mouth may pass into breast milk. As long as the daily dose is relatively low (Prednisone or Prednisolone less than 20 mg; Methylprednisolone less than 8 mg) and the medicine is being taken for a short time, the amount of drug that appears in breast milk is usually negligible. Nursing mothers taking doses in this range should either consider bottle-feeding their babies or wait 3 to 4 hours after each corticosteroid dose to nurse or collect breast milk. Those taking larger corticosteroid doses should bottle-feed their babies.

Seniors

Lower doses may be more desirable in older adults because they are as effective and cause fewer problems. Older adults are more likely to develop high blood pressure while taking an oral corticosteroid. Also, older women are more susceptible to osteoporosis (bone degeneration) associated with large doses of corticosteroids.

Type of Drug

Corticosteroid Eyedrops

Brand Names

Generic Name: Fluorometholone

Flarex	FML Forte
Fluor-Op	FML S.O.P.
FML	

Generic Name: Medrysone

HMS

Generic Name: Prednisolone

AK-Pred*	Inflamase Mild*
Econopred*	Pred Mild
Inflamase Forte*	Pred Forte

Generic Name: Dexamethasone

AK-Dex Solution/Ointment*	Maxidex Suspension/ Ointment*

Generic Name: Rimexolone

Vexol Suspension

(*Also available in generic form)

Prescribed for

Allergic and inflammatory conditions of the eye.

General Information

Corticosteroids produce a generalized reduction in inflammation throughout the body. When applied directly to the eye, they provide uniform relief of symptoms and are prescribed for general relief of allergies and inflammations. Very severe eye conditions that don't respond to eyedrops or ointments may require treatment with corticosteroid drugs taken by mouth. Fluorometholone, Medrysone, and Prednisolone (up to 0.125%) are preferred for long-term treatment because they are least likely to raise eye pressure.

Cautions and Warnings

Do not use these products if you are **allergic** or **sensitive** to them. Corticosteroid eyedrops should be used with care if you have a **fungus infection, herpes, tuberculosis,** or **virus infection** in the eye, or if you have **cataracts, glaucoma,** or **diabetes.**

Possible Side Effects

▼ Rare: watery eyes; glaucoma; optic nerve damage; gradual blurring or reduction or loss of vision; eye pain; nausea; vomiting; eye infections; and eye burning, stinging, or redness.

Drug Interactions

• Corticosteroids may, when applied to the eye, interfere with the effect of antiglaucoma drugs.
• The risk of raising pressure in the eye is increased when corticosteroid eyedrops are taken with anticholinergic drugs, especially Atropine, over a long period of time.

Food Interactions

None.

Usual Dose

Eyedrops
1 to 2 drops several times a day.

Eye Ointment
Place a thin strip of ointment into the affected eye(s) several times a day.

Overdosage:

Generally, swallowing a container of corticosteroid eyedrops or ointment does not produce serious effects. Call your doctor or your local poison center for information in the event of an accidental overdose.

Special Information

If you forget a dose of corticosteroid eyedrops or ointment, apply it as soon as you remember. If it is almost time for your next dose, skip the one you forgot and continue with your regular schedule.

To administer eyedrops, lie down or tilt your head backward and look at the ceiling. Hold the dropper above your eye and drop the medicine inside your lower lid while looking up. To prevent infection, keep the dropper from touching your fingers, eyelids, or any surface. Release the lower lid and keep your eye open. Don't blink for about 30 seconds. Press gently on the bridge of your nose at the inside corner of your eye for about 1 minute. This will help circulate the medicine around your eye. Wait at least 5 minutes before using any other eyedrops.

To use an eye ointment, tilt your head back and, with your index finger, gently pull your lower eyelid away from the eye to make a small space. Squeeze a thin strip of the ointment into the space; usually, about 1/3 inch is enough. Let go of the lower lid and close your eye for 1 to 2 minutes to allow the medicine to move around your eye.

Special Populations

Pregnancy/Breast-feeding

Problems have not been found in women using a corticosteroid eye product during their pregnancy. However, babies born to mothers who used large amounts of corticosteroid eyedrops during pregnancy should be watched for possible effects on the babies' adrenal gland. Consult your doctor.

Nursing mothers have used corticosteroid eyedrops without problems.

Seniors

Older adults may use these products without special precaution.

Type of Drug

Corticosteroid Inhalers

Brand Names

Generic Name: Beclomethasone

Beclovent Aerosol
Vanceril Aerosol

Generic Name: Dexamethasone Sodium Phosphate

Decadron Phosphate Respihaler

Generic Name: Flunisolide

AeroBid
AeroBid-M

Generic Name: Triamcinolone Acetonide

Azmacort Aerosol

Prescribed for

Chronic asthma and bronchial disease.

General Information

Corticosteroid inhalers relieve the symptoms associated with bronchial asthma and disease by reducing inflammation of the mucosal lining of the bronchi, making it easier to breathe. Asthma experts have come to recognize these drugs as essential to asthma treatment because all asthma is, in part, an inflammatory disease. Many believe that virtually all people with asthma should be taking an inhaled corticosteroid as part of their regular treatment. Corticosteroid inhalers produce the same effect as taking steroid tablets by mouth, with some important differences. These medicines are applied specifically to the area where they are needed. So you can get the same effect with a much smaller dose and without affecting other parts of the body, with the exception of a small portion of the medicine that is absorbed into the bloodstream. Corticosteroid inhalers are meant to be taken regularly to prevent an asthma attack; they will not relieve an acute asthma attack.

Cautions and Warnings

Do not use these drugs if you are **allergic** to any corticosteroid. Corticosteroid inhalers cannot be used as the primary treatment of **severe asthma**. They are intended only for people who take Prednisone (or other adrenal corticosteroids) by mouth and those who do not respond to other asthma drugs.

Combining Prednisone (or another oral corticosteroid) with a corticosteroid inhaler may cause **pituitary gland suppression**. The **combination of oral and nasal steroids** should be taken with caution.

Even though these drugs are inhaled directly into the lungs, they are potent adrenal corticosteroids. During periods of **severe stress,** you may have to go back to taking corticosteroids by mouth if the inhaler does not control your asthma.

Death because of **adrenal gland failure** has occurred in asthma patients during and after having been switched from oral corticosteroids to an aerosol product. Switching from oral to aerosol corticosteroid therapy requires several months to restore the body's natural corticosteroid production system.

Corticosteroid inhalers may be associated with **immediate or delayed drug reactions** (including breathing difficulty, rash, and bronchospasm).

During periods of **stress** or a **severe asthmatic attack,** people who have stopped using their inhaler should **contact their doctor** to find out about taking an oral corticosteroid.

Possible Side Effects

▼ Most common: dry mouth and hoarseness. Corticosteroid inhalers can also cause skin rash or bronchospasm.

▼ Other: cough, wheezing, and facial swelling. Corticosteroid inhaler-related cough and wheezing are probably caused by an ingredient in the product other than the corticosteroid itself. A chemical added to help disperse the drug around the lungs has been implicated as the cause of this side effect. Newer administration systems that omit this ingredient may minimize this problem.

Possible Side Effects *(continued)*

Deaths caused by adrenal gland failure have occurred in people who took adrenal corticosteroid tablets or syrup and were switched to Beclomethasone by inhalation. This is a rare complication and usually results from stopping the liquid or tablets too quickly. They must be stopped gradually over a long period of time. Adrenal gland suppression has occurred in people taking 38 puffs of Beclomethasone or 40 puffs of Triamcinolone a day for 1 month, or recommended doses of these drugs for 6 to 12 weeks.

Drug and Food Interactions

None known.

Usual Dose

Beclomethasone

Adult and Adolescent (age 13 and older): 2 inhalations (84 micrograms) 3 or 4 times a day, or 4 inhalations twice a day. People with severe asthma may take up to 16 inhalations a day.

Child (age 6 to 12): 1 or 2 inhalations 3 to 4 times a day.

Dexamethasone

Adult and Adolescent (age 13 and older): 3 inhalations (252 micrograms) 3 or 4 times a day.

Child (age 6 to 12): 2 inhalations (168 micrograms) 3 or 4 times a day.

Flunisolide

Adult and Adolescent (age 16 and older): 2 inhalations (500 micrograms) morning and evening. Do not take more than 8 inhalations a day.

Child (age 6 to 15): 2 inhalations (500 micrograms) morning and evening. Do not take more than 4 inhalations a day.

Triamcinolone

Adult and Adolescent (age 13 and older): 2 inhalations (200 micrograms) 3 or 4 times a day. Do not take more than 16 inhalations a day unless specifically directed to do so by your doctor.

Child (age 6 to 12): 1 or 2 inhalations (100 to 200 micrograms) 3 or 4 times a day. Do not take more than 12 inhalations a day.

Overdosage

Serious adverse effects are unlikely after swallowing an inhaled corticosteroid. Excessive use or large amounts of these products may require gradual product discontinuation and, in extreme situations, could parallel symptoms of overdose of oral corticosteroids. Call your local poison control center or hospital emergency room for more information.

Special Information

People using both one of these drugs and a bronchodilator, such as Albuterol, should use the bronchodilator first, wait a few minutes, then use the corticosteroid inhaler. This will allow more corticosteroid to be absorbed.

These drugs are for preventive therapy only and will not affect an asthma attack. Inhaled corticosteroids must be taken regularly, as directed. Wait at least 1 minute between inhalations.

To properly use this product, thoroughly shake the inhaler, if yours is one that must be shaken. Take a drink of water to moisten your throat. Place the inhaler two finger-widths away from your mouth and tilt your head back slightly. While activating your inhaler, take a slow deep breath for 3 to 5 seconds, then hold your breath for about 10 seconds and breathe out slowly. Allow at least 1 minute between puffs. Rinse your mouth after each use to reduce dry mouth and hoarseness.

If you forget a dose of your inhaler, take it as soon as you remember. If it is almost time for your next dose, skip the forgotten dose and continue with your regular schedule. Do not take a double dose.

Special Populations

Pregnancy/Breast-feeding

Using large amounts of corticosteroids during pregnancy may slow fetal growth. Corticosteroids may cause birth defects or interfere with fetal development. Check with your doctor before taking any of these if you are, or might be, pregnant.

Taken by mouth, corticosteroids may pass into breast milk and cause unwanted effects in nursing infants. It is not known if inhaled corticosteroids find their way into breast milk.

Seniors

Older adults may use corticosteroid inhalers without special restriction. Be sure your doctor knows if you suffer from bone disease, bowel disease, colitis, diabetes, glaucoma, fungal or herpes infections, high blood pressure, high blood cholesterol, an underactive thyroid, or heart, kidney, or liver disease.

Type of Drug

Corticosteroids, Nasal

Brand Names

Generic Name: Beclomethasone

| Beconase Intranasal Aerosol | Beconase AQ Nasal Spray | Vancenase AQ Nasal Spray |

Generic Name: Budesonide

Rhinocort

Generic Name: Dexamethasone Sodium Phosphate

Decadron Phosphate Turbinaire

Generic Name: Flunisolide

Nasalide
Nasarel

Generic Name: Fluticasone

Flonase

Generic Name: Triamcinolone Acetonide

Nasacort

Prescribed for

Seasonal or chronic (allergic or other) nasal inflammation; preventing the recurrence of nasal polyps after surgery; nonallergic nasal passage inflammation.

General Information

Nasal corticosteroids are specially formulated for use as a nasal spray. They are prescribed to treat severe symptoms of seasonal allergy when other product types (decongestants, etc) are not working. They work by reducing inflammation of the mucosal lining of the nasal passages, making it easier to breathe. These medications may take several days to have an effect. Do not use them continuously for more than 3 weeks unless they have produced a definite benefit for you. Fluticasone and Triamcinolone are approved only for allergic rhinitis. Other products are approved for both allergic and nonallergic uses.

Cautions and Warnings

Do not use a nasal corticosteroid if you are **allergic** to any of its ingredients. On rare occasions, serious and life-threatening drug-sensitivity reactions have occurred.

If your nose is **severely congested,** you may need to use a nasal decongestant before using your nasal steroid to get the best effect.

Combining Prednisone (or another oral corticosteroid) with a nasal corticosteroid may cause **pituitary gland suppression,** though nasal steroids by themselves rarely cause this problem. The combination of oral and nasal steroids should be taken with caution and only under your doctor's care.

On rare occasions, *Candida* **infections (yeast)** of the nose and throat may develop. If this happens, your steroid may be discontinued and other therapy may be prescribed.

Even though these drugs are taken by direct inhalation into the nose, they should be considered potent adrenal corticosteroid drugs. During periods of **severe stress,** you may have to go back to taking an oral corticosteroid drug if the nasal product does not control your symptoms.

Possible Side Effects

▼ Most common: mild irritation of the nose, nasal passages and throat, burning, stinging, dryness, and headache.

▼ Less common: light-headedness, nausea, nosebleeds or bloody mucus, unusual nasal congestion, bronchial asthma, sneezing attacks, runny nose, throat discomfort, and loss of the sense of taste.

▼ Rare: ulcers of the nasal passages, watery eyes, sore throat, vomiting, drug-hypersensitivity reactions (itching, rash, swelling, bronchospasms, and breathing difficulty), nasal infections, wheezing, perforation of the septal wall between your nostrils, and increased eye pressure.

Very rarely, deaths caused by failure of the adrenal gland have occurred in people taking adrenal corticosteroid tablets or syrup who were switched to a nasal corticosteroid and probably stopped taking the liquid or tablets too quickly; they must be stopped gradually over a long period of time.

Drug and Food Interactions

None known.

Usual Dose

Beclomethasone

Adult and Adolescent (age 13 and older): 1 spray (42 micrograms) in each nostril 2 to 4 times a day.

Child (age 6 to 12): 1 spray (42 micrograms) in each nostril 3 times a day.

Budesonide

Adult and Child (age 6 and older): 2 sprays (32 micrograms) in each nostril morning and evening, or 4 sprays in the morning.

Dexamethasone

Adult and Adolescent (age 13 and older): 2 sprays (168 micrograms) in each nostril 3 times a day; not more than 12 sprays a day.

Child (age 6 to 12): 1 or 2 sprays (84 to 168 micrograms) into each nostril 2 times a day; not more than 8 sprays a day.

Flunisolide

Adult and Adolescent (age 15 and older): 2 sprays (50 micrograms) in each nostril, 2 times a day to start. Dose may be increased up to 8 sprays a day in each nostril.

Child (age 6 to 14): 1 spray (25 micrograms) in each nostril 3 times a day, or 2 sprays in each nostril 2 times a day.

Fluticasone

Adult: two sprays in each nostril (50 micrograms each) once a day, or divided in two doses, to start. Dosage may be reduced in half in a few days, if tolerated.

Adolescent (age 12 and older): one spray per nostril once a day. Dosage may be increased if needed to 2 sprays per nostril a day.

Child (under age 12): not recommended.

Triamcinolone

Adult and Adolescent (age 13 and older): 2 sprays (220 micrograms) in each nostril once per day. Dose may be increased to 4 sprays per day in each nostril. Relief may be felt as soon as 12 hours after you start using this product, but the rate of response widely varies.

Child (age 12 and under): not recommended.

Overdosage

Serious adverse effects are unlikely after swallowing a nasal corticosteroid. Excessive use of large amounts of nasal corticosteroids may require gradual product discontinuation. Call your local poison control center or hospital emergency room for more information.

Special Information

It may be necessary to clear your nasal passages with a nasal decongestant before using one of these medicines to allow it to reach your nasal mucosa.

Some of these products must be used for 10 to 14 days before they start working. Beclomethasone, Budesonide, and Triamcinolone work faster, in 3 to 7 days. Flunisolide may take up to 3 weeks.

If you are applying more than one puff at a time, wait at least 1 minute between inhalations.

Nasal corticosteroids can cause irritation and drying of the nasal mucosa. Call your doctor if this effect persists or if your symptoms get worse.

Rarely, nasal *Candida* (yeast) infections have developed in people taking a nasal steroid. Such an infection may require treatment with an antifungal medicine and discontinuing your nasal steroid treatments.

People using nasal corticosteroids to prevent the return of nasal polyps after surgery may experience some nosebleeds because the steroids can slow the wound-healing process.

If you forget a dose of nasal corticosteroid, take it as soon as you remember. If it is almost time for your next dose, skip the forgotten dose and continue with your regular schedule. Do not take a double dose.

Special Populations

Pregnancy/Breast-feeding
Taking large amounts of corticosteroids during pregnancy may slow fetal growth. The small amount of medicine absorbed into the blood after nasal application is unlikely to have any effect. Nevertheless, talk with your doctor before taking any medicine if you are, or might be, pregnant.

Dexamethasone passes into breast milk. Nursing mothers who are using it should bottle-feed their babies. It is not known if other nasal steroids pass into breast milk. Nursing mothers should be cautious about using these drugs.

Seniors
Seniors may use these drugs without special restriction. Be sure your doctor knows if you suffer from bone disease, bowel disease, colitis, diabetes, glaucoma, fungal or herpes infections, high blood pressure, high blood cholesterol, an underactive thyroid, or heart, kidney, or liver disease.

Type of Drug

Corticosteroids, Topical

Brand Names

Generic Name: Aclometasone Dipropionate

Aclovate Cream/Ointment

Generic Name: Amcinonide

Cyclocort Cream/Lotion/Ointment

Generic Name: Augmented Betamethasone Dipropionate

Diprolene Cream/Gel/Lotion/Ointment
Diprolene AF

Generic Name: Betamethasone*

Alphatrex Cream/ Lotion/ Ointment	Diprosone Aerosol/Cream/ Lotion/Ointment	Uticort Cream/Gel/ Lotion
Betatrex Cream/ Lotion/Ointment	Maxivate Cream/ Lotion/Ointment	Valisone Cream/ Lotion/Ointment
Beta-Val Cream/ Lotion/Ointment	Teladar Cream	Valisone Reduced Strength Cream

Generic Name: Clobetasol Propionate*

Embeline
Temovate Cream/Ointment/Scalp Application

Generic Name: Clocortolone Pivalate

Cloderm Cream

Generic Name: Desonide

Desonide Cream
DesOwen Cream/Lotion/Ointment
Tridesilon Cream/Ointment/Otic Solution

Generic Name: Desoximetasone*

Topicort Emollient Cream/Gel/Ointment
Topicort LP Emollient Cream

Generic Name: Dexamethasone

Aeroseb-Dex Aerosol
Decadron Cream
Decaspray Aerosol

Generic Name: Diflorasone Diacetate

Florone Cream/	Maxiflor Cream/	Psorcon Cream/
Ointment	Ointment	Ointment
Florone E Cream		

Generic Name: Fluocinolone Acetonide*

Derma-Smoothe/	Flurosyn Cream/	Synalar Cream/
FS Oil	Ointment	Ointment/Topical
Fluonid Topical	FS Shampoo	Solution
Solution		Synalar-HP Cream
		Synemol Cream

Generic Name: Fluocinonide*

Fluonex Cream Lidex Cream/Gel/Ointment/Solution
Lidex-E Cream

Generic Name: Flurandrenolide*

Cordran Lotion/Ointment/Tape
Cordran SP Cream

Generic Name: Fluticasone Propionate

Cutivate Cream/Ointment

Generic Name: Halcinonide

Halog Cream/Ointment/Solution
Halog-E Cream

Generic Name: Halobetasol Propionate

Ultravate Cream/Ointment

Generic Name: Hydrocortisone*

1% HC Ointment	Ala-Cort Cream/	Anucort-HC
Acticort 100 Lotion	Lotion	Suppositories
Aeroseb-HC	Ala-Scalp Lotion	Anumed HC
Aerosol	Analpram HC	Anusol-HC Cream/
	Cream	Suppositories

Bactine
  Hydrocortisone
  Cream
CaldeCort
  Aerosol/Cream
CaldeCort Light
  Cream with Aloe
  Cream
Cetacort Lotion
CortaGel
Cortaid Spray
Cortaid with Aloe
  Cream/Ointment
Cortenema
Cort-Dome Cream/
  Lotion
Cortef Feminine
  Itch Cream
Corticaine Cream
Cortizone-5
  Cream/Ointment
Cortifoam
Cortizone-10
  Ointment

Dermacort Cream/
  Lotion
Dermol HC
  Ointment/Cream
Dermolate Cream
Dermtex HC with
  Aloe Cream
Gynecort Cream
Hydrocort Cream
Hemril HC
  Uniserts
Hi-Cor Cream
Hycort Cream/
  Lotion/Ointment
Hydro-Tex Cream
Hytone Cream/
  Lotion/Ointment
Lacticare-HC
  Lotion
Lanacort Cream/
  Ointment
Maximum
  Strength
  Bactine Cream

Maximum
  Strength Cortaid
  Cream
Gynecort
Lanacort Cream
  Pramoxine HC
Nutracort Cream/
  Lotion
Proctocort Cream
Penecort Cream/
  Lotion
Proctocream HC
Proctofoam-HC
Synacort
S-T Cort Lotion
Tegrin HC
  Ointment
Texacort Solution
U-Cort Cream
Westcort Cream/
  Ointment

Generic Name: Methylprednisolone

Medrol Acetate Topical Ointment

Generic Name: Mometasone Furoate

Elocon Cream/Lotion/Ointment

Generic Name: Prednicarbate

Dermatop Cream

Generic Name: Triamcinolone Acetonide

Aristocort Cream/
  Ointment
Aristocort A
  Cream/Ointment
Delta-Tritex

Flutex Cream/
  Ointment
Kenalog Aerosol/
  Cream/Lotion/
  Ointment

Kenalog-H Cream
Triacet Cream
Triderm Cream
Kenonel Cream/
  Ointment

(*Also available in generic form)

Prescribed for

Temporary relief of inflammation, itching, or other local skin (dermatologic) problems. These products may also be prescribed to treat psoriasis, severe diaper rash, and other conditions.

General Information

Topical (applied to the skin) corticosteroids are used to relieve the symptoms of skin rash, itching, or inflammation; they do not treat the underlying cause of the skin problem. They do this by interfering with the natural body mechanisms that produce the rash, itching, or inflammation. If you use one of these drugs without finding the cause of the problem, the condition may return after you stop using the drug. You should not use a topical corticosteroid without your doctor's knowledge because it could cover an important reaction, one that may be valuable to your doctor in deciding what is wrong or treating you.

Some generic versions of topical corticosteroids vary in their potency from their brand-name cousins. Check with your doctor or pharmacist for more information on the interchangeability of these products.

Cautions and Warnings

Do not use a topical corticosteroid as the only treatment for a **viral disease** of the skin (such as herpes), **fungal infections** of the skin (such as athlete's foot), or **tuberculosis** of the skin. These drugs should not be used in the ear if the eardrum has been perforated. Do not use one of these drugs if you have a history of **allergies** to a component of the aerosol, cream, gel, lotion, ointment, or topical solution.

Rectal corticosteroid products should not be used if you have a **bowel perforation, obstruction, abscess, systemic fungus infection,** or **other serious bowel condition**.

The **rectal foam is not expelled** after it has been applied and may lead to more drug absorption than rectal enema products. Systemic side effects are possible because of drug absorbed into the blood. If there is no improvement after 2 or 3 weeks of a rectal product, see your doctor.

Using a topical corticosteroid around the eyes for prolonged periods can cause **cataracts** or **glaucoma**.

Children may be more susceptible to serious side effects of these products, especially if they are applied to large areas of the body over long periods. **Augmented Betamethasone Propionate, Clobetasol, Desoximetasone, Fluticasone,** and **Halobetasol** are not recommended for use on children.

Possible Side Effects

▼ Most common: burning sensation, itching, irritation, acne, skin dryness and cracking, skin tightening, secondary infection, and skin discoloration. These happen more often if the product is covered with an occlusive bandage (one that shuts out water and air).

Large amounts of corticosteroid may be absorbed through the skin into the bloodstream if large amounts are applied over a period of time. This results in systemic effects and can result in serious problems, particularly in people with liver disease.

Drug and Food Interactions

None known.

Usual Dose

Cream/Ointment/Aerosol
Apply to the skin 2 to 4 times a day.

Rectal Enema
100 mg nightly for 21 days.

Rectal Foam
One applicatorful 1 or 2 times a day for 2 to 3 weeks.

Overdosage

Excess topical steroid may be simply washed off the skin. In extreme situations, it may be necessary to gradually discontinue product usage. Serious adverse effects are unlikely after swallowing a topical corticosteroid product. Call your local poison control center or hospital emergency room for more information.

Special Information

Clean the skin before applying a topical corticosteroid to prevent secondary infection. Apply in a very thin film and rub in gently (effectiveness is based on contact area and not on the thickness of the layer applied).

To use a lotion, solution, or gel on your scalp, part your hair, apply a small amount of the product to the affected area, and rub in gently.

Do not wash, rub, or put clothing on the area until the medication has dried.

Flurandrenolide tape comes with specific directions for use; follow them carefully.

If your doctor instructs you to apply plastic wrap or another occlusive dressing on top of the corticosteroid product, be sure to follow those directions. These dressings can increase the penetration of the product into your skin by as much as 10 times, which may be a crucial element in the effectiveness of the product. Occlusive dressings should not be used with augmented Betamethasone, Betamethasone Proprionate, Clobetasol, Halobetasol, or Mometasone.

If you are using one of these products for diaper rash, do not use tight-fitting diapers or plastic pants, which may cause too much drug to be absorbed through the skin into the blood.

Your doctor may prescribe a specific form of the product for a specific reason. Do not change forms without your doctor's knowledge, as a different form may not be as effective.

If you forget to apply a dose of a topical corticosteroid, do so as soon as you remember. If it is almost time for your next dose, skip the one you forgot and continue with your regular schedule. Do not apply a double dose.

Special Populations

Pregnancy/Breast-feeding

Corticosteroids applied to the skin in large amounts or over long periods of time have been linked to birth defects. Pregnant women should not use this medicine except under a doctor's care. Nonprescription hydrocortisone products should not be used for more than a few days without your doctor's knowledge.

Corticosteroid drugs taken by mouth pass into breast milk, and large drug doses may interfere with the growth of a nursing infant. Steroids applied to the skin are not likely to cause problems, but you should not use the medicine unless you're under a doctor's care. If you must apply this medicine to the nipple area, be sure to completely clean that area prior to nursing. Nursing mothers should not use Clobetasol.

Seniors

Older adults are more likely to develop high blood pressure and are more susceptible to osteoporosis (bone degeneration) associated with large doses of corticosteroid taken by mouth. However, these effects are unlikely with a steroid applied to the skin, unless a high-potency product is used over a large area for an extended period.

Brand Name

Cortisporin Otic Solution

Ingredients

Hydrocortisone
Neomycin Sulfate
Polymyxin B Sulfate

Other Brand Names

AK-Spore H.C. Otic	Otic-Care
AntibiOtic	OtiTricin
Cortatrigen Ear Drops	Pediotic
Octicair	UAD Otic

(Also available in generic form)

Type of Drug

Antibiotic-corticosteroid combination.

Prescribed for

Superficial infections; ear inflammation or itching; other problems involving the outer ear.

General Information

Cortisporin Otic contains a corticosteroid drug to reduce

inflammation and 2 antibiotics to treat local infections. This combination can be quite useful for local ear problems because of its dual method of action and its relatively broad, nonspecific applicability.

Cortisporin eyedrops do not contain the antibiotic Polymyxin B that is included in the eardrops and, more importantly, they are made for use only in the eye.

Cautions and Warnings

Do not use this product if you are **sensitive** or **allergic** to any of its ingredients.

Cortisporin Otic is specifically designed to be used in the ear. It can be very **damaging** if accidentally placed into your **eye**.

Possible Side Effects

▼ Local irritation such as itching or burning can occur if you are sensitive or allergic to one of the ingredients in this drug.

Drug and Food Interactions

None known.

Usual Dose

2 to 4 drops in the affected ear 3 to 4 times a day.

Overdosage

The amount of medicine contained in each bottle of Cortisporin Otic is too small to cause serious problems. Call your doctor, hospital emergency room, or local poison control center for more information.

Special Information

Use only when specifically prescribed by a physician. Overuse of this or similar products can result in the growth of other organisms such as fungi.

If new infections or new problems appear during the time

you are using this medication, stop using the drug and contact your doctor.

When using eardrops, wash your hands, then hold the closed bottle in your hand for a few minutes to warm it to body temperature. Shake well for 10 seconds to mix the suspended antibiotic in the solution. For best results, drops should not be self-administered; they should be given by another person. The person receiving the drops should lie on his or her side with the affected ear facing upward. Fill the dropper and instill the required number of drops directly in the ear canal.

If the drops are being given to an infant, hold the earlobe *down* and back to allow the drops to run in. If the drops are being given to an older child or adult, hold the earlobe *up* and back to allow them to run in. Do not put the dropper into the ear or allow it to touch any part of the ear or bottle. Keep the ear tilted for about 2 minutes after the drops have been put in or insert a soft cotton plug, whichever is recommended by your doctor.

If you forget a dose of Cortisporin Otic Drops, take it as soon as you remember. If it is almost time for your next regularly scheduled dose, skip the forgotten dose and continue with your regular schedule. Do not apply a double dose.

Special Populations

Pregnancy/Breast-feeding
Pregnant and breast-feeding women may use this product without special restriction.

Seniors
Older adults may use this product without special restriction.

Coumadin

see **Warfarin Sodium**, page 1173

Generic Name

Cromolyn Sodium

Brand Names

Crolom 4% Ophthalmic Solution
Intal Capsules/Inhaler/Nebulizer Solution
Nasalcrom Nasal Solution
Gastrocrom Capsules

(Also available in generic form)

Type of Drug

Allergy preventive; antiasthmatic.

Prescribed for

Prevention of severe allergic reactions, including various types of asthma, runny nose, and mastocytosis. Cromolyn is also used to treat food allergies, eczema, dermatitis, chronic itching, and hay fever. It may be used to treat and prevent chronic inflammatory bowel disease; however, other drug products are more effective for this use. Cromolyn eyedrops are used to treat conjunctivitis ("pink eye") and other eye irritations.

General Information

Cromolyn prevents allergy, asthma, and other conditions by stabilizing mast cells, which are a key component to developing any allergic reaction because they release histamine. Cromolyn prevents the release of histamine and other potent chemicals from mast cells in your body. This is a normal part of the allergic process. The drug works only in the areas to which it is applied; very little is absorbed into the blood (7 to 8 percent of an inhaled dose and 1 percent of a swallowed capsule). Even the oral capsules, which one would normally expect to be absorbed into the blood, are swallowed to treat only gastrointestinal-tract allergies. Cromolyn products must be used on a regular basis to be effective in reducing the frequency and intensity of allergic reactions and their consequences.

Cautions and Warnings

Cromolyn should **never** be used to treat an **acute allergy attack**. It is intended only **to prevent or reduce the number of allergic attacks** and their intensity. Once the proper dosage level has been established for you, your attacks may return if your dosage is reduced below that level.

On rare occasions, people have experienced severe **allergic attacks** after taking Cromolyn. People allergic to Cromolyn should not take any product containing that ingredient.

People with **kidney or liver disease** should take reduced dosages of this drug.

Cough or bronchial spasm may occasionally occur after the inhalation of a Cromolyn dose. Severe bronchospasm is rare.

Cromolyn aerosol should be used with caution in people with **abnormal heart rhythms** or **diseased coronary blood vessels** because of a possible reaction to the propellants used in the product.

Possible Side Effects

▼ Most common: skin rash and itching.

▼ Other: reactions to the inhaler, nasal solution, and eyedrops include local irritation (nasal stinging or sneezing, tearing, cough, stuffed nose), urinary difficulty, dizziness, headache, joint swelling, a bad taste in the mouth, nosebleeds, abdominal pain, and nausea.

▼ Rare: Severe drug reactions, consisting of coughing, difficulty swallowing, hives, itching, difficulty breathing, or swelling of the eyelids, lips, or face.

Most reactions reported after the oral capsules are minor and could be symptoms of the disease; headache and diarrhea are the most common. A variety of other side effects to oral Cromolyn capsules have been reported but could not be conclusively tied to the drug.

Drug Interactions

None known.

Food Interactions

Inhaled or swallowed Cromolyn products should not be

mixed with any food, juice, or milk. The nasal and eye products may be taken without regard to food or meals.

Usual Dose

Inhaled capsules or solution:

Adult and child (age 2 and over): 20 mg 4 times a day to start. (Children under age 5 may inhale Cromolyn powder if their allergies are severe.) The solution must be given with a power-operated nebulizer and face mask. Handheld nebulizers are not adequate. To prevent exercise asthma, 20 mg may be inhaled up to 1 hour before exercise.

Aerosol:

Adult and child (age 5 and over): up to 2 sprays 4 times a day, spaced equally throughout the day. The contents of a single capsule or 2 aerosol puffs may be inhaled up to 1 hour before exercise to prevent exercise asthma.

Nasal solution:

Adult and child (age 6 and over): 1 spray in each nostril 3 to 6 times a day at regular intervals. Blow your nose first, and inhale the solution through your nose.

Oral capsules:

Adult: 2 capsules a half hour before meals and at bedtime.

Child (under age 2): about 10 mg per pound of body weight per day divided into 4 equal doses. This product is recommended in infants and young children only if absolutely necessary.

Child (age 2 to 12): 1 capsule (100 mg) 4 times per day a half hour before meals and at bedtime, up to about 15 to 20 mg per pound of body weight per day in 4 equal doses.

Eyedrops:

Adult and child (age 4 and over): 1 to 2 drops in each eye 4 to 6 times a day at regular intervals.

Overdosage

No action is necessary other than medical observation. Call your local poison control center or hospital emergency room for more information.

Special Information

Cromolyn is taken to prevent or minimize severe allergic

reactions. It is imperative that you take Cromolyn products on a regular basis to provide equal protection throughout the day.

If you are taking Cromolyn to prevent seasonal allergic problems, it is essential that you start taking the medicine before you come into contact with the cause of the allergy and continue treatment throughout the period during which you will be exposed to the allergy source.

Cromolyn oral capsules should be opened and mixed with about 4 ounces of hot water. Stir until the solution is completely clear (powder has dissolved) and fill the rest of the glass with cold water. Drink the full glass without mixing the solution with food, juice, or milk.

People should not wear soft contact lenses while using Cromolyn eyedrops. The lenses may be replaced a few hours after you stop taking the drug.

Call your doctor if you develop wheezing, coughing, severe drug reaction (see *Possible Side Effects*), or skin rash. Other side effects should be reported if they are severe or particularly bothersome.

Call your doctor if your symptoms do not improve or get worse while you are taking this drug.

The effectiveness of this drug depends on taking it regularly. If you forget a dose of Cromolyn, take it as soon as you remember and space the remaining doses equally throughout the rest of the day. Do not take a double dose of this drug. Call your doctor if symptoms of your condition return because you have skipped too many doses.

Special Populations

Pregnancy/Breast-feeding

There are no reports of birth defects in animal studies with Cromolyn or of individual cases of birth defects associated with this drug. Animal studies with very large doses of Cromolyn administered directly into a vein have shown some potential for damage to the developing fetus. Pregnant women, or those who might become pregnant while taking the drug, should not use Cromolyn unless its advantages have been carefully weighed against the possible dangers of taking it while pregnant.

It is not known if Cromolyn passes into breast milk. No drug-related problems have been known to occur, but nursing mothers who use Cromolyn should exercise caution.

Seniors

No problems have been reported in older adults. However, older adults are likely to have age-related reduction in kidney and/or liver function. Your doctor should take this factor into account when determining your Cromolyn dosage.

Generic Name

Cyclobenzaprine

Brand Name

Flexeril

(Also available in generic form)

Type of Drug

Muscle relaxant.

Prescribed for

Serious muscle spasms and acute muscle pain. May also be prescribed for fibrositis (muscular rheumatism) characterized by pain, stiffness, and tenderness.

General Information

This drug is used as a part of the treatment for severe muscle spasms. It is not effective for spastic movements associated with spinal cord or brain disease. Physical therapy, rest, and other medical measures may also be used. It starts working an hour after you take it and reaches maximum effect after 1 to 2 weeks of continuous use.

Cautions and Warnings

Do not take Cyclobenzaprine if you are **allergic** to it. This drug should not be taken for several weeks following a **heart attack** or by people with **abnormal heart rhythms, heart failure, heart block,** or **hyperthyroidism** (an overactive thyroid).

Cyclobenzaprine should be avoided by people with **urinary retention, glaucoma,** or **increased eye pressure.** It inhibits the flow of saliva and may increase the chances for **dental cavities or gum disease.**

Cyclobenzaprine is intended only for **short-term use** (2 to 3 weeks). Painful muscle spasm is usually a short-term condition; treatment beyond 2 to 3 weeks is usually not needed.

Cyclobenzaprine is chemically similar to tricyclic antidepressants and can produce some of the more serious side effects associated with those drugs. Abruptly stopping Cyclobenzaprine can cause **nausea, headache,** and a **feeling of ill health;** this is not a sign of addiction.

Possible Side Effects

▼ Most common: dry mouth, drowsiness, and dizziness.

▼ Less common: muscle weakness, fatigue, nausea, constipation, upset stomach, unpleasant taste, blurred vision, headache, nervousness, and confusion.

▼ Rare: rapid heartbeat, fainting, low blood pressure, abnormal heart rhythms, heart palpitations, disorientation, sleeplessness, depression, unusual sensation, anxiety, agitation, abnormal thoughts and dreams, hallucinations, excitement, vomiting, loss of appetite, stomach irritation and pains, diarrhea, stomach gas, thirst, temporary loss of taste sensation, urinary changes, hepatitis, yellowing of the eyes or skin, sweating, skin rash, itching, muscle twitching, local weakness, and swelling of the face or tongue.

Many other side effects have been reported by people taking Cyclobenzaprine, but their relationship to the drug has never been established. Report anything unusual to your doctor.

Drug Interactions

• The effects of alcohol, sedatives, or other nervous-system depressants may be increased by Cyclobenzaprine.

• Cyclobenzaprine may increase some side effects of Atropine, Ipratropium, and other anticholinergic drugs. These include blurred vision, constipation, urinary difficulty, dry mouth, confusion, and drowsiness.

• The combination of Cyclobenzaprine with a monoamine oxidase (MAO) inhibitor type of antidepressant can produce very high fever, convulsions, and possibly death. Do not take these drugs within 14 days of each other.

• Cyclobenzaprine may increase the effects of Haloperidol, Loxapine, Molindone, Pimozide, anticoagulant (blood-thinning) drugs, anticonvulsants, thyroid hormones, antithyroid drugs, phenothiazines, and thioxanthenes. The effects of nasal decongestants such as Naphazoline, Oxymetazoline, Phenylephrine, and Xylometazoline may be increased by Cyclobenzaprine.

• Barbiturates and Carbamazepine may counteract the effects of Cyclobenzaprine.

• Fluoxetine, Ranitidine, Cimetidine, Methylphenidate, Estramustine, estrogens, and oral contraceptives may increase the effects and side effects of Cyclobenzaprine.

• Cyclobenzaprine may counteract the effects of Clonidine, Guanadrel, and Guanethidine.

Food Interactions

Cyclobenzaprine may be taken without regard to food.

Usual Dose

Adult and Adolescent (age 15 and older): 10 mg 3 times a day. May be increased up to 60 mg a day.
Child (under age 15): do not use.

Overdosage

Overdoses can cause confusion, loss of concentration, hallucinations, agitation, overactive reflexes, fever or vomiting, rigid muscles, and other drug side effects.

Overdose may also cause drowsiness, low body temperature, rapid or irregular heartbeat and other kinds of abnormal heart rhythms, heart failure, dilated pupils, convulsions, very low blood pressure, stupor, and coma. Sweating has been reported. Overdose victims must be taken to a hospital emergency room. ALWAYS bring the medicine bottle with you.

Special Information

Cyclobenzaprine causes drowsiness, dizziness, or blurred vision in more than 40 percent of people who take it. These side effects can interfere with your ability to perform complex tasks like driving or operating complicated equipment. Avoid alcohol, sedatives, and other nervous-system depressants because they can enhance these effects.

Call your doctor if you develop any of the following symptoms: skin rash, hives, or itching; urinary problems; clumsiness; confusion; depression; convulsions; yellowing of the eyes or skin; swelling of the face, lips, or tongue; or other persistent or bothersome side effects.

If you take Cyclobenzaprine once a day and forget to take a dose, take it as soon as you remember. If it is almost time for your next dose, skip the one you forgot and continue with your regular schedule. Do not take a double dose.

If you take Cyclobenzaprine twice a day and forget to take a dose, take it as soon as you remember. If it is almost time for your next dose, take one dose as soon as you remember and another in 5 or 6 hours, then go back to your regular schedule. Do not take a double dose.

If you take Cyclobenzaprine 3 times a day and forget to take a dose, take it as soon as you remember. If it is almost time for your next dose, take one dose as soon as you remember and another in 3 or 4 hours, then go back to your regular schedule. Do not take a double dose.

Special Populations

Pregnancy/Breast-feeding
Animal studies have shown no evidence that Cyclobenzaprine harms a developing fetus. Nevertheless, it should be avoided by pregnant women unless the potential benefits clearly outweigh the risks.

It is not known if Cyclobenzaprine passes into breast milk, but antidepressants with a similar chemical structure do pass into breast milk. Nursing mothers who must take this drug should consider bottle-feeding.

Seniors
Older adults are more likely to be sensitive to the effects of Cyclobenzaprine. Be sure to report any unusual or bothersome side effects to your doctor.

Generic Name

Cyclosporine

Brand Names

Sandimmune Capsules/Oral Solution/Injection
Neoral Capsules/Oral Solution

Type of Drug

Immunosuppressant.

Prescribed for

Preventing the rejection of a transplanted kidney, heart, or liver. Cyclosporine is also used for bone-marrow, heart, lung, and pancreas transplants. It has been prescribed for patchy hair loss, rheumatoid arthritis, aplastic anemia, atopic dermatitis, Behçet's disease, cirrhosis of the liver related to bile-duct blockade, ulcerative colitis, dermatomyositis, eye symptoms of Graves' disease, insulin-dependent diabetes, kidney inflammation associated with lupus and other kidney diseases, multiple sclerosis, severe psoriasis and arthritis associated with psoriasis, myasthenia gravis, pemphigus, sarcoidosis of the lung, pyoderma gangrenosum, and others. The drug is not FDA-approved for treating these conditions.

General Information

Cyclosporine was the first drug approved in the United States to prevent rejection of transplanted organs. A product of fungus metabolism, Cyclosporine was proven to be a potent immunosuppressant in 1972, and it was first given to human kidney- and bone-marrow-transplant patients in 1978. It selectively inhibits cells known as *T-lymphocytes*, which, as an integral part of the body's defense mechanism, destroy invading cells. Cyclosporine also prevents the production of a compound known as *Interleukin-II*, which activates T-lymphocyte cells. In 1995, a new form of Cyclosporine, a microemulsion, was introduced. This form is as safe and effective as the original product but requires less medicine to achieve the same effect. Thus, your dose of the newer product will be less than that of the original form of Cyclosporine and must be adjusted by your doctor if you already have been taking Cyclosporine.

Cautions and Warnings

This drug should be prescribed only by doctors experienced in immunosuppressive therapy and the care of organ-transplant patients. It is always used with **adrenal corticosteroid drugs**. Cyclosporine should **not** be **given with other immunosuppressants** because oversuppression of the immune system can result in lymphoma or extreme susceptibility to infection.

The original oral form of Cyclosporine is poorly absorbed into the bloodstream; it must be taken in doses 3 times larger than the injectable dose. People taking this drug orally over a period of time should have their blood checked for Cyclosporine levels so that the dose can be adjusted if necessary.

More of the newer microemulsion form of Cyclosporine **is absorbed into the blood,** and you will probably need less of the newer medicine. When you first start taking the microemulsion form, your dosage will be about the same as with the older oral liquid, but will then be reduced according to the amount of Cyclosporine in your blood. Follow your doctor's directions about drug dosage.

Cyclosporine causes **kidney toxicity** in 25 to 35 percent of people taking it to prevent organ transplant rejection. Mild symptoms usually start after about 2 or 3 months of treatment. This effect may be controlled by reducing drug dosage. In one study, Clonidine skin patches used before and after surgery decreased the chance of kidney toxicity.

Liver toxicity is seen in about 5 percent of organ-transplant patients taking Cyclosporine. This usually happens in the first month and can be controlled by reducing the dose.

Cyclosporine may cause **elevations in blood potassium** and/or **uric acid levels**.

In one study, Cyclosporine increased the level of **cholesterol** and **other blood fats**. It is not known how this affects people who take the medicine on a long-term basis.

The exact way in which Cyclosporine affects sugar in the body is not known. **Kidney-transplant patients** taking the drug have **developed insulin-dependent diabetes,** which is related to the dose of Cyclosporine, and which reverses itself when you stop taking the drug. On the other hand, this medicine preserves the function of insulin-producing cells in the pancreas and has allowed many insulin-dependent diabetics to live without taking Insulin.

Possible Side Effects

▼ Most common: Cyclosporine is known to be toxic to the kidneys. Your doctor will carefully monitor your kidneys while you are taking Cyclosporine.

▼ Common: high blood pressure, increased hair growth, growth of the gums. Lymphoma may develop in people whose immune systems are excessively suppressed. Almost 85 percent of people treated with this medicine will develop an infection, compared with 94 percent taking other immune system suppressants.

▼ Less common: tremors, cramps, acne, brittle hair or fingernails, convulsions, headache, confusion, diarrhea, nausea or vomiting, tingling in the hands or feet, facial flushing, reduction in blood counts of white cells and platelets, sinus inflammation, swollen and painful male breasts, drug allergy, conjunctivitis ("pink-eye"), fluid retention and swelling, ringing or buzzing in the ears, hearing loss, high blood sugar, and muscle pains.

▼ Rare: blood in the urine, heart attack, itching, anxiety, depression, lethargy, weakness, mouth sores, difficulty swallowing, intestinal bleeding, constipation, pancreas inflammation, night sweats, chest pain, joint pains, visual disturbances, and weight loss.

Drug Interactions

• Cyclosporine should be used carefully with other kidney-toxic drugs, including Gentamicin, Tobramycin, Vancomycin, Trimethoprim-Sulfamethoxazole, Melphalan, Amphotericin B, Ketoconazole, Azapropazon, Diclofenac, Cimetidine, Ranitidine, and Tacrolimus.

• Drugs that can increase blood levels of Cyclosporine are: Diltiazem, Micardipine, Verapamil, Fluconazole, Itraconazole, Clarithromycin, Erythromycin, Methylprednisolone, Allopurinol, Bromocriptine, Danazol, and Metoclopramide. Sometimes, this drug interaction may be intentionally used by your doctor to reduce the amount of Cyclosporine you must take to prevent organ rejection.

• Drugs that decrease Cyclosporine levels are: Nafcillin, Rifampin, Carbamazepine, Phenobarbital, Phenytoin, Octreotide, and Ticlopidine. Rifabutin may also have this effect, but it has not been studied in combination with Cyclosporine.

• Cyclosporine interferes with the body's ability to clear Digoxin, Prednisolone, and Lovastatin. People taking any of these medicines who start on Cyclosporine must have their drug dose reduced.

• Cyclosporine increases blood potassium. Excessive blood-potassium levels can be reached if Cyclosporine is taken with Enalapril, Lisinopril, a potassium-sparing diuretic (like Spironolactone), salt substitutes, Potassium supplements, or high-potassium (low-sodium) food.

• Cyclosporine prevents the normal body response to live vaccines. People taking Cyclosporine should be vaccinated only after specific discussions with their doctor. You must wait for a period of several months to several years after stopping the medicine before vaccination can be considered again.

Food Interactions

The original oral liquid form of this drug comes in a base made from castor oil. The newer product is in a microemulsion to make it taste a little better. Still, you should mix it in a glass (not a paper or plastic cup) with room-temperature orange or apple juice to make it taste better. DO NOT USE GRAPEFRUIT JUICE, BECAUSE IT AFFECTS THE BREAKDOWN OF CYCLOSPORINE. Drink immediately after mixing, then pour more juice in the glass and drink it to be sure that the entire dose has been taken. Cyclosporine microemulsion should not be taken with milk; it may be unpalatable. Cyclosporine (old or new) capsules may be taken with no special procedures.

Cyclosporine may be taken with food if it upsets your stomach.

Usual Dose

Adult and Adolescent: The usual oral dose of Cyclosporine is 6 to 8 mg per pound of body weight per day, given 4 to 12 hours before the transplant operation or immediately after surgery. This dosage is continued after the operation for 1 or 2 weeks and then slowly reduced to 2.25 to 4.5 mg per pound of body weight. Cyclosporine microemulsion doses are usually lower than old Cyclosporine dose levels because the newer form of the drug is better absorbed.

Child: Larger and more frequent doses may be required; children tend to release the drug from their bodies faster than adolescents or adults.

In general, the usual dose of Neoral is lower than that of Sandimmune, but dose adjustments must be made by your doctor. Injectable Cyclosporine is given to people who can't take or tolerate either the capsules or liquid in 1/3 of the oral dose.

Overdosage

Overdose victims can be expected to develop drug side effects and symptoms of extreme immunosuppression. Suspected victims must be made to vomit with Syrup of Ipecac (available at any pharmacy) to remove any remaining drug from the stomach. Call your doctor or a poison control center before doing this. If you must go to a hospital emergency room, ALWAYS bring the medicine bottle with you.

Special Information

Call your doctor at the first sign of fever; sore throat; tiredness; weakness; nervousness; unusual bleeding or bruising; tender or swollen gums; convulsions; irregular heartbeat; confusion; numbness or tingling of your hands, feet, or lips; difficulty breathing; severe stomach pains with nausea; or bloody urine. Other drug effects (shaking or trembling of the hands, increased hair growth, acne, headache, leg cramps, nausea, or vomiting) are less serious but should be brought to your doctor's attention, particularly if they are unusually bothersome or persistent.

It is important to maintain good dental hygiene while taking Cyclosporine and to use extra care when using your toothbrush or dental floss, because of the chance that the drug will make you more susceptible to dental infections. Cyclosporine can cause swollen gums and suppresses the normal body systems that fight infection. See your dentist regularly while taking this medicine.

This medicine should be continued as long as prescribed by your doctor. Do not stop taking it because of side effects or other problems. If you cannot tolerate the oral form, this drug can be given by injection.

Do not keep the oral liquid in the refrigerator. After the bottle is opened, use the medicine within 2 months.

If you forget to take a dose of Cyclosporine, take it as soon as you remember if it is within 12 hours of your regular dose. If not, skip the forgotten dose and continue with your regular schedule. Do not take a double dose.

Special Populations

Pregnancy/Breast-feeding

Pregnant women and those who might become pregnant should not take Cyclosporine. In those situations where it is deemed essential by your doctor, its potential benefits must be carefully weighed against its risks.

Cyclosporine passes into breast milk. Nursing mothers who must take this medicine should bottle-feed their babies.

Seniors

Older adults are likely to have age-related decreases in kidney function and may, therefore, be more susceptible to the kidney toxicity associated with this drug. Otherwise, older adults can take Cyclosporine without special restrictions.

Cycrin

see *Medroxyprogesterone Acetate*, page 665

Darvocet-N 100

see *Propoxyphene*, page 955

Daypro

see *Oxaprozin*, page 843

Deltasone

see **Corticosteroids**, page 269

Depakote

see **Valproic Acid**, page 1161

Generic Name

Desipramine

Brand Names

Norpramin Tablets

(Also available in generic form)

Type of Drug

Tricyclic antidepressant.

Prescribed for

Depression, cocaine withdrawal, panic disorder, and bulimia nervosa.

General Information

Desipramine is one of the tricyclic antidepressant drugs, which block the movement of certain stimulant chemicals in and out of nerve endings, have a sedative effect, and counteract the effects of a hormone called *acetylcholine* (which makes them anticholinergic drugs). They prevent the reuptake of important neurohormones (norepinephrine or serotonin) at the nerve ending. Theory says that people with depression have a chemical imbalance in their brains and that drugs such as Desipramine work to reestablish a proper balance. Although Desipramine and similar antidepressants immediately block neurohormones, it takes 2 to 4 weeks for their clinical antidepressant effect to come into play. Call your doctor if you're not better after 6 to 8 weeks.

Tricyclic antidepressants can also elevate mood, increase physical activity and mental alertness, and improve appetite and sleep patterns in a depressed patient. They are mild sedatives and are useful in treating mild forms of depression associated with anxiety. These drugs are broken down in the liver.

Cautions and Warnings

Do not take Desipramine if you are **allergic** or **sensitive** to it or other **tricyclic antidepressants**. None of these drugs should be used if you are recovering from a **heart attack**.

If you have a history of **epilepsy** or other **convulsive disorders, difficulty in urination, glaucoma, heart disease, liver disease,** or **hyperthyroidism,** Desipramine should be taken with caution. People who are **schizophrenic** or **paranoid** may get worse if given a tricyclic antidepressant, and manic-depressive people may switch phase. This can also happen if they are changing or stopping antidepressants. Desipramine and other antidepressants can be **lethal if taken in large quantities. Severely depressed** people should be allowed to keep only small numbers of pills on hand.

Possible Side Effects

Desipramine is generally safer than other tricyclic antidepressants.

▼ Most common: sedation and anticholinergic effects (blurred vision, disorientation, confusion, hallucinations, muscle spasms or tremors, seizures and/or convulsions, dry mouth, constipation [especially in older adults], difficult urination, worsening glaucoma, sensitivity to bright light or sunlight).

▼ Less common: blood-pressure changes, abnormal heart rates, heart attack, anxiety, restlessness, excitement, numbness and tingling in the extremities, poor coordination, rash, itching, retention of fluids, fever, allergy, changes in composition of blood, nausea, vomiting, loss of appetite, stomach upset, diarrhea, enlargement of the

Possible Side Effects *(continued)*

breasts (both sexes), changes in sex drive, and blood-sugar changes.

▼ Rare: agitation, inability to sleep, nightmares, feeling of panic, a peculiar taste in the mouth, stomach cramps, black discoloration of the tongue, yellowing of the eyes and/or skin, changes in liver function, increased or decreased weight, excessive perspiration, flushing, frequent urination, drowsiness, dizziness, weakness, headache, loss of hair, nausea, and not feeling well.

Drug Interactions

• Taking Desipramine with monoamine oxidase (MAO) inhibitors can cause high fevers, convulsions, and occasionally death. Don't take MAO inhibitors until at least 2 weeks after Desipramine has been discontinued. Patients who must take both Desipramine and an MAO inhibitor require close medical observation.

• Desipramine interacts with Guanethidine and Clonidine. Be sure to tell your doctor if you are taking **any** high-blood-pressure medicine.

• Desipramine increases the effects of barbiturates, tranquilizers, other sedative drugs, and alcohol. Also, barbiturates may decrease the effectiveness of Desipramine.

• Taking Desipramine and thyroid medicine together will enhance the effects of both medicines, possibly causing abnormal heart rhythms. The combination of Desipramine and Reserpine may cause overstimulation.

• Oral contraceptives can reduce the effect of Desipramine, as can smoking. Charcoal tablets can prevent Desipramine's absorption into the bloodstream. Estrogens can increase or decrease the effect of Desipramine.

• Drugs such as Bicarbonate of Soda, Acetazolamide, Quinidine, or Procainamide will increase the effect of Desipramine. Cimetidine, Methylphenidate, and Phenothiazine drugs (like Thorazine and Compazine) block the liver metabolism of Desipramine, causing it to stay in the body longer, which can cause severe drug side effects.

Food Interactions

Take Desipramine with food if it upsets your stomach.

Usual Dose

Adult: 75 to 300 mg per day. Your dosage must be tailored to your needs. People taking high doses of this drug should have regular heart examinations to check for side effects.

Adolescent and Senior: lower doses are recommended, usually 25 to 150 mg per day.

Child (under age 12): do not use.

Overdosage

Symptoms of overdosage are confusion, inability to concentrate, hallucinations, drowsiness, lowered body temperature, abnormal heart rate, heart failure, enlarged pupils of the eyes, convulsions, severely lowered blood pressure, stupor, and coma. Agitation, stiffening of body muscles, vomiting, and high fever may also occur. The overdose victim should be taken to a hospital emergency room immediately. ALWAYS bring the medicine bottle.

Special Information

Avoid alcohol and other depressants while taking this drug. Do not stop taking this medicine unless your doctor specifically tells you to do so. Abruptly stopping this medicine may cause nausea, headache, and a sickly feeling.

This medicine can cause drowsiness, dizziness, and blurred vision. Be careful when driving or operating hazardous machinery. Avoid prolonged exposure to the sun or sun lamps.

Call your doctor at once if you develop seizures, difficult or rapid breathing, fever and sweating, blood-pressure changes, muscle stiffness, loss of bladder control, or unusual tiredness or weakness. Dry mouth may lead to an increase in dental cavities, gum bleeding and disease. People taking Desipramine should pay special attention to dental hygiene.

If you forget a dose of Desipramine, skip it and go back to your regular schedule. Do not take a double dose.

Special Populations

Pregnancy/Breast-feeding

Desipramine crosses into your developing baby's circulation.

Birth defects have been reported when this drug was taken during the first 3 months of pregnancy. There have been reports of newborn infants suffering from heart, breathing, and urinary problems after their mothers had taken a tricyclyc antidepressant immediately before delivery. Avoid this medication while pregnant.

Small amounts of tricyclic antidepressants pass into breast milk and sedate the baby. Nursing mothers taking Desipramine should consider bottle-feeding.

Seniors

Older adults are more sensitive to the effects of this drug, especially abnormal rhythms and other heart side effects, and often require a lower dose to achieve the same effects. Follow your doctor's directions and report any side effects at once.

Desogen

see **Contraceptives**, page 262

DiaBeta

see **Antidiabetes Drugs (Oral Sulfonylureas)**, page 72

Generic Name

Diazepam

Brand Names

| Valium Tablets and Solution Ⓢ* | Valrelease Capsules* | Zetran* |

The information contained in this drug profile also applies to the following products:

Generic Name	Brand Name
Halazepam	Paxipam
Oxazepam	Serax*
Prazepam	Centrax*

(*Also available in generic form)

Type of Drug

Benzodiazepine tranquilizer.

Prescribed for

Relief of anxiety, tension, fatigue, agitation, muscle spasm, and seizures; irritable bowel syndrome; panic attacks.

General Information

Diazepam and the other drugs named above are *benzodiazepines*, used as antianxiety agents, anticonvulsants, or sedatives. Some are more suited to a specific role because of differences in chemical makeup that give them greater activity in a certain area or characteristics that make them more desirable for a certain function. Often, individual drugs are limited by the applications for which their research has been sponsored. Benzodiazepines directly affect the brain. In doing so, they can relax you and make you either more tranquil or sleepier, or can slow nervous system transmissions in such a way as to act as an anticonvulsant, depending on which drug you use and your dosage. Many doctors prefer the benzodiazepines to other drugs that can be used for similar effects because they tend to be safer, have fewer side effects, and are usually as, if not more, effective.

Cautions and Warnings

Do not take Diazepam if you know you are **sensitive** or **allergic** to it or to another benzodiazepine drug, including Clonazepam.

Diazepam can aggravate **narrow-angle glaucoma**. However, if you have open-angle glaucoma, you may take it. Check with your doctor.

Other **conditions where Diazepam should be avoided** are severe depression, severe lung disease, sleep apnea (intermittent breathing while sleeping), liver disease, drunkenness, and kidney disease. In all of these conditions, the depressive effects of Diazepam may be enhanced and/or could be detrimental to your overall condition.

Diazepam should **not be taken by psychotic patients**, because it doesn't work for them and can cause unusual excitement, stimulation, and rage.

Diazepam is **not intended for more than 3 to 4 months of continuous use**. Your condition should be reassessed before continuing your medicine beyond that time.

Diazepam may be **addictive**, and you can experience drug-withdrawal symptoms if you suddenly stop taking it after as little as 4 to 6 weeks of treatment. Withdrawal symptoms are increased anxiety, tingling in the extremities, sensitivity to bright light or the sun, long periods of sleep or sleeplessness, a metallic taste, flulike illness, fatigue, difficulty concentrating, restlessness, loss of appetite, nausea, irritability, headache, dizziness, sweating, muscle tension or cramps, tremors, and feeling uncomfortable. Other major symptoms are confusion, abnormal perception of movement, depersonalization, paranoid delusions, hallucinations, psychotic reactions, muscle twitching, seizures, and memory loss.

Possible Side Effects

▼ Most common: mild drowsiness during the first few days of therapy. Weakness and confusion may also occur, especially in seniors and those who are more sickly. If these effects persist, contact your doctor.

▼ Less common: depression, lethargy, disorientation, headache, inactivity, slurred speech, stupor, dizziness, tremors, constipation, dry mouth, nausea, inability to control urination, sexual difficulties, irregular menstrual cycle, changes in heart rhythm, lowered blood pressure, fluid retention, blurred or double vision, itching, rash, hiccups, nervousness, inability to fall asleep, and occasional liver dysfunction. If you have any of these symptoms, stop taking the medicine, and contact your doctor at once.

▼ Other: diarrhea, coated tongue, sore gums, vomiting, appetite changes, swallowing difficulty, increased salivation, upset stomach, changes in sex drive, urinary difficulties, changes in heart rate, palpitations, swelling,

Possible Side Effects *(continued)*

stuffy nose, hearing difficulty, hair loss or gain, sweating, fever, tingling in the hands or feet, breast pain, muscle disturbances, breathing difficulty, changes in blood components, and joint pain.

Drug Interactions

• Diazepam is a central-nervous-system depressant. Avoid alcohol, other tranquilizers, narcotics, barbiturates, monoamine oxidase (MAO) inhibitors, antihistamines, and antidepressants. Taking Diazepam with these drugs may result in excessive depression, drowsiness, or difficulty breathing.

• Smoking may reduce the effectiveness of Diazepam by increasing the rate at which it is broken down by the body.

• The effects of Diazepam may be prolonged when taken with Cimetidine, oral contraceptives, Disulfiram, Fluoxetine, Isoniazid, Ketoconazole, Rifampin, Metoprolol, Probenecid, Propoxyphene, Propranolol, and Valproic Acid.

• Theophylline may reduce the sedative effects of Diazepam.

• If you take antacids, separate them from your Diazepam dose by at least 1 hour to prevent them from interfering with the passage of Diazepam into the bloodstream.

• Diazepam may increase blood levels of Digoxin and the chances for Digoxin toxicity.

• Levodopa's effect may be decreased if it is taken with Diazepam.

• Phenytoin blood concentrations may be increased if taken with Diazepam, resulting in possible Phenytoin toxicity.

Food Interactions

Diazepam is best taken on an empty stomach, but it may be taken with food if it upsets your stomach.

Usual Dose

Adult: 2 to 40 mg per day. The dose must be adjusted to individual response for maximum effect.

Senior: less of the drug is usually required to control tension and anxiety.

Child (6 months and older): 1 to 2.5 mg, 3 or 4 times per day; more may be needed to control anxiety and tension.
Infant (under 6 months): do not use.

Overdosage

Symptoms of overdosage are confusion, sleepiness, poor coordination, lack of response to pain (such as a pin prick), loss of reflexes, shallow breathing, low blood pressure, and coma. The victim should be taken to a hospital emergency room. ALWAYS bring the medicine bottle with you.

Special Information

Diazepam can cause tiredness, drowsiness, inability to concentrate, or similar symptoms. Be careful if you are driving, operating machinery, or performing other activities that require concentration.

People taking Diazepam for more than 3 or 4 months at a time may develop drug-withdrawal reactions if the medication is stopped suddenly (see *Cautions and Warnings*).

If you forget a dose of Diazepam, take it as soon as you remember. If it is almost time for your next dose, skip the forgotten one and continue with your regular schedule. Do not take a double dose.

Special Populations

Pregnancy/Breast-feeding

Diazepam may cross into the developing fetal circulation and may cause birth defects if taken during the first 3 months of pregnancy. Avoid taking any benzodiazepine if you are or think you might be pregnant.

Diazepam may pass into breast milk. Since infants break the drug down more slowly than adults, the medicine may accumulate and have an undesirable effect on the baby. Nursing mothers who must take this drug should bottle-feed their babies.

Seniors

Older adults, especially those with liver or kidney disease, are more sensitive to the effects of Diazepam and generally require smaller doses to achieve the same effect. Follow your doctor's directions, and report any side effects at once.

Generic Name

Diclofenac

Brand Names

Cataflam
Voltaren Tablets/Eyedrops

(Also available in generic form)

Type of Drug

Nonsteroidal anti-inflammatory drug (NSAID).

Prescribed for

Rheumatoid arthritis, osteoarthritis, ankylosing spondylitis, mild to moderate pain, juvenile rheumatoid arthritis, shoulder pain, menstrual pain and cramps, sunburn relief, preventing eye inflammation after cataract surgery (eyedrops only).

General Information

Diclofenac is one of 16 NSAIDs used for their ability to reduce pain and inflammation. Cataflam, a newer version of Diclofenac, does not contain sodium and is the preferred form for menstrual pain and cramps. Since Voltaren, the older version of Diclofenac, does contain sodium, women taking Cataflam for menstrual problems should not switch to Voltaren. NSAID eyedrops are used during eye surgery (to prevent movement of the eye muscles) and for itching and redness due to seasonal allergies. We do not know exactly how NSAIDs work, but part of their action may be due to an ability to inhibit the body's production of a hormone called *prostaglandin* and to inhibit the action of other body chemicals, including cyclo-oxygenase, lipoxygenase, leukotrienes, lysosomal enzymes, and a host of other factors. NSAIDs are generally absorbed into the bloodstream fairly quickly. Pain relief generally comes within an hour after taking the first dose, but the NSAID's anti-inflammatory effect generally takes a lot longer (several days to 2 weeks) to become apparent, and may take a month or more to reach its maximum effect. Diclofenac is broken down in the liver and eliminated through the kidneys.

Cautions and Warnings

People **allergic** to Diclofenac (or any other NSAID) and those with a history of **asthma attacks** brought on by another NSAID, **Iodides,** or **Aspirin** should not take Diclofenac.

Diclofenac can cause **gastrointestinal (GI) bleeding, ulcers,** and **stomach perforation.** This can occur at any time, with or without warning, in people who take chronic Diclofenac treatment. People with a history of **active GI bleeding** should be cautious about taking any NSAID. **Minor stomach upset, distress,** or **gas** is common during the first few days of treatment with Diclofenac. People who develop **bleeding** or **ulcers** and continue treatment should be aware of the possibility of developing more serious drug toxicity.

Diclofenac can affect **platelets** and **blood clotting** at high doses, and should be avoided by people with **clotting problems** and by those taking **Warfarin.**

People with **heart problems** who use Diclofenac may experience swelling in their arms, legs, or feet.

Diclofenac can cause severe toxic effects to the **kidney.** Report any unusual side effects to your doctor, who may need to periodically test your kidney function.

Diclofenac can make you **unusually sensitive to the effects of the sun** (photosensitivity).

People taking this drug on a regular basis should have their **liver function** checked periodically.

Possible Side Effects

▼ Most common: diarrhea, nausea, vomiting, constipation, stomach gas, stomach upset or irritation, and loss of appetite (tablets); temporary burning, stinging, or other minor eye irritation (eyedrops).

▼ Less common: stomach ulcers, GI bleeding, hepatitis, gallbladder attacks, painful urination, poor kidney function, kidney inflammation, blood and protein in the urine, dizziness, fainting, nervousness, depression, hallucinations, confusion, disorientation, tingling in the hands or feet, light-headedness, itching, increased sweating, dry nose and mouth, heart palpitations, chest pain, difficulty breathing, and muscle cramps (tablets); nausea, vomiting, viral infections, and eye allergies (longer-lasting eye redness, burning, itching, or tearing) (eyedrops).

Possible Side Effects *(continued)*

▼ Rare: severe allergic reactions, including closing of the throat, fever and chills, changes in liver function, jaundice (yellowing of the skin or eyes), and kidney failure. People who experience such effects must be promptly treated in a hospital emergency room or doctor's office.

NSAIDs have caused severe skin reactions; if this happens to you, see your doctor immediately.

The risk of developing bleeding problems or other body-wide side effects with Diclofenac is small, because only a small amount of this drug is absorbed into the bloodstream.

Drug Interactions

• Diclofenac can increase the effects of oral anticoagulant (blood-thinning) drugs such as Warfarin. You may take this combination, but your doctor may have to reduce your anticoagulant dose.

• Taking Diclofenac with Cyclosporine may increase the toxic kidney effects of both drugs. Methotrexate toxicity may be increased in people also taking Diclofenac.

• Diclofenac may reduce the blood-pressure-lowering effect of beta blockers and loop diuretic drugs.

• Diclofenac may increase blood levels of Phenytoin, leading to increased Phenytoin side effects. Blood-Lithium levels may be increased in people taking Diclofenac.

• Diclofenac blood levels may be affected by Cimetidine because of that drug's effect on the liver.

• Probenecid may interfere with the elimination of Diclofenac from the body, increasing the chances for Diclofenac toxic reactions.

• Aspirin and other salicylates may decrease the amount of Diclofenac in your blood. These medicines should never be taken at the same time.

• No drug interactions have been reported with Diclofenac eyedrops.

Food Interactions

Take Diclofenac with food or a magnesium/aluminum antacid if it upsets your stomach.

Usual Dose

Tablets

Adult: 100 to 200 mg per day divided into 2, 3, or 4 doses.
Senior: probably should start with 1/3 to 1/2 the usual dose.

Eyedrops

One drop 4 times per day beginning 24 hours after cataract surgery and continuing for 2 weeks.

Overdosage

People have died from NSAID overdoses. The most common signs of overdosage are drowsiness, nausea, vomiting, diarrhea, abdominal pain, rapid breathing, rapid heartbeat, increased sweating, ringing or buzzing in the ears, confusion, disorientation, stupor, and coma.

Take the victim to a hospital emergency room at once. ALWAYS bring the medicine bottle.

Special Information

Diclofenac can make you drowsy and/or tired: Be careful when driving or operating hazardous equipment. Do not take any nonprescription products with Acetaminophen or Aspirin while taking this drug; also, avoid alcoholic beverages.

If you are taking Cataflam for menstrual problems, be sure not to substitute Voltaren, which contains sodium.

Take each dose with a full glass of water and don't lie down for 15 to 30 minutes after you take the medicine.

Contact your doctor if you develop skin rash or itching, visual disturbances, weight gain, breathing difficulty, fluid retention, hallucinations, black or tarry stools, persistent headache, or any unusual or intolerable side effects.

If you forget to take a dose of oral Diclofenac, take it as soon as you remember. If you take several doses a day, and it is within 4 hours of your next dose, skip the one you forgot and continue with your regular schedule. Do not take a double dose.

To self-administer the eyedrops, lie down or tilt your head

backward. Hold the dropper above your eye and drop the medicine inside your lower lid while looking up. To prevent possible infection, don't allow the dropper to touch your fingers or eyelids, or any surface. Release the lower lid and keep your eye open. Don't blink for about 30 seconds. Press gently on the bridge of your nose at the inside corner of your eye for about a minute. This will help circulate the medicine around your eye. Wait at least 5 minutes before using any other eyedrops.

If you forget a dose of eyedrops, take it as soon as you remember. If it is almost time for your next dose, skip the one you missed and continue with your regular schedule. Do not take a double dose.

Special Populations

Pregnancy/Breast-feeding

NSAIDs may cross into the fetal blood circulation. They have not been found to cause birth defects, but may affect a developing fetal heart during the second half of pregnancy; animal studies indicate a possible effect. Women who are or who might become pregnant should not take Diclofenac without their doctors' approval; pregnant women should be particularly cautious about using this drug during the last 3 months of their pregnancy. When the drug is considered essential by your doctor, its potential benefits must be carefully weighed against its risks.

NSAIDs may pass into breast milk, but have caused no problems among breast-fed infants, except for seizures in a baby whose mother was taking Indomethacin. Other NSAIDs have caused problems in animal studies. There is a possibility that a nursing mother taking Diclofenac could affect her baby's heart or cardiovascular system. If you must take Diclofenac, bottle-feed your baby.

Seniors

Older adults may be more susceptible to Diclofenac side effects, especially ulcer disease.

Generic Name

Dicyclomine Hydrochloride

Brand Names

Bemote
Bentyl
Byclomine
Di-Spaz

(Also available in generic form)

Type of Drug

Antispasmodic, anticholinergic.

Prescribed for

Dicyclomine is prescribed for irritable bowel, spastic colon, and similar digestive problems.

General Information

Dicyclomine is a member of a very large class of drugs that have been used for many years to calm "nervous stomachs." It was once widely prescribed for morning sickness during pregnancy. Dicyclomine and other anticholinergics work by inhibiting the effects of a neurohormone called *acetylcholine* in the stomach and intestines (GI tract). This effect directly reduces the mobility of the GI tract and slows the production of enzymes and other secretions. Dicyclomine and other members of this drug class may also cause dry mouth, reduce sweating, and cause dilation of the pupil, making it more difficult for you to become used to sudden bright light.

Cautions and Warnings

Do not take Dicyclomine if you are **allergic** to it or to any other **belladonna-related drug.** This drug should be used with caution if you have **heart disease, Down syndrome, reduced mobility of the stomach and lower esophagus, fever, stomach obstruction, glaucoma, acute bleeding, hiatal hernia, intestinal paralysis, myasthenia gravis, kidney** or **liver dysfunction, rapid heartbeat, high blood pressure,** or **ulcerative**

colitis. Because this drug reduces your ability to sweat, its use in **hot weather** may cause heat exhaustion.

Possible Side Effects

▼ Common: constipation, decreased sweating, and dry mouth, throat, or skin.

▼ Less common: reduced breast-milk flow, difficulty swallowing, blurred vision, and sensitivity to bright light.

▼ Rare: drug allergy (skin rash or hives), confusion, eye pain, dizziness when rising quickly from a sitting or lying position, a bloated feeling, difficult or painful urination, drowsiness, unusual tiredness or weakness, headache, memory loss, and nausea or vomiting.

Drug Interactions

• Antacids containing calcium and/or magnesium, citrates, sodium bicarbonate, and carbonic anhydrase inhibitor drugs may slow the rate at which Dicyclomine is released from the blood, increasing its therapeutic effect and possible side effects.

• Do not mix Dicyclomine with other anticholinergic drugs, including Atropine, Belladonna, Clidinium, Glycopyrrolate, Hyoscyamine, Isopropamide, Propantheline, Scopolamine, and others because of the possibility of intensifying drug side effects.

• Dicyclomine can reduce stomach acidity and reduce the amount of Ketoconazole, an antifungal drug, absorbed into the blood after it is taken by mouth.

• Dicyclomine may counteract the effect of Metoclopramide in reducing nausea and vomiting.

• Taking Dicyclomine together with a narcotic pain reliever can increase the chances of severe constipation.

• Taking this drug or any other drug that slows the movement of stomach and intestinal muscles together with a potassium chloride supplement (especially one that comes in wax-matrix tablet form) can lead to excessive irritation of the stomach.

Food Interactions

Take Dicyclomine on an empty stomach, 1/2 hour before to 2 hours after a meal.

Usual Dose

Adult: 30 to 160 mg a day.

Child (age 2 and older): 10 mg 3 or 4 times a day.

Child (age 6 months to 2 years): 5 to 10 mg 3 or 4 times a day.

Child (under 6 months): not recommended.

Senior: older adults should begin with the lowest possible dose and increase their dosage only as needed.

Overdosage

The principal signs of overdose are blurred vision; clumsiness; confusion; difficulty breathing; dizziness; drowsiness; dry mouth, nose, or throat; rapid heartbeat; fever; hallucinations; weakness; slurred speech; excitement, restlessness, or irritability; warmth; and dry or flushed skin. Overdose victims should be taken to a hospital emergency room at once for treatment. ALWAYS bring the medicine bottle with you.

Special Information

Children taking Dicyclomine may be more likely to develop high body temperature in hot weather and other drug side effects and should be carefully watched for side effects.

Call your doctor if you develop skin rash, flushing, or eye pain or if you develop other side effects such as dry mouth, urinary difficulty, constipation, or unusual sensitivity to light that are persistent or bothersome.

Brush and floss your teeth regularly while taking this drug. Because Dicyclomine can cause dry mouth, you may be more likely to develop cavities or other dental problems while you are taking it. Ice or hard candy can be used to relieve this side effect.

Constipation can be treated by using a stool-softening laxative.

Dicyclomine may make you drowsy or tired and can cause blurred vision. Be careful when driving or doing other tasks that require concentration and coordination.

If you forget to take a dose of Dicyclomine, take it as soon as you remember. If it is almost time for your next dose, skip the forgotten dose and continue with your regular schedule.

Special Populations

Pregnancy/Breast-feeding
A few cases of human malformations were linked to Dicyclomine, but studies have shown that the drug has no effect on the developing baby. As with all other drug products, Dicyclomine should be used during pregnancy only when absolutely necessary.

Dicyclomine should not be used by nursing mothers because like other drugs in its group, it may reduce the amount of milk produced. Also, a few infants less than 3 months of age who were given Dicyclomine drops developed breathing difficulty that went away on its own after 20 to 30 minutes.

Seniors
Older adults may be more susceptible to the side effects of this drug, especially memory loss, mental changes, and glaucoma, and may need less medicine to get a beneficial effect than a younger adult. Report any problems to your doctor at once.

Generic Name

Didanosine

Brand Name

Videx/Tablets/Solution Powder

(Also known as ddI or Dideoxyinosine)

Type of Drug

Antiviral

Prescribed for

HIV infection (AIDS)

General Information

Didanosine is approved for people with AIDS who have been

on long-term Zidovudine treatment and whose disease is continuing to worsen. It is also approved for children aged 6 months and older with AIDS who cannot tolerate or respond to Zidovudine.

Didanosine interferes with the reproduction of the HIV virus by interrupting its internal DNA manufacturing process. DNA carries the essential genetic message that directs all life processes, in this case interfering with the life of the HIV virus. Didanosine was tested in patients with advanced AIDS. It was approved because of its ability to prolong life or extend the time until patients developed a new AIDS-related opportunistic infection or another AIDS-defining event. Didanosine also was able to increase blood levels of CD4 cells. CD4 cells are considered important indicators of the severity of an AIDS infection because they represent the level of immune function.

Cautions and Warnings

The most serious (and possibly fatal) side effects of Didanosine are nervous system inflammation and inflammation of the pancreas.

Up to half of patients who take Didanosine experience symptoms of **nervous system inflammation** and about 1/3 may need to reduce their dosage of Didanosine to control these symptoms. It generally comes in the form of numbness, tingling and pain in the hands and feet. People who already have signs of this kind of nerve damage should not take Didanosine.

Possibly fatal **inflammation of the pancreas** has developed in up to 3 percent of people taking Didanosine. A third of people with a history of pancreatic inflammation who take Didanosine are likely to develop this problem. Some symptoms of inflammation of the pancreas are major changes in **blood sugar levels,** rising levels of **triglycerides** in the blood, a drop in **blood calcium, nausea, vomiting** or **abdominal pain.** People who develop pancreas inflammation must stop taking Didanosine.

Liver failure may develop in people taking this medicine. Fifteen to 20 percent of people taking Didanosine will develop abnormal liver function tests and a small number may go on to fatal liver disease.

Four children taking this drug developed **severe eye dis-**

ease, causing some loss of sight. The progress of the eye disease slowed or stopped when dosage was reduced. Children taking this medicine should undergo **eye examinations** every 6 months or if vision starts to worsen.

Didanosine has caused **muscle toxicities** in animals. This has not been seen in humans, but can occur with other AIDS antiviral medicines.

Kidney and **liver disease** can interfere with the elimination of Didanosine from your body. Dosage reduction may be needed to accommodate these situations.

Do not take Didanosine if you are **allergic** to it or any ingredient in the Didanosine tablet.

Possible Side Effects

▼ Most common: diarrhea, nervous system inflammation, fever and chills, itching, rash, abdominal pain, weakness, pains, headache, nausea and vomiting, infection, pneumonia, pancreas inflammation.

▼ Less common: tumors, muscle pain, appetite loss, dry mouth, convulsions, abnormal thought patterns, breathing difficulty, drug allergy, anxiety, nervousness, twitching, confusion, depression and blood component abnormalities.

▼ Rare: abscesses, skin infections, cysts, dehydration, flu-like symptoms, hernia, neck rigidity, numbness of the hands or feet, chest pain, blood pressure changes, heart palpitations, migraines, dizziness, coldness in the hands or feet, leg pains, colitis, stomach gas, stomach inflammation, ulcers or bleeding, oral fungus infections, personality changes, memory loss, convulsions, dizziness, muscle stiffness, loss of muscle control, poor coordination, loss of bowel control, stroke, feelings of ill health, paranoia, paralysis, psychosis, sleep disturbances, speech difficulties, tremors, joint inflammation or pains, swelling in the legs or arms, asthma, bronchitis, cough, nosebleeds, laryngitis, pneumonia, respiratory difficulties, blurred vision, double vision, conjunctivitis, dry eyes, hearing abnormalities, glaucoma, herpes infections of the skin, sweating,

Almost all children who take Didanosine experience drug side effects. They are likely to experience many of

---

Possible Side Effects *(continued)*

the same reactions as adults but most commonly develop chills, fever, weakness, appetite loss, nausea and vomiting, diarrhea, liver dysfunction, pains, headache, nervousness, sleeplessness, cough, runny nose, asthma or difficulty breathing, rashes, skin problems, and feelings of ill health.

Drug Interactions

• Other drugs that can cause inflammation of the nervous system such as Chloramphenicol, Cisplatin, Dapsone, Disulfiram, Ethionamide, Glutethimide, Gold, Hydralazine, Isoniazid, Metronidazole, Nitrofurantoin, Ribavirin, and Vincristine should be avoided while you are taking Didanosine.

• Didanosine should not be taken together with Zalcitabine.

• Drugs that can cause inflammation of the pancreas (including intravenous Pentamidine) should not be taken with Didanosine.

• Quinolone anti-infectives, tetracycline antibiotics and other drugs whose absorption into the bloodstream can be affected by antacids should not be taken within 2 hours of Didanosine because of its high magnesium and aluminum content.

Food Interactions

Food can prevent the absorption of up to ½ of a dose of Didanosine. Take Didanosine on an empty stomach.

Usual Dose

Adult: 167 to 250 mg every 12 hours.
Child: 50 to 250 mg per day.
Drug dosage should be adjusted to the patient's level of kidney and liver function.

Overdosage

Didanosine overdose causes many of the drug's usual side effects, especially inflammation of the nervous system or pancreas, diarrhea and liver failure. There is little experience with Didanosine overdose and victims should be taken to a hospital emergency room for testing and monitoring. ALWAYS remember to bring the prescription bottle with you.

Special Information

Didanosine is not an AIDS cure, nor will it prevent you from transmitting the HIV virus to another person. Patients may still develop AIDS-related opportunistic infections while taking this medicine.

Didanosine can affect components of the blood system. Your doctor will perform blood tests to check for any changes.

People taking Didanosine should take care of their teeth and gums to minimize the possibility of oral infections.

Call your doctor if you develop any of the following symptoms of Didanosine drug toxicity: numbness and pain in the hands and feet, nausea, vomiting or abdominal pain.

If you forget to take a dose of Didanosine, take it as soon as you remember. If it is almost time for your next dose, space the missed dose and your next dose by 4 to 8 hours, then continue your regular schedule. Call your doctor for more specific advice if you forget to take several doses.

How to Take Didanosine

Chewable Tablets: Thoroughly chew the tablets or completely dissolve them in about ¼ cup of water. Drink the entire mixture immediately. Don't mix with juice or any other acidic drink.

Powder for Solution: Pour the entire contents of a packet into ½ cup of water, stir until dissolved, and drink immediately. Don't mix with fruit juice or another acidic drink. For children, your pharmacist will prepare a mixture consisting of 10 mg per milliliter of Didanosine and an equal amount of Mylanta Double Strength Antacid or Maalox TC Antacid. This mixture must be stored in a refrigerator and can be kept for 30 days. Shake well before using.

Spilled Didanosine should be cleaned immediately to prevent accidental poisoning.

Special Populations

Pregnancy/Breast-feeding

Didanosine was slightly toxic to pregnant animals receiving doses 12 times human levels. There are no studies of pregnant women taking this medication; however, women who are, or might become, pregnant should only take Didanosine if absolutely necessary and should use effective contraception to avoid passing on the virus.

It is not known if Didanosine passes into breast milk. HIV-infected women who must take this medication should not nurse their infants, but use another method of feeding.

Seniors

People with reduced kidney or liver function, including older adults, should receive smaller doses of Didanosine than those with normal functioning.

Generic Name

Diflunisal

Brand Name

Dolobid

(Also available in generic form)

Type of Drug

Nonsteroidal anti-inflammatory drug (NSAID).

Prescribed for

Rheumatoid arthritis; osteoarthritis; mild to moderate pain.

General Information

Diflunisal is chemically related to Aspirin but is considered to be a nonsteroidal anti-inflammatory drug (NSAID), similar to the others that are used to relieve pain and inflammation. We do not know exactly how NSAIDs work, but part of their action may be caused by an ability to inhibit the body's production of a hormone called *prostaglandin* and to inhibit the action of other body chemicals, including cyclo-oxygenase, lipoxygenase, leukotrienes, lysosomal enzymes, and a host of other factors. Diflunisal is absorbed into the bloodstream fairly rapidly. Pain relief comes within 1 hour after taking the first dose, but the drug's anti-inflammatory effect takes a lot longer (several days to 2 weeks) to become apparent and may take several months to reach its maximum.

Cautions and Warnings

People who are **allergic** to Diflunisal (or any other NSAID) and those with a history of **asthma attacks** brought on by another NSAID, by **Iodides,** or by **Aspirin** should not take Diflunisal.

This medicine can cause **gastrointestinal (GI) bleeding, ulcers,** and **perforation.** This can occur at any time with or without warning in people who take chronic Diflunisal treatment. People with a history of **active GI bleeding** should be cautious about taking any NSAID. **Minor stomach upset, gas,** or **distress** is common during the first few days of treatment with Diflunisal. People who develop bleeding or ulcers and continue their NSAID treatment should be aware of the possibility of developing more serious drug toxicity.

Diflunisal can affect **platelets** and **blood clotting** at high doses and should be avoided by people with clotting problems and those taking Warfarin.

People with **heart problems** who use Diflunisal may find that their arms and legs or feet become swollen.

Diflunisal can cause severe toxic side effects to the **kidney.** Report any unusual side effects to your doctor, who may need to periodically test your kidney function.

Diflunisal can make you **unusually sensitive to the effects of the sun.**

Because Diflunisal is related to Aspirin, it should be used with caution in **children** and **adolescents** because of the possibility of Reye's syndrome.

Possible Side Effects

▼ Most common: diarrhea, nausea, vomiting, constipation, stomach gas, stomach upset or irritation, and loss of appetite.

▼ Less common: stomach ulcers, GI bleeding, hepatitis, gallbladder attacks, painful urination, poor kidney function, kidney inflammation, blood and protein in the urine, dizziness, fainting, nervousness, depression, hallucinations, confusion, disorientation, tingling in the hands or feet, light-headedness, itching, increased sweating, dry nose and mouth, heart palpitations, chest pain, difficulty breathing, and muscle cramps.

▼ Rare: severe allergic reactions, including closing of the throat, fever and chills, changes in liver function,

---

Possible Side Effects *(continued)*

jaundice (yellowing of the skin or eyes), and kidney failure. People who experience such effects must be promptly treated in a hospital emergency room or doctor's office.

NSAIDs have caused severe skin reactions; if this happens to you, see your doctor immediately.

Drug Interactions

• Diflunisal can increase the effects of oral anticoagulant (blood-thinning) drugs such as Warfarin. You may take this combination, but your doctor may have to reduce your anticoagulant dose to take this effect into account.

• Diflunisal may increase Acetaminophen blood levels by as much as 50 percent. This can be a problem for people with liver disease.

• Diflunisal increases the blood levels and effects of Thiazide diuretics.

• Combining Diflunisal with Indomethacin can cause GI bleeding, which can be fatal. Do not take this combination.

Food Interactions

Take Diflunisal with food or a magnesium/aluminum antacid if it upsets your stomach.

Usual Dose

500 mg to 1000 mg to start, then 250 mg to 500 mg every 8 to 12 hours. Do not take more than 1500 mg a day. Take each dose with a full glass of water and don't lie down for 15 to 30 minutes after you take the medicine. Do not crush or chew Diflunisal tablets.

Overdosage

People have died from Diflunisal overdoses. The most common overdose signs are drowsiness, nausea, vomiting, diarrhea, abdominal pain, rapid breathing, rapid heartbeat, increased sweating, ringing or buzzing in the ears, confusion, disorientation, stupor, and coma.

Take the victim to a hospital emergency room at once. ALWAYS bring the medicine bottle with you.

Special Information

Diflunisal can make you drowsy and/or tired: Be careful when driving or operating hazardous equipment.

Do not take any nonprescription products with Acetaminophen or Aspirin while taking Diflunisal; also, avoid alcoholic beverages.

Contact your doctor if you develop skin rash, itching, visual disturbances, weight gain, breathing difficulty, fluid retention, hallucinations, black stools, or persistent headache. Call your doctor if you develop any unusual side effects or if side effects become intolerable.

If you forget to take a dose of Diflunisal, take it as soon as you remember. If you take several Diflunisal doses a day and it is within 4 hours of your next dose, skip the one you forgot and continue with your regular schedule. If you take Diflunisal once a day, and it is within 8 hours of your next dose, skip the missed dose and continue with your regular schedule. Do not take a double dose.

Special Populations

Pregnancy/Breast-feeding

Diflunisal may cross into the fetal blood circulation. It has not been found to cause birth defects, but may affect a developing fetal heart during the last 3 months of pregnancy. Pregnant women and those who might become pregnant should not take Diflunisal without their doctors' approval; pregnant women should be particularly cautious about using this drug during the last 3 months of their pregnancy. When the drug is considered essential by your doctor, its potential benefits must be carefully weighed against its risks.

Diflunisal passes into breast milk. There is a possibility that a nursing mother taking Diflunisal could affect her baby's heart or cardiovascular system. Nursing mothers who must take this drug should bottle-feed their babies.

Seniors

Older adults may be more susceptible to Diflunisal side effects, especially ulcer disease.

Type of Drug

Digitalis Glycosides

Generic Name	**Brand Name**
Digitoxin	Crystodigin*
Digoxin	Lanoxicaps*
	Lanoxin*

(*Also available in generic form)

Prescribed for

Congestive heart failure; other heart conditions.

General Information

Digitalis glycosides directly affect the heart muscle, depending on the dose you are taking. They improve the heart's pumping ability or help to control its beating rhythm. People with heart failure very often develop swelling of the lower legs, feet, and ankles: Digitalis drugs improve these symptoms by improving blood circulation. Digitoxin is more useful than Digoxin for people who have kidney problems, because Digitoxin is removed mostly by the liver, not the kidneys.

These medications are generally used as part of the lifelong treatment of congestive heart failure.

Cautions and Warnings

Do not use these drugs if you know you are **allergic** or **sensitive** to them. Digitalis allergies are rare, and are often limited to only one member of the group; another digitalis drug may work in its place.

Digitalis drugs have been used as part of a treatment for obesity. The possibility of developing **fatal heart rhythms** while undergoing such treatment makes Digitalis extremely dangerous as a **weight-loss medicine.**

Many **symptoms of heart disease** can also be associated with Digitalis toxicity. **Report** any unusual side effects to your doctor at once.

Kidney disease can increase blood levels of all Digitalis drugs, except Digitoxin. **Liver disease** can increase blood levels of Digitoxin. Your dosage may need adjusting.

Long-term use of a Digitalis drug can cause the body to lose potassium, especially since these drugs are generally used in combination with diuretics. For this reason, be sure to eat a **well-balanced diet** emphasizing foods that are high in **potassium,** such as bananas, citrus fruits, melons, and tomatoes.

Digitalis requirements vary with **thyroid status.** If you are taking Digitalis and your thyroid status changes, your doctor will have to change your Digitalis dosage.

Possible Side Effects

▼ Most common: loss of appetite, nausea, vomiting, diarrhea, and blurred or disturbed vision. If you experience any of these problems, discuss them with your doctor immediately.

▼ Less common: headache, weakness, apathy, drowsiness, blurred or yellow vision, seeing halos or spots around bright lights, mental depression, psychoses, confusion or disorientation, restlessness, hallucinations, delirium, seizures, nerve pain, abnormal heart rhythms, and slow pulse.

▼ Rare: enlargement of the breasts (reported after long-term use of a Digitalis drug). Allergy or sensitivity to Digitalis drugs is also uncommon.

Children respond differently than adults to Digitalis. They are more likely to develop abnormal heart rhythms before they see yellow or green halos or spots and before they develop nausea, vomiting, diarrhea or stomach pains. Any abnormal rhythm that develops while a child is taking Digitalis should be assumed to be drug-related.

Drug Interactions

• Barbiturates, Phenytoin and related antiseizure drugs, Phenylbutazone, and Rifampin will counteract the effectiveness of a Digitalis drug by stimulating its breakdown by the liver.

• The absorption of a Digitalis drug into the bloodstream is reduced by taking it together with antacids, Aminosalicylic Acid, Cholestyramine, Colestipol, anticancer combinations, Kaolin-pectin mixtures, and Sulfasalazine. Other drugs that can prevent Digitalis drugs from being absorbed are oral Kanamycin, Metoclopramide, and oral Neomycin.

• Drugs that may increase the effect of a Digitalis drug are Aminoglycoside antibiotics, Amiodarone, Anticholinergic drugs, Benzodiazepines, Captopril, Diltiazem, Erythromycin, Esmolol, Flecainide, Hydroxychloroquine, Ibuprofen, Indomethacin, Nifedipine, Quinine, Tetracycline, Tolbutamide, and Verapamil.

• Quinidine may increase the amount of Digoxin or Digitoxin in the blood by 2 to 3 times, beginning 1 to 3 days after the Quinidine is started.

• Disopyramide may alter the effects of Digoxin, although the exact interaction is not well understood.

• Low blood potassium, a common side effect of Thiazide diuretics, Bumetanide, Ethacrynic Acid, and Furosemide, will increase a Digitalis drug's effect and increase the chance of developing a toxic side effect.

• Spironolactone can either increase or decrease the effect of a Digitalis drug. Its effect is unpredictable.

• Amiloride may decrease the effectiveness of Digoxin.

• Triamterene may increase the effects of Digoxin.

• The effects of a Digitalis drug on your heart may be additive to those of the Ephedrine, Epinephrine, and other stimulants, beta blockers, calcium salts, Procainamide, and Rauwolfia drugs.

• Thyroid drugs will change your Digitalis drug requirement. Your doctor will have to adjust your Digitalis dosage.

Food Interactions

Take each day's dose at the same time for consistency. Many people take their medicine after the morning meal.

Usual Dose

Digitoxin

Adult: The first dose—known as the digitalizing or loading dose—is 2 mg over about 3 days, or 0.4 mg per day for 4 days. Digitalization may also be accomplished with lower doses over 10 to 14 days. Maintenance dose ranges from 0.05 mg to 0.03 mg daily.

Senior: lower doses are required because of increased sensitivity to adverse effects.

Infant and Child: usually not recommended.

Digoxin

Adult: The first dose—known as the digitalizing or loading dose—is about 4 to 7 micrograms per pound of body weight. Digitalization may also be accomplished with lower doses over 7 days. Maintenance dose ranges from 0.125 mg to 0.5 mg and must be corrected for kidney function.

Senior: lower doses required, because of increased sensitivity to adverse effects.

Infant and Child (up to age 10): loading dose is 5 to 30 micrograms per pound of body weight. Doses do not vary in direct proportion to age because of variations in the ability of children to handle this medicine. For instance, children under age 2 will receive 2 to 4 times more medicine than a 10-year-old. The daily maintenance dose is 20 to 35 percent of the loading dose. Careful measurement of your child's Digoxin dose is crucial to safe and effective treatment.

Overdosage

An early sign of overdose in children is change in heart rhythm. Vomiting, diarrhea, and eye trouble are frequently seen in older people. General symptoms of overdosage are loss of appetite, nausea, vomiting, diarrhea, headache, weakness, apathy, blurred vision, yellow or green spots or halos before the eyes, yellowing of the skin and eyes, or changes in heartbeat. Contact your doctor immediately if any of these symptoms appear. Overdose victims must be taken to an emergency room for treatment. ALWAYS bring the medicine bottle with you.

Special Information

Do not stop taking this drug unless your doctor tells you to.

Avoid nonprescription medicines that contain stimulants. Ask your pharmacist if you have questions.

Call your doctor at once if you develop drug side effects.

There may be some variation among Digitalis drug tablets made by different manufacturers. Do not change drug brands without telling your doctor.

Check your pulse every day (your doctor will teach you how to do this) and call your doctor if it drops below 60 beats a minute.

If you forget to take a dose of a Digitalis drug and remember at least 12 hours before your next dose, take it right away.

If you do not remember until it is less than 12 hours to your next dose, skip the forgotten dose and go back to your regular schedule. Do not take a double dose. Call your doctor if you forget to take your medicine for 2 or more days.

Special Populations

Pregnancy/Breast-feeding
Digitalis drugs cross into the fetal blood circulation, but they have not been found to cause birth defects. In fact, fetal heart disease has been treated by giving the mother Digoxin. Nevertheless, pregnant women and those who might become pregnant should not take any Digitalis drug without their doctors' approval. When the drug is considered essential by your doctor, its potential benefits must be carefully weighed against any risks.

Small amounts of Digoxin pass into breast milk, but it has caused no problems among breast-fed infants. It is not known if Digitoxin passes into breast milk. You must consider the possible effect on the nursing infant if breast-feeding while taking one of these medicines.

Seniors
Older adults are more sensitive to the effects of Digitalis drugs, especially loss of appetite. Follow your doctor's directions and report any side effects at once.

Dilantin

see **Phenytoin**, page 893

Generic Name
Diltiazem Hydrochloride

Brand Names

Cardizem	Cardizem SR
Cardizem CD	Dilacor XR

(Also available in generic form, except for Cardizem CD)

Type of Drug

Calcium channel blocker.

Prescribed for

Angina pectoris, Raynaud's disease, prevention of second heart attacks, and tardive dyskinesia (severe side effects associated with some antipsychotic and other medicines). Long-acting Diltiazem products may be used to treat high blood pressure.

General Information

Diltiazem Hydrochloride is one of several calcium channel blockers, which work by slowing the passage of calcium into muscle cells. This causes muscles in the blood vessels that supply your heart to open wider (dilate), allowing more blood to reach heart tissues. The drugs also decrease muscle spasm in those blood vessels. Diltiazem also reduces the speed at which electrical impulses are carried through heart tissue, adding to its ability to slow the heart and prevent the pain of angina (chest pain). Diltiazem Hydrochloride, especially when combined with a diuretic (water-pill), beta-blocker, or other blood-pressure-lowering drug, can help to reduce high blood pressure by causing blood vessels to dilate, which allows blood to flow more easily. Other calcium channel blockers are used for abnormal heart rhythms, migraine headache, heart failure, and cardiomyopathy.

Cautions and Warnings

Diltiazem can **slow your heart** and interfere with normal electrical conduction. For people with a condition called **sick sinus syndrome**, this can result in temporary heart stoppage; most people will not develop this effect.

Diltiazem should not be taken if you are having a **heart attack** or if you have **lung congestion**. It should be taken with caution by people with **heart failure** because Diltiazem can worsen that condition.

Low blood pressure may occur, especially in people also taking a **beta blocker.**

Diltiazem can cause severe **liver damage** and should be taken with caution if you have had **hepatitis** or any other **liver condition.**

Caution should also be exercised if you have a history of **kidney problems,** although no clear tendency toward causing kidney damage is seen with this medicine.

Possible Side Effects

Diltiazem's side effects are generally mild, and rarely cause people to stop taking it.

▼ Common: dizziness, light-headedness, weakness, headache, and fluid accumulation in the hands, legs, or feet.

▼ Less common: low blood pressure, fainting, changes in heart rate (increase or decrease), abnormal heart rhythms, heart failure, nervousness, fatigue, nausea, rash, tingling in the hands or feet, hallucinations, temporary memory loss, difficulty sleeping, diarrhea, vomiting, constipation, upset stomach, itching, unusual sensitivity to sunlight, painful or stiff joints, liver inflammation, and increased urination, especially at night.

Drug Interactions

• Diltiazem taken with a beta-blocking drug for high blood pressure is usually well tolerated, but may lead to heart failure in people with already weakened hearts.

• Calcium channel blockers, including Diltiazem, may add to the effects of Digoxin, although this effect is not observed with any consistency and only affects people with a large amount of Digoxin already in their systems.

• Cimetidine and Ranitidine increase the amount of Diltiazem in the bloodstream and may account for a slight increase in the drug's effect.

• Diltiazem may increase blood levels of Cyclosporine, Carbamazepine, Encainide, and Theophylline, and thus increase the chance of side effects from these drugs.

• Diltiazem may cause a decrease in blood-Lithium levels, leading to a loss of antimanic control in people taking Lithium.

Food Interactions

Diltiazem is best taken on an empty stomach, at least 1 hour before, or 2 hours after meals.

Usual Dose

Tablets
Diltiazem
30 to 60 mg 4 times per day.

Sustained Release Capsules
Cardizem SR
60 to 180 mg twice per day.

Cardizem CD
120 to 480 mg once per day.

Dilacor XR
240 to 480 mg once per day.

Overdosage

The major symptoms of Diltiazem overdose are very low blood pressure and reduced heart rate. Overdose victims must be made to vomit within 30 minutes of taking the dose with Syrup of Ipecac (available at any pharmacy) to remove the drug from the stomach. **DO NOT INDUCE VOMITING IF THE VICTIM HAS FAINTED OR CONVULSED.** If overdose symptoms have developed or more than 30 minutes have passed, vomiting is of little value. Take the victim to a hospital emergency room immediately for treatment. ALWAYS bring the medicine bottle with you.

Special Information

Call your doctor if you develop any of the following symptoms: swelling of the hands, legs, or feet; severe dizziness; constipation or nausea; or very low blood pressure.

Do not open, chew, or crush sustained-release capsules of Dilacor XR. They must be swallowed whole.

If you take your Diltiazem 3 or 4 times per day and forget a dose, take it as soon as you remember. Space the remaining doses of medicine throughout the remaining hours of the day. Do not take a double dose.

If you take Diltiazem once or twice a day and forget to take a dose, take it as soon as you remember. If it is almost time for your next dose, skip the one you forgot and continue with your regular schedule. Do not take a double dose.

Special Populations

Pregnancy/Breast-feeding

Animal studies with Diltiazem at doses greater than the usual human dose have revealed a definite potential for harming a developing fetus. With increased dosages, adverse effects become more frequent and more severe. Diltiazem Hydrochloride should not be taken by pregnant women or by women who may become pregnant while using it. In situations in which this drug is deemed essential, the potential benefit must be carefully weighed against the risk.

Because Diltiazem passes into breast milk, nursing mothers taking this drug should bottle-feed their infants. Diltiazem's safety in children has not been established.

Seniors

Older adults may be more sensitive to the effects of this drug because it takes longer to pass out of their bodies. Follow your doctor's directions and report any side effects at once.

Generic Name

Dimenhydrinate

Brand Names

Calm-X	Dramamine,
Dimetabs	Children's
Dramamine	Triptone Caplets

(Also available in generic form)

Note: The information in this profile also applies to:

Generic Name

Meclizine

Brand Names

Antivert	Dizmiss	Ru-Vert-M
Antrizine		
Bonine		

(Also available in generic form)

Type of Drug

Antihistamine; antiemetic.

Prescribed for

Preventing and treating the nausea, vomiting, and dizziness associated with motion sickness.

General Information

Dimenhydrinate is a mixture of Diphenhydramine (an antihistamine) and another ingredient, although the antihistamine is believed to be the active ingredient. Dimenhydrinate depresses middle-ear function, but the way in which it actually prevents nausea, vomiting, or dizziness is not known. Dimenhydrinate tablets and liquid are available without a prescription. Meclizine is an antihistamine used to treat or prevent nausea, vomiting, and motion sickness. It takes a little longer to start working than Dimenhydrinate, but its effects last much longer. The specific method by which Meclizine acts on the brain to prevent nausea and dizziness is not fully understood. In general, Meclizine does a better job of preventing motion sickness than treating the symptoms once they are present. It takes 1/2 to 1 hour to work and lasts for 12 to 24 hours.

Cautions and Warnings

People with a **prostate condition**, some types of **stomach ulcers, bladder problems, difficulty urinating, glaucoma, asthma,** or **abnormal heart rhythms** should use Dimenhydrinate or Meclizine only while under a doctor's care. Newborn babies and people who are **allergic** or **sensitive** to Dimenhydrinate or Meclizine should not be given this medicine.

Because they control nausea and vomiting, Dimenhydrinate or Meclizine can hide the symptoms of **appendicitis** and **overdoses of other medicines.** Your doctor may have difficulty reaching an accurate diagnosis in these conditions unless he or she knows you are taking one of these drugs.

Possible Side Effects

▼ Most common: drowsiness.
▼ Less common: confusion; nervousness; excitation;

Possible Side Effects *(continued)*

restlessness; headache; sleeplessness (especially in children); tingling; heavy or weak hands; fainting; dizziness; tiredness; rapid heartbeat; low blood pressure; heart palpitations; blurred or double vision; difficult or painful urination; increased sensitivity to the sun; loss of appetite; nausea; vomiting; diarrhea; upset stomach; constipation; nightmares; rash; drug reactions (wheezing, skin reactions, etc.); ringing or buzzing in the ears; dry mouth, nose, or throat; stuffed nose; wheezing; and increased chest phlegm or chest tightness.

Drug Interactions

• Taking Dimenhydrinate or Meclizine together with alcoholic beverages, other antihistamines, tranquilizers, or other nervous-system depressants can cause excessive dizziness, drowsiness, or other signs of nervous-system depression.

• When taken with drugs that cause dizziness or other ear-related side effects, these drugs can mask early signs of these side effects, especially in infants and children.

Food Interactions

Take either of these medicines with food or milk if it upsets your stomach.

Usual Dose

Dimenhydrinate

Adult and Adolescent (age 13 and older): 50 to 100 mg (1 or 2 tablets, or 4 to 8 teaspoons) every 4 to 6 hours; not more than 400 mg per day.

Child (age 6 to 12): 25 to 50 mg (1/2 or 1 tablet, or 2 to 4 teaspoons) every 6 to 8 hours; not more than 150 mg.

Child (age 2 to 5): up to 25 mg (1/2 tablet, or 2 teaspoons) every 6 to 8 hours; not more than 3 doses per day.

Child (under age 2): consult your doctor.

Meclizine

Adult and Adolescent (age 13 and older): 25 to 50 mg 1 hour before travel; repeat every 24 hours for duration of journey.

Up to 100 mg may be needed to control dizziness from other causes.

Child: not recommended.

Overdosage

The usual overdose signs are drowsiness, clumsiness, or unsteadiness. A faint feeling, facial flushing, and dry mouth, nose, and throat can also occur. Convulsions, coma, and breathing difficulty can develop after a massive overdose. Overdose victims should be taken to a hospital emergency room for treatment. ALWAYS bring the medicine bottle.

Special Information

For maximum effectiveness against motion sickness, take the medicine 1 to 2 hours before traveling; it may still be effective if taken 30 minutes before traveling.

These drugs can cause dry mouth, nose, or throat. Sugarless candy, gum, or ice chips can usually relieve these symptoms. Constant dry mouth can make you more likely to develop tooth decay or gum disease. Pay special attention to oral hygiene while you are taking this medicine, and contact your doctor if excessive mouth dryness lasts more than 2 weeks.

If you forget to take a dose of Dimenhydrinate or Meclizine, take it as soon as you remember. If it is almost time for your next dose, skip the one you forgot and continue with your regular schedule. Do not take a double dose.

Special Populations

Pregnancy/Breast-feeding

Dimenhydrinate has not been proven to cause birth defects or other significant problems in pregnant women, although studies in animals have shown that Meclizine may cause birth defects. Do not take any antihistamine without your doctor's knowledge.

Small amounts of Dimenhydrinate or Meclizine may pass into breast milk and may affect a nursing infant. Either drug may also slow milk production. Nursing mothers should avoid antihistamines or bottle-feed their babies while taking these drugs.

Seniors

Seniors are more sensitive to antihistamine side effects. Take the lowest effective dose of this drug and call your doctor if side effects are bothersome or unusual.

Generic Name

Diphenhydramine Hydrochloride

Brand Names

AllerMax	Genahist	Nytol
Banophen	Hydramine	Phendry Children's
Belix	Nervine Nighttime	Allergy Medicine
Benadryl	Sleep-Aid	Sleep-Eze 3
Diphen Cough	Nidryl	Sominex 2
Dormarex-2	Nordryl	Twilite

(Also available in generic form)

Type of Drug

Antihistamine.

Prescribed for

Seasonal allergy; stuffed and runny nose; itchy eyes; scratchy throat caused by allergy; and other allergic symptoms such as itching, rash, or hives. In addition, Diphenhydramine Hydrochloride has been used for motion sickness and as a nighttime sleep aid because of its potent depressant effect. Diphenhydramine may also be prescribed as part of the treatment for Parkinson's disease.

General Information

Antihistamines are truly versatile. They work by antagonizing histamine at the site of the H_1 histamine receptor and drying up the secretions of the nose, throat, and eyes. They relieve itch and will help you go to sleep.

Cautions and Warnings

Diphenhydramine Hydrochloride should not be used if you

are **allergic** to it. This drug should be avoided or used with extreme care if you have **narrow-angle glaucoma (pressure in the eye), stomach ulcer** or other **stomach problems, enlarged prostate,** or **problems passing urine.** It should not be used by people who have deep-breathing problems such as **asthma.** Use with care if you have a history of **thyroid disease, heart disease, high blood pressure,** or **diabetes.**

Possible Side Effects

▼ Common: itching, rash, sensitivity to bright light, perspiration, chills, lowering of blood pressure, headache, rapid heartbeat, sleeplessness, dizziness, disturbed coordination, confusion, restlessness, nervousness, irritability, euphoria (feeling "high"), tingling and weakness of the hands or feet, blurred or double vision, ringing in the ears, stomach upset, loss of appetite, nausea, vomiting, constipation, diarrhea, difficulty in urination, thickening of lung secretions, tightness of the chest, wheezing, nasal stuffiness, and dry mouth, nose, or throat.

Drug Interactions

• Diphenhydramine Hydrochloride should not be taken with monoamine oxidase (MAO) inhibitors.

• Interaction with tranquilizers, sedatives, and sleeping medication will increase the effects of these drugs; it is extremely important that you discuss this with your doctor so that doses of these drugs can be properly adjusted.

• Diphenhydramine will enhance the intoxicating and sedating effects of alcohol. Be careful with this combination.

Food Interactions

Take this drug with food if it upsets your stomach.

Usual Dose

Adult: 25 mg to 50 mg 3 to 4 times a day; as a sleep aid, 25 mg to 50 mg at bedtime.

Child (over 20 pounds): 12.5 mg to 25 mg 3 to 4 times a day.

Overdosage

Symptoms of overdosage are depression or stimulation (especially in children), dry mouth, fixed or dilated pupils, flushing of the skin, and stomach upset. Overdose victims should be made to vomit with Syrup of Ipecac (available at any pharmacy). Follow the directions on the bottle or call your local poison control center. Take the overdose victim to a hospital emergency room immediately, if you cannot make him or her vomit. ALWAYS bring the medicine bottle with you.

Special Information

Diphenhydramine Hydrochloride produces a depressant effect: Be extremely cautious when driving or operating heavy equipment.

If you forget to take a dose, take it as soon as you remember. If it is almost time for your next dose, skip the one you forgot and continue with your regular schedule. Do not take a double dose.

Special Populations

Pregnancy/Breast-feeding

Antihistamines have not been proven to be a cause of birth defects or other problems in pregnant women. However, studies in animals have shown that some antihistamines may cause birth defects. Do not take any antihistamine without your doctor's knowledge.

Small amounts of antihistamine medicines pass into breast milk and may affect a nursing infant. Nursing mothers should avoid Diphenhydramine or use alternative feeding methods while taking the medicine.

Seniors

Seniors are more sensitive to antihistamine side effects, especially confusion, difficult or painful urination, dizziness, drowsiness, a faint feeling, nightmares, excitement, nervousness, restlessness, irritability, and dry mouth, nose, or throat.

Generic Name

Dipivefrin

Brand Name

Propine Eyedrops

Type of Drug

Sympathomimetic.

Prescribed for

Glaucoma.

General Information

When applied to the eye, Dipivefrin is converted to Epineph-rine, one of the cornerstone drugs of glaucoma treatment. It provides the same effect on glaucoma as Epinephrine, but has fewer side effects. Epinephrine decreases the production of the fluid inside the eye and opens the channels by which the eye fluid naturally drains. These two actions combine to reduce fluid pressure inside the eye, treating glaucoma. Dipivefrin may be used in combination with Pilocarpine Ophthalmic Solution or a beta-blocker eyedrop to produce an even greater drop in eye pressure. The drug starts working about a half hour after it is applied and has its maximum effect at about 1 hour.

Cautions and Warnings

Use this product with care if you have **reacted to Dipivefrin** in the past. Interestingly, people who have reacted to **Epineph-rine eyedrops** in the past are not likely to react to Dipivefrin and can probably use this product; this is because of the con-version step that must take place (see *General Information*).

Dipivefrin eyedrops contain sulfite preservatives. If you are sensitive to **sulfites,** this drug might cause irritation or allergic reactions.

Possible Side Effects

▼ Common: burning or stinging upon applying the eyedrops.

▼ Rare: conjunctivitis, drug allergies, rapid heartbeat, abnormal heart rhythms, and high blood pressure.

Drug Interactions

• Dipivefrin eyedrops may be taken with other antiglaucoma eyedrops.

Food Interactions

None known.

Usual Dose

One drop in the affected eye every 12 hours.

Overdosage

Possible symptoms of overdosage are rapid heartbeat, excitement, or sleeplessness. Call your local poison control center or hospital emergency room for more information.

Special Information

To administer eyedrops, lie down or tilt your head backward and look at the ceiling. Hold the dropper above your eye, hold out your lower lid to make a small pouch, and drop the medicine inside while looking up. Release the lower lid and keep your eye open. Don't blink for about 30 seconds. Press gently on the bridge of your nose at the inside corner of your eye for about a minute to help circulate the medicine around your eye. To prevent infection, don't touch the dropper tip to your finger or eyelid. Wait 5 minutes before using any other eyedrop or ointment.

If you forget a dose of Dipivefrin, take it as soon as you remember. If it is almost time for your next dose, take one dose as soon as you remember and then go back to your regular schedule. Do not take a double dose.

Special Populations

Pregnancy/Breast-feeding

As with all drug products, pregnant women should not use Dipivefrin unless the advantages of the product have been carefully weighed against the possible dangers of taking it while pregnant.

It is not known if this drug passes into breast milk. No drug-related problems have been known to occur. Nursing mothers who use Dipivefrin should exercise caution.

Seniors

Older adults may use Dipivefrin without any special precautions. Some older adults may have weaker eyelid muscles. This creates a small reservoir for the eyedrops and may actually increase the drug's effect by keeping it in contact with the eye for a longer period. Your doctor may take this into account when determining the proper drug dosage.

Generic Name

Dirithromycin

Brand Name

Dynabac

Type of Drug

Macrolide antibiotic.

Prescribed for

Infections caused by streptococcus, straphylococcus, and other susceptible bacteria when a Penicillin- or Tetracycline-type antibiotic cannot be used. Virtually any part of the body can be affected by one of these infections. Dirithromycin has been studied specifically in bronchitis, sore throat, pneumonia, tonsillitis, and Legionnaires' disease.

General Information

Dirithromycin is a member of the group of antibiotics known as *macrolides*, but it has no antimicrobial activity of its own. The macrolide group, which also includes Azithromycin,

Clarithromycin, and Erythromycin, are either bactericidal
(they kill the bacteria directly) or bacteriostatic (they slow the
bacteria's growth so that the body's natural protective mechanisms can kill them). Whether these drugs are bacteriostatic
or bactericidal depends on the organism in question and the
amount of antibiotic present in the blood or other body fluid.

After you swallow a Dirithromycin tablet, it is converted in the
intestine to an active antimicrobial form called Erythromycylamine. Erythromycylamine quickly distributes throughout the
body into blood and a variety of different tissues. It is not
broken down by the liver and passes out of the body primarily
through the stool.

Since the action of this antibiotic depends on its concentration in the infected tissues, it is important for you to take
Dirithromycin as directed. The effectiveness of any antibiotic
can be severely reduced if you do not follow directions.

Cautions and Warnings

Do not take Dirithromycin if you're **allergic** to it or to any
macrolide antibiotic.

Dirithromycin should not be taken for **serious blood infections** because not enough of the drug gets into the bloodstream. It does not work against and should not be used for
complications of *H. influenzae*, a contagious infection that
often affects children in daycare centers and their families.
Instead, a drug with specific action against this agent should
be used.

Higher blood levels of Dirithromycin are possible in people
with mild **liver disease,** but no dosage changes are needed.
This medicine has not been studied in people with more
severe liver disease. No dosage change is required in people
with kidney disease.

A form of **colitis** (bowel inflammation) can be associated
with all antibiotics, including Dirithromycin. Diarrhea may be
an indication of this problem.

Possible Side Effects

▼ Most common: abdominal pain, headache, nausea,
and diarrhea.

▼ Less common: increased blood platelet count, vomiting, upset stomach, increased blood potassium, dizziness,

Possible Side Effects (continued)

fainting, pain (no specific source), weakness, stomach disorders, increasing cough, stomach gas, difficulty breathing, itching, rash, and sleeplessness. Some blood tests can also be affected.

▼ Rare: abnormal stools, allergic reactions, dim vision, appetite loss, anxiety, constipation, dehydration, depression, dry mouth, painful menstruation, flushing, swelling in the hands or feet, nosebleeds, eye disorders, fever, flu symptoms, stomach and intestinal irritation, vomiting blood, rapid breathing, feelings of ill health, mouth sores, muscle aches, neck pain, nervousness, heart palpitations, tingling in the hands or feet, tiredness, sweating, taste changes, thirst, ringing or buzzing in the ears, tremors, frequent urination, vaginal fungus infections, and vaginal irritation.

Drug Interactions

• When Dirithromycin is taken right after an antacid or histamine H_2 antagonist (Cimetidine, Famotidine, Nizatidine, or Ranitidine—most of which can be bought without a prescription), the amount of drug absorbed is increased.

• Other macrolide antibiotics interfere with the elimination of Theophylline from the body, but this does not seem to be the case with Dirithromycin. Your doctor may want to check blood Theophylline levels when you start on this medicine.

• Erythromycin and other macrolide antibiotics interact with Terfenadine, a nonsedating antihistamine, to produce potentially fatal abnormal heart rhythms. However, studies do not show an interaction between Dirithromycin and Terfenadine.

Foot Interactions

Take with food or within 1 hour of meals. Food increases the amount of antibiotic absorbed into the blood.

Usual Dose

Adult and child (age 12 and older): 500 mg per day for 7 to 10 days.

Child (under age 12): not recommended.

Overdosage

Dirithromycin overdose may result in nausea, vomiting, stomach cramps, and diarrhea. Call your local poison control center or hospital emergency room for more information.

Special Information

Although Dirithromycin is a relatively safe antibiotic, it is not the antibiotic of choice for severe infections.

Do not crush, cut, or chew Dirithromycin tablets.

Call your doctor if you develop nausea, vomiting, diarrhea, stomach cramps, severe abdominal pain, or other severe or persistent side effects.

If you forget a dose of Dirithromycin, take it as soon as you remember. If you don't remember until the next day, skip the forgotten dose and go back to your regular schedule. Call your doctor if you forget to take more than 1 dose.

Remember to complete the full course of therapy as prescribed by your doctor, even if you feel perfectly well after only a few days of taking Dirithromycin.

Special Populations

Pregnancy/Breast-feeding

In studies with pregnant laboratory animals, Dirithromycin affected the developing fetus. There is no information on the use of this drug in pregnant women, but it should be taken only if the possible risks and benefits and alternative antibiotics have been considered.

Other macrolide antibiotics pass into human breast milk, but it is not known if Dirithromycin or Erythromycylamine act similarly. Nursing mothers who must take this drug should watch for possible side effects in their infants.

Seniors

Older adults may use this product without special restriction.

Generic Name

Disopyramide

Brand Names

Norpace
Norpace CR

(Also available in generic form)

Type of Drug

Antiarrhythmic.

Prescribed for

Abnormal heart rhythms.

General Information

Disopyramide slows the rate at which nerve impulses are carried through heart muscle, reducing the response of heart muscle to those impulses. It acts on the heart similarly to the more widely used antiarrhythmic medicines, namely, Procainamide Hydrochloride and Quinidine Sulfate. Disopyramide is often prescribed for people who do not respond to other antiarrhythmic drugs. It also may be prescribed for people who have had an infarction (heart attack) because it helps infarcted areas to respond more like adjacent, healthy heart tissue to nerve impulses.

Cautions and Warnings

This drug can worsen **heart failure** or produce **severe lowering of blood pressure**. It should be used **only in combination** with another antiarrhythmic agent or beta blocker (such as Propranolol Hydrochloride), **when single-drug treatment has not been effective** or the arrhythmia may be life-threatening.

In rare instances, Disopyramide has caused a reduction in **blood-sugar levels**. Therefore, the drug should be used with caution by **diabetics, older adults** (who are more susceptible to this effect), and people with **poor kidney** or **liver function.** Blood-sugar levels should be **measured periodically** in people with **heart failure** or **liver or kidney disease**, those who are **malnourished**, and those taking a **beta-blocking drug**.

Because of its anticholinergic effects, Disopyramide should be used with caution by people who have **severe difficulty urinating** (especially men with a severe prostate condition), **glaucoma**, or **myasthenia gravis**.

People with **liver or kidney disease** must take a reduced dose of Disopyramide.

Possible Side Effects

▼ Most common: heart failure, low blood pressure, and urinary difficulty.

▼ Common: dry mouth, throat or nose, constipation, and blurred vision.

▼ Less common: urination, dizziness, fatigue, headache, nervousness, difficulty breathing, chest pain, nausea, stomach bloating, gas, stomach pain, loss of appetite, diarrhea, vomiting, itching, rashes, muscle weakness, generalized aches and pains, feelings of ill health, low blood-potassium levels, increases in blood-cholesterol and triglyceride levels, and dry eyes.

▼ Rare: male impotence, painful urination, stomach pain, reduced heart activity, anemia (reduced levels of blood hemoglobin and hematocrit), reduced white-blood-cell counts, sleeplessness, depression, psychotic reactions, liver inflammation and jaundice, numbness and tingling in the hands or feet, elevated blood urea nitrogen (BUN) and creatinine (blood tests for kidney function), low blood sugar, fever, swollen and painful male breasts, drug allergy, and glaucoma.

Drug Interactions

• Phenytoin and Rifampin may increase the rate at which the body removes Disopyramide from the blood. Your Disopyramide dose may need alteration if this combination is used. Other drugs known to increase drug breakdown by the liver (such as barbiturates and Primidone) may also have this effect.

• Other antiarrhythmic drugs (Procainamide, Quinidine,

etc,) may increase the effect of Disopyramide, making dosage reduction necessary. At the same time, Disopyramide may reduce the effectiveness of Quinidine.

• Disopyramide, when taken together with a beta-blocking drug, may produce increased Disopyramide effects, additive effects, or depression of heart function.

• Erythromycin may increase the amount of Disopyramide in your blood, causing abnormal heart rhythms or other cardiac effects.

• Disopyramide may reduce the effectiveness of oral anti-coagulant (blood-thinning) drugs. Your doctor should check your anticoagulant dosage to be sure you are getting the right amount.

• Disopyramide may increase the amount of Digoxin in your blood, though the amount of the increase is not likely to affect your heart.

Food Interactions

Disopyramide should be taken on an empty stomach or at least 1 hour before or 2 hours after meals.

Disopyramide may cause symptoms of low blood sugar: anxiety, chills, cold sweats, drowsiness, excessive hunger, nausea, nervousness, rapid pulse, shakiness, unusual weakness, tiredness, or cool, pale skin. If this happens to you, eat some chocolate, candy, or other high-sugar food, and call your doctor at once.

Usual Dose

Adult: 400 mg to 600 mg per day, divided into 2 or 4 doses. In severe cases, 400 mg every 6 hours may be required. The long-acting preparation is taken every 12 hours.

Reduced kidney function: reduced dosage, depending on the degree of kidney function present.

People with liver failure: 400 mg per day.

Child (age 13 to 18): 2.5 mg to 7 mg per pound per day.

Child (age 5 to 12): 4.5 mg to 7 mg per pound per day.

Child (age 1 to 4): 4.5 mg to 9 mg per pound per day.

Child (under age 1): 4.5 mg to 13.5 mg per pound per day.

Overdosage

Symptoms of overdosage are breathing difficulty, abnormal

heart rhythms, and unconsciousness. In severe cases, overdosage can lead to death. Overdose victims should be made
to vomit with Syrup of Ipecac (available at any pharmacy) to
remove any remaining drug from the stomach. Call your
doctor or poison control center before doing this. If you must
go to a hospital emergency room, ALWAYS bring the medicine bottle with you. Prompt and vigorous treatment can
mean the difference between life and death in severe overdosage.

Special Information

Disopyramide can cause dry mouth, urinary difficulty, constipation, or blurred vision. Call your doctor if these symptoms
become severe or intolerable, but don't stop taking the
medicine without your doctor's approval.

If Disopyramide is required for a child, and capsules are not
appropriate, your pharmacist, with your doctor's permission,
can make a liquid product. (Do not do this at home, because
this medication requires special preparation.) The liquid should
be refrigerated and protected from light and should be
thrown away after 30 days.

If you forget to take a dose of Disopyramide, take it as soon
as possible. However, if it is within 4 hours of your next dose,
skip the forgotten dose and go back to your regular schedule.
Do not take a double dose.

Special Populations

Pregnancy/Breast-feeding

Do not take this drug if you are pregnant or planning to
become pregnant while using it, because it will pass into the
developing fetus and may affect its development. Also, Disopyramide can, if you are pregnant, cause your uterus to
contract. If Disopyramide is considered essential, discuss the
potential risks of taking it with your doctor.

Nursing women should not take Disopyramide because it
passes into breast milk. If you must take this medicine,
bottle-feed your baby.

Seniors

Older adults, especially those with liver or kidney disease, are
more sensitive to the effects of this drug, especially urinary
difficulty and dry mouth. Follow your doctor's directions and
report any side effects at once.

Brand Name

Donnatal Capsules/Elixir/Tablets/Extentabs

Ingredients

Atropine Sulfate

Hyoscyamine Sulfate

Phenobarbital

Scopolamine Hydrobromide

(Liquids also contain 23% alcohol)

Other Brand Names

Barophen Elixir

Donnamar Elixir

Donnapine Tablets

Hyosophen Elixir/Tablets

Malatal Tablets

Relaxadon Tablets

Spasmophen Elixir

Susano Elixir/Tablets

(Also available in generic form)

The following products contain the same ingredients in different concentrations and are also available in generic form:

Barbidonna Elixir/Tablets

Kinesed Tablets

Spasmophen Elixir/Tablets

Type of Drug

Anticholinergic combination.

Prescribed for

Symptomatic relief of stomach spasm and other forms of gastrointestinal cramps. Donnatal may also be prescribed for the treatment of motion sickness. There is considerable doubt among medical experts that this drug lives up to its claims.

General Information

Donnatal is a mild antispasmodic sedative drug. Its principal action is to counteract the effect of acetylcholine, an important neurohormone. It is used only to relieve symptoms, not to treat the cause of the symptoms. In addition to the brand names listed above, there are about 50 other anticholinergic combinations with similar properties. All are used to relieve cramps, and all are about equally effective. Some have additional ingredients to reduce or absorb excess gas in the stomach, to coat the stomach, or to control diarrhea. Donnatal and products like it should not be used for more than the temporary relief of symptoms.

Cautions and Warnings

Donnatal should not be used by people with **glaucoma, rapid heartbeat, severe intestinal disease** such as ulcerative colitis, **serious kidney or liver disease,** or a history of **allergy** to any of the ingredients of this drug. Donnatal and other drugs of this class can reduce your **ability to sweat**. Therefore, if you take this type of medication, avoid extended **heavy exercise** and the excessive **high temperatures** of summer.

Possible Side Effects

▼ Most common: blurred vision, dry mouth, difficulty in urination, flushing, and dry skin.

▼ Infrequent: rapid or unusual heartbeat, increased-sensitivity to bright light, loss of taste sensation, headache, nervousness, tiredness, weakness, dizziness, inability to sleep, nausea, vomiting, fever, stuffy nose, heartburn, loss of sex drive, decreased sweating, constipation, bloated feeling, and allergic reactions (such as fever and rash).

Drug Interactions

• Although Donnatal contains only a small amount of Phenobarbital, it is wise to avoid large amounts of alcohol or other sedative drugs. Other Phenobarbital interactions are probably not important, but are possible with anticoagulants, adrenal corticosteroids, tranquilizers, narcotics, sleeping pills, Digitalis or other cardiac glycosides, and antihistamines.

• Some Phenothiazine drugs, tranquilizers, tricyclic antidepressants, and narcotics may increase the side effects of the Atropine Sulfate contained in Donnatal, causing dry mouth, difficulty in urination, and constipation.

Food Interactions

Take this drug 30 to 60 minutes before meals.

Usual Dose

Adult and Adolescent (age 13 and older): 1 to 2 tablets, capsules, or teaspoons 3 to 4 times a day.
Child (age 2 to 12): 1/2 the adult dose.
Child (under age 2): do not use.

Overdosage

Symptoms of overdosage are dry mouth; difficulty in swallowing; thirst; blurred vision; sensitivity to bright light; flushed, hot, dry skin; rash; fever; abnormal heart rate; high blood pressure; difficulty in urination; restlessness; confusion; delirium; and difficulty in breathing. The victim should be taken to a hospital emergency room immediately. ALWAYS bring the medicine bottle with you.

Special Information

Dry mouth from Donnatal usually can be relieved by chewing gum or sucking hard candy or ice chips; constipation can be treated with a stool-softening laxative.

Donnatal can reduce the amount of saliva in your mouth, making it easier for bacteria to grow in your mouth. This means you need to pay special attention to dental hygiene while taking this medicine to prevent extra cavities and/or gum disease from developing.

Donnatal can cause sedation and blurred vision. Be careful when driving or operating hazardous equipment.

If you forget to take a dose of Donnatal, take it as soon as you remember. If it is almost time for your next dose, skip the one you forgot and continue with your regular schedule. Do not take a double dose.

Special Populations

Pregnancy/Breast-feeding

This drug should be used with caution by pregnant women. Check with your doctor before taking it if you are, or might be, pregnant. Regular use of Donnatal during the last 3 months of pregnancy may lead to moderate drug dependency of the newborn. Labor may be prolonged, delivery may be delayed, and the newborn may have breathing problems if it is used.

Breast-feeding while using Donnatal may cause your baby to be more tired, short of breath, or have a slower than normal heartbeat. Donnatal may reduce the flow of breast milk. Nursing mothers who must take this medicine should consider bottle-feeding their babies.

Seniors

Older adults are often more sensitive to the effects of this drug, especially excitement, confusion, drowsiness, agitation, constipation, dry mouth, and urinary problems. Memory may be impaired and glaucoma worsened. Follow your doctor's directions and report any side effects at once.

Generic Name

Dorzolamide

Brand Name

Trusopt Eyedrops

Type of Drug

Carbonic-anhydrase inhibitor.

Prescribed for

Glaucoma.

General Information

Dorzolamide is similar to Acetazolamide, a carbonic-anhydrase inhibitor taken by mouth, except that it has been put in eyedrop form. Carbonic anhydrase is an enzyme found in many parts of the body, including the eye. When you put Dorzolamide into your eye, it slows the formation of fluid in the eye, reducing eye pressure. In glaucoma, pressure inside the eye is higher than normal.

Cautions and Warnings

Do not take Dorzolamide if you are **sensitive** or **allergic** to it or to other drugs in its group (**sulfa drugs**). Small amounts of any drug placed into your eye find their way into the blood-stream. Rarely, people using this eyedrop will experience sulfa drug side effects or allergies.

Dorzolamide has not been studied in people with severe loss of kidney function. Since Dorzolamide is released from the body through the kidney, another glaucoma medicine should be used in people with **impaired kidney function**.

Possible Side Effects

▼ Most common: burning, stinging, or discomfort in the eye and a bitter taste immediately after you put drops into your eyes.

▼ Less common: allergic reactions, blurred vision, tearing, dryness, and unusual sensitivity to bright light.

▼ Other: headache, nausea, weakness, tiredness, skin rash, and kidney stones. The same types of side effects seen with other forms of sulfa drugs may also be seen with Dorzolamide, but this is unlikely. Be sure to report anything unusual to your doctor at once.

Drug Interactions

• If you are using other eyedrops besides Dorzolamide, make sure to wait at least 10 minutes between putting the different medicines into your eyes.

Food Interactions

None.

Usual Dose

Adult: One drop in the affected eye(s) 3 times a day.

Overdosage

Anyone who swallows a bottle of Dorzolamide should be taken to a hospital emergency room for treatment because of possible effects on potassium and other blood electrolytes. ALWAYS bring the medicine bottle with you.

Special Information

Dorzolamide is a sulfa drug; people allergic to sulfa drugs

should avoid this drug. Report anything unusual to your doctor.

Call your doctor and stop using the eyedrops if you develop any unusual eye reaction or condition, including swollen eyelids or pink-eye (conjunctivitis).

To administer Dorzolamide eyedrops, lie down or tilt your head backward and look at the ceiling. Hold the dropper above your eye and drop the medicine inside your lower lid while looking up. To prevent possible infection, don't allow the dropper to touch your fingers, eyelids, or any surface. Release the lower lid and keep your eye open. Don't blink for about 30 seconds. Press gently on the bridge of your nose at the inside corner of your eye for about a minute. This will help circulate the medicine around your eye. Wait at least 10 minutes before using any other eyedrops.

If you forget to take a dose of Dorzolamide eyedrops, take it as soon as you remember. If it is almost time for your next regularly scheduled dose, skip the one you forgot and continue with your regular schedule. Do not take a double dose.

Special Populations

Pregnancy/Breast-feeding
Pregnant rabbits receiving 31 times the human dose of Dorzolamide developed birth malformations. The chance of Dorzolamide causing birth defects is small, but pregnant women should not use this eyedrop without first discussing it thoroughly with their doctor.

In animal studies, Dorzolamide was found to cause developmental problems in doses 94 times the human dose. It is not known if Dorzolamide passes into breast milk, but nursing mothers should talk this over with their doctor before using Dorzolamide eyedrops.

Seniors
Older adults may be more sensitive to the side effects of this drug than younger adults.

Generic Name

Doxazosin Mesylate

Brand Name
Cardura

Type of Drug

Antihypertensive.

Prescribed for

High blood pressure and benign prostatic hypertrophy (BPH). Doxazosin has also been prescribed with Digoxin and diuretic drugs for congestive heart failure.

General Information

Doxazosin is one of several alpha-adrenergic-blocking agents, which work by opening blood vessels and reducing pressure in them. Alpha blockers like Doxazosin block nerve endings known as *alpha$_1$ receptors.* Other blood-pressure-lowering drugs block beta receptors, interfere with the movement of calcium in blood-vessel muscle cells, affect salt and electrolyte balance in the body, or interfere with the process for manufacturing norepinephrine in the body. The maximum blood-pressure-lowering effect of Doxazosin is seen between 2 and 6 hours after taking a single dose. In BPH, Doxazosin works by relaxing smooth muscles in the prostate and neck of the bladder. Here, too, this effect is produced by blockade of alpha receptors in the affected muscles. Despite the fact that Doxazosin reduces the symptoms of BPH, the drug's long-term effect on complications of BPH or the need for urinary surgery is not known. Drug response is not affected by age or race. Doxazosin's effect lasts for 24 hours. It is broken down in the liver, and little passes out of the body via the kidneys.

Cautions and Warnings

Doxazosin can cause **dizziness** and **fainting,** especially with the first few doses. This is known as a *first-dose effect.* It can be minimized by limiting the first dose to 1 mg at bedtime. The first-dose effect occurs in about 1 percent of people taking an alpha blocker and can recur if the drug is stopped for a few days and then restarted.

Doxazosin should be taken with caution if you have **liver disease,** because the drug is eliminated from your system almost exclusively via the liver.

People **allergic** or **sensitive** to any of the alpha blockers should avoid Doxazosin because of the chance that they will react to it as well.

Doxazosin may slightly **reduce cholesterol levels** and **increase the HDL/LDL** (important blood fats) **ratio,** a positive step for people with a blood-cholesterol problem. People with an already high blood-cholesterol level should discuss this situation with their doctor.

In animals, Doxazosin is toxic to the heart and causes loss of testicular function. These effects have not been seen in humans.

Red- and white-blood-cell counts may be slightly decreased in people taking Doxazosin.

Possible Side Effects

▼ Most common: headache, dizziness, and weakness.

▼ Less common: heart palpitations, abnormal heart rhythms, chest pain, nausea, diarrhea, constipation, abdominal pain or discomfort, stomach gas, breathing difficulty, nosebleeds, sore throat, runny nose, muscle or joint pains, visual disturbances, conjunctivitis ("pinkeye"), ringing in the ears, fainting, depression, decreased sex drive or sexual function, tingling in the hands or feet, nervousness, tiredness, anxiety, sleeplessness, poor muscle coordination, muscle stiffness, poor urinary bladder control, frequent urination, itching, rash, sweating, fluid retention, facial swelling and flushing, and back, neck, shoulder, arm, or leg pains.

▼ Rare: vomiting, dry mouth, sinus irritation, bronchitis, cold or flu symptoms, worsening of asthma, coughing, hair loss, weight gain, and fever.

Drug Interactions

• Doxazosin may interact with beta-blocking drugs to produce a higher rate of dizziness or fainting after taking the first dose of Doxazosin.

• The blood-pressure-lowering effect of Doxazosin may be reduced by Indomethacin.

• When taken with other blood-pressure-lowering drugs, Doxazosin produces an exaggerated reduction of blood pressure.

• The blood-pressure-lowering effect of Clonidine may be reduced by Doxazosin.

• This drug does not affect the results of the prostate-specific antigen (PSA) test, often used to monitor the progress of BPH.

Food Interactions

Doxazosin may be taken without regard to food or meals.

Usual Dose

The usual starting dose of Doxazosin is 1 mg at bedtime. The dosage may be increased to a total of 16 mg per day. It may be taken once or twice per day.

Overdosage

Doxazosin overdose may produce drowsiness, poor reflexes, and very low blood pressure. Overdose victims should be taken to a hospital emergency room at once. ALWAYS bring the medicine bottle with you.

Special Information

Take Doxazosin exactly as prescribed. Do not stop taking it unless directed to do so by your doctor. Avoid nonprescription drugs that contain stimulants because they can increase your blood pressure. Your pharmacist will be able to tell you what you can and cannot take.

Doxazosin can cause dizziness, headache, and drowsiness, especially 2 to 6 hours after you take your first drug dose, although these effects can persist after the first few doses.

Call your doctor if you develop severe dizziness, heart palpitations, or other bothersome or persistent side effects.

Before driving or doing anything that requires intense concentration, wait 12 to 24 hours after taking the first dose of Doxazosin. You may take this medication at bedtime to minimize this problem.

If you forget to take a dose of Doxazosin and you take it once a day, take it as soon as you remember. If it is almost time for your next dose, skip the forgotten dose and continue with your regular schedule. Do not take a double dose.

Special Populations

Pregnancy/Breast-feeding

There have been no studies of Doxazosin in pregnant women, and its safety for use during pregnancy is not known.

Small amounts of Doxazosin pass into breast milk. Nursing mothers who must take this medication should bottle-feed their babies.

Seniors

Older adults, especially those with liver disease, may be more sensitive to the effects and side effects of Doxazosin. Report any unusual side effects to your doctor.

Generic Name

Doxepin

Brand Names

Adapin Capsules
Sinequan Capsules and Concentrate

(Also available in generic form)

Type of Drug

Tricyclic antidepressant.

Prescribed for

Depression (with or without anxiety or sleep disturbance), anxiety, peptic ulcer disease, chronic pain (from migraines, tension headaches, diabetic disease, tic douloureux, cancer, herpes lesions, arthritis, and other sources), panic disorder, and chronic skin disorders.

General Information

Doxepin and other members of this group block the movement of certain stimulant chemicals in and out of nerve endings, have a sedative effect, and counteract the effects of a hormone called *acetylcholine* (which makes them anticholinergic). They prevent the reuptake of important neurohormones (norepinephrine or serotonin) at the nerve ending.

Theory says that people with depression have a chemical imbalance in their brains and that drugs such as Doxepin work to reestablish a proper balance. Although Doxepin and similar antidepressants immediately block neurohormones, it takes 2 to 4 weeks for their clinical antidepressant effect to come into play. Call your doctor if you don't get better after 6 to 8 weeks. Doxepin can also elevate mood, increase physical activity and mental alertness, and improve appetite and sleep patterns in a depressed patient. These drugs are mild sedatives and are useful in treating mild forms of depression associated with anxiety. Occasionally Doxepin and other tricyclic antidepressants have been used in treating nighttime bed-wetting in young children, but they do not produce long-lasting relief. Tricyclic antidepressants are broken down in the liver.

Cautions and Warnings

Do not take Doxepin if you are **allergic** or **sensitive** to it or another **tricyclic antidepressant**. Doxepin should not be used if you are recovering from a **heart attack**.

If you have a history of **epilepsy** or other **convulsive disorders, difficulty in urination, glaucoma, heart disease, liver disease,** or **hyperthyroidism,** you may take Doxepin, but use caution. People who are **schizophrenic** or **paranoid** may get worse if given a tricyclic antidepressant, and **manic-depressive** people may switch phase. This can also happen if they are stopping or changing antidepressants. **Suicide** is always a possibility in severely depressed people, who should be allowed to have only **minimal quantities** of medication in their possession at any time.

Possible Side Effects

▼ Most common: sedation and anticholinergic effects (blurred vision, disorientation, confusion, hallucinations, muscle spasms or tremors, seizures and/or convulsions, dry mouth, constipation [especially in older adults], difficult urination, worsening glaucoma, sensitivity to bright light or sunlight).

▼ Less common: blood-pressure changes, abnormal heart rates, heart attack, anxiety, restlessness, excitement, numbness or tingling in the extremities, poor coordination, rash, itching, retention of fluids, fever, allergy, changes in blood composition, nausea, vomiting, loss of appetite, stomach upset, diarrhea, enlargement of

Possible Side Effects *(continued)*

the breasts (both sexes), changes in sex drive, and blood-sugar changes.

▼ Rare: agitation, inability to sleep, nightmares, feeling of panic, a peculiar taste in the mouth, stomach cramps, black discoloration of the tongue, yellowing of the eyes and/or skin, changes in liver function, increased or decreased weight, excessive perspiration, flushing, frequent urination, drowsiness, dizziness, weakness, headache, loss of hair, nausea, and not feeling well.

Drug Interactions

• Interaction with monoamine oxidase (MAO) inhibitors can cause high fevers, convulsions, and occasionally death. Don't take MAO inhibitors until at least 2 weeks after Doxepin has been discontinued. People who take Doxepin with an MAO inhibitor require close medical observation.

• Doxepin interacts with Guanethidine and Clonidine. Be sure to tell your doctor if you are taking **any** high blood pressure medicine.

• Doxepin increases the effects of barbiturates, tranquilizers, other sedative drugs, and alcohol. Also, barbiturates may decrease the effectiveness of Doxepin.

• Taking Doxepin and thyroid medicine together will enhance the effects of both medicines, possibly causing abnormal heart rhythms. The combination of Doxepin and Reserpine may cause overstimulation.

• Oral contraceptives can reduce the effect of Doxepin, as can smoking. Charcoal tablets can prevent Doxepin's absorption into the blood. Estrogens can increase or decrease the effect of Doxepin.

• Drugs such as Bicarbonate of Soda, Acetazolamide, Quinidine, or Procainamide will increase the effect of Doxepin. Cimetidine, Methylphenidate, and phenothiazine drugs (like Thorazine and Compazine) block the liver metabolism of Doxepin, causing it to stay in the body longer, which can cause severe drug side effects.

Food Interactions

You may take Doxepin with food if it upsets your stomach.

Usual Dose

Adult: initial dose, about 75 mg per day in divided doses; then increased or decreased as necessary. The final dose may be less than 75 or up to 200 mg. Long-term patients being treated for depression may be given extended-acting medicine daily at bedtime or several times per day.

Adolescent and Senior: initial dose, 30 or 40 mg per day. Maintenance dose is usually less than 100 mg daily.

Child: 25 mg per day (age 6 and over), given 1 hour before bedtime, for nighttime bed-wetting. If relief of bed-wetting does not occur within 1 week, the daily dose is increased to 50 or 75 mg, depending on age; dosages are often in midafternoon and at bedtime (more than 75 mg a day increases side effects without increasing effectiveness). The medication should be gradually tapered off, which may reduce the probability that the bed-wetting will return. This drug, when used for nighttime bed-wetting, is often ineffective or of questionable value.

Overdosage

Symptoms are confusion, inability to concentrate, hallucinations, drowsiness, lowered body temperature, abnormal heart rate, heart failure, enlarged pupils, convulsions, severely lowered blood pressure, stupor, and coma. Agitation, stiffening of body muscles, vomiting, and high fever may also occur. The victim should be taken to a hospital emergency room immediately. ALWAYS bring the medicine bottle.

Special Information

Avoid alcohol and other depressants while taking Doxepin. Do not stop taking this drug unless your doctor has specifically told you to do so. Abruptly stopping this medicine may cause nausea, headache, and a sickly feeling.

This medicine can cause drowsiness, dizziness, and blurred vision. Be careful when driving or operating hazardous machinery. Avoid prolonged exposure to the sun or sunlamps.

Call your doctor at once if you develop seizures, difficult or rapid breathing, fever and sweating, blood-pressure changes, muscle stiffness, loss of bladder control, or unusual tiredness or weakness. Dry mouth may lead to an increase in dental cavities, gum bleeding and gum disease. People taking Doxepin should pay special attention to dental hygiene.

If you forget to take a dose of Doxepin, skip it and go back to your regular schedule. Do not take a double dose.

Special Populations

Pregnancy/Breast-feeding
Doxepin, like other antidepressants, crosses into your developing baby's circulation, and birth defects have been reported if the drug taken during the first 3 months of pregnancy. There have been reports of newborn infants suffering from heart, breathing, and urinary problems after their mothers had taken an antidepressant of this type immediately before delivery. Avoid taking this medication while pregnant.

Tricyclic antidepressants pass into breast milk in low concentrations, and sedate the baby. Nursing mothers taking Doxepin should bottle-feed their babies.

Seniors
Older adults are more sensitive to the effects of this drug, especially abnormal rhythms and other heart side effects, and often require a lower dose to achieve the same effect. Follow your doctor's directions and report any side effects at once.

Generic Name

Dronabinol

Brand Name
Marinol

Type of Drug
Antinauseant.

Prescribed for
Relief of nausea and vomiting associated with cancer chemotherapy; appetite stimulation and weight loss prevention in people with AIDS. It has been studied as a treatment for glaucoma.

General Information
Dronabinol is the first legal form of marijuana available to the American public. The psychoactive chemical ingredient in

marijuana is also known as *delta-9-THC*. Dronabinol has all of the psychological effects of marijuana and is therefore considered to be a highly abusable drug. Its ability to cause personality changes, feelings of detachment, hallucinations, and euphoria (feeling "high") has made Dronabinol relatively unacceptable among older adults and those who feel they must be in control of their environment. Younger adults have reported a greater success rate with Dronabinol, probably because they are better able to tolerate these effects.

Most people start on Dronabinol while in the hospital because the doctor needs to monitor closely their response to the medication and possible adverse effects.

Cautions and Warnings

Dronabinol **should not be used to treat nausea and vomiting caused by anything other than cancer chemotherapy**. It should not be used by people who are **allergic** to it, to **marijuana,** or to **sesame oil.** Dronabinol has a profound effect on its users' **mental status;** it will impair your ability to operate complex equipment, or engage in any activity that requires intense concentration, sound judgment, and coordination (such as driving a car).

Like other abusable drugs, Dronabinol produces a definite set of **withdrawal symptoms** when the drug is stopped. **Tolerance** to the drug's effects develops after a month of use. Withdrawal symptoms can develop within 12 hours of the drug's discontinuation and include **restlessness, sleeplessness,** and **irritability.** Within a day after the drug has been stopped, **stuffy nose, hot flashes, sweating, loose stools, hiccups,** and **appetite loss** may occur. The symptoms usually subside within a few days.

Dronabinol should be used with caution by people with a **manic-depressive** or **schizophrenic** history because of the chance that it will aggravate the underlying disease.

In animal studies, Dronabinol actually reduced the **number of sperm produced** and the number of cells from which sperm are made.

Possible Side Effects

▼ Most common: drowsiness, euphoria (feeling "high"), dizziness, anxiety, muddled thinking, perceptual difficul-

Possible Side Effects *(continued)*

ties, poor coordination, irritability, a weird feeling, depression, weakness, sluggishness, headache, hallucinations, memory lapses, loss of muscle coordination, unsteadiness, paranoia, depersonalization, disorientation and confusion, rapid heartbeat, and dizziness when rising from a sitting or lying position.

▼ Less common: difficulty talking or speech slurring, facial flushing, excessive perspiration, nightmares, ringing or buzzing in the ears, fainting, diarrhea, loss of ability to control bowel movement, and muscle pains.

Drug Interactions

• Dronabinol will increase the psychological effects of alcoholic beverages, tranquilizers, sleeping pills, sedatives, and other depressants. It will also enhance the effects of other psychoactive drugs, including tricyclic antidepressants, amphetamines, cocaine, and other stimulants.

• Dronabinol may increase the effects of Fluoxetine and Disulfiram.

• The effects of Theophylline drugs are reduced by Dronabinol because it stimulates the liver to break down Theophylline more quickly.

Food Interactions

This drug may be taken without regard to food or meals, though, as an appetite stimulant, it is often taken before meals.

Usual Dose

Antiemetic

5 mg to 15 mg, 1 to 3 hours before starting chemotherapy treatment, repeated every 2 to 4 hours after chemotherapy has been given, for a total of 4 to 6 doses a day. The dose may be increased up to 30 mg a day if needed, but psychiatric side effects increase greatly at higher doses.

Appetite Stimulant

2.5 mg before lunch and/or dinner or at bedtime. Dosage may be increased to 20 mg per day.

Overdosage

Overdosage symptoms can occur at usual doses or at higher doses if the drug is being abused. The primary symptoms of overdosage are the psychological symptoms listed under *Possible Side Effects*. In some cases, overdose may lead to panic reactions or seizures. No deaths have been reported with either marijuana or Dronabinol overdose. Dronabinol therapy may be restarted at lower doses if other medicines are ineffective.

Special Information

Dronabinol may impair your ability to drive a car or perform complex tasks. Avoid alcohol and other nervous-system depressants while taking Dronabinol.

Dronabinol can cause acute psychiatric or psychological effects. Be sure to remain in close contact with your doctor and call him or her if any such side effects develop.

Dronabinol capsules must be stored in the refrigerator.

If you forget to take a dose of Dronabinol, take it as soon as you remember. If it is almost time for your next dose, skip the one you forgot and continue with your regular schedule. Do not take a double dose.

Special Populations

Pregnancy/Breast-feeding

Studies of Dronabinol in pregnant animals taking doses 10 to 400 times the human dose have shown no adverse effects on fetal development. However, Dronabinol should not be taken by a pregnant woman unless it is absolutely necessary.

Dronabinol passes into breast milk and can affect a nursing infant. Nursing mothers who must take this medicine should bottle-feed their infants.

Seniors

Older adults are more sensitive to this drug, especially its psychological effects. Follow your doctor's directions and report any side effects at once.

Duricef

see Cephalosporin Antibiotics, page 171

Brand Name

Dyazide

Ingredients

Hydrochlorothiazide
Triamterene

Brand Name

Maxzide

This product contains the same ingredients in different concentrations. (Both Dyazide and Maxzide are also available in generic form.)

Similar combinations of a thiazide diuretic and a potassium-sparing diuretic are also available by prescription, including:

Brand Names

Ingredients: Amiloride + Hydrochlorothiazide

Moduretic

Ingredients: Spironolactone + Hydrochlorothiazide

Aldactazide

Type of Drug

Diuretic.

Prescribed for

High blood pressure or any condition where it is desirable to eliminate excess water from the body.

General Information

Dyazide is a combination of 2 diuretics and is a convenient, effective approach for the treatment of diseases where the elimination of excess water is required. One of the ingredients, Triamterene, has the ability to hold potassium in the body while producing a diuretic effect. This balances the other ingredient, Hydrochlorothiazide, which normally causes a loss of body potassium. Combination drugs like Dyazide should be used only when you need the exact amounts of ingredients in the product and when your doctor feels you would benefit from taking fewer pills each day.

Cautions and Warnings

Do not use Dyazide if you have **nonfunctioning kidneys,** if you may be **allergic** to this drug or any **sulfa drug,** or if you have a history of **allergy** or **bronchial asthma.**

Do not take any **potassium supplements** together with Dyazide unless specifically directed to do so by your doctor.

Possible Side Effects

▼ Most common: loss of appetite, drowsiness, lethargy, headache, gastrointestinal upset, cramping, and diarrhea.

▼ Less common: rash, mental confusion, fever, feelings of ill health, inability to achieve or maintain erection in males, bright red tongue, burning sensation in the tongue, headache, tingling in the toes and fingers, restlessness, anemia or other effects on components of the blood, unusual sensitivity to sunlight, and dizziness when rising quickly from a sitting position. Dyazide can also produce muscle spasms, gout, weakness, and blurred vision.

Drug Interactions

• Dyazide increases the action of other blood-pressure-lowering drugs. This is good and is the reason why people with high blood pressure often take more than one medicine.

• The possibility of developing imbalances in body fluids (electrolytes) is increased if you take medications such as Digitalis drugs, Amphotericin B, and adrenal corticosteroids while taking Dyazide. If you are taking Insulin or an oral antidiabetic drug and begin taking Dyazide, the Insulin or antidiabetic dose may have to be modified.

• Concurrent use of Dyazide and Allopurinol may increase the chances of experiencing Allopurinol side effects.

• Dyazide may decrease the effects of oral anticoagulant (blood-thinning) drugs.

• Antigout drug dosage may have to be modified since Dyazide raises blood-uric-acid levels.

• Dyazide may prolong the white-blood-cell-reducing effects of chemotherapy drugs.

• Dyazide may increase the effects of Diazoxide, leading to symptoms of diabetes.

• Dyazide should not be taken together with loop diuretics because the combination can lead to an extreme diuretic effect and an extreme effect on blood electrolyte (salt) levels.

• Dyazide can increase the biological actions of Vitamin D, leading to a possibility of high blood calcium levels.

• Propantheline and other anticholinergics may increase diuretic effect by increasing the amount of drug absorbed.

• Lithium Carbonate taken with Dyazide should be monitored carefully by a doctor because there may be an increased risk of Lithium toxicity.

• Cholestyramine and Colestipol bind Dyazide and prevent it from being absorbed into the blood. Dyazide should be taken more than 2 hours before taking Cholestyramine or Colestipol.

• Methenamine and other urinary agents may reduce the effect of Dyazide by reducing urinary acidity.

• Some nonsteroidal anti-inflammatory drugs (NSAIDs), particularly Indomethacin, may reduce the effect of Dyazide. Sulindac, another NSAID, may increase the effect of Dyazide.

Food Interactions

Take this drug with food if it upsets your stomach.

Usual Dose

1 or 2 capsules or tablets per day.

Overdosage

Signs of overdose can be tingling in the arms or legs, weakness, fatigue, changes in your heartbeat, a sickly feeling, dry mouth, restlessness, muscle pains or cramps, urinary difficulty, nausea, or vomiting. Take the overdose victim to a hospital emergency room immediately. ALWAYS bring the prescription bottle and any remaining medicine.

Special Information

Dyazide will cause excess urination at first, but that will

subside after several weeks of taking the medicine. Ordinarily, diuretics are taken early in the day to prevent excessive nighttime urination from interfering with your sleep.

This drug can make you drowsy. Be careful when driving or operating hazardous machinery.

Call your doctor if you develop muscle pain, sudden joint pain, weakness, cramps, nausea, vomiting, restlessness, excessive thirst, tiredness, drowsiness, increased heart or pulse rate, diarrhea, dizziness, headache, or rash.

Diabetic patients may experience an increased blood-sugar level and a need for dosage adjustments of their antidiabetic medicines.

Avoid alcohol and other medicines while taking Dyazide unless otherwise directed by your doctor.

If you are taking Dyazide for the treatment of high blood pressure or congestive heart failure, avoid over-the-counter medicines for the treatment of coughs, colds, and allergies; such medicines may contain stimulants. If you are unsure about them, ask your pharmacist.

If you forget to take a dose of Dyazide, take it as soon as you remember. If it is almost time for your next regularly scheduled dose, skip the one you forgot and continue with your regular schedule. Do not take a double dose.

Take Dyazide exactly as prescribed. Be aware that all Triamterene-Hydrochlorothiazide products are not equal to each other and should not be freely substituted for each other. Check with your doctor and pharmacist before switching brands.

Special Populations

Pregnancy/Breast-feeding
Dyazide may be used to treat specific conditions in pregnant women, but the decision to use this medication by pregnant women should be weighed carefully because the drug may cross the placental barrier into the blood of the unborn child.

Dyazide may appear in the breast milk of nursing mothers. Be sure your baby's doctor knows you are taking Dyazide.

Seniors
Older adults are more sensitive to the effects of this drug. Closely follow your doctor's directions and report any side effects at once.

Generic Name

Econazole Nitrate

Brand Name
Spectazole Cream

Type of Drug
Antifungal.

Prescribed for
Fungal infections of the skin, including athlete's foot, jock itch, and many other common infections.

General Information
This drug is similar to another antifungal agent, *Miconazole Nitrate.* However, unlike Miconazole Nitrate, Econazole Nitrate is available only as a cream for application to the skin. Very small amounts of Econazole Nitrate are absorbed into the bloodstream, but quite a bit of the drug penetrates to the middle and inner layers of the skin, where it can kill fungal organisms that may have penetrated to deeper layers.

Cautions and Warnings
Do not use Econazole Nitrate if you have had an **allergic** reaction to it or any other ingredient in this product. **Do not apply Econazole Nitrate cream in or near your eyes.**
    This product is generally safe, but it belongs to a family of drugs known to cause **liver damage.** Therefore, long-term application of this product to large areas of skin might produce an adverse effect on the liver.

Possible Side Effects

▼ Most common: burning, itching, stinging, and redness in the areas to which the cream has been applied.

Drug and Food Interactions
None known.

Usual Dose

Apply enough of the cream to cover affected areas with a thin layer once or twice a day.

Overdosage

This cream should not be swallowed. If it is swallowed, the victim may be nauseated and have an upset stomach. Other possible effects are drowsiness and liver inflammation and damage. Little is known about Econazole Nitrate overdose; call your local poison control center for more information.

Special Information

Clean the affected areas before applying Econazole Nitrate cream, unless otherwise directed by your doctor.

Call your doctor if the treated area burns, stings, or becomes red.

This product is quite effective and can be expected to relieve symptoms within a day or two after you begin using it. Follow your doctor's directions for the complete 2- to 4-week course of treatment to gain maximum benefit from the product. Stopping it too soon may not completely eliminate the fungus and can lead to a relapse.

If you forget to take a dose of Econazole Nitrate, apply it as soon as you remember. If it is almost time for your next regularly scheduled dose, skip the one you forgot and continue with your regular schedule. Do not apply a double dose.

Special Populations

Pregnancy/Breast-feeding

When given by mouth to pregnant animals in doses 10 to 40 times the amount normally applied to the skin, Econazole Nitrate was found to be toxic to the developing fetus. It should be strictly avoided during the first 3 months of pregnancy. During the last 6 months of pregnancy, it should be used only if absolutely necessary.

It is not known if Econazole Nitrate passes into human breast milk. Animal studies show passage of the drug and its breakdown products into breast milk. Nursing mothers should be cautious about using this medicine.

Seniors

Seniors may take this drug without special restriction.

Brand Name

EMLA Cream/Patch

Ingredients

Lidocaine + Prilocaine

Type of Drug

Topical anesthetic.

Prescribed for

Prevention of skin pain. EMLA Cream has also been studied for its effects on relieving the pain of intravenous catheter placement, minor plastic and skin surgery, shingles, and injections (such as vaccinations and blood donation).

General information

EMLA (which stands for Eutectic Mixture of Local Anesthetics) is a mixture of two anesthetics which, when mixed in a certain way, turn to liquid when applied to the skin. The anesthetics penetrate all layers of skin, deadening nerve endings and providing an anesthetic effect that is as good as that achieved by injecting local anesthetics under the skin. EMLA is effective in preventing virtually any kind of pain that is associated with the skin. It can be used on people of virtually all ages and offers the advantage of preventing pain without injection. The cream must be applied under an occlusive bandage (one that completely shuts out all contact with air or water), which intensifies the contact between the skin and the anesthetic cream. It works after staying on the surface of the skin for at least 1 hour, but may work more effectively if left on for 2 or 3 hours. The anesthetic effect remains for 2 hours after the cream has been removed from the surface of the skin.

Cautions and Warnings

Do not use EMLA Cream if you are allergic to either of the anesthetics in the mixture. People with *methemoglobinemia*, a rare blood condition, should not use EMLA.

  Do not apply EMLA Cream beyond the area prescribed by

your doctor. Excessive application of EMLA could put too much local anesthetic in your blood and expose you to the possibility of anesthetic-related side effects. Do not put EMLA in your eyes or ears.

People with severe liver disease should use EMLA with caution because they may have difficulty removing the absorbed anesthetics from their bloodstream.

Possible Side Effects

▼ Most common: irritation, redness, and swelling of the area to which it is applied.

▼ Common: skin pallor, patches of white skin, itching, rash, and changes in how you sense skin temperature.

▼ Rare: severe allergic reactions (itching, rash, swelling, difficulty breathing, and shock) can occur with this product.

In rare cases when too much EMLA is applied, is used too often, or too much anesthetic is absorbed, the following reactions may occur: nervous system excitation, nervousness, apprehension, light-headedness, euphoria (feeling "high"), confusion, dizziness, drowsiness, ringing or buzzing in the ears, blurred or double vision, vomiting, feelings of heat, cold, or numbness, twitching, tremors, convulsions, unconsciousness, or a very slow breathing rate or stopped breathing.

Drug Interactions

• Drugs associated with causing methemoglobinemia, should not be taken together with EMLA. This interaction is generally limited to children under 1 year. Some of these drugs are Acetaminophen, sulfa drugs, oral antidiabetes drugs, thiazide diuretics, Phenacetin, Phenobarbital, Phenytoin, Primaquine, and Quinine. Check with your doctor or pharmacist for more information about other methemoglobinemia-causing drugs.

Food Interactions

None known.

Usual Dose

Cream

Adult and Child (over age 1 month): Apply a thick layer (2 1/2 grams or 1/2 teaspoonful) and cover with the dressing provided in the package or some other occlusive bandage. Leave in place for at least 1 to 2 hours. The cream should be wiped away immediately before the surgical procedure or injection is done.

Senior: Avoid multiple uses over a short period of time because of the possibility of drug-induced side effects.

Patch

Apply to designated area and leave in place for at least 1 to 2 hours before removing.

Overdosage

EMLA overdose may affect the heart by making it less efficient. This is directly attributable to the depressant effects of the local anesthetics on the nerves within the heart. This would be more likely only if someone were to swallow an entire tube of EMLA. Call your local poison control center or hospital emergency room for more information. If you go for treatment, ALWAYS bring the medicine container with you.

Special Information

EMLA provides total loss of all feeling from the affected skin. Since there is no feeling in the skin, be careful not to accidentally scratch or burn yourself after the product has been applied.

When you apply the cream, place the entire dose in the center of the area you want to make pain-free. Then cover it with the occlusive dressing and allow the pressure of the dressing to spread the cream around.

Call your doctor if you develop severe, persistent, or unusually bothersome side effects from this product.

If you forget to apply EMLA, do so as soon as you can. But remember, it will still take at least 1 hour from the time you put the cream on your skin to make it numb. Don't expect any pain relief before then.

Special Populations

Pregnancy/Breast-feeding

There is no evidence that EMLA Cream interferes in any way

with fetal development. Nevertheless, you should not use this product during pregnancy unless you have first discussed it with your doctor.

The anesthetics in EMLA Cream pass into breast milk. Watch your infant for possible drug effects if you use EMLA Cream while you are nursing.

Seniors

Seniors may be more sensitive to the effects of drug side effects than younger adults, especially if repeated applications of EMLA are used.

Generic Name

Enalapril

Brand Name

Vasotec

Type of Drug

Angiotensin-converting-enzyme (ACE) inhibitor.

Combination Product

Enalapril + Hydrochlorothiazide

(Vaseretic used to treat high blood pressure)

Prescribed for

Hypertension and congestive heart failure. Enalapril may also be prescribed for diabetic kidney disease, childhood high blood pressure and high blood pressure related to sclero-derma disease, and post-heart attack treatment when the function of the left ventricle is affected.

General Information

Enalapril belongs to the class of drugs known as *angiotensin-converting-enzyme (ACE) inhibitors.* ACE inhibitors work by preventing the conversion of a hormone called *angiotensin I* to another hormone called *angiotensin II*, a potent blood-vessel constrictor. Preventing this conversion relaxes blood vessels and helps to reduce blood pressure and relieve the symptoms of heart failure by making it easier for a failing heart to pump blood through the body. The production of other hormones and enzymes that participate in the regulation of blood-vessel dilation is also affected by Enalapril and probably plays a role in the effectiveness of this medicine. Enalapril begins working about 1 hour after you take it and continues to work for 24 hours.

Some people who start taking Enalapril after they are already on a diuretic (water pill) experience a rapid blood-pressure drop after their first dose or when their dose is increased. To prevent this from happening, your doctor may tell you to stop taking your diuretic 2 or 3 days before starting Enalapril or increase your salt intake during that time. The diuretic may then be restarted gradually. Heart-failure patients generally have been on Digoxin and a diuretic before beginning Enalapril treatment.

Cautions and Warnings

Do not take Enalapril if you have had an **allergic** reaction to it. It can (rarely) cause **very low blood pressure**. It may also affect your **kidneys,** especially if you have **congestive heart failure.** Your doctor should **check your urine** for protein content during the first few months of treatment.

Enalapril may cause a decline in **kidney function.** Dosage adjustment of Enalapril is necessary if you have reduced kidney function because this drug is generally eliminated from the body via the kidneys.

Enalapril can affect **white-blood-cell counts,** possibly increasing your **susceptibility to infection.** Your doctor should **monitor your blood counts** periodically.

Possible Side Effects

▼ Most common: dizziness, fatigue, headache, nausea, and chronic cough. The cough usually goes away a few days after you stop taking the medicine.

▼ Less common: angina (chest tightness/pain), dizziness when rising from a sitting or lying position, fainting, abdominal pain, nausea, vomiting, diarrhea, bronchitis, urinary tract infection, breathing difficulty, weakness, and skin rash.

▼ Other: itching; fever; heart attack; stroke; abdomi-

Possible Side Effects *(continued)*

nal pain; abnormal heart rhythms; heart palpitations; sleeping difficulty; tingling in the hands or feet; appetite loss; odd taste perception; hepatitis and jaundice; blood in the stool; hair loss; unusual skin sensitivity to the sun; flushing; anxiety; nervousness; reduced sex drive; impotence; muscle cramps or weakness; muscle aches; arthritis; asthma; respiratory infections; sinus irritation; depression; feelings of ill health; sweating; kidney problems; anemia; blurred vision; swelling of the arms, legs, lips, tongue, face, and throat; upset stomach; and inflammation of the pancreas.

Drug Interactions

• The blood-pressure-lowering effect of Enalapril is additive with diuretic drugs and beta blockers. Any other drug that causes a rapid blood-pressure drop should be used with caution if you are taking Enalapril.

• Enalapril may increase blood-potassium levels, especially when taken with Dyazide or other potassium-sparing diuretics.

• Enalapril may increase the effects of Lithium; this combination should be used with caution.

• Antacids may reduce the amount of Enalapril absorbed into the blood. Separate doses of these by at least 2 hours.

• Capsaicin may cause or aggravate the cough associated with Enalapril therapy.

• Indomethacin may reduce the blood-pressure-lowering effects of Enalapril.

• Phenothiazine tranquilizers and antiemetics may increase the effects of Enalapril.

• Rifampin may reduce the effects of Enalapril.

• The combination of Allopurinol and Enalapril increases the chance of an adverse drug reaction. Avoid this combination.

• Enalapril increases blood levels of Digoxin, which possibly increases the chance of Digoxin-related side effects.

Food Interactions

Enalapril's action is not affected by food. You may take it with food if it upsets your stomach.

Usual Dose

2.5 to 40 mg, once per day. Some people may take their total daily dosage in 2 divided doses. People with poor kidney function need less medicine to achieve reduced blood pressure.

Overdosage

The principal effect of Enalapril overdose is a rapid drop in blood pressure, as evidenced by dizziness or fainting. Take the overdose victim to a hospital emergency room immediately. ALWAYS bring the medicine bottle.

Special Information

Enalapril can cause swelling of the face, lips, hands, or feet. This swelling can also affect the larynx (throat) or tongue and interfere with breathing. If this happens, go to a hospital emergency room at once. Call your doctor if you develop a sore throat, mouth sores, abnormal heartbeat, chest pain, a persistent rash, or loss of taste perception.

You may get dizzy if you rise to your feet too quickly from a sitting or lying position. Avoid strenuous exercise and/or very hot weather because heavy sweating or dehydration can cause a rapid blood-pressure drop.

Avoid nonprescription diet pills, decongestants, and stimulants that can raise blood pressure while taking Enalapril.

If you take Enalapril once a day and forget to take a dose, take it a soon as you remember. If it is within 8 hours of your next dose, skip the one you forgot and continue with your regular schedule.

If you take Enalapril twice a day and miss a dose, take it right away. If it is within 4 hours of your next dose, take 1 dose and then another in 5 or 6 hours, then go back to your regular schedule. Do not take a double dose.

Special Populations

Pregnancy/Breast-feeding

ACE inhibitors have caused low blood pressure, kidney failure, slow skull formation, and death in developing fetuses when taken during the last 6 months of pregnancy. Women who are or who may become pregnant should not take any ACE inhibitors. Sexually active women of childbearing age who must take Enalapril must use an effective contraceptive method to prevent pregnancy or use a different medicine. If you become pregnant, stop taking the medicine and call your doctor immediately.

Relatively small amounts of Enalapril pass into breast milk, and the effect on a nursing infant is likely to be minimal. However, nursing mothers who must take this drug should consider an alternative feeding method because infants, especially newborns, are more susceptible to this medicine's effects than adults.

Seniors

Older adults may be more sensitive to the effects of this drug because of normal age-related declines in kidney or liver function. Dosage must be individualized to your needs.

Generic Name

Enoxacin

Brand Name

Penetrex

Type of Drug

Fluoroquinolone anti-infective.

Prescribed for

Urinary infections and sexually transmitted diseases. Enoxacin does not work against syphilis.

General Information

The fluoroquinolones are widely used and work against many organisms that traditional antibiotic treatments have trouble killing. In addition to the above uses, fluoroquinolone anti-infectives can be used for the lower respiratory tract, skin, bones and joints, lung infections in people with cystic fibrosis, bronchitis, pneumonia, prostate infection, and traveler's diarrhea and infectious diarrhea. Fluoroquinolone medications are chemically related to an older antibacterial called *Nalidixic Acid*, but work better than that drug against urinary infections. Enoxacin does not work against the common cold, flu, or other viral infections.

Cautions and Warnings

Do not take Enoxacin if you have had an **allergic** reaction to it or another fluoroquinolone in the past, or if you have had a reaction to related medications like Nalidixic Acid. **Severe, possibly fatal, allergic reactions** can occur even after the very first dose; these include **cardiovascular collapse, loss of consciousness, tingling, swelling of the face or throat, breathing difficulty, itching,** or **rash. Stop taking the drug** if this happens and **seek medical help** at once.

Enoxacin dosage must be adjusted in the presence of **kidney failure**.

Enoxacin may cause increased pressure on parts of the brain, leading to **convulsions** and **psychotic reactions**. Other adverse effects include tremors, restlessness, confusion, lightheadedness, and hallucinations. Enoxacin should be used with caution in people with **seizure disorders** or other **conditions of the nervous system**.

People taking fluoroquinolone medicines can be **unusually sensitive to direct or indirect sunlight** (photosensitivity). Avoid the sun while taking this drug and for several days following therapy, *even if you are using a sunscreen!*

As with any other anti-infective, people taking Enoxacin may develop **colitis** that could range from mild to very serious. See your doctor if you develop **diarrhea** or **cramps** while taking this drug.

Prolonged use of Enoxacin, as with any other anti-infective, can lead to **fungal overgrowth**. Follow your doctor's directions exactly.

At very high doses, Enoxacin may cause **decreased sperm production** and **reduce male fertility**.

Possible Side Effects

  ▼ Most common: nausea and vomiting.
  ▼ Less common: abdominal pain, heartburn, upset

Possible Side Effects *(continued)*

stomach, diarrhea, itching, headache, sleeplessness, dizziness, and taste changes.

▼ Rare: constipation; gas; colitis; appetite loss; fatigue or drowsiness; not feeling well; seizures; confusion; tingling in the hands or feet; sensitivity to the sun; rash; sweating; fungal infections of the skin; skin peeling; nervousness; agitation; anxiety; tremors; weakness; muscle stiffness; muscle or joint pain in the back or chest; depersonalization; visual disturbances; ringing or buzzing in the ears; pink-eye; cough; nosebleeds; vaginal irritation or infection; kidney failure; heart palpitations; fainting; chills; fever; swollen legs, arms, or ankles; liver irritation; and black-and-blue marks.

Drug Interactions

• Antacids, Didanosine, Bismuth Subsalicylate (the active ingredient in Pepto-Bismol), Iron supplements, Sucralfate, and Zinc will decrease the amount of Enoxacin absorbed into the bloodstream. If you must take any of these products, separate them from your Enoxacin dosage by at least 2 hours.

• Anticancer drugs may also reduce the amount of Enoxacin in your bloodstream.

• Probenecid and Cimetidine interfere with the release of Enoxacin from your body, and may increase the chance of drug side effects.

• Enoxacin may increase the effects of oral anticoagulant (blood-thinning) drugs. Your anticoagulant dose may have to be adjusted.

• Enoxacin may increase the toxic effects of Cyclosporine (for organ transplants) on your kidneys.

• Enoxacin may reduce the rate at which Theophylline is released from your body, increasing blood levels of the drug and the chance for Theophylline-related drug side effects.

• Enoxacin decreases the clearance of Caffeine from your body, possibly increasing its effect on your system.

• Enoxacin increases blood levels of Digoxin. Your doctor may have to alter your Digoxin dose if you are taking this combination.

Food Interactions

Enoxacin is best taken at least 1 hour before or 2 hours after a meal.

Usual Dose

400 to 800 mg a day. Dosage is adjusted in the presence of kidney failure.

Overdosage

The symptoms of Enoxacin overdose are the same as those found under *Possible Side Effects*. One person experienced kidney failure following an overdose of Ciprofloxacin, another fluoroquinolone. Overdose victims should be taken to a hospital emergency room for treatment of those symptoms. ALWAYS bring the medicine bottle. You may induce vomiting with Syrup of Ipecac (available at any pharmacy) to remove excess medication from the victim's stomach. Consult your local poison control center or hospital emergency room for specific instructions.

Special Information

Take each dose with a full glass of water. Be sure to drink at least 8 glasses of water per day while taking Enoxacin to promote removal of the drug from your system and to help avoid side effects.

If you are taking an antacid, an Iron or Zinc supplement, Didanosine, or Sucralfate while taking Enoxacin, be sure to separate the doses by at least 2 hours to avoid a drug interaction.

Drug sensitivity reactions can develop even after only one dose of this medicine! Stop taking it and get immediate medical attention if you faint or if you develop itching, rash, facial swelling, difficulty breathing, convulsions, depression, visual disturbances, dizziness, headache, light-headedness, or any sign of a drug reaction.

Colitis can be caused by any anti-infective drug. If diarrhea develops after taking Enoxacin, call your doctor at once.

Avoid excessive sunlight or exposure to a sunlamp while taking Enoxacin and call your doctor if you become unusually sensitive to the sun.

It is essential that you take Enoxacin according to your doctor's directions. Do not stop taking it even if you feel better after a few days, unless directed to do so by your doctor.

If you forget to take a dose of Enoxacin, take it as soon as you remember. If it is almost time for your next dose, skip the forgotten dose and continue with your regular schedule. Do not take a double dose.

Special Populations

Pregnancy/Breast-feeding

Pregnant women should not take Enoxacin unless its benefits have been carefully weighed against its risks. Animal studies have shown that Enoxacin may reduce the chance for a successful pregnancy or cause damage to a developing fetus.

It is not known if Enoxacin passes into breast milk. Nursing mothers who must take Enoxacin should bottle-feed their babies.

Seniors

Enoxacin blood levels are 50 percent higher in seniors than in younger adults. Daily drug dosage may be reduced if your kidney function is compromised.

Brand Name

Entex LA Capsules/Liquid

Ingredients

Guaifenesin
Phenylpropanolamine
Phenylephrine (in liquids only)

Other Brand Names

Ami-Tex LA	Partuss LA
Contuss Liquid	Phenylfenesin LA
Despec Capsules/Liquid	Rymed-TR
Exgest LA	ULR-LA
Guaipax SR	Vanex-LA

The following products contain the same types of ingredients in different concentrations:

Codimal Expectorant Liquid
Conex Syrup
Dura-Vent
Entex Syrup/Entex
GuiaCough PE Liquid
Guaifed Syrup
Histalet X Syrup
Myminic Expectorant Liquid

Naldecon EX Children's
  Syrup/Pediatric Granules
Robitussin PE Syrup
Snaplets-EX Granules
Theramine Expectorant
  Liquid
Triaminic Expectorant Liquid
Triphenyl Expectorant Liquid

The following products contain similar ingredients (Caramiphen Edisylate and Phenylpropanolamine Hydrochloride) and can be used for the same purpose as Entex LA:

Ordrine AT Capsules
Rescaps-D S.R. Capsules
Tuss-Allergine Modified T.D. Capsules
Tussogest Capsules
Tuss-Ornade Spansules/Liquid

(Also available in generic form)

Type of Drug

Decongestant-expectorant combination.

Prescribed for

Relief of some symptoms of the common cold, allergy, or other upper-respiratory conditions, including nasal congestion, stuffiness, and runny nose. Guaifenesin is supposed to help loosen thick mucus that may contribute to your feeling of chest congestion, but the effectiveness of this and other expectorant drugs has not been established.

General Information

Entex LA and the other products listed in this section are only a few of the several hundred cold and allergy remedies available on either a prescription-only or nonprescription basis. There is a variety of formulas in these products, such as the combination used in Entex LA. The decongestant ingre-

dient, Phenylpropanolamine, dramatically reduces congestion and stuffiness. The expectorant, Guaifenesin, may help
relieve chest congestion. There are other products on the
market using this same general formula—an expectorant
plus a decongestant—but they use different decongestants
or a combination of decongestants plus the expectorant
Guaifenesin.

These products should not be used over extended periods
to treat a persistent or chronic cough, especially one that may
be caused by cigarette smoking, asthma, or emphysema.
Information on other decongestant-expectorant combinations
can be obtained from your pharmacist.

Since nothing can cure a cold or an allergy, the best you can
hope to achieve from taking this or any other cold or allergy
remedy is symptom relief.

Cautions and Warnings

These combination products can cause you to become **over-
anxious** or **nervous** and may **interfere with your sleep.**

Do not use these products if you have **diabetes, heart
disease, high blood pressure, thyroid disease, glaucoma,** or a
prostate condition.

Possible Side Effects

▼ Most common: fear, anxiety, restlessness, sleeplessness, tenseness, excitation, nervousness, dizziness,
drowsiness, hallucinations, headaches, psychological
disturbances, tremors, and convulsions.

▼ Less common: nausea, vomiting, upset stomach,
low blood pressure, heart palpitations, chest pain, rapid
heartbeat, abnormal heart rhythms, irritability, euphoria
(feeling "high"), eye irritation and tearing, hysterical
reactions, reduced appetite, difficulty urinating in men
with a prostate condition, weakness, loss of facial color,
and breathing difficulty.

Drug Interactions

• These products should be avoided if you are taking a
monoamine oxidase (MAO) inhibitor for depression or high

blood pressure because the MAO inhibitor may cause a very rapid rise in blood pressure or increase some side effects (dry mouth or nose, blurred vision, abnormal heart rhythms).

• The decongestant in these products may interfere with the normal effects of blood-pressure-lowering medicines. It can aggravate diabetes, heart disease, hyperthyroid disease, high blood pressure, a prostate condition, or stomach ulcers; it can also cause urinary blockage.

Food Interactions

Take these medicines with food if they upset your stomach.

Usual Dose

Capsules
1 twice per day.

Liquid
2 teaspoons 4 times a day.

Overdosage

The main symptoms of overdosage are sedation, sleepiness, increased sweating, and increased blood pressure. Hallucinations, convulsions, and nervous-system depression are particularly prominent in older adults, and breathing may become more difficult. Most cases of overdosage are not severe. Victims must be made to vomit with Syrup of Ipecac (available at any pharmacy) to remove any remaining drug from the stomach. Call your doctor or poison control center before doing this. If you must go to a hospital emergency room, ALWAYS bring the medicine bottle.

Special Information

Call your doctor if your side effects are severe or gradually become intolerable.

If you forget to take a dose of one of these combination products, take it as soon as you remember. If it is almost time for your next dose, skip the one you forgot and continue with your regular schedule. Do not take a double dose.

Special Populations

Pregnancy/Breast-feeding
These products should be avoided by pregnant women and

those who may become pregnant while using it. Discuss the potential risks with your doctor.

Nursing mothers should use caution when taking one of these products because the decongestant may pass into breast milk.

Seniors

Seniors are more sensitive to the effects of these drugs. Follow your doctor's directions. Report any side effects at once.

Brand Name

Equagesic

(Also available in generic form)

Ingredients

Aspirin + Meprobamate

Type of Drug

Analgesic combination.

Prescribed for

Pain from muscle spasms, sprains, strains, or bad backs.

General Information

Equagesic is one of several combination products containing a tranquilizer and an analgesic; it is used to relieve pain associated with muscle spasms. The Meprobamate in this product opens it to many drug interactions, especially with other tranquilizers or depressant drugs, which can lead to habituation and possible drug dependence. These combinations may be effective in providing temporary relief from pain and muscle spasm. Follow all of your doctor's instructions to help treat the basic problem.

Cautions and Warnings

Do not take this combination if you are **allergic** to any of its ingredients or to other **salicylates** or **Carisoprodol**.

Aspirin can worsen **kidney function** in people who already have a kidney condition, and Meprobamate should be used with caution by people with **liver** or **kidney disease**. **Aspirin** can irritate your stomach and should be avoided by people with gastritis or ulcers. Also, Aspirin should be used with caution by people with **mild diabetes** or **bleeding tendencies**.

People taking Meprobamate may become **dependent** on it. Avoid using this product for more than a few weeks at a time. Abruptly stopping this medicine can lead to **drug withdrawal** (anxiety, appetite loss, insomnia, vomiting, tremors, muscle weakness or twitching, confusion, and hallucinations) or recurrence of symptoms. The dose should be **gradually reduced** over a period of 1 to 2 weeks.

Possible Side Effects

▼ Most common: nausea, vomiting, stomach upset, dizziness, and drowsiness.

▼ Less common: allergy, itching, rash, fever, swelling in the arms and/or legs, occasional fainting spells, and bronchial spasms leading to difficulty breathing.

▼ Rare: changes in blood components and blurred vision.

Drug Interactions

• The Meprobamate in these products can cause sleepiness, drowsiness, or difficulty breathing (in high doses). Avoid taking them with other nervous-system depressants, including alcohol, barbiturates, narcotics, sleeping pills, tranquilizers, and some antihistamines.

• If you are taking an anticoagulant (blood-thinning medication) and have been given a new prescription for one of these combination products, be sure that your doctor knows they contain Aspirin. Aspirin affects the ability of your blood to clot and can necessitate a change in the dose of your anticoagulant.

Food Interactions

These drugs may be taken with food if they upset your stomach.

Usual Dose

1 or 2 tablets 3 to 4 times per day.

Overdosage

Overdoses are serious. Symptoms are drowsiness, light-headedness, desire to go to sleep, nausea, and vomiting. Victims should be taken to a hospital emergency room immediately. ALWAYS bring the medicine bottle.

Special Information

Be careful when driving or performing complex tasks while taking one of these products.

Call your doctor if drug side effects become bothersome or persistent. If you forget to take a dose of one of these combinations, take it as soon as you remember. If it is almost time for your next dose, skip the one you forgot and continue with your regular schedule. Do not take a double dose.

Special Populations

Pregnancy/Breast-feeding

These drugs cross into the fetal blood circulation. They have not caused birth defects, although Meprobamate has been known to increase the chance of birth defects if taken during the first 3 months of pregnancy. When such a drug is considered essential by your doctor, its potential benefits must be carefully weighed against its risks.

These drugs pass into breast milk. Nursing mothers taking this product should consider bottle-feeding their babies.

Seniors

Older adults are more sensitive to the effects of these combination products, especially drowsiness or sleepiness.

Generic Name

Ergoloid Mesylates

Brand Names

Gerimal
Hydergine
Hydergine LC

(Also available in generic form)

Type of Drug

Psychotherapeutic agent.

Prescribed for

Age-related decline in mental capacity in people over age 60 that cannot be traced to known causes. People who respond to this drug are likely to have Alzheimer's disease or some other primary cause of dementia or age-related condition.

General Information

Nobody knows exactly how Ergoloid Mesylates produces its effect, but it improves the supply of blood to the brain in test animals and reduces heart rate and muscle tone in blood vessels. Some studies have shown the drug to be very effective in relieving mild symptoms of mental impairment, while others have found it to be only moderately effective. It has been most beneficial in patients whose symptoms are due to the effects of high blood pressure in the brain. This medicine should not be used for any condition that is treatable with another medicine or that may be reversible. Your doctor should check periodically to be sure that this medicine is still needed and that it is working for you. It must be taken for 6 months before your doctor will be able to decide if it is working or not.

Cautions and Warnings

Ergoloid Mesylates should not be taken if you are **allergic** or **sensitive** to it or if you have any **psychotic symptoms** or **psychosis**.

Possible Side Effects

▼ Common: Ergoloid Mesylates does not produce serious side effects. If taking this drug under the tongue, you may experience some irritation, nausea, or stomach upset. Some other side effects are drowsiness, slow heartbeat, and rash.

Food Interactions

Do not eat, drink, or smoke while you have one of these pills under your tongue.

Usual Dose

1 mg 3 times per day. Doses may be raised to 12 mg a day.

Overdosage

Symptoms of overdosage are blurred vision, dizziness, fainting, flushing, headache, loss of appetite, nausea, vomiting, stomach cramps, and stuffed nose. Take the victim to a hospital emergency room for treatment. ALWAYS bring the medicine bottle.

Special Information

The effects of this drug are gradual and are frequently not seen for up to 6 months.

Dissolve sublingual tablets under the tongue. Do not chew or crush them; they are not effective if swallowed whole.

If you forget to take a dose of Ergoloid Mesylates, skip the missed dose and go back to your regular schedule. Do not take a double dose. Call your doctor if you forget to take two or more consecutive doses.

Special Populations

Pregnancy/Breast-feeding

This drug may interfere with fetal development. Check with your doctor before taking it if you are, or might be, pregnant.

Nursing mothers who must take this medication should bottle-feed their babies.

Seniors
Older adults are more likely to develop drug side effects,
especially hypothermia (low body temperature).

Ery-Tab

see **Erythromycin**, page 406

Generic Name
Erythromycin

Brand Names

Erythromycin Base*

E-Base Caplets and Tablets	Ery-Tab	PCE Dispertab
E-Mycin	Erythromycin Filmtabs	Robimycin
ERYC		Robitabs

Erythromycin Estolate*

Ilosone

Erythromycin Ethylsuccinate*

E.E.S. Tablets/Suspension/Drops
EryPed

Erythromycin Stearate*

Eramycin	Erythrocin Stearate	Wyamycin S

Erythromycin Eye Ointments*

AK-Mycin
Ilotycin

Erythromycin Topical Ointments and Solutions

Akne-Mycin Ointment and Solution	Erycette Solution Eryderm 2 Solution	E-Solve 2 Solution ETS-2% Solution Staticin Solution
A/T/S Solution	Erygel	T-Stat 2 Solution
C-Solve 2 Solution	Erymax Solution	

(*Also available in generic form)

Type of Drug

Macrolide antibiotic.

Prescribed for

Infections of virtually any part of the body: upper and lower respiratory tract infections; some sexually transmitted diseases; urinary tract infections; infections of the mouth, gums, and teeth; and infections of the nose, ears, and sinuses. It is prescribed for acne and may be used for mild to moderate skin infections, but is not considered the antibiotic of choice. Erythromycin is effective against diphtheria as well as amoeba infections in the intestinal tract, which cause dysentery. It is also prescribed for Legionnaires' disease, rheumatic fever, bacterial endocarditis, and a variety of other infections.

Erythromycin eye ointment is used to prevent newborn gonococcal or chlamydial infections of the eye. Erythromycin topical solution and ointment are used to control acne.

General Information

Erythromycin is a member of the group of antibiotics known as macrolides. This group of medicines, which also includes Azithromycin and Clarithromycin, are either bacteriocidal (they kill the bacteria directly) or bacteriostatic (they slow the bacteria's growth so that the body's natural protective mechanisms can kill them). Whether these drugs are bacteriostatic or bacteriocidal depends on the organism in question and the amount of antibiotic present in the blood or other body fluid. They are effective against all varieties of organisms, with each of the macrolide antibiotics working against a somewhat different profile of bacteria.

Erythromycin is absorbed from the gastrointestinal tract, but it is deactivated by the acid content of the stomach.

Because of this, the tablet form of this drug is formulated to bypass the stomach and dissolve in the intestine.

Since the action of this antibiotic depends on its concentration within the invading bacteria, it is imperative that you follow the doctor's directions regarding the spacing of the doses as well as the number of days you should continue taking Erythromycin. The effectiveness of this antibiotic can be severely reduced if these instructions are not followed.

Cautions and Warnings

Do not take Erythromycin if you are **allergic** to it or to any of the macrolide antibiotics.

Erythromycin is excreted primarily through the liver. People with **liver disease** or **damage** should exercise caution and consult their doctors. Those on long-term therapy with Erythromycin are advised to have **periodic blood tests**.

Erythromycin is available in a variety of types and formulations. Erythromycin Estolate has occasionally produced **liver difficulties,** including fatigue, nausea, vomiting, abdominal cramps, and fever. If you are susceptible to **stomach problems,** Erythromycin may cause mild to moderate stomach upset. Discontinuing the drug will reverse this condition. If you restart Erythromycin after having experienced liver damage, it is likely that symptoms will recur within 48 hours.

A form of **colitis** (bowel inflammation) can be associated with all antibiotics, including Erythromycin. **Diarrhea** associated with the antibiotic may be an indication of this problem.

Possible Side Effects

▼ Most common: nausea, vomiting, stomach cramps, and diarrhea. Colitis may develop after taking Erythromycin.

▼ Less common: hairy tongue, itching, and irritation of the anal and/or vaginal region. If any of these symptoms appear, consult your physician immediately.

▼ Rare: hearing loss (which reverses itself after the drug is stopped and occurs most often in people with liver and kidney problems) and abnormal heart rhythms.

Erythromycin should not be given to people with known sensitivity to this antibiotic. It may cause yellow-

Possible Side Effects *(continued)*

ing of the skin and eyes. If this occurs, discontinue the drug and notify your doctor immediately.

Drug Interactions

• Erythromycin may slow the breakdown of Carbamazepine (for seizures) and Theophylline (for asthma). People taking these medicines should not use Erythromycin.

• Erythromycin may neutralize Penicillin and the antibiotics Lincomycin and Clindamycin; avoid these combinations.

• Erythromycin interferes with the elimination of Theophylline from the body, which may cause toxic effects of Theophylline overdose. It can also increase the effects of Caffeine, which is chemically related to Theophylline, on your body.

• Erythromycin may increase blood levels of Astemizole and Terfenadine, two nonsedating antihistamines broken down in the liver. This drug interaction may lead to serious cardiac toxicity and should be avoided.

• Erythromycin may increase blood levels of Alfentanil (an injectable pain reliever), Bromocriptine, Digoxin, Disopyramide, Ergotamine, Cyclosporine, Methylprednisolone (a corticosteroid), and Triazolam, resulting in an increase in drug effects as well as toxicities.

• Erythromycin Estolate may increase the toxic side effects of other drugs that can affect the liver.

• Erythromycin may increase the anticoagulant (blood-thinning) effects of Warfarin in people who take it regularly, especially older adults. People taking anticoagulant drugs who must also take Erythromycin may need their anticoagulant dose adjusted.

Food Interactions

Food in the stomach will decrease the absorption rate of Erythromycin Base and Erythromycin Stearate products. They are best taken on an empty stomach or 1 hour before or 2 hours after meals, but may be taken with food if they cause stomach upset. Other forms of Erythromycin can be taken without regard to food or meals. Check with your pharmacist for specific directions.

Usual Dose

Tablets

Adult: 250 to 500 mg every 6 hours.

Child: 50 to 200 mg per pound of body weight per day in divided doses, depending upon age, weight, and severity of infection.

Eye Ointment

½-inch ribbon, 2 to 3 times per day.

Topical Solution

Apply morning and night.

Doses of Erythromycin Ethylsuccinate and Wyamycin are 60 percent higher due to differences in chemical composition.

Overdosage

Erythromycin overdose may result in exaggerated side effects, especially nausea, vomiting, stomach cramps, and diarrhea. Mild hearing loss, ringing or buzzing in the ears, or fainting may also occur. Call your local poison control center or hospital emergency room for more information.

Special Information

Erythromycin is a relatively safe antibiotic. It is used instead of Penicillin for mild to moderate infections in people who are allergic to the Penicillin class of antibiotics. Erythromycin is not the antibiotic of choice for severe infections.

Erythromycin products should be stored at room temperature, except for oral liquids and topical liquids, which should be kept in the refrigerator.

Take each dose of Erythromycin with 6 to 8 ounces of water.

Call your doctor if you develop any of the following: nausea; vomiting; diarrhea; stomach cramps; severe abdominal pain; skin rash, itching or redness; dark or amber-colored urine; yellowing of the skin or eyes; or other severe or persistent side effects.

If you forget a dose of oral Erythromycin, take it as soon as you remember. If it is almost time for your next dose, space the next 2 doses over 4 to 6 hours, then go back to your regular schedule.

Remember to complete the full course of therapy prescribed by your doctor, even if you feel perfectly well after only a few days of antibiotic.

Special Populations

Pregnancy/Breast-feeding

Erythromycin passes into the circulation of the developing fetus. Erythromycin Estolate has caused mild liver inflammation in about 10 percent of pregnant women and should not be used if you are, or may become, pregnant. Other forms of Erythromycin have been used safely without difficulty.

Erythromycin passes into breast milk. Nursing mothers who are taking the drug should watch for side effects in their nursing infants, although this happens only rarely.

Seniors

Older adults, except those with liver disease, may generally use this product without restriction.

Generic Name

Estazolam

Brand Name

ProSom

Type of Drug

Benzodiazepine sedative.

Prescribed for

Short-term treatment of insomnia or sleeplessness, difficulty falling asleep, frequent nighttime awakening, and waking too early in the morning.

General Information

Estazolam is a member of the group of drugs known as *benzodiazepines*. All have some activity as either antianxiety agents, anticonvulsants, or sedatives. Benzodiazepines work

by a direct effect on the brain. Benzodiazepines make it easier
to go to sleep and decrease the number of times you wake up
during the night.

The principal differences between these medicines lie in
how long they work on your body. They all take about 2 hours
to reach maximum blood level but some remain in your body
longer, so they work for a longer period of time. Estazolam is
considered an intermediate-acting sedative and generally
remains in your body long enough to give you a good night's
sleep with minimal "hangover." Often, sleeplessness is a
reflection of another disorder that would be untreated by one
of these medicines.

Cautions and Warnings

People with **respiratory disease** taking Estazolam may experience **sleep apnea** (intermittent breathing while sleeping).

People with **kidney** or **liver disease** should be carefully
monitored while taking Estazolam. Take the lowest possible
dose to help you sleep.

Clinical depression may be increased by Estazolam, which
can depress the nervous system. Intentional overdosage is
more common among depressed people who take sleeping
pills than those who do not.

All benzodiazepines **can be abused** if taken for long periods
of time, and it is possible for a person taking a benzodiazepine to develop drug-withdrawal symptoms if the drug is
suddenly discontinued.

Withdrawal symptoms include convulsions, tremors, muscle
cramps, insomnia, agitation, diarrhea, vomiting, sweating,
and convulsions.

Possible Side Effects

▼ Common: drowsiness, headache, dizziness, talkativeness, nervousness, apprehension, poor muscle coordination, light-headedness, daytime tiredness, muscle
weakness, slowness of movements, hangover, and euphoria (feeling "high").

▼ Less common: nausea, vomiting, rapid heartbeat,
confusion, temporary memory loss, upset stomach,
stomach cramps and pain, depression, blurred or double
vision and other visual disturbances, constipation, changes

Possible Side Effects *(continued)*

in taste perception, appetite changes, stuffy nose, nose-bleeds, common cold symptoms, asthma, sore throat, cough, breathing problems, diarrhea, dry mouth, allergic reactions, fainting, abnormal heart rhythms, itching, acne, dry skin, sensitivity to bright light or the sun, rash, nightmares or strange dreams, difficulty sleeping, tingling in the hands or feet, ringing or buzzing in the ears, ear or eye pains, menstrual cramps, frequent urination and other urinary difficulties, blood in the urine, discharge from the penis or vagina, lower back and joint pains, muscle spasms and pain, fever, swollen breasts, and weight changes.

Drug Interactions

• As with all benzodiazepines, the effects of Estazolam are enhanced if it is taken with an alcoholic beverage, antihistamine, tranquilizer, barbiturate, anticonvulsant medicine, antidepressant, or monoamine oxidase (MAO) inhibitor drug (most often prescribed for severe depression).

• Oral contraceptives, Cimetidine, Disulfiram, and Isoniazid may increase the effect of Estazolam by interfering with the drug's breakdown in the liver. Probenecid also increases Estazolam's effects.

• Cigarette smoking, Rifampin, and Theophylline may reduce the effect of Estazolam.

• Levodopa's effectiveness may be decreased by Estazolam.

• Estazolam may increase the amount of Zidovudine, Phenytoin, or Digoxin in your bloodstream, increasing the chances of drug toxicity.

• The combination of Clozapine and benzodiazepines has led to respiratory collapse in a few people. Estazolam should be stopped at least 1 week before starting Clozapine treatment.

Food Interactions

Estazolam may be taken with food if it upsets your stomach.

Usual Dose

Adult (age 18 and older): 1 to 2 mg about 60 minutes before you want to go to sleep.

Senior: 0.5 to 1 mg to start. Dosage should be increased cautiously.

Child: not recommended.

Overdosage

The most common symptoms of overdose are confusion, sleepiness, depression, loss of muscle coordination, and slurred speech. Coma may develop if the overdose is particularly large. Overdose symptoms can develop if a single dose of only 4 times the maximum daily dose is taken. Patients who take an overdose of this drug must be made to vomit with Syrup of Ipecac (available at any pharmacy) to remove any remaining drug from the stomach. Call your doctor or a poison control center before doing this. If 30 minutes have passed since the overdose was taken or symptoms have begun to develop, the victim must be taken immediately to a hospital emergency room for treatment. ALWAYS bring the medicine bottle.

Special Information

Never take more Estazolam than your doctor has prescribed.

Avoid alcoholic beverages and other nervous-system depressants while taking Estazolam.

People taking this drug must be careful when performing tasks requiring concentration and coordination because of the chance that the drug will make them tired, dizzy, or light-headed.

If you take Estazolam daily for 3 or more weeks, you may experience some withdrawal symptoms when you stop taking the drug. Talk with your doctor about the best way to discontinue the drug.

If you forget to take a dose of Estazolam and remember within about an hour of your regular time, take it as soon as you remember. If you do not remember until later, skip the forgotten dose and go back to your regular schedule. Do not take a double dose.

Special Populations

Pregnancy/Breast-feeding

Estazolam should absolutely not be used by pregnant women or women who may become pregnant. Animal studies have shown that Estazolam passes easily into the fetal blood system and can affect fetal development.

Estazolam passes into breast milk and can affect a nursing infant. The drug should not be taken by nursing mothers.

Seniors
Older adults are more susceptible to the effects of Estazolam and should take the lowest possible dosage.

Estrace

see Estrogen, page 415

Estraderm

see Estrogen, page 415

Type of Drug
Estrogen

Generic Name	Brand Name
Chlorotrianisene	TACE Capsules
Conjugated Estrogens	Premarin Tablets/Vaginal Cream
Conjugated Estrogens plus Medroxyprogesterone	Prempro
	Premphase
Dienestrol	DV Vaginal Cream
	Ortho Dienestrol Cream
Diethylstilbestrol	Diethylstilbestrol Tablets
Esterified Estrogens	Estrab
	Menest Tablets
Estradiol	Climara
	Estrace Tablets/Vaginal Cream
	Estraderm Transdermal System
Estropipate	Ogen Tablets/Vaginal Cream
	Ortho-Est
Ethinyl Estradiol	Estinyl Tablets
	Feminone Tablets
Quinestrol	Estrovis

Prescribed for

Moderate to severe menopausal symptoms and preventing postmenopausal osteoporosis. Estrogen drugs are also prescribed for ovarian failure, breast cancer (in selected women and men), advanced cancer of the prostate, osteoporosis, abnormal bleeding of the uterus, vaginal irritation, female castration, and Turner's syndrome. Estrogens may also be prescribed for birth control. Diethylstilbestrol is an effective "morning after" contraceptive, but should only be used as an emergency treatment because of the damage it causes to developing fetuses.

There is no evidence that Estrogens work for nervous symptoms or depression occurring during menopause. They should not be used to treat these conditions; they should be used only to replace estrogen that is naturally absent after menopause.

General information

Six different estrogenic substances have been identified in women, but only three are actually present in large amounts: estradiol, estrone, and estriol. Estradiol is the most potent of the three and is the major estrogen produced by the ovaries. Estradiol is naturally modified to estrone, which is then turned into estriol, the least potent of the three. All of the Estrogens listed in this section will produce equal effects and side effects when their doses are equal, taking their various potencies into account. More potent medicines require a smaller dose to produce the same effect.

Estrogens are natural body substances with specific effects on the human body, including growth and maintenance of the female reproductive system and all female sex characteristics. They promote growth and development of all parts of the reproductive system and breasts; they affect the release of hormones from the pituitary (master) gland that controls the opening of the capillaries (the smallest blood vessels); they can cause fluid retention; they affect protein breakdown in the body; they prevent ovulation and breast engorgement in women after giving birth; and they continue in the shaping and maintenance of the skeleton through their influence on calcium in the body.

The differences between the various products lie in the specific estrogenic substances they contain, their dose, and, in some cases, the fact that they affect one part of the body more than another. For the most part, however, estrogen products are interchangeable, as long as differences in dosage are taken into account.

Cautions and Warnings

Estrogens have been reported to increase the risk of **endometrial cancer in postmenopausal women** taking them without a progestin for prolonged periods of time by a factor of 5 to 10 times; the risk depends upon the duration of treatment and the dose of the Estrogen being taken. When long-term Estrogen therapy is needed for the treatment of menopausal symptoms, **taking a Progestin product** such as Medroxyprogesterone reduces the chance of endometrial cancer and other problems. In women who have had a **hysterectomy,** there is no need for Progestin treatment.

Estrogens have been prescribed as **"morning-after" contraceptives,** primarily in emergencies such as rape or incest, but they are dangerous because of the way they affect the developing fetus. Combination oral contraceptives containing Norgestrel and Ethinyl Estradiol are more commonly prescribed for this use.

Postmenopausal women taking Estrogens have a 2 to 3 times greater chance of developing **gallbladder disease**.

If you are taking an Estrogen product and experience recurrent, abnormal, or **persistent vaginal bleeding,** contact your doctor immediately.

If you have active **thrombophlebitis** or any other disorder associated with the **formation of blood clots,** you probably should not take this drug. If you feel that you have a disorder associated with blood clots, and you are taking an Estrogen or a similar product, contact your doctor immediately.

Estrogens should **not be used to treat painful breast engorgement with milk** that sometimes develops after giving birth. This condition usually responds to pain relievers and other treatments.

Animal studies have shown that prolonged continuous administration of Estrogen substances can increase the frequency of cancer (breast, cervix, testis, uterus, vagina, kidney, and liver). The question of whether Estrogens increase the **risk of breast cancer** has not been answered. Some studies have reported an increased risk, but others have not verified that result. Estrogens should be taken with caution by women with a **strong family history of breast cancer** and by those who have **breast nodules, fibrocystic disease of the breast,** or **abnormal mammograms**.

It is possible that women taking Estrogens for extended periods of time may experience some of the same **long-term side effects** as women who have taken oral contraceptives for extended periods of time. These long-term problems may include the development of blood-clotting disorders, liver cancer or other liver tumors, high blood pressure, glucose intolerance (symptoms similar to diabetes) or worsening of the disease in diabetic patients, unusual sensitivity to the sun, and high blood levels of calcium.

Vaginal Estrogen creams may stimulate **bleeding of the uterus.** They can also cause **breast tenderness, vaginal discharge,** and **withdrawal bleeding** (if the product is suddenly stopped). Women with **endometriosis** may experience heavy vaginal bleeding.

Possible Side Effects

▼ Most common: breast enlargement or tenderness (both sexes), ankle and leg swelling, loss of appetite, weight changes, retention of water, nausea, vomiting, abdominal cramps, and feeling of bloatedness. The estrogen patch can cause skin rash, irritation, and redness at the patch site.

▼ Less common: bleeding gums, breakthrough vaginal bleeding, vaginal spotting, changes in menstrual flow, painful menstruation, premenstrual syndrome, no menstrual period during and after Estrogen use, enlargement of uterine fibroids, vaginal infection with *Candida*, a cystitis-like syndrome, mild diarrhea, jaundice or yellowing of the skin or whites of the eyes, rash, loss of scalp hair, and development of new hairy areas. Lesions of the eye and contact-lens intolerance have also been associated with estrogen therapy. You may experience migraine headache, mild dizziness, depression, and increased sex drive (women) or decreased sex drive (men).

▼ Rare: stroke, blood-clot formation, dribbling or sudden passage of urine, loss of coordination, chest pains,

---

Possible Side Effects *(continued)*

leg pains, difficulty breathing, slurred speech, and vision changes. Men who receive large Estrogen doses as part of the treatment of prostate cancer are at a greater risk for heart attack, phlebitis, and blood clots in the lungs.

Drug Interactions

• Phenytoin, Ethotoin, and Mephenytoin may interfere with Estrogen effects. Estrogens may reduce your requirement for oral anticoagulant (blood-thinning) drugs, an adjustment your doctor can make after a simple blood test.

• Estrogens increase the amount of calcium absorbed from the stomach. This interaction is used to help women with osteoporosis to increase their calcium levels.

• Estrogens may increase the side effects of antidepressants and Phenothiazine tranquilizers. Low estrogen doses may increase Phenothiazine effectiveness.

• Estrogens may increase the amount of Cyclosporine and adrenal corticosteroid drugs in your blood. Dosage adjustments of the nonEstrogen drugs may be needed.

• Estrogen increases the toxic effects of other drugs on the liver, especially in women over 35 and people with preexisting liver disease.

• Rifampin, barbiturates, and other drugs that stimulate the liver to break down drugs may reduce the amount of Estrogen in the blood.

• Estrogens may interfere with the actions of Tamoxifen and Bromocriptine.

• Women, especially those over 35, who smoke cigarettes and take an Estrogen have a much greater chance of developing stroke, hardening of the arteries, or blood clots in the lungs. The risk increases as age and tobacco use increase.

• Estrogens interfere with many diagnostic tests. Make sure your doctor knows that you are taking an Estrogen before doing any blood tests or other diagnostic procedures.

Food Interactions

Estrogens may be taken with food to reduce nausea and stomach upset. Avoid drinking grapefruit juice if you are taking this medicine.

Usual Dose

Estrogen dosage depends on the condition being treated and the individual's response. All of these products, including the Estradiol skin patch, can be taken continuously or on a cyclic schedule of 3 weeks on, 1 week off.

Tablet

Chlorotrianisene: 12 to 200 mg.
Conjugated Estrogens: 0.3 to 7.5 mg.
Diethylstilbestrol: 1 to 15 mg.
Esterified Estrogens: 0.3 to 30 mg.
Estradiol: 1 to 60 mg.
Estropipate: 0.625 to 7.5 mg.
Ethinyl Estradiol: 0.02 to 2.0 mg.
Quinestrol: 100 micrograms once per day for 7 days, then 100 to 200 micrograms per week.

Skin Patches

Estradiol: 1 (0.05 or 0.1 mg) patch twice a week for 3 weeks; stop for 1 week, then start again. May be used continuously in some cases.

Vaginal Cream

Use the lowest possible dosage. Your doctor should reevaluate your need for an Estrogen vaginal cream every 3 to 6 months. Don't stop using the medicine suddenly, because this can increase your chance of developing unpredicted or breakthrough vaginal bleeding.

Conjugated Estrogens: 2 to 4 grams per day for 3 weeks; stop for 1 week, then start again.

Dienestrol: 1 applicatorful 1 or 2 times per day for 1 to 2 weeks, then half the original dose for 1 or 2 weeks, then 1 applicatorful 1 to 3 times per week.

Estradiol: 2 to 4 grams per day for 2 weeks, half the starting dose for another 2 weeks, then 1 gram 1 to 3 times per week.

Estropipate: 2 to 4 grams per day for 3 weeks; stop for 1 week, then start again.

Overdosage

Overdose may cause nausea and withdrawal bleeding in adult women. Accidental overdoses in children have not resulted in serious adverse side effects. Call your local poison control center or hospital emergency room for information. ALWAYS bring the medicine container with you if you go to a hospital emergency room for treatment.

Special Information

Call your doctor if you develop breast pain or tenderness, swelling of the feet and lower legs, rapid weight gain, chest pain, difficulty breathing, pain in the groin or calves, unusual vaginal bleeding, missed menstrual period, lumps in the breast, sudden severe headaches, dizziness or fainting, disturbances in speech or vision, weakness or numbness in the arms or legs, abdominal pains, depression, yellowing of the skin or whites of the eyes, or jerky or involuntary muscle movements. Call your doctor if you think you are pregnant.

Women using a vaginal Estrogen cream who start to bleed or develop breast tenderness or other vaginal discharge should contact their doctors at once.

Women who smoke cigarettes and take Estrogens have a greater chance of cardiovascular side effects, including stroke and blood clotting.

Estrogen skin patches should be applied to a clean, dry, nonoily, hairless area of intact skin, preferably on the abdomen. Do not apply to your breasts, waist, or other area where tight-fitting clothes can loosen the patch from your skin. The application site should be rotated to prevent irritation, and each site should have a 7-day patch-free period.

It is important to maintain good dental hygiene while taking Estrogen products, and to use extra care when using your toothbrush or dental floss because of the chance that your Estrogen will make you more susceptible to some infections. Dental work should be completed prior to starting on any Estrogen medication.

Vaginal Estrogen creams should be inserted high into the vagina, about two-thirds of the length of the applicator.

Some of these products contain Tartrazine, a dye widely used to color pharmaceutical products. Avoid Tartrazine-containing products if you are allergic to it or have asthma. Check with your pharmacist to find out if your Estrogen product contains Tartrazine.

If you forget your Estrogen, take it as soon as you remember. If it is almost time for your next dose, skip the forgotten dose and continue with your regular schedule. Do not take a double dose.

Special Populations

Pregnancy/Breast-feeding
Estrogens should not be used during pregnancy to prevent a possible miscarriage; they don't work for this purpose and are dangerous to the fetus.

Estrogens may reduce the flow of breast milk. The effects of Estrogens on nursing infants are not predictable. Either avoid the drug while breast-feeding or bottle-feed your baby.

Seniors
Estrogens may be taken without special precaution by most seniors, but the risk of some side effects increases with age, especially if you smoke.

Generic Name

Etodolac

Brand Name
Lodine

Type of Drug
Nonsteroidal anti-inflammatory drug (NSAID).

Prescribed for
Osteoarthritis. Can also be prescribed for rheumatoid arthritis, ankylosing spondylitis, mild to moderate pain, tendinitis, bursitis, painful shoulder, and gout.

General information
Etodolac is one of 16 NSAIDs used to relieve pain and inflammation. We do not know exactly how NSAIDs work, but part of their action may be due to an ability to inhibit the body's production of a hormone called *prostaglandin* and to inhibit the action of other body chemicals, including cyclo-oxygenase, lipoxygenase, leukotrienes, lysosomal enzymes, and a host of other factors. NSAIDs are generally absorbed

into the bloodstream fairly quickly. Etodolac starts relieving pain in about 30 minutes, and its effects last for 4 to 12 hours. Etodolac is broken down in the liver and eliminated through the kidneys.

Cautions and Warnings

People who are **allergic** to Etodolac (or any other NSAID) and those with a history of **asthma attacks** brought on by another NSAID, by **Iodides,** or by **Aspirin** should not take Etodolac.

Etodolac can cause **gastrointestinal (GI) bleeding, ulcers,** and **stomach perforation.** This can occur at any time, with or without warning, in people who take chronic Etodolac treatment. People with a history of **active GI bleeding** should be cautious about taking any NSAID. **Minor stomach upset, distress,** or **gas** is common during the first few days of treatment with Etodolac. People who develop **bleeding** or **ulcers** and continue treatment should be aware of the possibility of developing more serious drug toxicity.

Etodolac can affect **platelets and blood clotting** at high doses, and should be avoided by people with **clotting problems** and by those taking **Warfarin.**

People with **heart problems** who use Etodolac may experience swelling in their arms, legs, or feet.

Etodolac can cause severe toxic effects to the **kidney.** Report any unusual side effects to your doctor, who may need to periodically test your kidney function.

Etodolac can make you **unusually sensitive to the effects of the sun** (photosensitivity).

Possible Side Effects

▼ Most common: diarrhea, nausea, vomiting, constipation, stomach gas, stomach upset or irritation, and loss of appetite.

▼ Less common: stomach ulcers, GI bleeding, hepatitis, gallbladder attacks, painful urination, poor kidney function, kidney inflammation, blood and protein in the urine, dizziness, fainting, nervousness, depression, hallucinations, confusion, disorientation, tingling in the hands or feet, light-headedness, itching, increased sweating, dry nose and mouth, heart palpitations, chest pain, difficulty breathing, and muscle cramps.

Possible Side Effects *(continued)*

▼ Rare: severe allergic reactions, including closing of the throat, fever and chills, changes in liver function, jaundice (yellowing of the skin or eyes), and kidney failure. People who experience such effects must be promptly treated in a hospital emergency room or doctor's office.

NSAIDs have caused severe skin reactions; if this happens to you, see your doctor immediately.

Drug Interactions

• Etodolac can increase the effects of oral anticoagulant (blood-thinning) drugs such as Warfarin. You may take this combination, but your doctor may have to reduce your anticoagulant dose.

• Taking Etodolac with Cyclosporine may increase the toxic kidney effects of both drugs. Methotrexate toxicity may be increased in people also taking Etodolac.

• Etodolac may increase blood levels of Phenytoin, leading to increased Phenytoin side effects. Blood-Lithium levels may be increased in people taking Etodolac.

• Etodolac blood levels may be affected by Cimetidine because of that drug's effect on the liver.

• Probenecid may interfere with the elimination of Etodolac from the body, increasing the chances for Etodolac toxic reactions.

• Aspirin and other salicylates may decrease the amount of Etodolac in your blood. These medicines should never be taken at the same time.

Food Interactions

Take Etodolac with food or a magnesium/aluminum antacid if it upsets your stomach.

Usual Dose

200 to 400 mg every 6 to 8 hours. Do not take more than 1200 mg per day. People weighing 132 pounds or less should not take more than 20 mg for every 2.2 pounds of body weight.

Take each dose with a full glass of water and don't lie down
for 15 to 30 minutes after you take the medicine.

Overdosage

People have died from NSAID overdoses. The most common
signs of overdosage are drowsiness, nausea, vomiting, diarrhea, abdominal pain, rapid breathing, rapid heartbeat, increased sweating, ringing or buzzing in the ears, confusion,
disorientation, stupor, and coma. Take the victim to a hospital
emergency room at once. ALWAYS bring the medicine bottle.

Special Information

Etodolac can make you drowsy and/or tired: Be careful when
driving or operating hazardous equipment. Do not take any
nonprescription products with Acetaminophen or Aspirin
while taking this drug; also, avoid alcoholic beverages.

Contact your doctor if you develop skin rash or itching,
visual disturbances, weight gain, breathing difficulty, fluid
retention, hallucinations, black or tarry stools, persistent
headache, or any unusual or intolerable side effects.

If you forget to take a dose of Etodolac, take it as soon as
you remember. If you take several Etodolac doses a day and
it is within 4 hours of your next dose, skip the one you forgot
and continue with your regular schedule. If you take Etodolac
once a day and it is within 8 hours of your next dose, skip the
missed dose and continue with your regular schedule. Do not
take a double dose.

Special Populations

Pregnancy/Breast-feeding

NSAIDs may cross into the fetal blood circulation. They have
not been found to cause birth defects, but may affect a
developing fetal heart during the second half of pregnancy;
animal studies indicate a possible effect. Women who are or
who might become pregnant should not take Etodolac without their doctors' approval; pregnant women should be
particularly cautious about using this drug during the last 3
months of their pregnancy. When the drug is considered
essential by your doctor, its potential benefits must be carefully weighed against its risks.

NSAIDs may pass into breast milk, but have caused no
problems among breast-fed infants, except for seizures in a

baby whose mother was taking Indomethacin. Other NSAIDs have caused problems in animal studies. There is a possibility that a nursing mother taking Etodolac could affect her baby's heart or cardiovascular system. If you must take Etodolac, bottle-feed your baby.

Seniors

Older adults may be more susceptible to Etodolac side effects, especially ulcer disease.

Generic Name

Famciclovir

Brand Name

Famvir

Type of Drug

Antiviral.

Prescribed for

Shingles (herpes zoster infections).

General Information

Famciclovir is the second antiviral product (after Acyclovir) to be approved for treatment of herpes zoster infection. Famciclovir also works against herpes simplex virus infections. After it is absorbed into the body, Famciclovir is converted into Penciclovir, which works against shingles by interfering with basic reproductive DNA in the viruses. Penciclovir does not work on DNA in uninfected body cells. Penciclovir is broken down in the liver and eliminated from the body through the kidneys.

Cautions and Warnings

People **sensitive** or **allergic** to Famciclovir should not take this drug.

People with a **loss of kidney function** should have their dosage adjusted accordingly. **Severe liver disease** also calls for a reduction in daily Famciclovir dosage.

Lab animals receiving 1½ times the maximum dosage of Famciclovir developed tumors and testicular toxicity (abnormal or reduced numbers of sperm). The implication of these findings for people is not known.

Possible Side Effects

In preliminary studies of this drug, side effects were about equal in people who received Famciclovir and those who took an inactive placebo.

▼ Most common: headache, nausea, and diarrhea.

▼ Less common: fever, fatigue, pain, vomiting, constipation, loss of appetite, dizziness, tingling in the hands or feet, sleepiness, sore throat, sinus irritation, itching, and signs of shingles.

▼ Rare: chills, abdominal pains, and back or joint pains.

Drug Interactions

• Probenecid interferes with the elimination of Penciclovir from the body, possibly leading to higher than expected levels of Penciclovir in the blood.

• People who took both Famciclovir and Digoxin together had more Digoxin in their blood than those who did not take Famciclovir.

Food Interactions

This drug may be taken without regard to food or meals.

Usual Dose

Adult (age 18 and older): 500 mg every 8 hours for 1 week. People with reduced kidney function may take it as infrequently as once a day.

Child (under age 18): not recommended.

Overdosage

There is little information available about the effects of Famciclovir overdose. Overdose victims should be taken to a hospital emergency room for treatment. ALWAYS bring the medicine bottle with you.

Special Information

This drug should be started as soon as shingles are diagnosed. Be sure to complete the full week of treatment to get the maximum benefit from this medicine.

Call your doctor if any unusual side effects develop or if your side effects become particularly intolerable.

If you forget a dose of Famciclovir, take it as soon as you remember. If it is almost time for your next dose, skip the forgotten dose. Do not take a double dose. Call your doctor if you forget to take more than 2 doses in a row.

Special Populations

Pregnancy/Breast-feeding

Famciclovir should be taken by a pregnant woman only if it is absolutely necessary and the possible benefits outweigh the possible risk to the developing baby.

In animal studies, Penciclovir passes into breast milk in high concentrations, but it is not known if this happens in people. Nursing mothers who must take this medicine should bottle-feed their babies.

Seniors

Older adults have more active Penciclovir in their blood after taking Famciclovir than younger people and should have their dosage adjusted according to kidney function.

Generic Name

Famotidine

Brand Name

Pepcid
Pepcid AC (nonprescription form)

Type of Drug

Histamine H_2 antagonist.

Prescribed for

Ulcers of the stomach and upper intestine (duodenum). It is also prescribed for gastroesophageal reflux disease (GERD), stress ulcers, and other conditions characterized by the production of large amounts of gastric fluids, to prevent bleeding in the upper intestines and stomach and formation of stress ulcers. A surgeon may prescribe Famotidine for a patient under anesthesia when it is desirable for the production of stomach acid to be stopped completely.

Famotidine is the first histamine H_2 antagonist to be approved for sale without a prescription in the US for heartburn.

General Information

Famotidine works in the same way as other histamine H_2 antagonists, by turning off the system that produces stomach acid, as well as other secretions.

Famotidine is effective in treating the symptoms of ulcer and preventing complications of the disease. However, since all of the histamine H_2 antagonists work in the exact same way, it is doubtful that an ulcer that does not respond to one will be effectively treated by another. Histamine H_2 antagonists differ only in their potency. Cimetidine is the least potent, with 1000 mg roughly equal to 300 mg of Nizatidine and Ranitidine and 40 mg of Famotidine. The ulcer healing rates of all of these drugs are roughly equivalent, as are the chances of drug side effects.

Cautions and Warnings

Do not take Famotidine if you have had an **allergic** reaction to it or another **H_2 antagonist** in the past. Caution must be exercised by people with **kidney and liver disease** who take Famotidine because one third of each dose is broken down in the liver; the rest passes out of the body through the kidneys.

Possible Side Effects

▼ Most common: headache.

▼ Less common: dizziness, mild diarrhea, and constipation.

▼ Rare: drowsiness, dry mouth or skin, joint or muscle pains, loss of appetite, depression, nausea or vomiting, abdominal discomfort, stomach pains, ringing or buzzing in the ears, skin rash or itching, temporary hair loss, changes in taste perception, fever, swelling of the eyelids,

---

Possible Side Effects *(continued)*

chest tightness, rapid heartbeat, unusual bleeding or bruising, unusual tiredness or weakness, confusion, hallucination, anxiety or agitation, sleeplessness, reduced platelet counts, and impotence or reduced sex drive.

Drug Interactions

• Enteric-coated tablets should not be taken with Famotidine. The change in stomach acidity will cause the tablets to disintegrate prematurely in the stomach.

• Antacids, anticholinergic drugs, and Metoclopramide may slightly reduce the amount of Famotidine absorbed into the blood. No special precaution is needed.

Food Interactions

Food may slightly increase the amount of drug absorbed, but this is of no consequence; it may be taken without regard to food or meals.

Usual Dose

The usual adult dosage is either 20 to 40 mg at bedtime, or 20 mg twice a day. Dosage should be reduced in people with severe kidney disease.

Nonprescription dose: Take 1 pill (10 mg) with water, up to 2 pills a day. To prevent heartburn, take 1 pill (10 mg) 1 hour before eating or drinking anything that gives you indigestion, no more than twice a day. Call your doctor if you don't feel better in 2 weeks.

Overdosage

There is little information on Famotidine overdosage. Overdose victims might be expected to show exaggerated side effect symptoms, but little else is known. Your local poison control center may advise giving the victim Syrup of Ipecac (available at any pharmacy) to cause vomiting as soon as possible. This should remove any remaining drug from the stomach. Victims who have definite symptoms should be taken to a hospital emergency room for observation and possible treatment. ALWAYS bring the prescription bottle.

Special Information

You must take this medicine exactly as directed and follow your doctor's instructions for diet and other treatments in order to get the maximum benefit from it. Antacids may be taken together with Famotidine, if needed.

Cigarettes are known to be associated with stomach ulcers and may reverse the effect of Famotidine on stomach acid.

Call your doctor at once if any unusual side effects develop, particularly unusual bleeding or bruising, unusual tiredness, diarrhea, dizziness, or rash. Black, tarry stools or vomiting "coffee-ground"-like material may indicate your ulcer is bleeding.

If you forget to take a dose of Famotidine, take it as soon as you remember. If it is almost time for your next regularly scheduled dose, skip the one you forgot and continue with your regular schedule. Do not take a double dose.

Special Populations

Pregnancy/Breast-feeding

Although studies with laboratory animals have revealed no damage to a developing fetus, Famotidine should be avoided by pregnant women and those who might become pregnant while using it. When it is essential, Famotidine's potential risk must be carefully weighed against any benefit it might produce.

Famotidine may pass into breast milk. No problems have been identified in nursing babies, but nursing mothers must consider possible drug effects.

Seniors

Older adults respond well to Famotidine but may need less medication than younger adults to achieve the desired response, because the drug is eliminated through the kidneys, and kidney function tends to decline with age. Seniors may be more susceptible to some drug side effects.

Generic Name

Felbamate

Brand Name

Felbatol

Type of Drug

Anticonvulsant.

Prescribed for

Partial seizures; Lennox-Gastaut syndrome in children.

General Information

Felbamate is related to the older tranquilizer/sedative Meprobamate (Miltown). The exact way it works is not known, but Felbamate raises the seizure threshold and prevents the spread of the seizure in the brain, similarly to other anticonvulsant medicines. Felbamate is well absorbed into the bloodstream. About half of each dose passes out of the body through the kidneys and the other half is eliminated from the body by being broken down in the liver. Because of the potential dangers associated with Felbamate, this medicine should only be used when other seizure medicines have failed.

Cautions and Warnings

More than 20 cases of **aplastic anemia** (severe reductions in white blood cell count)—including 3 deaths—occurred in people taking Felbamate for 5 weeks or more. Ordinarily, this is a rare side effect, happening in only 2 to 5 per 1 million people. **This drug should not be used unless it is essential for your treatment and its benefits outweigh its risks.**

Dosages of Felbamate should be only gradually reduced or replaced by other anticonvulsant medicines; this drug should **never be suddenly stopped** because seizures may become more frequent.

People who are **allergic** to Felbamate or related medicines should not take this drug.

Felbamate may **increase your sensitivity to the sun.** Wear protective clothing and use sunscreen while taking this drug.

People with **severe liver** or **kidney disease** may require lower doses of Felbamate.

Possible Side Effects

▼ Most common: sleeplessness, fatigue, headache, anxiety, dizziness, nervousness, tremors, depression, unusual walk, upset stomach, nausea, vomiting, diarrhea,

Possible Side Effects *(continued)*

constipation, weight loss, fever, liver inflammation, taste changes, loss of appetite, hiccups, upper respiratory infection, runny nose, sore throat, coughing, double vision, middle ear infections, loss of urine control, black-and-blue marks, abnormal thinking, emotional instability, and pinpointed pupils.

▼ Less common: facial swelling, chest pain, generalized pain, tingling in the hands or feet, weakness, dry mouth, stupor, blurred or abnormal vision, sinus inflammation, bleeding between menstrual periods, urinary tract infections, muscle aches, and poor muscle control or coordination.

▼ Rare: weight gain and appetite increase, feelings of ill health, flulike symptoms, drug allergies, heart palpitations, rapid heartbeat, euphoria (feeling "high"), suicidal tendencies, migraines, inflammation of the esophagus, swollen lymph glands, reduced levels of white blood cells and blood platelets, reduced body sodium and/or potassium, itching, rash, swollen skin eruptions, swelling of tissue inside the mouth, Stevens-Johnson syndrome, unusual muscle movements, and unusual sensitivity to the sun.

Drug Interactions

• Felbamate increases the breakdown of Carbamazepine by the liver (by as much as 40 percent). This increased breakdown becomes obvious within the first 2 to 4 weeks after you start taking Felbamate. Carbamazepine dose adjustment is necessary. When this combination is taken together, the amount of Felbamate in the blood is also reduced by almost 50 percent because the drug is cleared from the body more quickly.

• Felbamate decreases the rate at which Phenytoin is broken down in the liver. Your daily Phenytoin dosage may have to be reduced by as much as 30 percent to account for this effect. When this combination is taken together, the amount of Felbamate in the blood is reduced by almost 50 percent because the drug is cleared from the body more quickly.

• Felbamate increases the amount of Valproic Acid in the blood. Unlike other anticonvulsants, Valproic Acid does not affect Felbamate.

Food Interactions

Felbamate is best taken on an empty stomach but may be taken with food if it upsets your stomach.

Usual Dose

Adult and Adolescent (age 14 and older): 1200 to 3600 mg per day divided into 3 or 4 doses.

Child (age 2 to 13): 6.8 to 20.5 mg per pound per day divided into 3 or 4 doses.

Overdosage

The only overdose effects that have been reported are upset stomach and increased heart rate. No serious effects have been seen, but one could expect usual drug side effects in overdose situations. Call your doctor, local poison control center, or hospital emergency room for more information. If you go to the emergency room for treatment, ALWAYS bring the medicine bottle.

Special Information

Do not take more Felbamate than your doctor has prescribed.

Felbamate can cause drowsiness; be careful when driving or performing complicated tasks.

Avoid long exposure to the sun while taking Felbamate.

Call your doctor if you develop any unusual or bothersome side effects.

It is important to maintain good dental hygiene while taking Felbamate and to use extra care when using your toothbrush or dental floss because this drug can cause swollen gums. See your dentist regularly while taking this medicine.

If you forget to take a dose of Felbamate, take it as soon as you remember. If it is almost time for your next dose, take one dose right away and another in 3 or 4 hours, then go back to your regular schedule. Do not take a double dose.

Special Populations

Pregnancy/Breast-feeding

This drug may cross into the fetal blood circulation. When the drug is considered essential by your doctor, its potential benefits must be carefully weighed against its risks.

Felbamate passes into breast milk, but its effect on nursing infants is not known. Consider bottle-feeding your baby because of possible effects on the nursing infant.

Seniors
Older adults, especially those with liver, kidney, or heart disease, may be more sensitive to the effects of this drug and should take doses in the low end of the usual dosing range.

Generic Name

Felodipine

Brand Name
Plendil

Type of Drug
Calcium channel blocker.

Prescribed for
High blood pressure.

General Information
Felodipine is a member of one of the most widely prescribed drug categories in the United States. Its once-daily dosage schedule makes Felodipine a natural for treating high blood pressure. It works by blocking the passage of calcium into heart and smooth-muscle tissue, especially the smooth muscle found in arteries. Since calcium is an essential factor in muscle contraction, any drug that affects calcium in this way will interfere with the contraction of these muscles. This causes the veins to dilate (open), reducing blood pressure. Also, the amount of oxygen used by the muscles is reduced. Therefore, Felodipine is also useful in the treatment of angina, a type of heart pain related to poor oxygen supply to the heart muscles. Felodipine also dilates the vessels that supply blood to the heart muscles and prevents spasm of these arteries. Felodipine affects the movement of calcium only into

muscle cells. It does not have any effect on calcium in the blood. Other calcium channel blockers are used for angina pains, abnormal heart rhythms, diseases involving blood vessel spasm (migraine headache, Raynaud's syndrome), heart failure, and cardiomyopathy.

Cautions and Warnings

Felodipine should not be taken if you have had an **allergic** reaction to it in the past.

On rare occasions, Felodipine may cause **very low blood pressure** in some people that may lead to stimulation of the heart and **rapid heartbeat** and can worsen **angina pains.** This reaction may happen when treatment is first started, when dosage is increased, or if the drug is rapidly withdrawn and can be avoided by gradual dosage reduction.

Studies have shown that people taking **calcium channel blockers** (usually those taken several times a day, not those taken only once daily) have a greater chance of having a **heart attack** than in people taking beta blockers or other medicines for the same purposes. Discuss this with your doctor to be sure you are receiving the best possible treatment.

Patients taking a **beta-blocking drug** who begin taking Felodipine may develop **heart failure** or **increased angina pain.** Angina pain may also increase when your Felodipine dosage is increased.

People with **severe liver disease** break down Felodipine much more slowly than people with less severe disease or normal livers. Your doctor should take this factor into account when determining your Felodipine dosage.

People taking Felodipine who have had a **heart attack** and have lung congestion may have **worsened heart failure,** since this drug can actually slow the force of each heartbeat.

Possible Side Effects

Calcium-channel-blocker side effects are generally mild and rarely cause people to stop taking them. Side effects are more common with higher doses and increasing age.

▼ Most common: swelling in the ankles, feet and legs, dizziness, light-headedness, muscle weakness or cramps, facial flushing, and headache.

Possible Side Effects *(continued)*

▼ Less common: respiratory infections, cough, tingling in the hands or feet, upset stomach, abdominal pains, chest pains, nausea, constipation, diarrhea, heart palpitations, sore throat, runny nose, back pain, and rash.

▼ Rare: facial swelling and a feeling of warmth, rapid heartbeat, heart attack, very low blood pressure, fainting, angina pains, abnormal heart rhythms, vomiting, dry mouth, stomach gas, anemia, muscle joint and bone pain, depression, anxiety, sleeplessness, irritability and nervousness, daytime tiredness, bronchitis, flu-like symptoms, sinus irritation, breathing difficulty, nosebleeds, sneezing, itching, redness, bruising, sweating, blurred vision, ringing or buzzing in the ears, swelling of the gums, decreased sex drive, loss of sexual ability, painful urination, and frequent and urgent urination.

Drug Interactions

• Felodipine may increase the amount of beta-blocking drug in the bloodstream. This can lead to heart failure, very low blood pressure, or an increased incidence of angina pain. However, in many cases these drugs have been taken together with no problem.

• Felodipine increases the effects of other blood-pressure-lowering drugs. Such drug combinations are often used to treat hypertension.

• Cimetidine and Ranitidine increase the amount of Felodipine in the blood and may account for a slight increase in the drug's effect.

• Phenytoin and other hydantoin antiseizure medicines, Carbamazepine, and barbiturate sleeping pills and sedatives may decrease the amount of Felodipine in the blood, reducing its effect on your body.

• Erythromycin may increase the side effects of Felodipine by slowing its release from the body.

• Felodipine may increase the effects of Digoxin, Theophylline (for asthma and other respiratory problems), and oral anticoagulant (blood-thinning) drugs.

• Felodipine may also interact with Quinidine (for abnormal heart rhythm) to produce low blood pressure, very slow heart rate, abnormal heart rhythms, and swelling in the arms or legs.

Food Interactions

Felodipine can be taken without regard to food or meals. You may take it with food if it upsets your stomach. Taking Felodipine with concentrated grapefruit juice doubles the amount of the drug normally absorbed into the blood; avoid this combination.

Usual Dose

5 to 10 mg per day. No patient should take more than 20 mg per day.

Do not stop taking Felodipine abruptly. The dosage should be gradually reduced over a period of time.

Overdosage

Felodipine overdose can cause low blood pressure. If you think you have taken an overdose of Felodipine, call your doctor or go to a hospital emergency room. ALWAYS bring the medicine bottle.

Special Information

Call your doctor if you develop constipation, nausea, very low blood pressure, difficulty breathing, increased heart pains, dizziness, or light-headedness, or if other side effects are particularly bothersome or persistent.

Swelling of the hands or feet may develop within 2 or 3 weeks of starting Felodipine. The chances of this happening depend both on your age and the Felodipine dosage: It occurs in less than 10 percent of people under age 50 taking 5 mg a day and more than 30 percent of those over age 60 taking 20 mg a day.

Be sure to continue taking your medicine and follow any instructions for diet restriction or other treatments to help maintain lower blood pressure. High blood pressure is a condition with few recognizable symptoms; it may seem to you that you are taking medicine for no good reason. Call your doctor or pharmacist if you have any questions.

Do not break or crush Felodipine tablets.

It is important to maintain good dental hygiene while taking Felodipine and to use extra care when using your toothbrush or dental floss because of the chance that the drug will make you more susceptible to some infections.

If you forget to take a dose of Felodipine, take it as soon as you remember. If it is almost time for your next regularly scheduled dose, skip the forgotten dose and continue with your regular schedule. Do not take a double dose of this medicine.

Special Populations

Pregnancy/Breast-feeding
Animal studies with Felodipine have shown that it crosses into the blood circulation of the developing fetus and has caused some birth defects. Women who are or who might become pregnant while taking this drug should not take it without their doctors' approval. The potential benefit of taking Felodipine must be carefully weighed against its risks.

It is not known if Felodipine passes into breast milk, but it has caused no problems among breast-fed infants. However, you must consider the potential effect on the nursing infant if you breast-feed while taking this medicine.

Seniors
Older adults, especially those with liver disease, are more sensitive to the effects of this drug because it takes longer to pass out of their bodies. Follow your doctor's directions and report any side effects at once.

Generic Name

Fenoprofen

Brand Name

Nalfon

(Also available in generic form)

Type of Drug

Nonsteroidal anti-inflammatory drug (NSAID).

Prescribed for

Rheumatoid arthritis, juvenile rheumatoid arthritis, osteoarthritis, mild to moderate pain, sunburn treatment, and migraine prevention and treatment.

General Information

Fenoprofen is one of 16 nonsteroidal anti-inflammatory drugs
(NSAIDs) that are used to relieve pain and inflammation. We
do not know exactly how NSAIDs work, but part of their
action may be due to an ability to inhibit the body's production of a hormone called *prostaglandin* and to inhibit the
action of other body chemicals, including cyclo-oxygenase,
lipoxygenase, leukotrienes, lysosomal enzymes, and a host of
other factors. NSAIDs are generally absorbed into the bloodstream fairly quickly. Fenoprofen starts relieving pain within
the first day it is used, but it takes about 2 days for its
anti-inflammatory effect to begin and 2 to 3 weeks to reach its
maximum effect. Fenoprofen is broken down in the liver and
eliminated through the kidneys.

Cautions and Warnings

People who are **allergic** to Fenoprofen (or any other NSAID)
and those with a history of **asthma attacks** brought on by
another **NSAID,** by **Iodides,** or by **Aspirin** should not take
Fenoprofen.

Fenoprofen can cause **gastrointestinal (GI) bleeding, ulcers,** and **stomach perforation.** This can occur at any time,
with or without warning, in people who take chronic Fenoprofen treatment. People with a history of **active GI bleeding**
should be cautious about taking any NSAID. **Minor stomach
upset, distress,** or **gas** is common during the first few days of
treatment with Fenoprofen. People who develop **bleeding** or
ulcers and continue treatment should be aware of the possibility of developing **more serious drug toxicity.**

Fenoprofen can affect **platelets and blood clotting** at high
doses, and should be avoided by people with **clotting problems** and by those taking **Warfarin.**

People with **heart problems** who use Fenoprofen may
experience swelling in their arms, legs, or feet.

People with **impaired hearing** may be affected by Fenoprofen and should be given periodic hearing tests.

Fenoprofen may actually cause **headaches.** If this happens, you may have to stop taking the medicine or switch to another NSAID.

Fenoprofen can cause severe toxic effects to the **kidney.** Report any unusual side effects to your doctor, who may need to periodically test your kidney function. People with **kidney disease** should not take Fenoprofen.

Fenoprofen can make you **unusually sensitive to the effects of the sun** (photosensitivity).

Possible Side Effects

▼ Most common: diarrhea, vomiting, nausea, constipation, stomach gas, stomach upset or irritation, and loss of appetite.

▼ Less common: stomach ulcers, GI bleeding, hepatitis, gallbladder attacks, painful urination, poor kidney function, kidney inflammation, blood and protein in the urine, dizziness, fainting, nervousness, depression, hallucinations, confusion, disorientation, tingling in the hands or feet, light-headedness, heart palpitations, chest pain, itching, increased sweating, dry nose and mouth, difficulty breathing, and muscle cramps.

▼ Rare: severe allergic reactions, including closing of the throat, fever and chills, changes in liver function, jaundice (yellowing of the skin or eyes), and kidney failure. People who experience such effects must be promptly treated in a hospital emergency room or doctor's office.

NSAIDs have caused severe skin reactions; if this happens to you, see your doctor immediately.

Drug Interactions

• Fenoprofen can increase the effects of oral anticoagulant (blood-thinning) drugs such as Warfarin. You may take this combination, but your doctor may have to reduce your anticoagulant dose.

• Taking Fenoprofen with Cyclosporine may increase the toxic kidney effects of both drugs. Methotrexate toxicity may be increased in people also taking Fenoprofen.

• Fenoprofen may reduce the blood-pressure-lowering effect of beta blockers and loop diuretic drugs.

• Fenoprofen may increase blood levels of Phenytoin, leading to increased Phenytoin side effects. Blood-Lithium levels may be increased in people taking Fenoprofen.

• Fenoprofen blood levels may be affected by Cimetidine because of that drug's effect on the liver.

• Probenecid may interfere with the elimination of Fenoprofen from the body, increasing the chances for Fenoprofen toxic reactions.

• Aspirin and other salicylates may decrease the amount of Fenoprofen in your blood. These medicines should never be taken at the same time.

Food Interactions

Take Fenoprofen with food or a magnesium/aluminum antacid if it upsets your stomach.

Usual Dose

Adult: 300 to 600 mg 4 times per day to start. *Mild to moderate pain:* 200 mg every 4 to 6 hours. *For arthritis:* 300 to 600 mg 3 to 4 times per day; up to 3200 mg per day.
Child: not recommended.

Overdosage

People have died from NSAID overdoses. The most common signs of overdosage are drowsiness, nausea, vomiting, diarrhea, abdominal pain, rapid breathing, rapid heartbeat, increased sweating, ringing or buzzing in the ears, confusion, disorientation, stupor, and coma. Take the victim to a hospital emergency room at once. ALWAYS bring the medicine bottle.

Special Information

Fenoprofen can make you drowsy and/or tired: Be careful when driving or operating hazardous equipment. Do not take any nonprescription products with Acetaminophen or Aspirin while taking this drug; also, avoid alcoholic beverages.

Take each dose with a full glass of water and don't lie down for 15 to 30 minutes after you take the medicine.

Contact your doctor if you develop skin rash or itching, ual disturbances, weight gain, breathing difficulty, fluid retention, hallucinations, black or tarry stools, persistent headache, or any unusual or intolerable side effects.

If you forget to take a dose of Fenoprofen, take it as soon as you remember. If you take several Fenoprofen doses a day and it is within 4 hours of your next dose, skip the one you forgot and continue with your regular schedule. If you take Fenoprofen once a day and it is within 8 hours of your next dose, skip the missed dose and continue with your regular schedule. Do not take a double dose.

Special Populations

Pregnancy/Breast-feeding
Fenoprofen may cross into the fetal blood circulation but has not been found to cause birth defects, though it may affect a developing fetal heart during the second half of pregnancy; animal studies indicate a possible effect. Women who are or who might become pregnant should not take Fenoprofen without their doctor's approval; be particularly cautious about using this drug during the last 3 months of your pregnancy. When the drug is considered essential by your doctor, its potential benefits must be carefully weighed against its risks.

Fenoprofen may pass into breast milk but has caused no problems among breast-fed infants, except for seizures in a baby whose mother was taking Indomethacin. Other NSAIDs have caused problems in animal studies. There is a possibility that a nursing mother taking Fenoprofen could affect her baby's heart or cardiovascular system. If you must take Fenoprofen, bottle-feed your baby.

Seniors
Older adults may be more susceptible to Fenoprofen side effects, especially ulcer disease.

Generic Name

Finasteride

Brand Name
Proscar

Type of Drug
Alpha-reductase inhibitor.

Prescribed for

Benign prostatic hypertrophy (BPH). Finasteride has also been studied as therapy following radical prostatectomy surgery and for the prevention of first-stage prostate cancer, male pattern baldness, acne, and unusual hairiness.

General Information

Progressive enlargement of the prostate gland generally occurs in men over age 50 and is associated with a gradual reduction in urine flow. (The number of men affected by BPH increases with advancing age.) Finasteride works by interfering with the action of the enzyme *alpha-reductase*, which is essential in the process of converting testosterone into a much more potent androgenic substance called *5α-dihydrotestosterone* (DHT). A single 5-mg dose of Finasteride produces a rapid drop in DHT levels, with the maximum reduction occurring 8 hours after taking the dose. DHT levels remain low for 24 hours and stay low as long as the drug is continued. Six to 12 months of Finasteride treatment may be needed to assess its effect.

There is no way to predict who will respond and who will not. In a clinical study of Finasteride, men experienced a significant regression in prostate size after 3 months, a reduction that was maintained throughout the 12-month study period. Also, study subjects experienced a significant improvement in urine flow. Extended studies showed that these improvements could be maintained up to 36 months.

Cautions and Warnings

Do not take Finasteride if you are **allergic** to any component of the product. This drug is **not meant to be taken by women or children.**

Finasteride only works in BPH. Other conditions that can mimic BPH, such as infection, prostate cancer, bladder or nerve disorders, or physical obstruction of the urinary tubes, will not be improved by this medicine.

Finasteride must be used with caution by people with **liver disease,** because that is where it is broken down in the body.

Animal studies have shown that Finasteride may increase the chance of **testicular cancer** and **reduce male fertility.** Finasteride may **mask prostate cancer** by causing a reduction in the level of prostate-specific antigen (PSA), an increasingly acknowledged indicator of prostate cancer. While a low PSA level does not necessarily exclude the possibility of prostate cancer, a higher one is definitely cause for further investigation.

Possible Side Effects

Finasteride side effects are generally mild and well tolerated.

▼ Most common: impotence, loss of sex drive, and decreased amount of semen.

Drug Interactions

• Finasteride increases the rate at which Theophylline and Aminophylline are broken down in the liver. These changes may not affect the amount of Theophylline or Aminophylline you need to control your asthma.

Food Interactions

You may take this drug with food if it upsets your stomach.

Usual Dose

Adult and Senior: 5 mg once per day.
Woman and Child: do not use.

Overdosage

People have taken single doses up to 400 mg and daily doses up to 80 mg for 3 months without any side effects. In animal studies, the drug was lethal at doses equal to 182 to 455 mg per pound of body weight. Call your local poison control center or hospital emergency room for more information. If you go to a hospital for treatment, ALWAYS bring the medicine bottle.

Special Information

Crushed Finasteride tablets should not be handled by women who are, or might become, pregnant because small amounts of the drug could be absorbed into the blood, possibly affecting a developing fetus.

If your sexual partner is, or may become, pregnant and you start taking this medicine, you must wear a condom to avoid directly exposing her to Finasteride-containing semen. Other options are to avoid sexual contact or stop the drug.

Semen volume may be decreased while on Finasteride, but this should not interfere with normal sexual function. Impotence or reduced sex drive is a possibility.

If you forget to take a dose of Finasteride, take it as soon as you remember. If it is almost time for your next dose, skip the forgotten dose and continue with your regular schedule. Do not take a double dose. Call your doctor if you forget to take this medicine for 2 or more days.

Special Populations

Pregnancy/Breast-feeding
Pregnant or nursing women must not take this drug because of the harm it could cause (see *Cautions and Warnings*).

Seniors
Seniors retain Finasteride in their bodies longer, but dosage adjustment is not required, nor is dose adjustment needed in people with kidney disease.

Brand Name

Fioricet

Ingredients

Acetaminophen + Butalbital + Caffeine

Other Brand Names

Amaphen	Esgic Plus	Repan
Anoquan	Femcet	Two-Dyne
Endolor	Medigesic	
Esgic		

(Also available in generic form)

Type of Drug

Nonnarcotic-analgesic combination.

Prescribed for

Migraine headaches and other types of pain.

General Information

Fioricet is one of many combination products containing a barbiturate (Butalbital) and an analgesic, or pain reliever (Acetaminophen). Products of this kind often also contain a tranquilizer or a narcotic. Other analgesic combinations, such as Fiorinal, substitute Aspirin for Acetaminophen.

Cautions and Warnings

Do not take Fioricet if you know you are allergic or sensitive to it. Use this drug with extreme caution if you suffer from asthma or other breathing problems or if you have kidney or liver disease or virus infections of the liver. Long-term use of Fioricet may lead to drug dependence or addiction.

Butalbital is a respiratory depressant and affects the central nervous system, producing drowsiness, tiredness, and/or inability to concentrate.

Possible Side Effects

▼ Most common: light-headedness, dizziness, sedation, nausea, vomiting, sweating, loss of appetite, and mild stimulation.

▼ Less common: weakness, headache, stomach upset, sleeplessness, agitation, tremor, uncoordinated muscle movements, mild hallucinations, disorientation, visual disturbances, euphoria (feeling "high"), dry mouth, constipation, flushing of the face, changes in heart rate, palpitations, faintness, difficulty in urination, skin rashes, itching, confusion, rapid breathing, and diarrhea.

Drug Interactions

• Mixing Fioricet with alcohol, tranquilizers, barbiturates, sleeping pills, or other nervous-system depressants can cause tiredness, drowsiness, and trouble concentrating.

Food Interactions

Fioricet is best taken on an empty stomach, but may be taken with food if it upsets your stomach.

Usual Dose

1 to 2 tablets or capsules every 4 hours or as needed, up to 6 doses a day.

Overdosage

Overdose symptoms are difficulty in breathing, nervousness progressing to stupor or coma, pinpointed pupils of the eyes, cold clammy skin and lowered heart rate and/or blood pressure, nausea, vomiting, dizziness, ringing in the ears, flushing, sweating, and thirst. The victim should be taken to a hospital emergency room immediately. ALWAYS bring the medicine bottle with you.

Special Information

Be careful if you are driving, operating hazardous machinery, or performing other functions requiring concentration. Alcohol may increase the chances of Acetaminophen-related liver toxicity and Butalbital-related drowsiness.

Call your doctor if you develop side effects that are unusual, persistent, or bothersome.

If you forget to take a dose of Fioricet, take it as soon as you remember. If it is almost time for your next dose, skip the one you forgot and continue with your regular schedule. Do not take a double dose.

Special Populations

Pregnancy/Breast-feeding

Fioricet should be avoided during pregnancy. There is an increased chance of birth defects when pregnant women use Fioricet. Regular use of Fioricet during the last 3 months of pregnancy may cause drug dependency of the newborn. Pregnant women using Fioricet may experience prolonged labor and delayed delivery, and breathing problems may afflict the newborn. Alternative therapies should be used if you are pregnant.

Breast-feeding while using Fioricet may cause the baby to become tired, short of breath, or have a slow heartbeat. If you must take Fioricet, consider bottle-feeding your baby.

Seniors
The Butalbital in this combination product may have a more exaggerated depressant effect on seniors than on younger adults. Other effects that may be more prominent are light-headedness or dizziness, or fainting when rising suddenly from a sitting or lying position.

Brand Name
Fiorinal

Ingredients
Aspirin + Butalbital + Caffeine

Other Brand Names

Butalbital Compound	Isollyl Improved
Fiorgen PF	Lanorinal

(Also available in generic form)

Type of Drug
Nonnarcotic-analgesic combination.

Prescribed for
Relief of migraine headache and other pain.

General Information
Fiorinal is one of many combination products containing a barbiturate (Butalbital) and an analgesic or pain reliever (Aspirin). Products of this kind often also contain a tranquilizer or a narcotic. Other analgesic combinations, such as Esgic and Fioricet, substitute Acetaminophen for Aspirin.

Cautions and Warnings

Do not take Fiorinal if you know you are **allergic** or **sensitive** to it or any of its ingredients. Use this drug with extreme caution if you suffer from **asthma** or other **breathing problems**. Long-term use of this drug may cause **drug dependence** or **addiction**. Butalbital is a respiratory depressant and affects the central nervous system, producing **drowsiness, tiredness,** and/or **inability to concentrate**.

Do not take this product if you are **allergic** to **Aspirin,** any **salicylate,** or any **nonsteroidal anti-inflammatory drug (NSAID)**. Check with your doctor or pharmacist if you are not sure. This and all other Aspirin-containing products should not be taken by children under age 17. People with **liver damage** should avoid Fiorinal.

Alcoholic beverages can aggravate the stomach irritation caused by Aspirin. The risk of Aspirin-related ulcers is increased by alcohol. Alcohol will also increase the nervous-system depression caused by Butalbital.

Do not take any Aspirin-containing product if you develop **dizziness, hearing loss,** or **ringing or buzzing in your ears**. Aspirin can interfere with **normal blood coagulation (clotting)** and should be avoided for 1 week before **surgery** for this reason. It would be wise to ask your surgeon or dentist for their recommendation before taking an Aspirin-containing product for pain after surgery.

Possible Side Effects

▼ Most common: light-headedness, dizziness, sedation, nausea, vomiting, sweating, stomach upset, loss of appetite, and mild stimulation.

▼ Less common: weakness, headache, sleeplessness, agitation, tremor, uncoordinated muscle movements, mild hallucinations, disorientation, visual disturbances, euphoria (feeling "high"), dry mouth, constipation, flushing of the face, changes in heart rate, palpitations, faintness, difficulty in urination, skin rashes, itching, confusion, rapid breathing, and diarrhea.

Drug Interactions

• Mixing this drug with alcohol, tranquilizers, barbiturates, sleeping pills, or other nervous-system depressants can cause tiredness, drowsiness, and trouble concentrating.

• Interaction with Prednisone, other steroids, Phenylbutazone, or alcohol can irritate your stomach and increase the chance of developing an ulcer.

• Your anticoagulant (blood-thinning) drug dose will have to be changed if you begin taking Fiorinal, which contains Aspirin.

• Fiorinal will counteract the uric acid-eliminating effect of Probenecid and Sulfinpyrazone. Fiorinal may counteract the blood-pressure-lowering effects of the angiotensin-converting-enzyme (ACE) inhibitor and beta-blocking drugs.

• Fiorinal may counteract the effects of some diuretics when given to people with severe liver disease.

• Fiorinal may increase blood levels of Methotrexate or Valproic Acid when taken together, leading to increased chances of drug toxicity.

• Combining Fiorinal and Nitroglycerin tablets may lead to an unexpected drop in blood pressure.

• Do not take Fiorinal together with an NSAID drug. There is no benefit to the combination, and the chance of side effects, especially stomach irritation, is vastly increased.

Food Interactions

Fiorinal is best taken on an empty stomach but may be taken with food if it upsets your stomach.

Usual Dose

1 to 2 tablets or capsules every 4 hours or as needed, up to 6 doses a day.

Overdosage

Overdose symptoms are difficulty in breathing, nervousness progressing to stupor or coma, pinpointed pupils, cold clammy skin and lowered heart rate and/or blood pressure, nausea, vomiting, dizziness, ringing in the ears, flushing, sweating, and thirst.

Symptoms of mild overdosage are rapid and deep breathing, nausea, vomiting, dizziness, ringing or buzzing in the ears, flushing, sweating, thirst, headache, drowsiness, diarrhea, and rapid heartbeat.

Severe overdose may cause fever, excitement, confusion, convulsions, liver or kidney failure, coma, or bleeding.

Any suspected overdose victim should be taken to a hospital emergency room immediately. ALWAYS bring the medicine bottle.

Special Information

This drug may cause drowsiness, affecting your ability to drive a car or operate complicated machinery.

Call your doctor if you develop side effects that are unusual, persistent, or bothersome.

If you forget to take a dose of Fiorinal, take it as soon as you remember. If it is almost time for your next dose, skip the one you forgot and continue with your regular schedule. Do not take a double dose.

Special Populations

Pregnancy/Breast-feeding

Fiorinal should be avoided during pregnancy. There is an increased chance of birth defects while using Fiorinal during pregnancy. Regular use of Fiorinal during the last 3 months of pregnancy may cause drug dependency of the newborn. Pregnant women using Fiorinal may experience prolonged labor and delayed delivery, and breathing problems may afflict the newborn. If taken during the last 2 weeks of pregnancy, Fiorinal may cause bleeding problems in the newborn child. Problems may also be seen in the mother, including bleeding. Alternative therapies should be used if you are pregnant.

Breast-feeding while using Fiorinal may cause the baby to be tired and short of breath, or have a slow heartbeat. If you must take Fiorinal, consider bottle-feeding your baby.

Seniors

The Butalbital in this combination product may have a more exaggerated depressant effect on seniors than on younger adults. Other effects that may be more prominent are light-headedness or dizziness or fainting when rising suddenly from a sitting or lying position.

Brand Name

Fiorinal with Codeine

Ingredients

Aspirin + Butalbital + Caffeine + Codeine Phosphate

(Also available in generic form)

Type of Drug

Narcotic-analgesic combination.

Prescribed for

Relief of migraine headaches or other pain.

General Information

Fiorinal with Codeine is one of many combination products containing a barbiturate (Butalbital), an analgesic or pain reliever (Aspirin), and a narcotic (Codeine). These products often also contain a tranquilizer, and Acetaminophen may be substituted for Aspirin.

Cautions and Warnings

Do not take Fiorinal with Codeine if you know you are **allergic** or **sensitive** to it. Use this drug with extreme caution if you suffer from **asthma** or other **breathing problems**. Long-term use of this drug may cause **drug dependence** or **addiction**. Fiorinal with Codeine is a respiratory depressant and affects the central nervous system, producing **sleepiness, tiredness,** and/or **inability to concentrate.**

Do not take this product if you are **allergic** to **Aspirin,** any **salicylate, or** any **nonsteroidal anti-inflammatory drug (NSAID).** Check with your doctor or pharmacist if you are not sure. This and all other Aspirin-containing products should not be taken by children under age 17. People with **liver damage** should avoid all the active ingredients in this product.

Alcoholic beverages can aggravate the stomach irritation caused by Aspirin. The risk of Aspirin-related ulcers is increased by alcohol. Alcohol will also increase the nervous-system depression caused by Codeine and Butalbital.

Do not use any Aspirin-containing product if you develop **dizziness, hearing loss,** or **ringing or buzzing in your ears.** Aspirin can interfere with **normal blood coagulation (clotting)** and should be avoided for 1 week before **surgery** for this reason. It would be wise to ask your surgeon or dentist for their recommendation before taking an Aspirin-containing product for pain after surgery.

Possible Side Effects

▼ Most common: light-headedness, dizziness, sleepiness, nausea, vomiting, loss of appetite, and sweating. If these occur, consider asking your doctor about lowering the dose you are taking. Usually the side effects disappear if you simply lie down.

▼ Less common: euphoria (feeling "high"), shallow breathing or difficulty in breathing, weakness, sleepiness, headache, agitation, uncoordinated muscle movement, minor hallucinations, disorientation and visual disturbances, dry mouth, constipation, flushing of the face, rapid heartbeat, palpitations, faintness, urinary difficulties or hesitancy, reduced sex drive and/or potency, itching, rashes, anemia, lowered blood sugar, and yellowing of the skin and/or whites of the eyes. Narcotic analgesics may aggravate convulsions in those who have had convulsions in the past.

Drug Interactions

• Interaction with alcohol, tranquilizers, barbiturates, sleeping pills, or other drugs that produce depression can cause tiredness, drowsiness, and trouble concentrating.

• Mixing this drug with Prednisone or other corticosteroids, alcohol, or Phenylbutazone can irritate your stomach.

• Your anticoagulant (blood-thinning) drug dose will have to be changed if you begin taking Fiorinal with Codeine, which contains Aspirin.

• This product will counteract the uric acid-eliminating effects of Probenecid and Sulfinpyrazone.

• Fiorinal with Codeine may counteract the blood-pressure-lowering effects of the angiotensin-converting-enzyme (ACE) inhibitor and beta-blocker drugs.

• Fiorinal with Codeine may counteract the effects of some diuretics when given to people with severe liver disease.

• Mixing this drug with Methotrexate or Valproic Acid may increase blood levels of those drugs, increasing the chances of drug side effects.

• Combining Fiorinal with Codeine and Nitroglycerin tablets may lead to an unexpected drop in blood pressure.

• Do not take this drug together with any NSAID drug. There is no benefit to the combination and the chance of side effects, especially stomach irritation, is vastly increased.

Food Interactions

Fiorinal with Codeine is best taken on an empty stomach, but you may take it with food if it upsets your stomach.

Usual Dose

1 to 2 tablets or capsules every 4 hours or as needed. Maximum of 6 doses per day.

Overdosage

Usual overdose symptoms are difficulty in breathing, nervousness progressing to stupor or coma, pinpointed pupils of the eyes, cold clammy skin and lowered heart rate and/or blood pressure, nausea, vomiting, dizziness, ringing in the ears, flushing, sweating, and thirst.

Symptoms of mild overdosage are rapid and deep breathing, nausea, vomiting, dizziness, ringing or buzzing in the ears, flushing, sweating, thirst, headache, drowsiness, diarrhea, and rapid heartbeat.

Severe overdose may cause fever, excitement, confusion, convulsions, liver or kidney failure, coma, or bleeding. The suspected overdose victim should be taken to a hospital emergency room immediately. ALWAYS bring the medicine bottle.

Special Information

Fiorinal with Codeine may cause drowsiness, affecting your ability to drive a car or operate complicated machinery.

Call your doctor if you develop any drug side effects that are unusual, bothersome, or persistent.

If you forget to take a dose of Fiorinal with Codeine, take it as soon as you remember. If it is almost time for your next regularly scheduled dose, skip the one you forgot and continue with your regular schedule. Do not take a double dose.

Special Populations

Pregnancy/Breast-feeding

Pregnant women should not take Fiorinal with Codeine because this drug carries an increased chance of birth defects. Regular use of Fiorinal with Codeine during the last 3 months of pregnancy may cause drug dependency of the newborn. Pregnant women using Fiorinal with Codeine may experience prolonged labor and delayed delivery, and breathing problems may afflict the newborn. If taken during the last 2 weeks of pregnancy, this drug may cause bleeding problems in the newborn child. Problems may also be seen in the mother, including bleeding.

Breast-feeding while using Fiorinal with Codeine may cause increased tiredness, shortness of breath, or a slow heartbeat in the baby. If you must take this medicine, consider bottle-feeding your baby.

Seniors

Both the Codeine and Butalbital in this combination product may have more of a depressant effect on seniors than on younger adults. Other effects that may be more prominent are dizziness, light-headedness, or fainting when rising suddenly from a sitting or lying position.

Generic Name

Flecainide

Brand Name

Tambocor

Type of Drug

Antiarrhythmic.

Prescribed for

Abnormal heart rhythm.

General Information

Flecainide is prescribed for situations where the abnormal rhythm is so severe as to be life-threatening and does not respond to other drug treatments. Like other antiarrhythmic drugs, Flecainide works by affecting the movement of nervous impulses within the heart.

Flecainide's effects may not become apparent for 3 to 4 days after you start taking it. Since Flecainide therapy is often started while you are in the hospital, especially if you are being switched from another antiarrhythmic drug to Flecainide, your doctor will be able to closely monitor how well the drug is working for you.

Cautions and Warnings

As with other antiarrhythmic drugs, there is **no proof** that Flecainide helps people **live longer or avoid sudden death**. Do not take Flecainide if you are **allergic** or **sensitive** to it or if you have **heart block** (unless you have a **cardiac pacemaker**).

Flecainide can cause new **arrhythmias** or worsen already existing ones in 7 percent of people who take it; this risk increases with certain kinds of **underlying heart disease** and higher doses of the drug. Flecainide may cause or worsen **heart failure** in about 5 percent of people taking it because it tends to reduce the force and rate of each heartbeat.

Flecainide is extensively broken down in the liver. People with **poor liver function** should not take Flecainide unless the benefits clearly outweigh the possible risks of drug toxicity.

Possible Side Effects

▼ Most common: dizziness, fainting, light-headedness, unsteadiness, visual disturbances (blurred vision, seeing spots before the eyes), difficulty breathing, headache, nausea, fatigue, heart palpitations, chest pain, tremors, weakness, constipation, bloating, and abdominal pain.

▼ Less common: new or worsened heart arrhythmias or heart failure, heart block, slowed heart rate, vomiting, diarrhea, upset stomach, loss of appetite, stomach gas, a bad taste in your mouth, dry mouth, tingling in the hands or feet, partial or temporary paralysis, loss of muscle control, flushing, sweating, ringing or buzzing in the ears,

---

Possible Side Effects *(continued)*

anxiety, sleeplessness, depression, feeling sick, twitching, weakness, convulsions, speech disorders, stupor, memory loss, personality loss, nightmares, a feeling of apathy, eye pain, unusual sensitivity to bright light, sagging eyelids, reduced white-blood-cell or blood-platelet counts, male impotence, reduced sex drive, frequent urination, urinary difficulty, itching, rash, fever, muscle aches, closing of the throat, and swollen lips, tongue, or mouth.

Drug Interactions

• The combination of Propranolol and Flecainide can cause an exaggerated lowering in heart rate. Other drugs that slow the heart may also interact with Flecainide to produce an excessive slowing of heart rate.

• The acidity of your urine affects the passing of Flecainide out of your body. Less acidity increases the amount of drug released, and more acidity, such as can occur with megadoses of vitamin C, decreases the amount you release. Extreme changes in urine acid content can expose you to more side effects (more acid) or fewer drug effects (less acid).

• The amount of Flecainide in your blood and its effect on your heart can be increased if it is taken together with Amiodarone, Cimetidine, Disopyramide, or Verapamil.

• Cigarette smoking increases the rate at which Flecainide is broken down in the liver. Smokers may need a larger dose than nonsmokers.

• Flecainide may increase the amount of Digoxin in the bloodstream, increasing the chance of drug side effects.

Food Interactions

Flecainide can be taken without regard to food or meals.

Usual Dose

The usual starting dose for all age groups is 50 to 100 mg every 12 hours. Your doctor can increase your dose by 50 mg each time every several days, if needed. The maximum dose of Flecainide depends on your response to the drug, your kidney function, and the specific arrhythmia being treated, but can go up to 600 mg per day.

Overdosage

Flecainide overdosage affects heart function, causing slower heart rate, low blood pressure, and possible death from respiratory failure. Victims of Flecainide overdose should be taken to a hospital emergency room for treatment. ALWAYS bring the medicine bottle.

Special Information

Flecainide can make you dizzy, light-headed, or disoriented. Take care while driving or performing any complex tasks.

Call your doctor if you develop chest pains, an abnormal heartbeat, difficulty breathing, bloating in your feet or legs, tremors, fever, chills, sore throat, unusual bleeding or bruising, yellowing of the whites of your eyes, or any other intolerable side effect.

If you forget to take a dose of Flecainide and remember within 6 hours, take it as soon as possible. If you don't remember until later, skip the forgotten dose and continue with your regular schedule. Do not take a double dose.

Special Populations

Pregnancy/Breast-feeding

Animal studies have shown that Flecainide at 4 times the normal human dose damages a developing fetus, but it is not known if the drug passes into fetal blood circulation. Pregnant women should discuss with their doctors the potential benefits of taking this drug versus its potential dangers.

Flecainide passes into mother's milk in concentrations about 2 1/2 times that found in blood. Nursing mothers who must take this drug should bottle-feed their infants.

Seniors

Seniors with reduced kidney or liver function are more likely to develop drug side effects and require a lower dosage.

Generic Name

Fluconazole

Brand Name

Diflucan Suspension/Tablets

Type of Drug

Antifungal.

Prescribed for

Infections of the blood, mouth, throat, vagina, or central nervous system due to *Candida*, *Aspergillus*, or *Cryptococcus*.

General Information

Fluconazole is an antifungal agent that is effective against a variety of fungal organisms, including *Aspergillus*, *Cryptococcus*, and *Candida*. It works by inhibiting important enzyme systems in the organisms it attacks. Fluconazole's effectiveness against *Candida* and *Cryptococcus* has made this drug an important contributor in the fight against the opportunistic fungal infections that afflict many people with AIDS.

Cautions and Warnings

Do not take Fluconazole if you are **allergic** to it. People who are allergic to **similar antifungals** (Ketoconazole, Miconazole, and Itraconazole) may also be allergic to Fluconazole, but cross-reactions are not common and serious allergic reaction is rare.

Rarely, Fluconazole causes **liver damage**. The drug should be used with caution in people with **pre-existing liver disease**. In studies with laboratory animals, Fluconazole caused an increase in liver tumors.

Skin rash may be an important sign of drug toxicity, especially in people with AIDS or others with compromised immune function. Report any skin rashes, especially ones that don't heal readily, to your doctor.

Possible Side Effects

Side effects are, generally, more common among AIDS patients, but they follow the same pattern for all people taking this drug.

▼ Most common: nausea, headache, skin rash, vomiting, abdominal pain, and diarrhea.

▼ Less common: Fluconazole may cause some liver toxicity, as measured by increases in specific lab tests. These changes in lab values are more common in people with AIDS or cancer, who are more likely to be taking several drugs, some of which may also be toxic to the liver; these include Rifampin, Phenytoin, Isoniazid, Valproic Acid, and oral antidiabetes agents. People with AIDS or cancer who take Fluconazole for fungal infections rarely develop severe liver or skin problems.

Drug Interactions

• Cimetidine and Rifampin may reduce blood levels of Fluconazole, but the importance of these interactions is not known.

• Fluconazole may increase the amount of the oral antidiabetes drugs Tolbutamide, Glyburide, and Glipizide in the blood, causing low blood sugar. Cyclosporine, Phenytoin, Theophylline, Warfarin, and Zidovudine are similarly affected. Dosage adjustments of these drugs may be required to offset the effect of Fluconazole.

• Fluconazole may interfere with the effectiveness of oral contraceptive drugs.

• Hydrochlorothiazide may increase blood levels of Fluconazole up to 40 percent.

Food Interactions

Fluconazole may be taken without regard to food or meals.

Usual Dose

Adult and Adolescent (age 14 and older): 100 to 400 mg, once a day.

Child (age 3 to 13): 1.3 to 2.6 mg per pound of body weight once a day.

Child (under age 3): not recommended.

Overdosage

Symptoms of a very large Fluconazole overdose may include breathing difficulty, lethargy, excess tearing, droopy eyelids, excess salivation, loss of bladder control, convulsions, and blue discoloration of the skin under the nails. Overdose victims should be taken to a hospital emergency room for treatment. ALWAYS bring the medicine bottle.

Special Information

Regular visits to your doctor are necessary to monitor your liver function and general progress.

Call your doctor if you develop reddening, loosening, blistering or peeling of the skin, darkening of the urine, yellowing of the skin or eyes, loss of appetite, or abdominal pain (especially on the right side). Other symptoms need be reported only if they are bothersome or persistent.

If you forget to take a dose of Fluconazole, take it as soon as you remember. If it is almost time for your next dose, skip the one you forgot and continue with your regular schedule. Do not take a double dose.

Special Populations

Pregnancy/Breast-feeding

Animal studies with Fluconazole show very specific effects on the developing fetus that have not been seen in humans. Nevertheless, pregnant women should not use Fluconazole unless the possible benefits clearly outweigh the risks.

Fluconazole passes into breast milk. Nursing mothers who must take this drug should bottle-feed their babies.

Seniors

Because seniors are more likely to have lost some kidney function, they may require a reduced dosage.

Generic Name

Flucytosine

Brand Name

Ancobon

Type of Drug

Antifungal.

Prescribed for

Serious blood-borne fungal infections.

General Information

Flucytosine is meant for fungal infections (*Candida*, *Chromo-mycoses*, and *Cryptococcus*) carried in the blood that affect the urinary tract, respiratory tract, central nervous system, heart, and other organs. It is not meant for fungal infections of the skin (such as common athlete's foot).

Cautions and Warnings

Do not take this drug if you are **allergic** to it. Flucytosine can worsen **bone-marrow depression** in people whose immune systems are already compromised. **Liver** and **kidney function** and **blood composition should be monitored** during the time you are taking this drug.

People with **kidney disease** who take this medicine should take extreme caution and must be closely monitored by their doctor. Daily dosage must be reduced.

Possible Side Effects

▼ Most common: unusual tiredness or weakness, liver inflammation, yellowing of the eyes or skin, abdominal pain, diarrhea, loss of appetite, nausea, vomiting, skin rash, redness, itching, sore throat, fever, and unusual bleeding or bruising.

▼ Less common: chest pains, breathing difficulties, sensitivity to the sun or bright light, dry mouth, duodenal

---

Possible Side Effects *(continued)*

ulcers, severe bowel irritation, stomach bleeding, interference with kidney function, kidney failure, reduced red-
and white-blood-cell counts or other changes in blood
composition, headache, hearing loss, confusion, dizziness, weakness, shaking, sedation or tiredness, psychosis, hallucinations, heart attack, and low blood-sugar and
-potassium levels.

Drug Interactions

• Amphotericin B increases Flucytosine's effectiveness; this
combination is generally used to produce better results.
• Flucytosine may interfere with some routine blood tests.

Food Interactions

Take Flucytosine with food if it upsets your stomach.

Usual Dose

22 to 66 mg per pound a day, in divided doses.

Overdosage

There is little experience with Flucytosine overdose, but it
would be usual for an overdose of Flucytosine to cause
exaggerated drug side effects.

Special Information

Take the capsules a few at a time over 15 minutes to avoid
nausea and vomiting, which can occur while taking your
regular dose of Flucytosine.

Call your doctor if any of the following symptoms develop:
unusual tiredness or weakness; yellowing of the skin or eyes;
skin rash, redness, or itching; sore throat or fever; unusual
bleeding or bruising; or any other persistent or intolerable
side effect.

It is important to maintain good dental hygiene while taking
Flucytosine and use extra care when using your toothbrush
or dental floss because of the chance that Flucytosine will

make you more susceptible to some infections. Dental work should be completed prior to starting on this drug.

If you forget a dose, take it as soon as you remember. If it is almost time for your next dose, take one dose right away and another in 3 or 4 hours, then go back to your regular schedule. Do not take a double dose.

Special Populations

Pregnancy/Breast-feeding

Flucytosine causes birth defects in rats and mice. It crosses the placenta, but no problems have been seen in pregnant women. However, Flucytosine should be used by pregnant women only when its potential benefits clearly outweigh its risks.

It is not known if Flucytosine passes into breast milk. Nursing mothers who must take this drug should bottle-feed their babies because of possible serious side effects in the nursing infant.

Seniors

Because older adults are likely to have some loss of kidney function, dosage adjustment may be required.

Generic Name

Fluoxetine Hydrochloride

Brand Name

Prozac

Type of Drug

Selective serotonin reuptake inhibitor (SSRI)-type antidepressant.

Prescribed for

Depression. Fluoxetine may also be prescribed for the treatment of bulimia (an eating disorder), obesity, and obsessive-compulsive disorder.

General Information

Fluoxetine Hydrochloride and the other SSRIs (Fluvoxamine,

Paroxetine, and Sertraline) are chemically unrelated to the older tricyclic and tetracyclic antidepressant medicines. They work by preventing the movement of a neurohormone called *serotonin* into nerve endings. This forces the serotonin to remain in the spaces surrounding nerve endings, where it works. The drug is effective in treating common symptoms of depression. It can help improve your mood and mental alertness, increase physical activity, and improve sleep patterns. The drug takes about 4 weeks to work and stays in the body for several weeks, even after you stop taking it. This may be important when your doctor starts or stops treatment.

Cautions and Warnings

Do not take **Fluoxetine** Hydrochloride if you are **allergic** to it. Some people have experienced serious drug reactions to Fluoxetine. Allergies to other antidepressants should not prevent you from taking Fluoxetine Hydrochloride because the drug is chemically different from other antidepressants.

About 1 of every 25 people taking Fluoxetine develop an **itching rash** so severe that they have to stop taking the drug. Other symptoms associated with this rash are **fever, joint pains, swelling, wrist and hand pains, breathing difficulty, swollen lymph glands,** and laboratory abnormalities. In most people, these symptoms resolve when they stop taking the drug and receive antihistamine or corticosteroid treatments.

People with severe **liver or kidney disease** should be cautious about taking this drug and should be treated with doses that are lower than normal.

Of every 100 people taking Fluoxetine, 10 to 15 experienced **anxiety, sleeplessness,** and **nervousness** and had to stop taking it.

Underweight depressed people who take this medicine may experience **weight loss.** About 9 percent experienced appetite loss, while 13 percent of Fluoxetine-treated patients experienced a weight loss of more than 5 percent of their body weight.

A few patients (fewer than 2 of every 1000) taking Fluoxetine experienced **seizures or convulsions.** This effect is similar to that seen with other antidepressants.

The possibility of **suicide** exists in severely depressed patients and may be present until the condition is significantly improved. Depressed patients should be allowed to carry only small quantities of Fluoxetine with them to limit the possibility of overdose.

Possible Side Effects

▼ Most common: headache, anxiety, nervousness, sleeplessness, drowsiness, tiredness, weakness, tremors, sweating, dizziness, light-headedness, dry mouth, upset or irritated stomach, appetite loss, nausea, vomiting, diarrhea, stomach gas, rash, and itching.

▼ Less common: changes in sex drive, abnormal ejaculation, impotence, abnormal dreams, difficulty concentrating, increased appetite, acne, hair loss, dry skin, chest pains, allergy, runny nose, bronchitis, abnormal heart rhythms, bleeding, blood pressure changes, headaches, fainting when rising suddenly from a sitting position, bone pain, bursitis, twitching, breast pain, fibrocystic disease of the breast, cystitis, urinary pain, double vision, eye or ear pain, conjunctivitis, anemia, swelling, low blood sugar, and low thyroid activity.

▼ Other: many other side effects affecting virtually every body system have been reported by people taking this medicine. They are too numerous to mention here, but are considered infrequent or rare and affect only a small number of people.

Be sure to report anything unusual to your doctor at once.

Drug Interactions

• At least **5 weeks** should elapse between stopping Fluoxetine Hydrochloride treatment and starting a monoamine oxidase (MAO) inhibitor drug. Two weeks should be allowed to elapse between stopping an MAO inhibitor drug and starting on Fluoxetine. Taking these drugs too close together or at the same time can cause serious, life-threatening reactions.

• Fluoxetine blood levels may be increased if taken together with a tricyclic antidepressant drug.

• Fluoxetine may increase blood levels of Lithium, leading to Lithium-related side effects. Lithium dosage adjustment may be needed.

- The effects of Fluoxetine may be reversed if it is taken together with Cyproheptadine, an antihistamine.
- Hallucinations have occurred when people have taken Fluoxetine together with Dextromethorphan, the most common nonprescription cough suppressant ingredient. Don't take this combination.
- People taking L-Tryptophan and Fluoxetine Hydrochloride together may develop agitation, restlessness, and upset stomach.
- Alcoholic beverages may increase tiredness and other nervous-system-depressant effects of Fluoxetine.
- Fluoxetine may reduce the effectiveness of Buspirone when these drugs are taken together. This has led to the worsening of obsessive-compulsive disorder (OCD) in people taking this combination to relieve OCD.
- Fluoxetine may raise blood levels of Carbamazepine, increasing the chances of Carbamazepine toxic effects.

Food Interactions

Fluoxetine Hydrochloride may be taken without regard to food or meals.

Usual Dose

20 to 80 mg per day. Seniors, people with kidney or liver disease, and those taking several different medicines should take a lower dosage.

Overdosage

Two people died after taking a Fluoxetine Hydrochloride overdose, and there have been about 35 reported cases of nonfatal overdoses. Symptoms of overdose may include seizures, nausea, vomiting, agitation, restlessness, and nervous-system excitation. There is no specific antidote for Fluoxetine Hydrochloride overdose. Any person suspected of having taken a Fluoxetine overdose should be taken to a hospital emergency room for treatment at once. ALWAYS take the medicine bottle with you.

Special Information

Fluoxetine Hydrochloride can make you dizzy or drowsy. Take

care when driving or doing other tasks that require alertness and concentration. Avoid alcoholic beverages.

Be sure your doctor knows if you are pregnant, breast-feeding, or taking other medications (including nonprescription drugs) while taking this drug.

Notify your doctor if any unusual side effects occur, if rash or hives develop, if you become excessively nervous or anxious while taking Fluoxetine Hydrochloride, or if you lose your appetite (especially if you are already underweight).

If you forget a dose of Fluoxetine Hydrochloride, take it as soon as you remember. If it is almost time for your next dose, skip the forgotten dose and continue with your regular schedule. Do not take a double dose.

Special Populations

Pregnancy/Breast-feeding
There is no information on Fluoxetine use during pregnancy. Do not take this medicine if you are, or might become, pregnant without first seeing your doctor and reviewing the benefits of Fluoxetine therapy against its risks.

Fluoxetine Hydrochloride passes into breast milk. Nursing mothers should be cautious about taking this medicine.

Seniors
Fluoxetine Hydrochloride has been studied in older adults. Several hundred seniors took the drug during its study phase without any unusual adverse effect, but any person with liver or kidney disease, problems that are more common among seniors, must receive a lower dose than an otherwise healthy person. Be sure to report any unusual side effects to your doctor.

Generic Name

Fluoxymesterone

Brand Name

Halotestin

(Also available in generic form)

Type of Drug

Androgenic (male) hormone.

Prescribed for

Male hormone replacement or augmentation; treating breast pain and fullness in women who have given birth; inoperable breast cancer in women; male menopause. Weekly androgen injections have also been used to provide safe, effective, and reversible male contraception for up to 12 months.

The information in this section also applies to:

Generic Name

Methyltestosterone

Brand Name

Oreton

(Also available in generic form)

Generic Name

Testosterone Transdermal System

Brand Name

Testoderm Transdermal Patch

Prescribed for

Male hormone replacement for men who are testosterone deficient.

General Information

These drugs are androgenic (male) hormones. Other androgenic hormones are Calusterone and Dromostanolone Propionate, which are used primarily to treat breast cancer in women. Androgens are responsible for the normal growth and development of male sex organs and for maintaining secondary sex characteristics, including growth of the prostate, penis and scrotum, beard and other male hair distribution, vocal cord thickening, muscle development, fat distribution, and adolescent growth spurts.

Cautions and Warnings

Although androgens have been used to improve athletic performance, they don't help and they expose you to serious side effects.

Women taking any androgenic drug should watch for deepening of the voice, oily skin, acne, hairiness, increased sex drive, menstrual irregularities, and effects related to the so-called virilizing **(masculinizing) effects** of these hormones. Virilization is a sign that the drug is starting to produce changes in secondary sex characteristics. These drugs should be avoided if possible by **young boys who have not gone through puberty.**

Fluoxymesterone and other androgens will aggravate **swollen or painful breasts** (gynecomastia) in men and women and should be avoided if you already have this problem.

Men with unusually **high blood levels of calcium, known or suspected cancer of the prostate** or **prostate destruction,** or **cancer of the breast** should not use this medication, nor should anyone with **severe liver, heart,** or **kidney disease.**

Long-term, high-dose androgen therapy can cause **severe liver disease** (including hepatitis and cancer), **reduced sperm count,** and **water retention. Blood cholesterol** may be altered by androgenic hormones.

Possible Side Effects

▼ Most common in men: inhibition of testicle function, impotence, chronic erection of the penis, and painful enlargement of the breast.

▼ Most common in women: unusual hairiness, baldness (in a pattern similar to that seen in men), deepening of the voice, and enlargement of the clitoris. These changes are usually irreversible once they have occurred. Females also experience increases in blood calcium and menstrual irregularities.

▼ Most common in both sexes: changes in sex drive, headache, anxiety, depression, a tingling feeling, sleep apnea (intermittent breathing while sleeping), flushing of the skin, rashes, acne, habituation, excitation, chills, sleeplessness, water retention, nausea, vomiting, diarrhea, hepatitis (yellowing of the skin or eyes), liver inflamma-

---

Possible Side Effects *(continued)*

tion, and liver cancer. Symptoms resembling a stomach ulcer may develop.

Drug Interactions

• This drug may increase the effect of an oral anticoagulant; dosage of the anticoagulant may have to be decreased. Androgens may have an effect on the glucose-tolerance test, a blood test used to screen for diabetes mellitus. They may also interfere with some tests of thyroid function.

• Androgens given together with tricyclic antidepressants (such as Imipramine) may result in severe paranoid reactions.

Food Interactions

Take oral androgens with meals if they upset your stomach.

Usual Dose

Fluoxymesterone:
2½ to 40 mg per day, depending upon the disease being treated and drug response.

Methyltestosterone:
10 to 200 mg per day, depending on the condition being treated.

Testosterone transdermal patches:
Apply patch to the scrotum and remove after 1 day. Skin should be clean and dry before application. Scrotal skin should be dry-shaved for maximum patch contact. Do not use chemical depilatories.

Overdosage

The acute effects of androgen overdose are likely to be nausea, vomiting, and diarrhea. Call your local poison control center or hospital emergency room for additional information.

Special Information

Androgens are potent drugs. They must be taken only under

the close supervision of your doctor and never used casually. The dosage and clinical effects of the drug vary widely and require constant monitoring. Call your doctor if you develop nausea or vomiting, swelling of the legs or feet, yellowing of the skin or eyes, or a painful or persistent erection. Women should call their doctor immediately if they develop a deep voice, hoarseness, acne, hairiness, male-pattern baldness, or menstrual irregularities.

If you forget to take a dose of this drug, take it as soon as you remember. If it is almost time for your next dose, skip the one you forgot and continue with your regular schedule. Do not take a double dose.

Special Populations

Pregnancy/Breast-feeding
This drug should never be taken by pregnant or nursing women. It may cause unwanted problems, including the masculinization of female babies.

Seniors
Older men treated with this medicine run an increased risk of prostate enlargement or prostate cancer. A marked increase in sex drive can also occur.

Generic Name

Flurazepam

Brand Name

Dalmane

(Also available in generic form)

Type of Drug

Benzodiazepine sedative.

Prescribed for

Short-term treatment of insomnia or sleeplessness, difficulty falling asleep, frequent nighttime awakening, and waking too early in the morning.

General Information

Flurazepam is a member of the group of drugs known as *benzodiazepines*. All have some activity as either antianxiety agents, anticonvulsants, or sedatives. Benzodiazepines work by a direct effect on the brain. They make it easier to go to sleep and decrease the number of times you wake up during the night.

The principal differences between these medicines lie in how long they work in your body. They all take about 2 hours to reach maximum blood level, but some remain in your body longer, so they work for a longer period of time. Flurazepam and Quazepam remain in your body the longest, so their effect lasts the longest, resulting in the greatest incidence of morning hangover.

Often, sleeplessness is a reflection of another disorder that would be untreated by one of these medicines.

Cautions and Warnings

People with **kidney or liver disease** should be carefully monitored while taking Flurazepam. Take the lowest possible dose to help you sleep.

People with **respiratory disease** may experience **sleep apnea** (intermittent breathing while sleeping) while taking Flurazepam.

Clinical depression may be increased by Flurazepam, which can depress the nervous system. Intentional **overdosage** is more common among depressed people who take sleeping pills than those who do not.

All benzodiazepines can be **abused** if taken for long periods of time, and it is possible for a person taking a benzodiazepine to develop **drug-withdrawal symptoms** if the drug is suddenly discontinued. Withdrawal symptoms include tremors, muscle cramps, insomnia, agitation, diarrhea, vomiting, sweating, and convulsions.

Possible Side Effects

▼ Common: drowsiness, headache, dizziness, talkativeness, nervousness, apprehension, poor muscle coordination, light-headedness, daytime tiredness, muscle

---

Possible Side Effects (continued)

weakness, slowness of movements, hangover, and euphoria (feeling "high").

▼ Less common: nausea, vomiting, rapid heartbeat, confusion, temporary memory loss, upset stomach, cramps and pain, depression, blurred or double vision and other visual disturbances, constipation, changes in taste perception, appetite changes, stuffy nose, nosebleeds, common cold symptoms, asthma, sore throat, cough, breathing problems, diarrhea, dry mouth, allergic reactions, fainting, abnormal heart rhythms, itching, rash, acne, dry skin, sensitivity to the sun, rash, nightmares or strange dreams, difficulty sleeping, tingling in the hands or feet, ringing or buzzing in the ears, ear or eye pains, menstrual cramps, frequent urination and other urinary difficulties, blood in the urine, discharge from the penis or vagina, lower back and other pains, muscle spasms and pain, fever, swollen breasts, and weight changes.

Drug Interactions

• As with all benzodiazepines, the effects of Flurazepam are enhanced if it is taken with an alcoholic beverage, antihistamine, tranquilizer, barbiturate, anticonvulsant medicine, antidepressant, or monoamine oxidase (MAO) inhibitor drug (most often prescribed for severe depression).

• Oral contraceptives, Cimetidine, Disulfiram, and Isoniazid may increase the effect of Flurazepam by reducing the drug's breakdown in the liver. Probenecid also increases Flurazepam's effects.

• Cigarette smoking, Rifampin, and Theophylline may reduce the effect of Flurazepam on your body by increasing the rate at which it is broken down by the liver.

• Levodopa's effectiveness may be decreased by Flurazepam.

• Flurazepam may increase the amount of Zidovudine, Phenytoin, or Digoxin in your blood, increasing the chances of drug toxicity.

• The combination of Clozapine and benzodiazepines has led to respiratory collapse in a few people. Flurazepam should be stopped at least 1 week before starting Clozapine treatment.

Food Interactions

Flurazepam may be taken with food if it upsets your stomach.

Usual Dose

Adult and Adolescent (age 15 and older): 15 to 30 mg at bedtime. Dosage must be individualized for maximum benefit.

Senior: begin treatment with 15 mg at bedtime.

Child: not recommended.

Overdosage

The most common symptoms of overdose are confusion, sleepiness, depression, loss of muscle coordination, and slurred speech. Coma may develop if the overdose is particularly large. Overdose symptoms can develop if a single dose of only 4 times the maximum daily dose is taken. Patients who overdose on this drug must be made to vomit with Syrup of Ipecac (available at any pharmacy) to remove any remaining drug from the stomach. Call your doctor or a poison control center before doing this. If 30 minutes have passed since the overdose was taken or symptoms have begun to develop, do not make the victim vomit: Take him or her to a hospital emergency room for treatment immediately. ALWAYS bring the medicine bottle.

Special Information

Never take more Flurazepam than your doctor has prescribed. Avoid alcoholic beverages and other nervous system depressants while taking Flurazepam.

People taking this drug must be careful when performing tasks requiring concentration and coordination because of the chance that the drug will make them tired, dizzy, or light-headed.

If you take Flurazepam daily for 3 or more weeks, you may experience some withdrawal symptoms when you stop taking the drug. Talk with your doctor about the best way to discontinue the drug.

If you forget to take Flurazepam and remember within an

hour of your regular time, take it as soon as you remember. If
you do not remember until later, skip the forgotten dose and
go back to your regular schedule. Do not take a double dose.

Special Populations

Pregnancy/Breast-feeding
Flurazepam should absolutely not be used by pregnant women
or women who may become pregnant. Animal studies have
shown that Flurazepam passes easily into the fetal blood
system and can affect fetal development.

Flurazepam passes into breast milk and can affect a nursing
infant. The drug should not be taken by nursing mothers.

Seniors
Seniors are more susceptible to the effects of Flurazepam and
should take the lowest possible dosage.

Generic Name

Flurbiprofen

Brand Names

Ansaid
Ocufen Eyedrops

(Also available in generic form)

Type of Drug

Nonsteroidal anti-inflammatory drug (NSAID).

Prescribed for

Rheumatoid arthritis, osteoarthritis, ankylosing spondylitis,
mild to moderate pain, menstrual pain, tendinitis, bursitis,
painful shoulder, gout, sunburn treatment, and migraine
treatment. The eyedrops are prescribed prior to eye surgery
to prevent movement of the eye muscles.

General Information

Flurbiprofen is one of 16 nonsteroidal anti-inflammatory

drugs (NSAIDs) that are used to relieve pain and inflammation. Other NSAID eyedrops are also prescribed for inflammation following cataract extraction (Diclofenac) and for itching and redness due to seasonal allergies (Ketorolac).

We do not know exactly how NSAIDs work, but part of their action may be due to an ability to inhibit the body's production of a hormone called *prostaglandin* and to inhibit the action of other body chemicals, including cyclo-oxygenase, lipoxygenase, leukotrienes, lysosomal enzymes, and a host of other factors. NSAIDs are generally absorbed into the bloodstream fairly quickly. Pain relief generally comes within an hour after taking the first dose, but the NSAID's anti-inflammatory effect generally takes a lot longer (several days to 2 weeks) to become apparent, and may take a month or more to reach its maximum effect. Flurbiprofen is broken down in the liver and eliminated through the kidneys.

Cautions and Warnings

People who are **allergic** to Flurbiprofen (or any other NSAID) and those with a history of **asthma attacks** brought on by an NSAID, **Iodides,** or Aspirin should not take this drug.

Flurbiprofen can cause **gastrointestinal (GI) bleeding, ulcers,** and **stomach perforation**. This can occur at any time, with or without warning, in people who take chronic Flurbiprofen treatment. People with a history of **active GI bleeding** should be cautious about taking any NSAID. **Minor stomach upset, distress,** or **gas** is common during the first few days of treatment with Flurbiprofen. People who develop **bleeding** or **ulcers** and continue treatment should be aware of the possibility of developing **more serious drug toxicity.**

Flurbiprofen can affect **platelets and blood clotting** at high doses, and should be avoided by people with **clotting problems** and by those taking **Warfarin.**

People with **heart problems** who use Flurbiprofen may experience swelling in their arms, legs, or feet.

Flurbiprofen can cause **toxic effects to the kidney.** Report any unusual side effects to your doctor, who may need to periodically test your kidney function.

Flurbiprofen can make you **unusually sensitive to the effects of the sun** (photosensitivity).

Possible Side Effects

▼ Most common: diarrhea, nausea, vomiting, constipation, stomach gas, stomach upset or irritation, and loss of appetite (tablets); temporary burning, stinging, or other minor eye irritation (eyedrops).

▼ Less common: stomach ulcers, GI bleeding, hepatitis, gallbladder attacks, painful urination, poor kidney function, kidney inflammation, blood and protein in the urine, dizziness, fainting, nervousness, depression, hallucinations, confusion, disorientation, tingling in the hands or feet, light-headedness, itching, increased sweating, dry nose and mouth, heart palpitations, chest pain, difficulty breathing, and muscle cramps (tablets); nausea, vomiting, viral infections, and eye allergies (longer-lasting eye redness, burning, itching, or tearing) (eyedrops).

▼ Rare: severe allergic reactions, including closing of the throat, fever and chills, changes in liver function, jaundice (yellowing of the skin or eyes), and kidney failure. People who experience such effects must be promptly treated in a hospital emergency room or doctor's office.

NSAIDs have caused severe skin reactions; if this happens to you, see your doctor immediately.

The risk of developing bleeding problems or other body-wide side effects with Flurbiprofen eyedrops is small because only a small amount of this drug is absorbed into the bloodstream.

Drug Interactions

• Flurbiprofen can increase the effects of oral anticoagulant (blood-thinning) drugs such as Warfarin. You may take this combination, but your doctor may have to reduce your anticoagulant dose.

• Taking Flurbiprofen with Cyclosporine may increase the toxic kidney effects of both drugs. Methotrexate toxicity may be increased in people also taking Flurbiprofen.

• Flurbiprofen may reduce the blood-pressure-lowering effect of beta blockers and loop diuretic drugs.

• Flurbiprofen may increase blood levels of Phenytoin,

leading to increased Phenytoin side effects. Blood-Lithium
levels may be increased in people taking Flurbiprofen.

• Flurbiprofen blood levels may be affected by Cimetidine
because of that drug's effect on the liver.

• Probenecid may interfere with the elimination of Flurbiprofen from the body, increasing the chances for Flurbiprofen
toxic reactions.

• Aspirin and other salicylates may decrease the amount of
Flurbiprofen in your blood. These medicines should never be
taken at the same time.

• Flurbiprofen eyedrops may inactivate Acetylcholine or
Carbachol eyedrops.

Food Interactions

Take Flurbiprofen with food or a magnesium/aluminum antacid if it upsets your stomach.

Usual Dose

Tablets
200 to 300 mg per day. Seniors and those with kidney
problems should start with a lower dose.

Eyedrops
1 drop every 1/2 hour for 2 hours before eye surgery.

Overdosage

People have died from NSAID overdoses. The most common
overdose signs are drowsiness, nausea, vomiting, diarrhea,
abdominal pain, rapid breathing, rapid heartbeat, increased
sweating, ringing or buzzing in the ears, confusion, disorientation, stupor, and coma. Take the victim to a hospital emergency room at once. ALWAYS bring the medicine bottle.

Special Information

Flurbiprofen can make you drowsy and/or tired: Be careful
when driving or operating hazardous equipment. Do not take
any nonprescription products with Acetaminophen or Aspirin
while taking this drug; also, avoid alcoholic beverages.

Take each dose with a full glass of water and don't lie down
for 15 to 30 minutes after you take the medicine.

Contact your doctor if you develop skin rash or itching,

visual disturbances, weight gain, breathing difficulty, fluid retention, hallucinations, black or tarry stools, persistent headache, or any unusual or intolerable side effects.

If you forget to take a dose of Flurbiprofen, take it as soon as you remember. If you take several Flurbiprofen doses a day and it is within 4 hours of your next dose, skip the one you forgot and continue with your regular schedule. If you take Flurbiprofen once a day and it is within 8 hours of your next dose, skip the missed dose and continue with your regular schedule. Do not take a double dose.

To self-administer the eyedrops, lie down or tilt your head backward. Hold the dropper above your eye and drop the medicine inside your lower lid while looking up. To prevent possible infection, don't allow the dropper to touch your fingers, eyelids, or any surface. Release the lower lid and keep your eye open. Don't blink for about 30 seconds. Press gently on the bridge of your nose at the inside corner of your eye for about a minute. This will help circulate the medicine around your eye. Wait at least 5 minutes before using any other eyedrops.

If you forget a dose of your eyedrops, take it as soon as you remember. If it is almost time for your next dose, skip the missed dose and continue with your regular schedule. Do not take a double dose.

Special Populations

Pregnancy/Breast-feeding

NSAIDs may cross into the fetal blood circulation. They have not been found to cause birth defects, but may affect a developing fetal heart during the second half of pregnancy; animal studies indicate a possible effect. Women who are or who might become pregnant should not take Flurbiprofen without their doctor's approval; be particularly cautious about using this drug during the last 3 months of pregnancy. When the drug is considered essential by your doctor, its potential benefits must be carefully weighed against its risks.

NSAIDs may pass into breast milk, but have caused no problems among breast-fed infants, except for seizures in a baby whose mother was taking Indomethacin. Other NSAIDs have caused problems in animal studies. There is a possibility that a nursing mother taking Flurbiprofen could affect her baby's heart or cardiovascular system. If you must take Flurbiprofen, consider bottle-feeding your baby.

Seniors
Older adults may be more susceptible to Flurbiprofen side effects, especially ulcer disease.

Generic Name

Fluvastatin

Brand Name
Lescol

Type of Drug
Cholesterol-lowering agent (HMG-CoA reductase inhibitor).

Prescribed for
High blood cholesterol, LDL cholesterol, and triglycerides levels, in conjunction with a low-cholesterol diet.

General Information
The HMG-CoA reductase inhibitors work by interfering with the natural body process for manufacturing cholesterol and converting the process to produce a harmless by-product. The value of drugs that reduce blood cholesterol lies in the assumption that reducing levels of blood fats reduces the chance of heart disease. Studies conducted by the National Heart, Lung, and Blood Institute have closely related high blood-fat levels (total blood cholesterol, LDL cholesterol, and triglycerides) to heart and blood-vessel disease. Drugs that can reduce the amounts of any of these blood fats and increase HDL cholesterol (the "good" cholesterol) reduce the risk of death and heart attacks.

The HMG-CoA reductase inhibitors (Fluvastatin, Lovastatin, Pravastatin, and Simvastatin) reduce total triglyceride, blood cholesterol, and LDL-cholesterol counts while raising HDL cholesterol. These drugs have similar profiles in that a very small amount of the drug you swallow actually reaches the body circulation; most is broken down in the liver. Ten to 20 percent of the drug is released from the body through your kidneys; the rest is eliminated by the liver. Blood fat levels start dropping after 1 to 2 weeks of treatment and reach their lowest levels within 4 to 6 weeks after you start taking Fluvastatin. Levels remain low as long as you continue to take the medicine.

Fluvastatin generally doesn't benefit anyone under age 30, so it is not usually recommended for children. It may, under special circumstances, be prescribed for teenagers in the same doses as adults.

Cautions and Warnings

Do not take Fluvastatin if you are **allergic** to it or to any other member of this group.

People with a history of **liver disease** and those who drink **large amounts of alcohol** should avoid these medications because of the possibility that the drug can aggravate or cause liver disease. Your doctor should take a blood sample to test your liver function every month or so during the first year of treatment to be sure that the drug is not adversely affecting you.

These medicines cause **muscle aches** and/or **muscle weakness** in a small number of people, which can be a sign of a more serious condition.

At doses between 50 and more than 100 times the maximum human dose, the HMG-CoA reductase inhibitors have caused central-nervous-system lesions, liver tumors, and male infertility in lab animals. The importance of this information for people is not known.

Possible Side Effects

Most people who take Fluvastatin tolerate it quite well, though it has more side effects than other cholesterol-lowering drugs.

▼ Most common: nausea, vomiting, headache, upper respiratory or flu-like infections, stuffy nose, cough, sore throat, sinusitis, bronchitis, allergy, itchiness, rash, fatigue, constipation, diarrhea, heartburn, stomach gas, upset stomach, muscle cramps and pain, back and joint pains, tooth disorders, abdominal pain or cramps, dizziness, clumsiness, and sleeplessness.

▼ Rare: rash and itching, hepatitis, inflammation of the pancreas, yellowing of the skin or eyes, appetite loss,

---

Possible Side Effects *(continued)*

blurred vision, changes in taste perception, respiratory infections, urinary abnormalities, changes in the lens of your eye, reduced sex drive, male impotence and/or breast pain, anxiety, tingling in the hands or feet, hair loss, swelling, and blood-cell changes.

Drug Interactions

• The cholesterol-lowering effects of Fluvastatin (or other HMG-CoA reductase inhibitors) and those of Colestipol or Cholestyramine are additive when the drugs are taken together.

• The anticoagulant effect of Warfarin may be increased by Fluvastatin. People taking both Warfarin and Fluvastatin (or any HMG-CoA reductase inhibitor) should be periodically monitored by their doctor for the blood-thinning effect of Warfarin.

• The combination of Cyclosporine, Erythromycin, Gemfibrozil, or Niacin with Fluvastatin (or any HMG-CoA reductase inhibitor) may cause severe muscle aches or degeneration or other muscle problems and should be avoided.

Food Interactions

Fluvastatin may be taken without regard to food or meals. Continue your low-cholesterol diet while taking this medicine.

Usual Dose

20 to 40 mg a day, taken in the evening.

Your daily dosage of Fluvastatin should be adjusted monthly, based on your doctor's assessment of how well the drug is working to reduce your blood cholesterol.

Overdosage

There are few reports of Fluvastatin overdose, and all those taking an overdose recovered. Persons suspected of having taken an overdose of Fluvastatin should be taken to a hospital emergency room for evaluation and treatment. The effects of overdose are not well understood.

Special Information

Call your doctor if you develop blurred vision or muscle aches, pain, tenderness, or weakness, especially if you are also feverish or feel sick.

These medicines are always prescribed in combination with a low-fat diet. Be sure to follow your doctor's dietary instructions, since both the diet and medicine are necessary to treat your condition.

Do not take more cholesterol-lowering medicine than your doctor has prescribed or stop taking the medicine without your doctor's knowledge.

If you forget to take a dose of Fluvastatin, take it as soon as you remember. If it is almost time for your next regularly scheduled dose, skip the one you forgot and continue with your regular schedule. Do not take a double dose.

Special Populations

Pregnancy/Breast-feeding

Pregnant women and those who might become pregnant ABSOLUTELY MUST NOT take Fluvastatin. Since hardening of the arteries is a long-term process, you should be able to stop this medication during pregnancy with no serious problems. If you become pregnant while taking any of these medicines, stop the drug immediately and call your doctor.

Fluvastatin passes into breast milk in twice the concentrations found in blood. Nursing mothers should bottle-feed their infants to avoid possible interference with the baby's development.

Seniors

People over age 65 have shown a greater cholesterol-lowering response to Fluvastatin than people under age 65 and may require less medicine than a younger adult to achieve the same response. Be sure to report any side effects to your doctor.

Generic Name

Fluvoxamine Maleate

Brand Name

Luvox

Type of Drug

Selective serotonin reuptake inhibitor (SSRI)-type antidepressant.

Prescribed for

Obsessive-compulsive disorder (OCD).

General Information

Fluvoxamine Maleate and the other SSRIs (Fluoxetine, Paroxetine, and Sertraline) are chemically unrelated to the older tricyclic and tetracyclic antidepressant medicines. They work by preventing the movement of a neurohormone (serotonin) into nerve endings, which forces the serotonin to remain in the spaces surrounding nerve endings, where it works. The drug is effective in treating common symptoms of OCD. It can help improve symptoms of OCD and allow people to function more reasonably without devoting time and effort to compulsive behaviors. The drug takes several weeks to work and stays in the body for several weeks, even after you stop taking it. This may be important when your doctor starts or stops treatment.

Cautions and Warnings

Do not take Fluvoxamine if you are **allergic** to it. Some people have experienced **serious drug reactions** to Fluvoxamine. Allergies to other antidepressants should not prevent you from taking Fluvoxamine because the drug is chemically different from other antidepressants.

People with **severe liver disease** should be cautious about taking this drug and should be treated with doses that are lower than normal.

Possible Side Effects

▼ Most common: headache, weakness, sleeplessness, tiredness, nervousness, dizziness, nausea, upset stomach, diarrhea, dry mouth, and constipation.

▼ Common: anxiety, tremors, upper respiratory infections, stomach gas, loss of appetite, vomiting, and excessive sweating.

▼ Less common: allergy or allergic reactions, flu-like-

Possible Side Effects *(continued)*

symptoms, chills, palpitations, flushing, dizziness when rising from a sitting or lying position, high blood pressure, fainting, rapid heartbeat, depression, reduced sex drive or function, muscle twitching, agitation, muscle stiffness, nervous system stimulation, fatigue, feelings of ill health, memory loss, emotional upset, apathy, mood changes, manic or psychotic reaction, swelling, weight changes, stomach irritation, tooth cavities or other tooth disorders, swallowing difficulty, liver inflammation, cough, sinus irritation, breathing difficulty, bronchitis, and yawning.

▼ Other: many other side effects affecting virtually every body system have been reported by people taking this medicine. They are too numerous to mention here, but are considered infrequent or rare and affect only a small population. Be sure to report anything unusual to your doctor at once.

Drug Interactions

• At least **5 weeks** should elapse between stopping Fluvoxamine Maleate treatment and starting a monoamine oxidase (MAO) inhibitor drug. Two weeks should be allowed to elapse between stopping an MAO inhibitor drug and starting Fluvoxamine. Taking these drugs too close together or at the same time can cause serious, life-threatening reactions.

• Fluvoxamine blood levels may be increased if taken together with a tricyclic antidepressant drug.

• Lithium may increase blood levels of Fluvoxamine, leading to Fluvoxamine side effects. Dosage adjustment may be needed.

• People taking L-Tryptophan and Fluvoxamine together may develop agitation, restlessness, and upset stomach.

• Alcoholic beverages may add to the tiredness associated with Fluvoxamine, as well as other nervous-system-depressant effects of the drug.

• Fluvoxamine may raise blood levels of Clozapine, Diltiazem, Methadone, Carbamazepine, or Theophylline, increasing the chances of toxic effects from those drugs. Dosage adjustment may be needed.

- Fluvoxamine may increase blood levels and the effects of the beta-adrenergic-blocking drugs Propranolol and Metoprolol. Atenolol blood levels were not affected by Fluvoxamine.
- Cigarette smoking can increase the rate at which the body breaks down Fluvoxamine by 25 percent.
- Blood levels of the nonsedating antihistamines Astemizole and Terfenadine may be increased if these drugs are taken with Fluvoxamine. This can increase the risk of cardiac reactions to the antihistamines, which can sometimes be fatal.
- Fluvoxamine may reduce the rate at which Diazepam and other benzodiazepines are cleared from the body, increasing the effect of those drugs.
- People taking Warfarin may experience an increase in that drug's anticoagulant (blood-thinning) effect if they start taking Fluvoxamine. Your doctor will need to re-evaluate your Warfarin dosage.

Food Interactions

Fluvoxamine may be taken without regard to food.

Usual Dose

50 to 300 mg at bedtime. Seniors, people with liver disease, and those taking several different medicines should start with a lower dosage.

Overdosage

Of more than 350 people who took a Fluvoxamine overdose, 19 have died. Symptoms of overdose may include drowsiness, diarrhea, vomiting, and dizziness. Other signs are coma, change in heart rate, low blood pressure, convulsions, and liver or cardiac abnormalities. There is no specific antidote for Fluvoxamine overdose.

Any person suspected of having taken a Fluvoxamine overdose should be taken to a hospital emergency room for treatment at once. ALWAYS take the medicine bottle with you.

Special Information

Fluvoxamine can make you dizzy or drowsy. Take care when

driving or doing other tasks that require alertness and concentration. Avoid alcoholic beverages.

Be sure your doctor knows if you are pregnant, breast-feeding, or taking other medications (including nonprescription drugs) while taking Fluvoxamine.

Notify your doctor if any unusual side effects occur, if rash or hives develop, if you become excessively nervous or anxious, or if you lose your appetite (especially if you are already underweight) while taking Fluvoxamine.

If you forget a dose of Fluvoxamine, take it as soon as you remember. If it is almost time for your next dose, skip the forgotten dose and continue with your regular schedule. Do not take a double dose.

Special Populations

Pregnancy/Breast-feeding

Animal studies indicate that Fluvoxamine may affect the developing fetus. Do not take this medicine if you are, or might become, pregnant without first seeing your doctor and reviewing the benefits of Fluvoxamine therapy against its risks.

Fluvoxamine passes into breast milk. Nursing mothers should be cautious if taking this medicine because its safety is unknown in infants and children and may want to consider bottle-feeding their infants.

Seniors

Older adults clear Fluvoxamine about half as efficiently as younger adults. Seniors should begin with a 25-mg dosage that is increased as needed every 4 to 7 days. Be sure to report any unusual side effects to your doctor.

Generic Name

Fosinopril

Brand Name

Monopril

Type of Drug

Angiotensin-converting-enzyme (ACE) inhibitor.

Prescribed for

High blood pressure.

General Information

The ACE inhibitors work by preventing the conversion of a hormone called *angiotensin I* to another hormone called *angiotensin II*. Angiotensin II is a potent blood-vessel constrictor. Preventing this conversion relaxes blood vessels and helps to reduce blood pressure and relieve the symptoms of heart failure by making it easier for a failing heart to pump blood around your body. The production of other hormones and enzymes that participate in the regulation of blood vessel dilation is also affected by the ACE inhibitors and probably plays a role in the effectiveness of these medicines. Fosinopril begins working 2 to 6 hours after you take it.

Some people who start taking an ACE inhibitor after they are already on a diuretic experience a rapid drop in blood pressure after their first dose or when the dose is increased. To prevent this from happening, you may be told to stop taking the diuretic 2 or 3 days before starting the ACE inhibitor or to increase your salt intake during that time. The diuretic may then be restarted gradually.

Cautions and Warnings

Do not take Fosinopril if you have had an **allergic** reaction to it in the past. It can, rarely, cause **very low blood pressure** or affect your **kidneys**. Your doctor should **check your urine** for changes during the first few months of treatment.

ACE inhibitors can affect **white-blood-cell count,** possibly increasing your **susceptibility to infection.** Blood counts should be checked periodically.

Possible Side Effects

▼ Most common: headache and chronic cough. The cough usually goes away a few days after you stop taking the medicine.

▼ Other: chest pain, low blood pressure, dizziness (especially when rising from a sitting or lying position), fatigue, diarrhea, vomiting, and nausea.

Possible Side Effects *(continued)*

▼ Rare: angina, low blood pressure, stroke, abnormal heart rhythms, heart palpitations, sleeping difficulty, tingling in the hands or feet, confusion, fainting, abdominal pain, constipation, dry mouth, hepatitis, pancreatitis, asthma, sinusitis, sweating, flushing, itching, rash, unusual sensitivity to the sun, reduced sex drive, muscle cramps or aches, joint pains, and ringing in the ears.

Drug Interactions

• The blood-pressure-lowering effect of Fosinopril is additive with diuretic drugs and beta-blockers. Any other drug that causes a rapid blood-pressure drop should be used with caution if you are taking an ACE inhibitor.

• Fosinopril may increase potassium levels in your blood, especially when taken with Dyazide or other potassium-sparing diuretics.

• Fosinopril may increase the effects of Lithium; this combination should be used with caution.

• Antacids may reduce the amount of Fosinopril absorbed into the blood. Separate doses of the two medicines by at least 2 hours.

• Capsaicin may cause or aggravate the cough associated with Fosinopril therapy.

• Indomethacin may reduce the blood-pressure-lowering effects of Fosinopril.

• Phenothiazine tranquilizers and antivomiting drugs may increase the effects of Fosinopril.

• The combination of Allopurinol and Fosinopril increases the chance of a drug reaction.

• ACE inhibitors increase blood levels of Digoxin, possibly increasing the chance of Digoxin-related side effects.

Food Interactions

Fosinopril is not affected by food in the stomach and may be taken without regard to food or meals. You may take it with food if it upsets your stomach.

Usual Dose

10 to 80 mg, once a day. People with liver disease may require less medicine. No adjustment is required for kidney disease.

Overdosage

The principal effect of ACE inhibitor overdose is a rapid drop in blood pressure, as evidenced by dizziness or fainting. Take the overdose victim to a hospital emergency room immediately. ALWAYS remember to bring the medicine bottle.

Special Information

Call your doctor if you develop swelling of the face or throat, if you have sudden difficulty breathing, or if you develop a sore throat, mouth sores, abnormal heartbeat, chest pain, a persistent rash, or loss of taste perception.

Unexplained swelling of the face, lips, hands, and feet can also affect the larynx (throat) and tongue and interfere with breathing. If this happens, the victim should be taken to a hospital emergency room at once for treatment.

You may get dizzy if you rise to your feet quickly from a sitting or lying position.

Avoid strenuous exercise and/or very hot weather, because heavy sweating or dehydration can cause a rapid decrease in blood pressure.

Avoid nonprescription diet pills, decongestants, and stimulants that can raise blood pressure.

If you forget to take a dose, take it as soon as you remember. If it is within 8 hours of your next dose, skip the one you forgot and continue with your regular schedule. Do not take a double dose.

Special Populations

Pregnancy/Breast-feeding

ACE inhibitors have caused low blood pressure, kidney failure, slow formation of the skull, and death in developing fetuses when taken during the last 6 months of pregnancy. Women who are pregnant should not take ACE inhibitors; women who may become pregnant should use an effective contraceptive method while taking an ACE inhibitor and stop the medicine if they do become pregnant.

Because large amounts of Fosinopril pass into breast milk, this drug should not be taken by nursing mothers. Nursing mothers who must take this drug should consider an alternative feeding method since infants, especially newborns, are more susceptible than adults to the effects of these medicines.

Seniors

Older adults are generally given the same Fosinopril dosage as younger adults, but may be more sensitive to the effects of Fosinopril.

Furosemide

see **Loop Diuretics**, page 617

Generic Name

Ganciclovir

Brand Name

Cytovene

Type of Drug

Antiviral.

Prescribed for

Cytomegalovirus (CMV) infection of the eye. It may also be prescribed for CMV infection in other parts of the body.

General Information

Ganciclovir works by preventing reproduction of the ganciclovir virus. Unlike other antiviral drugs, it does not have any effect against other viruses. The capsule form of this drug is used only as follow-up treatment in people who have received intravenous treatment for CMV infections. It must be converted to an active form in the body before it can work. Only 5 to 9 percent of the medicine in each capsule is actually absorbed into your blood. The medicine is eliminated through your kidneys.

Intravenous Ganciclovir has been given to a small number of children under age 12 with mixed results. Side effects were similar to those experienced by adults taking the drug.

Studies of Ganciclovir in African-Americans, Hispanics, and

Caucasians showed a trend toward more drug in the blood of Caucasians than in other groups. Though most often used for CMV retinitis (eye infections), Ganciclovir has also been used for CMV infection of the urine, blood, throat, and semen. In heart or bone marrow transplant patients, Ganciclovir has been helpful in controlling CMV infection.

Cautions and Warnings

Ganciclovir causes **anemia, reduced white-blood-cell count,** and **blood platelet loss** and, in animal studies, caused **cancer, birth defects,** and **reduced sperm production.** Regular blood and platelet counts are recommended while taking this drug.

Taking oral Ganciclovir is linked to a faster progression of **CMV retinitis infection** than taking **intravenous medicine** for CMV infection. The risk of rapid progression should be balanced against the benefit of taking oral Ganciclovir.

People **allergic** to Acyclovir or Ganciclovir should not use this drug.

Ganciclovir should not be taken by people who are not immunocompromised. It is not intended to treat or prevent **CMV infections** in **newborns.**

Detachment of the **retina** has been noted in people taking Ganciclovir, as well as in people with CMV who have not taken the drug. The relationship between the drug and this effect is not well understood.

Ganciclovir causes unusual **sensitivity** to the **sun;** use a sunscreen and/or wear protective clothing when going outside.

Possible Side Effects

▼ Most common: fever, diarrhea, abdominal pain, reduced white-blood-cell counts, anemia, rash, sweating, nausea, vomiting, and appetite loss.

▼ Common: infection; chills; stomach gas; low platelet counts (bleeding or oozing blood); tingling; burning; numbness or pain in the hands, arms, legs, or feet; itching; pneumonia; weakness; and headache.

Many other less common side effects can occur and can affect almost any other part of the body. Report anything unusual to your doctor.

Drug Interactions

• Dapsone, Pentamidine, Flucytosine, Vincristine, Vinblastine, Adriamycin, Amphotericin B, Trimethoprim/Sulfamethoxazole, and other antiviral medicines can increase the toxic effects of Ganciclovir and should be used together only if absolutely necessary and the potential benefits outweigh the risks.

• People taking Imipenem-Cilastatin together with Ganciclovir have experienced generalized seizures. Avoid this combination.

• Mixing Ganciclovir with other drugs that can be damaging to the kidney can increase the rate and extent of the damage.

• Probenecid interferes with Ganciclovir release through the kidneys and substantially increases blood levels of Ganciclovir.

• Mixing Ganciclovir with Didanosine or Zidovudine (for HIV) can increase Didanosine or Zidovudine levels and reduce Ganciclovir levels. Because Zidovudine and Ganciclovir both cause anemia and low-white-cell counts, many people cannot tolerate this combination.

Food Interactions

High-fat, high-calorie meals can increase the amount of Ganciclovir absorbed into the blood. Take this drug with food.

Usual Dose

Adult and Child (age 13 and older): 3000 mg a day, divided into 3 or 6 equal doses. People with reduced kidney function will have their dosage reduced accordingly by their doctor to as little as 500 mg 3 times a week.

Child (age 12 and younger): not recommended.

Overdosage

No overdoses have been reported with Ganciclovir capsules. As much as 6000 mg a day has been taken with only temporary lowering of white-blood-cell count. Call your hospital emergency room for instructions if someone accidentally takes a Ganciclovir overdose.

Special Information

Ganciclovir does not cure CMV retinitis, and immunocompromised people taking this medicine may continue to experience worsening of their disease. Dosage reductions or drug discontinuance may be needed if white-blood-cell or platelet counts get too low.

Ganciclovir can cause infertility in men and women. Also, pregnant women should use effective contraception while taking this drug; men should use a condom while taking the drug and for at least 90 days after stopping treatment to avoid passing the drug to their partner.

Good dental hygiene is important while taking this drug to minimize the chances of infection. If you have dental work while taking this drug, expect the healing process to take longer.

Regular blood tests are necessary to watch for white-blood-cell or platelet-level alterations.

It is very important to take this medicine exactly as directed. If you forget a dose of Ganciclovir, take it as soon as you remember, and continue with your regular schedule. If you take the medicine 3 times a day and it is almost time for your next dose, take one dose now and another in 6 hours, and then continue with your regular schedule. If you take it 6 times a day and it is almost time for your next dose, skip the forgotten dose and continue with your regular schedule.

Special Populations

Pregnancy/Breast-feeding
Ganciclovir has been shown to be toxic to the developing fetus in animal studies. There is no reliable information about its effect in pregnant women, but it should be used only when the possible benefits outweigh the dangers. Women who are likely to become pregnant while taking this drug should use reliable contraception.

It is not known if Ganciclovir passes into breast milk, but the possible toxic effects of this drug on a nursing infant should be kept in mind. Nursing mothers who must take this drug should bottle-feed their babies.

Seniors
Older adults often have reduced kidney function, and dosage adjustments may be needed to take this into account.

Generic Name

Gemfibrozil

Brand Name

Lopid

(Also available in generic form)

Type of Drug

Antihyperlipidemic (blood-fat reducer).

Prescribed for

Excessively high levels of blood triglycerides.

General Information

Gemfibrozil consistently reduces blood-triglyceride levels, but is usually prescribed only for people with very high blood-fat levels who have not responded to dietary changes or other therapies. Normal triglyceride levels range between 50 and 200 mg. People with very high levels (1000 to 2000 mg) are likely to have severe abdominal pains and pancreas inflammation. Gemfibrozil usually has little effect on blood-cholesterol levels, although it may reduce blood cholesterol in some people.

Gemfibrozil works by affecting the breakdown of body fats and by reducing the amount of triglyceride manufactured by the liver. It is not known if these two mechanisms are solely responsible for the drug's effect on triglyceride levels.

Cautions and Warnings

Gemfibrozil should not be taken by people with **severe liver or kidney disease** or by those who have had **allergic reactions** to it in the past. Gemfibrozil users may have an increased chance of developing **gallbladder disease** and should realize that this drug, like other blood-fat reducers (including Clofibrate and Probucol), has **not been proven to directly reduce the chance of a fatal heart attack.**

Long-term studies in which male rats were given between 1 and 10 times the maximum human dose showed an increase in **liver tumors** (both cancerous and noncancerous). Other studies of male rats, in which 3 to 10 times the human dose was given for 10 weeks, showed that the drug reduced sperm activity, although this effect **has not been reported in humans**.

Estrogens can cause massive **increases** in **triglyceride levels** and may have to be discontinued in addition to Gemfibrozil treatment in some women. Other diseases such as thyroid disease and diabetes should also be considered as causes of high blood triglycerides.

People taking this drug may be more susceptible to the common cold or other viral or bacterial infections.

Possible Side Effects

▼ Most common: abdominal and stomach pains, gas, diarrhea, nausea, and vomiting.

▼ Less common: rash or itching, dizziness, blurred vision, anemia, reduced levels of certain white blood cells, increased blood sugar, and muscle pains (especially in the arms or legs).

▼ Other: dry mouth, constipation, loss of appetite, upset stomach, sleeplessness, tingling in the hands or feet, ringing or buzzing in the ears, back pains, painful muscles and/or joints, swollen joints, fatigue, feelings of ill health, reduction in blood potassium, and abnormal liver function.

Drug Interactions

• Gemfibrozil increases the effects of oral anticoagulant (blood-thinning) drugs; your doctor will have to reduce your anticoagulant dosage when Gemfibrozil treatment is started.

• Taking Gemfibrozil and Lovastatin together has been associated with severe drug side effects. These effects can begin as soon as 3 weeks after you start taking the combination or may not appear for months.

Food Interactions

Gemfibrozil is best taken on an empty stomach 30 minutes before meals, but may be taken with food if it upsets your stomach. It is important that you follow your doctor's diet instructions.

Usual Dose

900 to 1500 mg per day, in 2 doses taken 30 minutes before breakfast and your evening meal.

Overdosage

There are no reports of Gemfibrozil overdosage, but victims might be expected to develop exaggerated side effects. Overdose victims must be made to vomit with Syrup of Ipecac (available at any pharmacy) to remove any remaining drug from the stomach. Call your doctor or poison control center before doing this. If you must go to a hospital emergency room, ALWAYS bring the medicine bottle.

Special Information

Your doctor should perform periodic blood counts during the first year of Gemfibrozil treatment to check for anemia or other blood effects. Liver-function tests are also necessary. Blood-sugar levels should be checked periodically while you are taking Gemfibrozil, especially if you are diabetic or have a family history of diabetes.

Gemfibrozil may cause dizziness or blurred vision. Use caution while driving or doing anything else that requires concentration and alertness.

Call your doctor if any drug side effects become severe or intolerable, especially diarrhea, nausea, vomiting, or stomach pains or gas. These may disappear if your doctor reduces the drug dose.

If you forget to take a dose of Gemfibrozil, take it as soon as you remember. If it is almost time for your next dose, skip the one you forgot and continue with your regular schedule. Do not take a double dose.

Special Populations

Pregnancy/Breast-feeding

There have been no Gemfibrozil studies involving pregnant women. However, this drug should be avoided by pregnant women and by those who may become pregnant. In situations where Gemfibrozil is considered essential, its potential benefits must be carefully weighed against its risks.

Because of the tumor-stimulating effect of Gemfibrozil, nursing mothers should bottle-feed their infants while taking this drug.

Seniors
Older adults may be more likely to develop drug side effects because the drug primarily passes out of the body through the kidneys, and kidney function declines with age.

Glipizide

*see **Antidiabetes Drugs (Oral Sulfonylureas)**, page 72*

Glyburide

*see **Antidiabetes Drugs (Oral Sulfonylureas)**, page 72*

Glynase PresTab

*see **Antidiabetes Drugs (Oral Sulfonylureas)**, page 72*

Generic Name
Granisetron

Brand Name
Kytril

Type of Drug
Antiemetic.

Prescribed for
Preventing nausea and vomiting after certain cancer chemotherapy treatments.

General Information

Granisetron, like Ondansetron, produces its effect in a unique way. It antagonizes the receptor for a special form of the neurohormone *serotonin* ($5HT_3$). Receptors of this type are found in both the part of the brain that controls vomiting (chemoreceptor trigger zone) and the vagus nerve in the stomach and intestines.

Women absorb more Granisetron faster than men, and they clear the drug more slowly from their bodies. This means that women will have more drug in their blood than men after taking the same dose of Granisetron, but these differences have not been reflected in any difference in response to the drug.

Granisetron is extremely effective in preventing nausea and vomiting and works in situations where many older antiemetics are ineffective.

Cautions and Warnings

Don't take Granisetron if you are **allergic or sensitive** to it. People with **liver failure** break the drug down about half as quickly as others, but dosage adjustment is generally not required.

Possible Side Effects

▼ Most common: headache, nausea, weakness, and constipation.

▼ Less common: abdominal pains, liver inflammation, vomiting, diarrhea, high blood pressure, dizziness, sleeplessness, anxiety, tiredness, fever, appetite reduction, anemia, low white-blood-cell and platelet counts, and hair loss.

▼ Rare: low blood pressure, angina pains, fainting, rapid heartbeat, and drug allergy (possibly including difficulty breathing, itching, rash, low blood pressure, and shock).

Drug Interactions

• Granisetron is broken down in the liver by the same

enzyme system responsible for breaking down many other drugs. It may be affected by other drugs that stimulate or inhibit these enzymes, but no interactions have been discovered to date.

Food Interactions

Food slightly decreases the amount of Granisetron absorbed but does not affect your Granisetron dose.

Usual Dose

Adult and Child (age 12 and older): 1 mg 2 times a day, given 1 hour before chemotherapy and then 12 hours later.
Child (age 11 and under): not recommended.

Overdosage

Little is known about Granisetron overdose. Call your local poison center or hospital emergency room for more information. If you go to the hospital for treatment, ALWAYS bring the medicine bottle with you.

Special Information

Call your doctor if you begin to have chest tightness, wheezing, trouble breathing, chest pains, or other unusual or severe side effects.

If you forget to take a dose of Granisetron, take it as soon as you remember. If it is almost time for your next dose, skip the dose you forgot and continue with the regular schedule. Forgetting more than 1 dose may increase your chances of vomiting.

Special Populations

Pregnancy/Breast-feeding

Animal studies with Granisetron have revealed no potential to cause birth defects. Nevertheless, pregnant women should not take this, or any other, drug unless the possible risks and benefits of taking it have been discussed with their doctors.

It is not known if Granisetron passes into breast milk. Nursing mothers who take this medicine should carefully observe their infants for possible drug side effects.

Seniors

Seniors may take this medicine without restriction.

Generic Name

Guanabenz Acetate

Brand Name

Wytensin

(Also available in generic form)

Type of Drug

Antihypertensive.

Prescribed for

High blood pressure.

General Information

Guanabenz Acetate works by stimulating certain central-nervous-system receptors. This results in a general reduction of the level at which the nervous system is stimulated by the brain. The immediate blood-pressure lowering occurs without a major effect on blood vessels. However, chronic use of Guanabenz can result in widening of blood vessels and a slight slowing of the pulse rate. Guanabenz can be taken alone or together with a thiazide diuretic.

Cautions and Warnings

Do not take Guanabenz if you are **sensitive** or **allergic** to it.

Possible Side Effects

▼ Most common: drowsiness, sedation, dry mouth, dizziness, weakness, and headache.

▼ Less common: chest pains, swelling (in the hands, legs, or feet), heart palpitations or abnormal heart rhythms, stomach or abdominal pain or discomfort, nausea, diarrhea, vomiting, constipation, anxiety, poor muscle control, anxiety, depression, difficulty sleeping, stuffy nose, blurred vision, muscle aches and pains, difficulty breathing, frequent urination, male impotence, unusual taste in the mouth, and swollen and painful male breasts.

Possible Side Effects *(continued)*

Side effects are more common and more severe as your dose of Guanabenz increases.

Drug Interactions

• The effect of this drug is increased by taking it together with other blood-pressure-lowering agents. Its sedating effects are increased by taking it with tranquilizers, sleeping pills, or other nervous-system depressants, including alcohol.

• People taking this drug for high blood pressure should avoid nonprescription medicines that might aggravate hypertension (e.g., decongestants, cold and allergy remedies, and diet pills, all of which may contain stimulants). If you are unsure about which medicines to avoid, ask your pharmacist.

Food Interactions

This drug is best taken on an empty stomach, but it may be taken with food if it upsets your stomach.

Usual Dose

4 mg twice a day to start, with a gradual increase to a maximum of 32 mg twice a day (doses this large are rarely needed).

Overdosage

Guanabenz overdose will cause sleepiness, lethargy, low blood pressure, irritability, pinpointed pupils, and reduced heart rate. Overdose victims must be made to vomit with Syrup of Ipecac (available at any pharmacy) to remove any remaining drug from the stomach. Call your doctor or poison control center before doing this. If you must go to a hospital emergency room, ALWAYS bring the medicine bottle with you.

Special Information

Take this drug exactly as prescribed for maximum benefit. If any side effects become severe or intolerable, contact your doctor, who may need to reduce your daily dosage.

Guanabenz often causes tiredness or dizziness; avoid alcohol when taking this drug because it tends to increase these effects. Take care when driving or doing anything else that requires intense concentration.

Do not stop taking this medicine without your doctor's approval. Suddenly stopping it can cause a rapid increase (or rebound) in blood pressure. The dosage must be gradually reduced by your doctor.

If you forget to take a dose of Guanabenz Acetate, take it as soon as you remember. If it is almost time for your next dose, skip the one you forgot and continue with your regular schedule. Do not take a double dose. Call your doctor if you miss 2 or more consecutive doses.

Special Populations

Pregnancy/Breast-feeding
Reports of the effects of this drug in pregnant women have yielded conflicting results. Because it may adversely affect a developing baby, Guanabenz should be avoided by pregnant women and by those who may become pregnant while using it. When Guanabenz is deemed essential, its potential benefits must be carefully weighed against its risks.

Nursing mothers should bottle-feed their babies if they must take Guanabenz.

Seniors
Older adults are more sensitive to the sedating and blood-pressure-lowering effects of this drug. Follow your doctor's directions, and report any side effects at once.

Generic Name

Guanfacine Hydrochloride

Brand Name

Tenex

(Also available in generic form)

Type of Drug

Antihypertensive.

Prescribed for

High blood pressure, heroin withdrawal, migraine head-aches, nausea, and vomiting.

General Information

Guanfacine works by stimulating a particular portion of the nervous system that dilates (widens) blood vessels. Because the studies of Guanfacine were conducted only in people taking a thiazide-type diuretic, the drug is recommended for use only in combination with one of those drugs. Guanfacine's effect is long-acting; it can be taken only once a day (usually at bedtime, to benefit from the drug's side effect of producing sleepiness).

Cautions and Warnings

Do not use Guanfacine if you are **allergic** to it. Guanfacine should be used with caution if you have **severe coronary insufficiency**, a **recent history of heart attack, blood vessel disease of the brain**, or **kidney or liver failure**. People with kidney disease should have their Guanfacine dosage adjusted by their doctor because the drug passes out of the body primarily through the kidneys.

Guanfacine causes **sedation,** especially when it is first taken. This sedation is greater with larger doses and is intensified by other nervous-system depressants, including phenothiazine antipsychotic medicines, benzodiazepine seda-tives and sleeping pills, and barbiturate sedatives and sleep-ing pills.

Abruptly stopping Guanfacine may result in a rebound reaction consisting of anxiety, nervousness, and occasional increases in blood pressure. When rebound reactions occur, they happen 2 to 4 days after the medicine is stopped. This is consistent with the fact that it takes longer for Guanfacine to leave the body than Clonidine or other similar drugs.

Possible Side Effects

Guanfacine may cause sedation, especially when treat-ment is first started. The frequency with which drowsi-ness occurs tends to increase with increased drug dosage

Possible Side Effects *(continued)*

and to become less severe as you continue to take the drug.

▼ Most common: drowsiness.

▼ Less common: heart palpitations, chest pain, slow heartbeat, abdominal pain, diarrhea, upset stomach, difficulty swallowing, nausea, memory loss, confusion, depression, loss of sex drive, runny nose, taste changes, ringing or buzzing in the ears, conjunctivitis ("pink-eye"), eye irritation, blurring and other visual disturbances, leg cramps, unusually slow movements, breathing difficulty, itching, rash, skin redness, sweating, testicle disorders, poor urinary control, feelings of ill health, and tingling in the hands or feet.

▼ Other: dry mouth, weakness, dizziness, headache, constipation, and sleeplessness.

Drug Interactions

• Alcohol or any other nervous-system depressant will increase the sedative effects of Guanfacine.

• Indomethacin, Ibuprofen, and other nonsteroidal anti-inflammatory pain relievers (NSAIDs) may decrease Guanfacine's effectiveness. Stimulants, including those used in nonprescription decongestants and diet pills, can antagonize Guanfacine's effect.

• Estrogen drugs may cause fluid retention, which increases blood pressure.

• Any medication that lowers blood pressure will increase the blood-pressure-lowering effect of Guanfacine.

Food Interactions

Guanfacine may be taken with food if it upsets your stomach.

Usual Dose

Adult and Adolescent (age 12 and older): 1 to 3 mg per day, taken at bedtime. Doses above 3 mg per day are rarely used because side effects increase, whereas effectiveness does not.

Child (less than age 12): not recommended.

Overdosage

Symptoms are likely to be drowsiness, slow heartbeat, low blood pressure, and weakness. Overdose victims should be taken to a hospital emergency room. ALWAYS bring the medicine bottle with you.

Special Information

High blood pressure is usually a symptomless condition. Be sure to continue taking your medicine even if you feel perfectly healthy. If the medicine causes problems, do not stop taking it unless your doctor so advises. Abruptly stopping Guanfacine treatment can result in a rebound increase in blood pressure after 2 to 4 days.

Call your doctor if you develop any of the following: breathing difficulty; slow heartbeat; extreme dizziness; dry mouth that lasts more than 2 weeks and is not relieved by gum, candy, or saliva substitutes; dry, itchy, or burning eyes; sex-drive loss; headache; nausea or vomiting; sleeping difficulty; unusual tiredness or weakness during the daytime; or other persistent or intolerable side effects.

People taking Guanfacine must be careful when performing tasks requiring concentration and coordination because it may make them tired, dizzy, or light-headed.

Visit your doctor regularly to check on your progress, and be sure to follow your doctor's directions for diet, salt restriction, and other lifestyle approaches to control your blood pressure.

Pay extra attention to dental hygiene while taking Guanfacine. The dry mouth caused by the drug can make it easier for you to develop cavities and gum disease.

This medicine is generally taken at bedtime. If you forget to take a dose, you may take it the following morning, but it can make you tired during the day. If you don't remember until it is almost time for your next dose, skip the one you forgot and continue with your regular schedule. Do not take a double dose. Call your doctor if you miss 2 or more consecutive doses.

Special Populations

Pregnancy/Breast-feeding

Animal studies indicate that high doses of Guanfacine may be toxic to a developing fetus. This drug is not recommended to treat high blood pressure during pregnancy. Consult your doctor.

Guanfacine passes into animal breast milk, but it is not known if this happens in humans. Nursing mothers who must take Guanfacine should exercise caution.

Seniors

Older adults may be more sensitive to the sedative and blood-pressure-lowering effects of Guanfacine because of usual age-related losses of kidney function. This factor should be taken into account by your doctor when determining your daily dosage of Guanfacine.

Generic Name

Haloperidol

Brand Name

Haldol

(Also available in generic form)

Type of Drug

Butyrophenone antipsychotic.

Prescribed for

Psychotic disorders (including Gilles de la Tourette's syndrome, sometimes used together with nicotine gum), severe behavioral problems in children, short-term treatment of hyperactive children, chronic schizophrenia, vomiting, treatment of acute psychiatric situations, PCP (phencyclidine) psychosis.

General Information

Haloperidol is one of many nonphenothiazine agents used in the treatment of psychosis. These drugs are generally equally effective when given in therapeutically equivalent doses. The major differences are in type and severity of side effects. Some people may respond well to one and not at all to another; this variability is not easily explained and is thought to result from inborn biochemical differences.

Haloperidol acts on a portion of the brain called the *hypo-thalamus.* It affects parts of the hypothalamus that control metabolism, body temperature, alertness, muscle tone, hormone balance, and vomiting and may be used to treat problems related to any of these functions. Haloperidol is available in liquid form for those who have trouble swallowing tablets.

Cautions and Warnings

Haloperidol should not be used by people who are **allergic** to it. Those with **very low blood pressure, Parkinson's disease, or blood, liver, or kidney disease** should avoid this drug.

If you have **glaucoma, epilepsy, ulcers, or difficulty passing urine,** Haloperidol should be used with caution and under strict supervision of your doctor.

Avoid exposure to **extreme heat** because this drug can upset your body's normal temperature-control mechanism.

Possible Side Effects

▼ Most common: drowsiness, especially during the first or second week of therapy. If the drowsiness becomes troublesome, contact your doctor.

▼ Less common: jaundice (yellowing of the whites of the eyes or skin), which usually occurs in the first 2 to 4 weeks. The jaundice usually goes away when the drug is discontinued, but there have been cases where it did not. If you notice this effect or develop fever, or generally do not feel well, contact your doctor immediately. Other less common side effects are changes in components of the blood (including anemias), raised or lowered blood pressure, abnormal heartbeat, heart attack, and feeling faint or dizzy.

▼ Other: extrapyramidal effects, such as spasms of the neck muscles, severe stiffness of the back muscles, rolling back of the eyes, convulsions, difficulty in swallowing, and symptoms associated with Parkinson's disease. These effects seem very serious but disappear after the drug has been withdrawn; however, symptoms of the face, tongue, or jaw may persist for years, especially in seniors with a long history of brain disease. If you

Possible Side Effects *(continued)*

experience any of these effects, contact your doctor immediately.

Haloperidol may cause an unusual increase in psychotic symptoms or may cause paranoid reactions, tiredness, lethargy, restlessness, hyperactivity, confusion at night, bizarre dreams, inability to sleep, depression, or euphoria (feeling "high"). Other reactions are itching, swelling, unusual sensitivity to bright light, red skin or rash, dry mouth, stuffy nose, headache, nausea, vomiting, loss of appetite, change in body temperature, loss of facial color, excessive salivation, excessive perspiration, constipation, diarrhea, changes in urine and bowel habits, worsening of glaucoma, blurred vision, weakening of eyelid muscles, and spasms of bronchial and other muscles, as well as increased appetite, fatigue, excessive thirst, and skin discoloration (particularly in sun-exposed areas). There have been cases of breast enlargement, false-positive pregnancy tests, changes in menstrual flow in females, and impotence and changes in sex drive in males.

Drug Interactions

• Be cautious about taking Haloperidol with barbiturates, sleeping pills, narcotics or other tranquilizers, alcohol, or any other medication that may produce a depressive effect.

• Anticholinergic drugs can reduce the effectiveness of Haloperidol and increase the chance of drug side effects.

• The blood-pressure-lowering effect of Guanethidine may be counteracted by Haloperidol.

• Taking Lithium together with Haloperidol may lead to disorientation or loss of consciousness. This combination may also cause uncontrolled muscle movements.

• Mixing Propranolol and Haloperidol may lead to unusually low blood pressure.

• Blood concentrations of tricyclic antidepressant drugs may increase if they are taken together with Haloperidol. This can lead to antidepressant side effects.

Food Interactions

This medicine is best taken on an empty stomach, but you may take it with food if it upsets your stomach.

Usual Dose

Adult: 0.5 to 2 mg 2 to 3 times per day to start. Your doctor may later increase your dose according to your need (up to 100 mg per day). Seniors generally need smaller doses.

Child (age 3 to 12 years, or 33 to 88 pounds): 0.5 mg per day to start. Dose may be increased in 0.5-mg steps every 5 to 7 days until a satisfactory effect is realized.

Child (under age 3): not recommended.

Overdosage

Symptoms of overdosage are depression, extreme weakness, tiredness, desire to sleep, coma, lowered blood pressure, uncontrolled muscle spasms, agitation, restlessness, convulsions, fever, dry mouth, and abnormal heart rhythms. The victim should be taken to a hospital emergency room immediately. ALWAYS bring the medicine bottle.

Special Information

This medication may cause drowsiness. Use caution when driving or operating hazardous equipment; also, avoid alcoholic beverages while taking the medicine.

The drug may cause unusual sensitivity to the sun. It can also turn your urine reddish-brown to pink.

If dizziness occurs, avoid sudden changes in posture and avoid climbing stairs. Use caution in hot weather. This medicine may make you more prone to heat stroke.

If you forget to take a dose of Haloperidol, take it as soon as you remember. Take the rest of the day's doses evenly spaced throughout the day. Do not take a double dose.

Special Populations

Pregnancy/Breast-feeding

Serious problems have been seen in pregnant animals given large amounts of Haloperidol. Although Haloperidol has not been studied in pregnant women, you should avoid this drug if you are pregnant.

Haloperidol passes into breast milk. Nursing mothers who

must use this medicine should bottle-feed their babies to avoid possible side effects in their infants.

Seniors

Older adults are more sensitive to the effects of this medication and usually require ½ to ¼ the usual adult dose to achieve the desired results. Also, seniors are more likely to develop drug side effects.

Humulin 70/30

see **Insulin Injection**, page 533

Humulin N

see **Insulin Injection**, page 533 .

Generic Name

Hydralazine Hydrochloride

Brand Names

Apresoline

(Also available in generic form)

Type of Drug

Antihypertensive.

Prescribed for

Hypertension (high blood pressure), aortic insufficiency after heart valve replacement, and congestive heart failure.

General Information

Although its mechanism of action is not completely understood, Hydralazine Hydrochloride is believed to lower blood pressure by enlarging the blood vessels throughout the body. This also helps to improve heart functions and blood flow to the kidneys and brain.

Cautions and Warnings

Long-term administration of **more than 200 mg per day** of Hydralazine may produce lupus erythematosus, an arthritis-like syndrome (muscle and joint pains, skin reactions, fever, anemia), although symptoms of this problem usually disappear when the drug is discontinued. Fever, chest pain, feelings of ill health, or other unexplained symptoms should be reported to your doctor. The chances of this happening increase as your dose of Hydralazine increases; 10 to 20 percent of people taking 400 mg per day of Hydralazine will develop lupus.

Hydralazine may actually improve kidney blood flow and kidney function in people who have below-normal function. It should be used with caution in people with **advanced kidney damage.**

Hydralazine may worsen specific heart problems and should be used with care in people with a history of **heart disease**. It can **cause angina pain** and has been thought to cause heart attacks.

Tingling in the hands or feet caused by Hydralazine may be relieved by taking vitamin B_6 (Pyridoxine).

People taking Hydralazine may develop reduced red-blood-cell counts and hemoglobin. Reduced white-blood-cell and platelet counts can also occur. **Periodic blood counts** are recommended while taking Hydralazine.

Possible Side Effects

▼ Most common: headache, loss of appetite, nausea, vomiting, diarrhea, rapid heartbeat, and chest pain.

▼ Less common: stuffy nose, flushing, tearing in the eyes, itching or redness of the eyes, numbness or tingling in the hands or feet, dizziness, tremors, muscle cramps, depression, disorientation, anxiety, itching, rash, fever, chills, occasional hepatitis (yellowing of the skin or eyes), constipation, difficulty in urination, and adverse effects on the normal composition of the blood.

Drug Interactions

• Taking Hydralazine with Metoprolol or Propranolol (beta blockers) can result in raised blood levels of any of the drugs.

• Indomethacin can reduce the effects of Hydralazine.

• Do not self-medicate with over-the-counter cough, cold, or allergy remedies whose stimulant ingredients can increase blood pressure.

Food Interactions

Hydralazine Hydrochloride may antagonize vitamin B_6 (pyridoxine), which can result in peripheral neuropathy (tremors or tingling and numbness of the fingers, toes, or other extremities). If these symptoms occur, your doctor may consider Pyridoxine supplementation.

Take Hydralazine Hydrochloride with food or meals.

Usual Dose

As with other antihypertensive drugs, dosage is tailored to your specific needs.

Adult: 40 mg per day for the first few days; increase to 100 mg per day for the rest of the first week. Dose increases until the maximum effect is seen.

Child: 0.34 mg per pound of body weight per day; increase up to 200 mg per day.

Overdosage

If symptoms of extreme lowering of blood pressure, rapid heartbeat, headache, generalized skin flushing, chest pains, or poor heart rhythms appear, contact your doctor immediately. If you go to a hospital emergency room for treatment, ALWAYS bring the medicine bottle with you.

Special Information

Take this medicine exactly as prescribed.

Call your doctor if you experience a prolonged period of unexplained tiredness, fever, muscle or joint aching, or chest pains while taking this drug.

If you forget to take a dose of Hydralazine Hydrochloride, take it as soon as you remember. If it is almost time for your next dose, skip the one you forgot and continue with your regular schedule. Do not take a double dose.

Special Populations

Pregnancy/Breast-feeding

Animal studies with high doses of Hydralazine have shown that it causes birth defects, although this has not been found in humans. Blood-related problems have been seen in newborns whose mothers took Hydralazine during pregnancy. These problems got better on their own in 1 to 3 weeks. Pregnant women and those who might become pregnant should not take this drug unless all the possible benefits and risks have been considered.

Hydralazine passes into breast milk but has caused no problems in breast-fed infants.

Seniors

Older adults are more sensitive to the side effects (especially low body temperature) and blood-pressure-lowering effects of this drug. Follow your doctor's directions, and report any side effects at once.

Hydrochlorothiazide

see **Thiazide Diuretics**, *page 1088*

Generic Name

Hydroxyzine

Brand Names

Anxanil Tablets
Atarax Tablets/Syrup
Hydroxyzine Paoate
  Capsules

Vistaril Capsules/
  Suspension

(Also available in generic form)

Type of Drug

Antihistamine.

Prescribed for

Nausea and vomiting; anxiety, tension, or agitation; itching caused by allergies; and sedation (before or after a general anesthetic). Hydroxyzine injection has been used to treat acute adult psychiatric emergencies (including acute alcoholism), for surgical sedation, and for sedation before or after delivering a baby.

General Information

Hydroxyzine is an antihistamine with muscle-relaxing, antiemetic, bronchial dilation, pain-relieving, and antispasm properties. As such, Hydroxyzine has been used in a variety of applications, including relieving temporary anxiety such as stress of dental or other minor surgical procedures, acute emotional problems, and the management of anxiety associated with stomach and digestive disorders, skin problems, and behavior difficulties in children. It is a relatively older medicine and has been passed by for newer medications by most doctors, but it still works in a wide variety of situations.

Cautions and Warnings

Hydroxyzine should not be used if you are **sensitive** or **allergic** to it.

Possible Side Effects

Wheezing, chest tightness, and breathing difficulty are signs of a drug-sensitivity reaction.

▼ Most common: dry mouth and drowsiness. These usually disappear after a few days of continuous use or when the dose is reduced.

▼ Infrequent: occasional tremors or convulsions at higher doses.

Drug Interactions

• Hydroxyzine has a depressive effect on the nervous system, producing drowsiness and sleepiness. It should not be used with alcohol, sedatives, tranquilizers, antihistamines, or other depressants. When Hydroxyzine is taken together with one of these drugs, the dose of the latter should be cut in half.

Food Interactions

Take this drug with food if it upsets your stomach.

Usual Dose

Adult: 25 to 100 mg 3 to 4 times per day.
Child (age 6 and older): 5 to 25 mg 3 to 4 times per day.
Child (under age 6): 5 to 10 mg 3 to 4 times per day.

Overdosage

The most common sign of overdose is sleepiness. Overdose victims should be taken to a hospital emergency room for treatment. ALWAYS bring the medicine bottle with you.

Special Information

Be aware of the depressive effect of Hydroxyzine: Be careful when driving, operating hazardous machinery, or doing anything that requires intense concentration.

The dry mouth associated with taking Hydroxyzine can increase your risk of dental cavities and decay. Pay attention to dental hygiene while taking this medicine.

If you develop drug-sensitivity reaction to Hydroxyzine (see *Possible Side Effects*), call your doctor.

If you forget to take a dose of Hydroxyzine, take it as soon as you remember. If it is almost time for your next dose, skip the one you forgot and continue with your regular schedule. Do not take a double dose.

Special Populations

Pregnancy/Breast-feeding

Antihistamines have not been proven to be a cause of birth defects or other problems in pregnant women. Animal studies have shown that regular treatment with Hydroxyzine can cause birth defects during the first months of pregnancy. Do not take any antihistamine without your doctor's knowledge.

Hydroxyzine can reduce the amount of breast milk you make. Also, small amounts of Hydroxyzine may pass into breast milk and can sedate a nursing infant. Nursing mothers taking Hydroxyzine should bottle-feed their babies.

Seniors
Older adults are more sensitive to antihistamine side effects,
particularly confusion, difficult or painful urination, drowsiness, dizziness, a faint feeling, nightmares or excitement,
nervousness, restlessness, irritability, and dry mouth, nose,
or throat.

Hytrin

see **Terazosin**, page 1065

Generic Name

Ibuprofen

Brand Names

Aches-n-Pains	IBU	Pamprin-IB
Advil	Ibuprin	PediaProfen
Children's Advil	Ibuprohm	Rufen
Children's Motrin	Medipren	Saleto-200
Excedrin-IB	Midol-200	Trendar
Genpril	Motrin	

(Also available in generic form)

Type of Drug

Nonsteroidal anti-inflammatory drug (NSAID).

Prescribed for

Rheumatoid arthritis, osteoarthritis, mild to moderate pain,
juvenile rheumatoid arthritis, sunburn treatment, menstrual
pain, fever.

General Information

NSAIDs are drugs that relieve pain and inflammation. We do
not know exactly how they work, but part of their action may
be due to an ability to inhibit the body's ability to make a

hormone called *prostaglandin* and inhibit the action of other body chemicals, including cyclo-oxygenase, lipoxygenase, leukotrienes, lysosomal enzymes, and a host of other factors. NSAIDs are generally absorbed into the bloodstream fairly rapidly, but some work more quickly than others. NSAIDs are generally broken down in the liver and eliminated through the kidneys. Over-the-counter doses of Ibuprofen provide pain relief but are below the level at which a significant anti-inflammatory response is usually seen. Anti-inflammatory doses are in the prescription range (400 mg per dose or more) and take a week or more to develop. Pain relief should come within 30 minutes or so of taking an over-the-counter dose.

Cautions and Warnings

People who are **allergic** to Ibuprofen (or to any other NSAID) and those with a history of **asthma attacks** brought on by another NSAID, by Iodides, or by Aspirin should not take these medicines.

NSAIDs can cause **gastrointestinal bleeding, ulcers,** and **perforation.** This can occur at any time, with or without warning, in people who take chronic NSAID treatment. People with a **history of active gastrointestinal bleeding** should be cautious about taking any NSAID. **Minor stomach upset, gas, or distress** is common during the first few days of treatment with the NSAIDs. People who develop these symptoms and continue their NSAID treatment should be aware of the possibility of developing more serious drug toxicity.

NSAIDs can affect **platelets and blood clotting** at high doses and should be avoided by people with clotting problems and those taking **Warfarin.**

People with **heart problems** who use an NSAID may find that their arms and legs or feet become swollen.

People taking Ibuprofen, especially those with a **collagen disease** such as **systemic lupus erythematosus,** may experience an unusually severe drug sensitivity reaction. **Report any unusual symptoms** to your doctor at once.

NSAIDs can cause severe toxic effects to the **kidney.** Report any unusual side effects to your doctor, who may need to periodically test your kidney function.

NSAIDs can make you **unusually sensitive to the effects of the sun** (photosensitivity).

Possible Side Effects

▼ Common: diarrhea, nausea, vomiting, constipation, stomach gas, upset stomach, and stomach irritation.

▼ Less common: stomach ulcers, gastrointestinal bleeding, loss of appetite, hepatitis, gallbladder attacks, painful urination, poor kidney function, kidney inflammation, blood and protein in the urine, dizziness, fainting, nervousness, depression, hallucinations, confusion, disorientation, tingling in the hands or feet, light-headedness, itching, sweating, dry nose and mouth, heart palpitations, chest pain, difficulty breathing, and muscle cramps.

▼ Rare: severe allergic reactions, including closing of the throat, fever and chills, changes in liver function, jaundice, and kidney failure. These people must be treated in a hospital emergency room or doctor's office.

Severe skin reactions have occurred while taking this medication; these should be treated promptly by a physician.

Drug Interactions

• NSAIDs can increase the effects of oral anticoagulant drugs, such as Warfarin. You may take this combination, but your doctor may have to adjust your anticoagulant dose to take this effect into account.

• The blood-pressure-lowering effect of beta blockers may be reduced by NSAIDs.

• Taking an NSAID together with Cyclosporine may increase the toxic effects of each drug on the kidney.

• Ibuprofen and Indomethacin may increase Digoxin levels in the blood.

• NSAIDs may increase blood levels of Phenytoin, leading to increased Phenytoin side effects.

• Blood-Lithium levels may be increased in people taking Lithium and an NSAID.

• Methotrexate toxicity may be increased in people taking Methotrexate and an NSAID.

• NSAID blood levels may be affected by Cimetidine because of that drug's effect on the liver.

• Probenecid may interfere with the elimination of NSAIDs

from the body, increasing the chances for NSAID toxic reactions.

• Aspirin and other salicylates may decrease the amount of NSAID in your blood. These medicines should never be taken at the same time.

Food Interactions

Take this medicine with food or a magnesium/aluminum antacid if it upsets your stomach.

Usual Dose

Adult: 200 to 800 mg 4 times per day, depending on the condition being treated. Follow your doctor's directions. If you are using an over-the-counter product, do not take more than 1200 mg (6 tablets) in 24 hours.

Mild to moderate pain: 200 mg every 4 to 6 hours.

Child: Juvenile arthritis: 9 to 18 mg per pound of body weight per day divided into several doses. If you are using an over-the-counter Ibuprofen product to treat a fever, the dose is 2 to 4.5 mg per pound of body weight, depending on the level of the fever, up to 4 doses a day. FOLLOW PACKAGE DIRECTIONS.

Overdosage

People have died from NSAID overdoses. The most common signs of overdose are drowsiness, nausea, vomiting, diarrhea, abdominal pain, rapid breathing, rapid heartbeat, sweating, ringing or buzzing in the ears, confusion, disorientation, stupor, and coma.

Take the victim to a hospital emergency room at once for treatment. ALWAYS bring the medicine bottle with you.

Special Information

Ibuprofen can make you drowsy and/or tired: Be careful when driving or operating equipment.

Do not take any nonprescription products with Acetaminophen or Aspirin while taking any NSAID.

Avoid alcoholic beverages while taking an NSAID.

Take each dose with a full glass of water, and don't lie down for 15 to 30 minutes after you take the medicine.

Contact your doctor if you develop skin rash, itching, visual disturbances, weight gain, breathing difficulty, fluid retention, hallucinations, black stools, persistent headache, or any unusual side effects, or if side effects become intolerable.

If you forget to take a dose of Ibuprofen, take it as soon as you remember. If you take several Ibuprofen doses a day and it is within 4 hours of your next regularly scheduled dose, skip the one you forgot and continue with your regular schedule. **Do not take a double dose.**

Special Populations

Pregnancy/Breast-feeding

NSAIDs may cross into the blood circulation of a developing fetus. They have not been found to cause birth defects, but animal studies have indicated a possible effect on the developing fetal heart if taken during the last half of pregnancy. Pregnant women or those who might become pregnant while taking Ibuprofen should not take it without their doctor's approval. When the drug is considered essential by your doctor, the potential risk of taking the medicine must be carefully weighed against the benefit it might produce.

NSAIDs may pass into breast milk but have caused no problems among breast-fed infants, except for seizures in a baby whose mother was taking Indomethacin. Other NSAIDs have caused problems in animal studies. There is a possibility that a nursing mother taking an NSAID could affect her baby's heart or cardiovascular system. If you must take Ibuprofen, use an alternative feeding method.

Seniors

Older adults, especially those with poor kidney or liver function, may be more susceptible to the side effects of the NSAIDs.

Generic Name

Imipramine

Brand Names

Janimine Tablets
Tofranil Tablets
Tofranil-PM Capsules

(Also available in generic form)

Type of Drug

Tricyclic antidepressant.

Prescribed for

Depression, panic disorder, childhood bed-wetting (older than age 6), chronic pain (from migraines, tension headaches, diabetic disease, tic douloureux, cancer, herpes lesions, arthritis, and other sources), and bulimia.

General Information

Imipramine, like other tricyclic antidepressants, blocks the movement of certain stimulant chemicals (norepinephrine or serotonin) in and out of nerve endings, has a sedative effect, and counteracts the effects of a hormone called *acetylcholine* (which makes it anticholinergic).

Theory says that people with depression have a chemical imbalance in their brains and that drugs such as Imipramine work to reestablish a proper balance. It usually takes 2 to 4 weeks for Imipramine's clinical antidepressant effect to come into play. Call your doctor if you don't improve after 6 to 8 weeks.

Imipramine can elevate mood, increase physical activity and mental alertness, and improve appetite and sleep patterns in depressed individuals. Imipramine is a mild sedative, and is therefore useful in treating mild forms of depression associated with anxiety. Occasionally, Imipramine and other tricyclic antidepressants have been used to treat nighttime bed-wetting in young children, but they do not produce long-lasting relief. Tricyclic antidepressants are broken down in the liver.

Cautions and Warnings

Do not take Imipramine if you are **allergic** or **sensitive** to it or another **tricyclic antidepressant**. Imipramine should not be used if you are recovering from a **heart attack**. If you have a history of **epilepsy** or other **convulsive disorders, difficulty in urination, glaucoma, heart disease, liver disease,** or **hyperthyroidism**, use caution if taking Imipramine. People who are **schizophrenic** or **paranoid** may get worse if given a tricyclic antidepressant, and **manic-depressive** people may switch phase. This can also happen if you are changing antidepressants or stopping them. Imipramine and other antidepressants can be lethal if taken in **large quantities. Severely depressed people** should have only small numbers of pills on hand.

Possible Side Effects

▼ Most common: sedation and anticholinergic effects (blurred vision, disorientation, confusion, hallucinations, muscle spasms or tremors, seizures and/or convulsions, dry mouth, constipation [especially in older adults], difficult urination, worsening glaucoma, sensitivity to bright light or sunlight).

▼ Less common: blood-pressure changes, abnormal heart rate, heart attack, anxiety, restlessness, excitement, numbness or tingling in the extremities, poor coordination, rash, itching, retention of fluids, fever, allergy, changes in composition of blood, nausea, vomiting, loss of appetite, stomach upset, diarrhea, enlargement of the breasts in males and females, changes in sex drive, and blood-sugar changes.

▼ Rare: agitation, inability to sleep, nightmares, feelings of panic, a peculiar taste sensation, stomach cramps, black discoloration of the tongue, yellowing of the eyes and/or skin, changes in liver function, increased or decreased weight, excessive perspiration, flushing, frequent urination, drowsiness, dizziness, weakness, headache, loss of hair, and feelings of ill health.

Drug Interactions

• Interaction with monoamine oxidase (MAO) inhibitors can cause high fever, convulsion, and occasionally death. Don't take any MAO inhibitor until at least 2 weeks after Imipramine has been discontinued. Those who must take Imipramine and an MAO inhibitor require close medical observation.

• Imipramine interacts with Guanethidine and Clonidine. Be sure to tell your doctor if you are taking **any** high-blood pressure medicine.

• Imipramine increases the effects of barbiturates, tranquilizers, other sedative drugs, and alcohol. Also, barbiturates may decrease the effectiveness of Imipramine.

• Taking Imipramine and thyroid medicine together will enhance the effects of both medicines, possibly causing abnormal heart rhythms. The combination of Imipramine and Reserpine may cause overstimulation.

• Oral contraceptives can reduce the effect of Imipramine, as can smoking. Charcoal tablets can prevent Imipramine's absorption into the bloodstream. Estrogens can increase or decrease the effect of Imipramine.

• Drugs such as Bicarbonate of Soda, Acetazolamide, Quinidine, or Procainamide will increase the effect of Imipramine. Cimetidine, Methylphenidate, and phenothiazine drugs (such as Thorazine and Compazine) block the liver metabolism of Imipramine, causing it to stay in the body longer, which can cause severe drug side effects.

Food Interactions

You may take Imipramine with food if it upsets your stomach.

Usual Dose

Adult: initial dose, about 75 mg per day in divided doses; then increased or decreased as necessary. The final dose may be less than 75 or up to 200 mg. Long-term patients being treated for depression may be given extended-acting medicine daily at bedtime or several times per day.

Adolescent and Senior: initial dose, 30 or 40 mg per day. Maintenance dose is usually less than 100 mg daily.

Child (age 6 and over): 25 mg per day, given 1 hour before bedtime, for nighttime bed-wetting. If relief of bed-wetting does not occur within 1 week, the daily dose is increased to 50 or 75 mg, depending on age; large doses are often given in midafternoon and at bedtime (more than 75 mg per day increases side effects without increasing effectiveness). The medication should be gradually tapered off; this may reduce the probability that the bed-wetting will return.

Overdosage

Symptoms of overdosage are confusion, inability to concentrate, hallucinations, drowsiness, lowered body temperature, abnormal heart rate, heart failure, enlarged pupils, convulsions, severely lowered blood pressure, stupor, and coma. Agitation, stiffening of body muscles, vomiting, and high fever may also occur. The overdose victim should be taken to a hospital emergency room immediately. ALWAYS bring the medicine bottle with you.

Special Information

Avoid alcohol and other depressants while taking Imipramine. Do not stop taking this medicine unless your doctor has specifically told you to do so: Abruptly stopping may cause nausea, headache, and a sickly feeling.

Imipramine can cause drowsiness, dizziness, and blurred vision. Be careful when driving or operating hazardous machinery. Avoid prolonged exposure to the sun or sunlamps.

Call your doctor at once if you develop seizures, difficult or rapid breathing, fever and sweating, blood-pressure changes, muscle stiffness, loss of bladder control, or unusual tiredness or weakness.

Dry mouth may lead to an increase in dental cavities, gum bleeding, and gum disease. People taking Imipramine should pay special attention to dental hygiene.

If you forget to take a dose of Imipramine, skip it and go back to your regular schedule. **Do not take a double dose.**

Special Populations

Pregnancy/Breast-feeding

Imipramine, like other antidepressants, crosses into your developing baby's circulation. Birth defects have been reported when this drug was taken during the first 3 months of pregnancy. There have been reports of newborn infants suffering from heart, breathing, and urinary problems after their mothers had taken an antidepressant of this type immediately before delivery. Avoid taking it while pregnant.

Tricyclic antidepressants pass into breast milk in low concentrations and sedate the baby. Nursing mothers should consider alternate feeding methods if taking Imipramine.

Seniors

Older adults are more sensitive to Imipramine's effects, especially abnormal rhythms and other heart side effects. Seniors often require lower dosages than younger adults to achieve the same effect. Follow your doctor's directions and report any side effects at once.

Generic Name

Indomethacin

Brand Names

Indocin Capsules/Suspension/Suppositories
Indocin SR
Indochron E-R

(Also available in generic form)

Type of Drug

Nonsteroidal anti-inflammatory drug (NSAID).

Prescribed for

Rheumatoid arthritis, osteoarthritis, ankylosing spondylitis, menstrual pain, tendinitis, bursitis, painful shoulder, gout (except Indocin SR), sunburn prevention and treatment (as a cream or lotion), and migraine and cluster headache prevention (except Indocin SR). Indomethacin can be used to prevent premature labor, but this can affect the development of the baby's heart and should be avoided. The drug is also used in place of surgery to treat a rare condition in premature infants called *patent ductus arteriosus*, where the baby's heart is not fully formed. Topical Indomethacin has been used as eyedrops to treat a severe and unusual inflammation of part of the retina.

General Information

Indomethacin is one of 16 nonsteroidal anti-inflammatory drugs (NSAIDs), which are used to relieve pain and inflammation. We do not know exactly how NSAIDs work, but part of their action may be due to an ability to inhibit the body's production of a hormone called *prostaglandin* and to inhibit the action of other body chemicals, including cyclo-oxygenase, lipoxygenase, leukotrienes, lysosomal enzymes, and a host of other factors. Indomethacin is absorbed into the bloodstream fairly quickly. Pain relief comes about 30 minutes after taking the first dose and lasts for 4 to 6 hours, but the drug's anti-inflammatory effect takes a week to become apparent, and may take 2 weeks to reach its maximum effect. Indomethacin is broken down in the liver and eliminated through the kidneys.

Cautions and Warnings

People who are **allergic** to Indomethacin (or any other NSAID) and those with a history of **asthma attacks** brought on by another NSAID, by Iodides, or by Aspirin should not take Indomethacin.

Indomethacin can cause **gastrointestinal (GI) bleeding, ulcers,** and **stomach perforation,** which can occur at any time, with or without warning, in people who take chronic Indomethacin treatment. People with a history of **active GI bleeding** should be cautious about taking any NSAID. **Minor stomach upset, distress,** or **gas** is common during the first few days of treatment with Indomethacin. People who develop bleeding or ulcers and continue treatment may develop more serious drug toxicity.

Indomethacin can affect **platelets** and **blood clotting** at high doses, and should be avoided by people with clotting problems and by those taking **Warfarin.**

People with **heart problems** who use Indomethacin may experience swelling in their arms, legs, or feet.

Indomethacin should not be used by people who have had **ulcers** or other **stomach lesions.**

Indomethacin may worsen **depression** or other **psychiatric disorders, epilepsy,** and **parkinsonism.**

Indomethacin should **never be used as "first therapy"** for any disorder (with the possible exception of ankylosing spondylitis), because of the severe side effects often associated with this medicine.

Indomethacin can cause **severe toxic effects to the kidney. Report any unusual side effects to your doctor,** who may need to periodically test your kidney function.

Indomethacin can make you **unusually sensitive to the effects of the sun** (photosensitivity).

Possible Side Effects

▼ Most common: diarrhea, nausea, vomiting, constipation, stomach gas, stomach upset or irritation, and loss of appetite.

▼ Less common: stomach ulcers, GI bleeding, hepatitis, gallbladder attacks, painful urination, poor kidney function, kidney inflammation, blood and protein in the urine, dizziness, fainting, nervousness, depression, hallucinations, confusion, disorientation, tingling in the hands or feet, light-headedness, itching, increased sweating, dry nose and mouth, heart palpitations, chest pain, difficulty breathing, and muscle cramps.

▼ Rare: severe allergic reactions, including closing of the throat, fever and chills, changes in liver function, jaundice (yellowing of the skin or eyes), and kidney failure. People who experience such effects must be promptly treated in a hospital emergency room or doctor's office.

NSAIDs have caused severe skin reactions; if this happens to you, see your doctor immediately.

Drug Interactions

• Indomethacin can increase the effects of oral anticoagulant (blood-thinning) drugs, such as Warfarin. You may take this combination, but your doctor may have to reduce your anticoagulant dose.

• The combination of Indomethacin and a thiazide diuretic affects the amount of diuretic in your blood. Indomethacin may reduce the effect of the diuretic.

• Diflunisal increases the amount of Indomethacin in your blood; the combination of Indomethacin and Diflunisal has resulted in a fatal GI hemorrhage.

• Indomethacin may reduce the blood-pressure-lowering effect of beta blockers, angiotensin-converting-enzyme (ACE) inhibitor drugs, and loop diuretics.

• Taking Indomethacin with Cyclosporine may increase the toxic kidney effects of both drugs. Methotrexate toxicity may be increased in people also taking Indomethacin.

• Indomethacin may increase Digoxin levels in the blood.

• Taking Indomethacin with Phenylpropanolamine (found in many over-the-counter drug products) may cause an increase in blood pressure.

• The combination of Indomethacin and Dipyridamole may increase your water retention.

• Indomethacin may increase blood levels of Phenytoin, leading to increased Phenytoin side effects. Blood-Lithium levels may be increased in people taking Indomethacin.

• Indomethacin blood levels may be affected by Cimetidine because of that drug's effect on the liver.

• Probenecid may interfere with Indomethacin's elimination from the body, increasing the chances for Indomethacin toxic reactions.

• Aspirin and other salicylates may decrease the amount of Indomethacin in your blood. These medicines should never be taken at the same time.

Food Interactions

Take Indomethacin with food or a magnesium/aluminum antacid if it upsets your stomach.

Usual Dose

Adult and Adolescent (age 14 and older): 50 to 200 mg per day, individualized to your needs.

Child (age 14 and under): Not recommended.

Overdosage

People have died from NSAID overdoses. The most common signs of overdosage are drowsiness, nausea, vomiting, diarrhea, abdominal pain, rapid breathing, rapid heartbeat, increased sweating, ringing or buzzing in the ears, confusion, disorientation, stupor, and coma.

Take the victim to a hospital emergency room at once. ALWAYS bring the medicine bottle with you.

Special Information

Indomethacin can make you drowsy and/or tired: Be careful when driving or operating hazardous equipment. Do not take any nonprescription products containing Acetaminophen or Aspirin while taking this drug; also, avoid alcoholic beverages.

Take each dose with a full glass of water, and don't lie down for 15 to 30 minutes after you take the medicine.

Contact your doctor if you develop skin rash or itching, visual disturbances, weight gain, breathing difficulty, fluid retention, hallucinations, black or tarry stools, persistent headache, or any unusual or intolerable side effects.

If you forget to take a dose of Indomethacin, take it as soon as you remember. If you take several Indomethacin doses a day and it is within 4 hours of your next dose, skip the one you forgot and continue with your regular schedule. If you take it once a day and it is within 8 hours of your next dose, skip the missed dose and continue with your regular schedule. Do not take a double dose.

Special Populations

Pregnancy/Breast-feeding

Indomethacin may cross into the fetal blood circulation. Although it has not been found to cause birth defects, Indomethacin should not be used during the second half of pregnancy, because it may affect the developing fetal heart. Women who are or who might become pregnant should not take Indomethacin without their doctor's approval. When the drug is considered essential by your doctor, its potential benefits must be carefully weighed against its risks.

Indomethacin may pass into breast milk but has caused few problems among breast-fed infants, except for seizures in a baby whose mother was taking it. However, there is also a possibility that a nursing mother taking Indomethacin could affect her baby's heart or cardiovascular system. If you must take Indomethacin, bottle-feed your baby.

Seniors

Older adults may be more susceptible to Indomethacin side effects, especially ulcer disease.

Generic Name

Insulin Injection

Brand Names

Insulin for Injection (Regular)

Concentrated Regular Iletin II (pork only)	Pork Regular Iletin II
	Regular Iletin I
Humulin R	Regular Insulin
Novolin R	Regular Purified Pork Insulin
Novolin R PenFill	Velosulin Human

Insulin Zinc Suspension (Lente)

Humulin L	Lente L (pork)
Lente Iletin I (beef & pork)	Lente Insulin (beef)
Lente Iletin II (pork)	Novolin L

Insulin Zinc Suspension, Extended (Ultralente)

Humulin U Ultralente
Ultralente U

Isophane Insulin Suspension and Insulin Injection

Humulin 70/30	Novolin 70/30
Humulin 50/50	Novolin 70/30 PenFill

Isophane Insulin Suspension (NPH)

Humulin N	NPH-N
Novolin N	NPH Insulin
Novolin N PenFill	NPH Purified
NPH Iletin I (beef & pork)	Pork NPH Iletin II

Protamine Zinc Insulin Suspension (PZI)

Protamine Zinc and Iletin I (beef and pork)
Protamine Zinc and Iletin II (beef)
Protamine Zinc and Iletin II (pork)

Type of Drug

Antidiabetic.

Prescribed for

Type I (Insulin-dependent) diabetes mellitus and Type II (non–Insulin-dependent) diabetes mellitus that cannot be controlled by diet. Insulin may also be used in a hospital, together with glucose injection, to treat hyperkalemia (high blood-potassium levels). It is also used for severe complications of diabetes, including ketoacidosis or diabetic coma.

General Information

Insulin is a complex hormone normally produced by the pancreas. Diabetes develops when the body does not make enough Insulin or when the Insulin does not work. At one time, most of the Insulin used as a drug was obtained from animals. Today, most of what is used is human Insulin manufactured by biosynthetic techniques. People whose diabetes is well controlled by Insulin derived from an animal source should not be automatically switched to a human Insulin product, but new diabetics are usually treated with highly purified synthetic human Insulin.

Synthetic human Insulin is identical in structure to the Insulin we make in our bodies. Insulin derived from pork is closer in chemical structure to our own Insulin than that derived from beef, and causes fewer reactions. So-called human Insulin products differ in slight, but significant, ways from animal-derived Insulin.

Human Insulin is the product of choice for (1) people allergic to other Insulin products, (2) all pregnant diabetic women, (3) people who need Insulin only for short periods (during surgery, etc.), and (4) all newly diagnosed diabetics. It causes fewer allergic reactions than the older Insulins manufactured from pork and/or beef sources. Human Insulins may also be produced by semisynthetic processes. These semisynthetic Insulins, however, start with an animal product and may contain some of the same impurities. Animal Insulin used for injection is the unmodified material derived from an animal source, usually beef or pork.

Regular Insulin starts to work quickly and lasts only 6 to 8 hours. People using only Insulin injection must take several injections per day. Pharmaceutical scientists have been able to add other chemical structures onto the Insulin molecule to extend the time over which the drug works. Prompt Insulin

Zinc Suspension (also called Semilente Insulin), like Insulin for injection, is considered rapid-acting. It starts to work in 30 to 60 minutes and lasts 12 to 16 hours.

The intermediate-acting Insulins (NPH or Isophane Insulin and Lente or Insulin Zinc Suspension) start working 1 to 2 1/2 hours after injection and continue to work for 24 hours. Long-acting Insulins (PZI or Protamine Zinc Insulin Suspension and Ultralente or Extended Insulin Zinc Suspension) begin working 4 to 8 hours after injection, and last for 36 hours or more. Other factors that have a definite influence on Insulin response include diet, exercise, and other drugs being used.

Insulin products derived from natural sources contain a number of normal contaminants. In the 1970s, processes were developed to remove many of these contaminants. The first process resulted in single-peak Insulin, making the action of the drug more predictable and safer. Today, all Insulin sold in the United States is single-peak, and most of that is identical to natural human Insulin. The second refinement resulted in purified Insulin, which produces fewer reactions at the injection site than single-peak Insulin.

Cautions and Warnings

Be sure to take the **exact dose** of Insulin that was prescribed. **Too much Insulin will excessively lower blood sugar, and too little will not control the diabetes. Do not change Insulin brands or types** unless you are under direct medical supervision. Diabetics taking Insulin *must* **follow their prescribed diet** and should **avoid alcoholic beverages.**

Low blood sugar (see *Overdosage* for symptoms) can result from taking too much Insulin, doing excess physical work or exercise without eating, or not absorbing food normally because meals are postponed or skipped, or because of illness with vomiting, fever, or diarrhea. Often, you can correct the situation by eating sugar or something with sugar in it. You can also use a commercial 40 percent glucose product, but they work in the same way as plain sugar or candy. The symptoms of low blood sugar are less pronounced if you are taking human Insulin rather than an animal Insulin, but the possible consequences are just as dire.

Possible Side Effects

▼ Most common: allergic reactions, breakdown of fat tissue at the site of injection (causing a depression in the skin), and accumulation of fat under the skin from using the same site for many Insulin injections.

Drug Interactions

• Your Insulin dosage may need to be raised if you are taking drugs that increase blood-sugar levels: These include corticosteroids, oral contraceptives, Dextrothyroxine, Diltiazem, Dobutamine, Epinephrine, cigarettes, thiazide-type diuretics, thyroid hormones, estrogens, Furosemide, Molindone, Phenytoin, and Ethacrynic Acid.

• Other medicines can lower blood sugar and may require a reduced insulin dosage. These medicines include alcohol, anabolic steroids, beta-blocking drugs, Clofibrate, Fenfluramine, Phenylbutazone, Sulfinpyrazone, Tetracycline, Guanethidine, monoamine oxidase (MAO) inhibitor antidepressants, and Aspirin (in large doses).

• Oral antidiabetes drugs also lower blood sugar and should be taken together with Insulin only if you are under the direct care of a doctor. Nonsteroidal anti-inflammatory drugs (NSAIDs) may also increase the blood-sugar-lowering effect of Insulin, but by a different mechanism.

• Beta-blocking drugs can mask the symptoms of low blood sugar and thus increase the risk of taking Insulin.

• Stopping smoking cigarettes, using a Nicotine patch or gum, or taking other smoking deterrents can also lower blood sugar by increasing the amount of Insulin that is absorbed after injection under the skin. Lowering of your Insulin dose may be necessary if you stop smoking.

• Insulin may affect blood-potassium levels and can affect Digitalis drugs.

Food Interactions

Follow your doctor's directions for diet restrictions. Diet is a key element in controlling your disease.

Usual Dose

The dose and kind of Insulin must be individualized to your

specific need. Insulin is generally injected half an hour before meals; the longer-acting forms are taken half an hour before breakfast. Since Insulin can be given only by injection, diabetics must learn to give themselves their Insulin subcutaneously (under the skin) or have a family member or friend give them injections. Hospitalized patients may receive Insulin injection directly into a vein.

One manufacturer has developed a device to aid in injecting Insulin. The device looks like a pen and is easily used. Another type of injection convenience device is the Insulin-infusion pump. The pump automatically administers a predetermined amount of regular Insulin. Consult your doctor or pharmacist for complete details on either of these devices.

Overdosage

If swallowed, Insulin has little or no effect, because it is not absorbed into the blood. Injecting too much Insulin will cause low blood sugar. Symptoms come suddenly and include weakness, fatigue, nervousness, confusion, headache, double vision, convulsions, dizziness, psychoses, unconsciousness, rapid shallow breathing, numbness or tingling around the mouth, hunger, nausea, loss of skin color, dry skin, and pulse changes. Overdose victims should eat chocolate, candy, or another sugar source at once to raise blood-sugar levels. Call your doctor immediately.

Special Information

Use the same brand and strength of Insulin and Insulin syringes or administration devices to avoid dosage errors. Rotate injection sites to prevent fat loss at the site.

Mix Insulins according to your doctor's directions; don't change the mixing method or the mixing order.

You may develop low blood sugar if you take too much Insulin, work or exercise more strenuously than usual, skip a meal, take Insulin too long before a meal, or vomit before a meal. Signs of low blood sugar may be fatigue, headache, drowsiness, nausea, tremulous feeling, sweating, or nervousness. If you develop any of these signs while taking Insulin, your blood sugar may be too low. The usual treatment for low blood sugar is eating a candy bar or lump of sugar, which diabetics should carry with them at all times. If the signs of low blood sugar do not clear up within 30 minutes, call your doctor. You may need further treatment.

Your Insulin requirements may change if you get sick, especially if you vomit or have a fever.

If your Insulin is in suspension form, you must evenly distribute the particles throughout the liquid before taking the dose out. Do this by gently rotating the vial and turning it over several times. Do not shake the vial.

Diabetics must pay special attention to dental hygiene because of their increased chance of developing oral infections. Also, your dentist may detect other signs of advancing diabetes during an examination. Be sure your dentist knows you have diabetes.

Have your eyes checked regularly. One of the primary complications of diabetes (blood-vessel disease) may be seen by an eye doctor during a routine eye examination.

Read and follow all patient information provided with the Insulin products you are using. Monitor your blood and urine regularly for sugar and ketones, using over-the-counter testing products.

Insulin products are generally stable at room temperature for about 2 years. They must be kept away from direct sunlight and extreme temperatures. Most manufacturers, however, still recommend that Insulin be stored in a refrigerator or a cool place whenever possible. Insulin should not be put in a freezer or exposed to very high temperatures; this can affect its stability. Partly used vials of Insulin should be thrown away after several weeks if not used. Do not use any Insulin that looks lumpy or grainy or that sticks to the bottle. Regular Insulin should be clear and colorless; do not use it if it is thick or cloudy.

Some Insulin products can be mixed. Mix 2 or more different Insulins only if you have been so directed by your doctor. Your pharmacist may also mix your Insulins to assure accuracy. Insulin for injection may be mixed with Isophane Insulin Suspension and Protamine Zinc Insulin in any proportion. Insulin Zinc Suspension, Insulin Zinc Suspension (Prompt), and Insulin Zinc Suspension (Extended) may also be mixed in any proportions. Insulin for injection and Insulin Zinc Suspension must be mixed immediately before using.

If you forget a dose of Insulin, take it as soon as you remember. If it is almost time for your next dose, or if you completely forget one or more doses, call your doctor for exact instructions.

Special Populations

Pregnancy/Breast-feeding

Insulin is the preferred method for controlling diabetes in pregnant women, though pregnancy usually complicates the process. Pregnant diabetic women must follow their doctor's directions for Insulin use exactly because Insulin requirements normally decrease during the first half of pregnancy and then increase to more than normal requirements during the second half. Pregnant women who must take Insulin injections should use human Insulin.

Insulin does not pass into breast milk. Breast-feeding can reduce your Insulin needs, despite the need for more calories. Your doctor should closely monitor your Insulin dosage during this period.

Seniors

Older adults may use Insulin without special restriction. Follow your doctor's directions for medication and diet.

Generic Name

Interferon beta-1b

Brand Name

Betaseron

Type of Drug

Multiple sclerosis therapy.

Prescribed for

Symptomatic relief of multiple sclerosis in patients with the "relapsing-remitting" form of the disease. Interferon beta-1b is also being studied for AIDS, Kaposi's sarcoma, metastatic renal-cell cancer, malignant melanoma, and acute non-A, non-B hepatitis.

General Information

Multiple sclerosis (MS) is an inflammatory disease in which

protective central-nervous-system myelin sheaths are broken down by immune system abnormalities. This leads to a gradual and progressive loss of muscle tone and function, progressive weakness, and paralysis. Exacerbations or episodes of MS in which the disease worsens develop slowly and may take weeks to months to resolve. About two thirds of MS sufferers have the relapsing-remitting form, in which stable periods are followed by periods of worsening disease. Until now, MS treatment has been aimed at controlling the symptoms of the disease. Interferon beta-1b is a biotechnological product that has been found to help reduce the number and severity of MS flare-ups in some patients. It shares antitumor, antiviral, and other actions with other Interferons, but it has much more of an effect on the immune system.

This medicine, the first to be approved for any form of MS, was studied in 372 patients for 2 years before its approval by the Food and Drug Administration. Studies will continue to investigate whether Interferon beta-1b can slow or prevent the worsening of MS over time. Nobody knows how this medicine produces its effect.

Cautions and Warnings

The **safety and benefit** of this drug in **chronic, progressive MS** have **not been proven.**

Potentially **severe depression** and **suicidal tendencies** have been experienced by patients taking Interferon beta-1b. Report any depressive feelings or tendencies to your doctor.

Half of patients who take this drug are likely to develop **flu-like symptoms,** including fever, chills, muscle aches, sweating, and feelings of ill health.

Interferon beta-1b can make you **unusually sensitive to the sun.** Wear protective clothing and use a sunscreen if you are taking this drug.

Possible Side Effects

▼ Most common: pain, burning or stinging at the injection site, sinusitis, headache, migraines, fever, weakness, chills, muscle aches, abdominal pain, flu-like symptoms, menstrual disorders, painful menstruation, diarrhea, con-

Possible Side Effects *(continued)*

stipation, vomiting, liver inflammation, sweating, and reduced white-blood-cell counts.

▼ Less common: swelling, pelvic pain, cyst, suicide attempt, thyroid goiter, heart palpitations, high blood pressure, rapid heartbeat, bleeding, laryngitis, difficulty breathing, stiffness, tiredness, speech problems, convulsions, uncontrolled movements, hair loss, visual disturbances, pink-eye, urinary urgency, cystitis, breast pain, and cystic breast disease.

▼ Rare: reactions affecting virtually every part of the body. Report any other reactions to your doctor.

Drug and Food Interactions

None known.

Usual Dose

8 million units every other day by subcutaneous injection. This medicine may be self-administered at home in much the same way that Insulin injections are taken.

Overdosage

The effects of Interferon beta-1b overdose are unknown. Symptoms are most likely to be exaggerated side effects. Call your doctor or poison control center for more information.

Special Information

Interferon beta-1b may be associated with severe depression. Mood swings or changes, lack of interest in daily activities, excessive sleep, and other possible signs of depression should be reported to your doctor at once.

Interferon beta-1b injections should be taken at the same time each day to establish them as part of your daily routine. If you forget to take a dose of Interferon beta-1b, take it as soon as you remember. If it is almost time for your next dose, skip the forgotten dose and continue with your regular schedule. Do not take a double dose.

Special Populations

Pregnancy/Breast-feeding

The effect of this product on pregnant women and nursing mothers is not known. Exercise caution with all medicines.

Seniors

Seniors may use this medicine without special restriction.

Generic Name

Ipratropium Bromide

Brand Name

Atrovent

Type of Drug

Bronchodilator.

Prescribed for

Maintenance treatment of bronchospasm associated with chronic lung disease, including bronchitis and emphysema.

General Information

Unlike most other bronchodilator products, Ipratropium is chemically related to *Atropine Sulfate*, an anticholinergic drug. Ipratropium works by inhibiting the action of acetylcholine in bronchial muscles. This results in a local effect that produces bronchial dilation, not a systemic one produced by drug circulating in the bloodstream. This is an advantage because it reduces the chances of drug side effects. Little drug is absorbed into the bloodstream; much of each dose that is inhaled is swallowed and passes out of the body in the stool.

Cautions and Warnings

Do not use Ipratropium if you are **allergic** to Atropine or to any related product. It should be used with caution if you have **glaucoma, prostate disease,** or **bladder obstruction.**

Ipratropium is not meant for the treatment of **acute bron-**

chospasm where rapid response is needed. This drug should be used only to prevent bronchospasm associated with chronic lung diseases.

Possible Side Effects

Generally, Ipratropium side effects are infrequent and mild.

▼ Most common: nervousness, dizziness, headache, nausea, upset stomach, blurred vision, sensitivity to bright light, dry mouth, throat irritation, cough, worsening of symptoms, heart palpitations, and rash. Mouth or throat irritation may also occur.

▼ Less common: rapid heartbeat, urinary difficulty, tingling in the hands or feet, poor coordination, itching, hives, flushing, loss of hair, constipation, tremors, fatigue or sleeplessness, and hoarseness.

▼ Rare: worsening of glaucoma, eye pain, low blood pressure, and severe skin reactions.

Drug Interactions

• Ipratropium has been used in combination with virtually all other kinds of bronchodilators without drug interaction.

Food Interactions

Do not inhale a dose of Ipratropium if you have any food in your mouth.

Usual Dose

Adult and Adolescent (age 12 or older): 2 inhalations (36 micrograms) 4 times per day, no more than 12 inhalations every 24 hours.

Child (under age 12): do not use.

Overdosage

The chance of overdose is small because so little Ipratropium is absorbed into the bloodstream. Ipratropium accidentally sprayed into the eye will cause blurred vision. ALWAYS bring the medicine container with you if you go for treatment.

Special Information

Use this product according to your doctor's instructions. Because long-term use of Ipratropium should reduce the number of bronchial attacks, you may feel that you have gotten better and no longer need the medicine. Do not stop taking Ipratropium without your doctor's approval. Call your doctor if you develop skin rash or hives, sores on the mouth or lips, blurred vision, and other side effects that are bothersome or persistent.

Call your doctor if you stop responding to your usual dose of Ipratropium, because this may be a sign that your bronchial disease has worsened and may require reevaluation.

Prolonged use of Ipratropium may decrease or stop the flow of saliva produced in your mouth. This can expose you to an increased chance of cavities, gum disease, oral infections, and other problems. Dry mouth can be relieved with hard candies or regular fluids. Increased attention to dental hygiene is important.

If you take a corticosteroid inhaler or Cromolyn Sodium with Ipratropium for your lung disease, use the Ipratropium about 5 minutes before the other inhaler.

If you take Ipratropium and Albuterol, Metaproterenol, or another beta-stimulating aerosol product for your bronchial disease, use the beta stimulator about 5 minutes before the Ipratropium, unless otherwise instructed by your doctor.

If you forget to take a dose of Ipratropium, take it as soon as you remember. If it is almost time for your next dose, skip the one you forgot and continue with your regular schedule. Do not take a double dose.

Special Populations

Pregnancy/Breast-feeding

Massive oral doses of Ipratropium have caused birth defects in animals, but there is no information to indicate that the drug would have such an effect if used by pregnant women. Ipratropium should be used during pregnancy only if clearly needed.

It is not known if Ipratropium passes into breast milk, but it is unlikely that enough Ipratropium will be absorbed to make a difference to a nursing infant. Nevertheless, nursing mothers who take this drug should observe their infants for drug side effects.

Seniors

Older adults, especially those with prostate disease, may be more sensitive to the side effects of this drug and require a dosage adjustment.

Type of Drug

Iron Supplement

_____

Brand Names

Ferrous Sulfate (20% iron)

Feosol	Fero-Gradumet	Ferra-TD
Feratab	Ferospace	Mol-Iron
Fer-In-Sol	Ferralyn	Slow FE
Fer-Iron		

Ferrous Gluconate (11.6% iron)

Fergon	Simron
Ferralet	

Ferrous Fumarate (33% iron)

Femiron	Ircon	Span-FF
Feostat	Hemocyte	
Fumerin	Nephro-Fer	
Fumasorb		

Polysaccharide Iron Complex

Hytinic	Nu-Iron	[S]
Niferex	[S]	

(All available in generic form)

Prescribed for

Prevention and treatment of iron-deficiency anemia.

General Information

All of these products are used to treat anemias due to iron deficiency. They are of no value in treating other kinds of anemias. They work by being incorporated into red blood cells, where oxygen is carried throughout the body. Iron is absorbed only in a small section of the gastrointestinal (GI) tract called the *duodenum* (the upper part of the small intestine). Sustained-release preparations of iron should be used only to help minimize the stomach discomfort that iron supplements can cause, since any drug that passes the duodenum cannot be absorbed.

Other iron-containing drugs may also provide a source of iron to treat iron-deficiency anemia. The iron in these products may be combined with other vitamins or with special extracts, as in the product Trinsicon, where iron is combined with vitamin B_{12}, Folic Acid, and Intrinsic Factor.

Cautions and Warnings

Do not take an iron supplement if you have **hemochromatosis, hemosiderosis,** or a **hemolytic anemia.**

Do not take iron supplements if you have a history of **stomach problems, peptic ulcer,** or **ulcerative colitis.** People with **normal iron balance** in their bodies should not take any iron product on a regular basis.

Possible Side Effects

▼ Common: stomach upset or irritation, nausea, diarrhea, constipation, appetite loss, and darkened stools.

Drug Interactions

• Iron and Tetracycline interfere with each other's absorption into the blood. Separate doses of these medicines by at least 2 hours.

• Iron interferes with the absorption of Levodopa, Methyldopa, Penicillamine, and quinolone antibacterials into the bloodstream.

• Antacids and Cimetidine will interfere with the absorption of iron.

• Ascorbic Acid (vitamin C) and Chloramphenicol increase the amount of iron absorbed into the bloodstream.

Food Interactions

Iron salts and iron-containing products are best absorbed on an empty stomach, but if they upset your stomach, take with some food or immediately after meals. Be aware that eggs and milk interfere with iron absorption. Coffee or tea taken with a meal or within an hour after the meal will interfere with the absorption of iron from your food. Taking iron and calcium supplements together with food can reduce the amount of iron absorbed by one-third.

Usual Dose

Iron dosage is the same regardless of the type of iron you take. In order to figure out how much iron you are receiving, you can use the percentage of iron content provided above or read the iron content in mg directly from the product's label.

Adult and Adolescent (age 13 and older): 0.9 to 1⅓ mg per pound of body weight each day.

Pregnant Women: 30 mg of iron daily. Do not take with food or meals.

Child (age 3 to 12): 1⅓ mg per pound of body weight per day.

Child (age 6 months to 2 years): up to 2¾ mg per pound of body weight per day.

Infant: 10 to 25 mg per day.

Overdosage

Overdosage symptoms usually appear after 30 minutes to several hours, and include lethargy (tiredness), vomiting, diarrhea, stomach upset, change in pulse to weak and rapid, and lowered blood pressure—or, after massive doses, shock, black and tarry stools (due to massive bleeding in the stomach or intestine), and pneumonia. Be sure to call a doctor before inducing vomiting. Quickly induce vomiting by giving Syrup of Ipecac (available in any pharmacy) and feed the victim eggs and milk until he or she can be taken to a hospital for stomach pumping. The victim must be taken to the hospital as soon as possible because stomach pumping should not be performed after the first hour of iron ingestion; otherwise, there is a danger of perforation of the stomach wall. In the hospital emergency room, measures to treat shock, loss of water, loss of blood, and respiratory failure may be necessary. ALWAYS bring the medicine bottle.

Special Information

Iron often causes black discoloration to stools and is slightly constipating. However, if stools become black or tarry in consistency, this may indicate some bleeding in the stomach or intestine. Discuss this with your doctor at once.

Do not chew or crush extended-release iron products. Liquid iron products may stain your teeth. Drink lots of water or juice with them and sip the iron through a straw to prevent tooth contact and staining.

If you forget to take a dose of iron, take it as soon as you remember. If it is almost time for your next dose, skip the one you forgot and continue with your regular schedule. Do not take a double dose.

Special Populations

Pregnancy/Breast-feeding
This drug has been found to be safe for use during pregnancy and breast-feeding and is generally prescribed for women in those states. But, if you are pregnant, you should check with your doctor before taking any medication.

Seniors
Seniors may require larger doses to correct an iron deficiency, because the ability to absorb iron decreases with age.

Generic Name

Isosorbide

Brand Names

Isosorbide Mononitrate

Imdur	ISMO	Monoket

Isosorbide Dinitrate

Dilatrate-SR	Isordil Titradose
Isordil Tembids	Sorbitrate

(Also available in generic form)

Type of Drug

Antianginal agent.

Prescribed for

Relief of heart or chest pain associated with angina pectoris. It is also used to control or prevent the recurrence of chest or heart pain and to reduce heart work in congestive heart failure and other similar conditions.

General Information

Isosorbide belongs to the class of drugs known as *nitrates*, which are used to treat pain associated with heart problems. The exact nature of their action is not fully understood. However, they are believed to relax muscles of veins and arteries. Isosorbide Dinitrate sublingual tablets begin working in 2 to 5 minutes and last for 1 to 3 hours. The regular tablets begin working in 20 to 40 minutes and continue for 4 to 6 hours. Sustained-release Isosorbide Dinitrate may take up to 4 hours to begin working and lasts for 6 to 8 hours. Isosorbide Mononitrate begins working in 30 to 60 minutes and lasts for an undetermined period of time.

Cautions and Warnings

If you know that you are **allergic** or **sensitive** to this drug or other drugs for heart pain, such as Nitroglycerin, do not use Isosorbide. Anyone who has a **head injury** or has recently had a head injury should use this drug with caution. Other conditions where the use of Isosorbide should be carefully considered are **severe anemia, glaucoma, severe liver disease, overactive thyroid, cardiomyopathy (disease of the heart muscle), low blood pressure, recent heart attack, severe kidney problems,** and **overactive gastrointestinal tract.**

Possible Side Effects

▼ Common: headache and flushing of the skin, which should disappear after your body gets used to the drug. You may experience dizziness and weakness in the process. There is a possibility of blurred vision and dry mouth; if this happens, stop taking the drug and call your physician.

▼ Less common: nausea, vomiting, weakness, sweating, rash with itching, redness, possible peeling. If these signs appear, discontinue the medication and consult your physician.

Drug Interactions

• If you take Isosorbide, do not self-medicate with over-the-counter cough and cold remedies, since many of them contain ingredients that may aggravate heart disease.

• Interaction with large amounts of whiskey, wine, or beer can cause rapid lowering of blood pressure, resulting in weakness, dizziness, and fainting.

• Nitrates raise the amount of Dihydroergotamine absorbed into the blood, either raising blood pressure or working against the effect of Isosorbide.

• Aspirin and calcium channel blockers can lead to higher Isosorbide blood levels and increased drug side effects.

Food Interactions

Take Isosorbide on an empty stomach with a glass of water unless you get a headache that cannot be controlled by the usual means. If this occurs, the drug can be taken with meals.

Usual Dose

Isosorbide Dinitrate

10 to 20 mg, 4 times per day. The drug may be given in doses from 5 to 40 mg, 4 times per day.

Sustained-release: 40 to 80 mg every 8 to 12 hours.

Isosorbide Mononitrate

20 mg twice a day, with the 2 doses taken 7 hours apart. Usually, the first dose is taken on arising and the second dose is taken 7 hours later.

Overdosage

Isosorbide overdose can result in low blood pressure; very rapid heartbeat; flushing; perspiration (later on, your skin can become cold, bluish, and clammy); headache; heart palpitations; blurring and other visual disturbances; dizziness; nausea; vomiting; difficult, slow breathing; slow pulse; confusion; moderate fever; and paralysis. Overdose victims should be taken to a hospital emergency room at once for treatment. ALWAYS bring the medicine bottle with you.

Special Information

If you take this drug sublingually (under the tongue), be sure the tablet is fully dissolved before you swallow the drug. Do not crush or chew sustained-release capsules or tablets.

Avoid alcoholic beverages while taking any of these drugs.

Do not switch brands of Isosorbide without discussing this with your doctor or pharmacist. All brands of Isosorbide may not be equivalent.

Call your doctor if you develop a persistent headache, dizziness, facial flushing, blurred vision, or dry mouth.

If you take regular Isosorbide and forget to take a dose, take it as soon as you remember, unless it is within 2 hours of your next scheduled dose. If that happens, skip the dose you forgot and continue with your regular schedule.

If you take long-acting Isosorbide and miss a dose, take it as soon as you remember, unless it is within 6 hours of your next dose. In that case, skip the dose you forgot and continue with your regular schedule. Do not take a double dose.

Special Populations

Pregnancy/Breast-feeding
This drug crosses into the blood circulation of a developing baby. It has not been found to cause birth defects. Nevertheless, pregnant women and those who might become pregnant should not take Isosorbide without their doctor's approval. When the drug is considered essential by your doctor, its potential benefits must be carefully weighed against its risks.

This drug passes into breast milk but has caused no problems among breast-fed infants.

Seniors
Older adults may take this medicine without special restriction. Be sure to follow your doctor's directions, and report any side effects.

Generic Name

Isotretinoin

Brand Name

Accutane

Type of Drug

Antiacne.

Prescribed for

Severe cystic acne that has not responded to other treatment, including medicines applied to the skin and antibiotics.

Isotretinoin has been used experimentally to treat a variety of other skin disorders involving the process of keratinization (hardening of skin cells), and a condition known as *mycosis fungoides* that begins in the skin and can progress to a form of leukemia. Isotretinoin is usually successful for these conditions, but relatively high doses are usually needed.

General Information

Isotretinoin was one of the first specialized products of vitamin research to be released for prescription by doctors. Researchers have long known that several vitamins, including A and D, have special properties that make them attractive treatments for specific conditions. However, the vitamins themselves are not appropriate treatments for these conditions, because of the side effects that would develop if you took the quantities needed to produce the desired effects.

It is not known exactly how Isotretinoin works in cases of severe cystic acne. It reduces the amount of sebum (the skin's natural oily lubricant) in the skin, shrink the skin glands that produce sebum, and inhibit the process of keratinization, in which skin cells become hardened and block the flow of sebum into the skin. Keratinization is key to the problem of severe acne because it leads to the buildup of sebum within skin follicles and causes the formation of closed comedones (whiteheads). Sebum production may be permanently reduced after Isotretinoin treatment, but no one knows why this happens.

Cautions and Warnings

People **allergic** or **sensitive to vitamin** A (or any vitamin A product), or to **Paraben preservatives** (used in **Accutane**), should not use Isotretinoin.

Isotretinoin has been associated with several cases of **increased fluid pressure inside the head.** The symptoms of this condition, known as *pseudotumor cerebri*, are **severe headaches, nausea, vomiting, and visual disturbances.**

Diabetics taking this drug may have their diabetes medicines reevaluated by their doctor. Some new cases of diabetes were found in people taking Isotretinoin, but no relationship to Isotretinoin drug therapy has been found.

Isotretinoin may cause temporary opaque spots on the cornea of your eye, causing **visual disturbances.** These generally go away by themselves within 2 months after the drug has been stopped.

Difficulty seeing at night can develop suddenly while taking Isotretinoin.

Several cases of **severe bowel inflammation** (abdominal discomfort and pain, severe diarrhea, or bleeding from the rectum) have developed in people taking Isotretinoin.

About 1 in 4 people (25 percent) who take this drug develop **high blood-triglyceride levels,** 15 percent develop a **reduction in HDL cholesterol** (so-called good cholesterol), and 7 percent develop an **increase in total cholesterol.**

Several cases of **hepatitis** have been linked to Isotretinoin, and 15 percent of people who take this drug develop signs of **liver inflammation.**

Occasionally, healing cystic acne lesions crust while healing, and **acne may actually worsen** when Isotretinoin treatment is first started.

Possible Side Effects

Side-effect frequency increases with daily dose. The most severe effects occur at doses above 0.45 mg per pound of body weight per day.

▼ Most common: dry, chapped, or inflamed lips; dry mouth; dry nose; nosebleeds; eye irritation and conjunctivitis; dry or flaky skin; rash; itching; skin peeling (from the face, palms, or soles); unusual skin sensitivity to the sun; temporary skin discoloration; dry mucous membranes (mouth or nose); brittle nails; inflammation of the nailbed or bone under the toe or fingernails; temporary hair thinning; nausea; vomiting; abdominal pains; tiredness; lethargy; sleeplessness; headache; tingling in the hands or feet; dizziness; protein, blood, or white blood cells in the urine; urinary difficulty; blurred vision; bone and joint aches or pains; and muscle pains or stiffness.

Isotretinoin causes extreme elevations of blood triglycerides and milder elevations of other blood fats, including cholesterol. It also can cause increased blood-

Possible Side Effects *(continued)*

sugar or uric-acid levels and can increase liver-function test values.

▼ Less common: crusting over wounds (caused by an exaggerated healing response stimulated by the drug), hair problems (other than thinning), loss of appetite, stomach upset or intestinal discomfort, severe bowel inflammation, stomach or intestinal bleeding, weight loss, visual disturbances, intolerance to contact lenses, pseudotumor cerebri (see *Cautions and Warnings* for symptoms), mild bleeding or easy bruising, fluid retention, and infections of the lungs or respiratory system. Several people taking Isotretinoin have developed widespread herpes simplex infections.

Drug Interactions

• Vitamin A supplements increase Isotretinoin side effects and must be avoided while you are taking this medicine. Also avoid alcohol because this combination can cause severe elevations of blood-triglyceride levels.

• People taking Isotretinoin who have developed pseudotumor cerebri have usually also been taking a Tetracycline antibiotic. Although the link has not been definitely established, avoid Tetracycline antibiotics while taking Isotretinoin.

Food Interactions

Isotretinoin should be taken with food or meals. However, avoid eating liver (beef or chicken) while taking Isotretinoin, because liver contains extremely large amounts of Vitamin A. Foods with moderate amounts of vitamin A that you need not avoid, but should limit your intake of, include apricots, broccoli, cantaloupe, carrots, endive, persimmons, pumpkin, spinach, and winter squash.

Usual Dose

0.22 to 0.9 mg per pound of body weight per day, in 2 divided doses for 15 to 20 weeks. Lower doses may be effective, but relapses are more common. Because Isotretinoin, like Vitamin A, dissolves in body fat, people weighing more than 155 pounds may need doses at the high end of the usual range.

If the total acne cyst count drops by 70 percent before 15 to 20 weeks, the drug may be stopped. You should stop taking this drug for 2 months after the 15- to 20-week treatment. A second course of treatment may be given if the acne does not clear up.

Overdosage

Isotretinoin overdose is likely to cause nausea, vomiting, lethargy, and other common drug side effects. Overdose victims must be made to vomit with Syrup of Ipecac (available at any pharmacy) to remove any remaining drug from the stomach. Call your doctor or poison control center before doing this. If you must go to a hospital emergency room, ALWAYS bring the medicine bottle with you.

Special Information

Your skin may become unusually sensitive to the sun while taking this drug. Use a sunscreen and wear protective clothing until your doctor can determine if you are likely to develop this effect.

Be sure your doctor knows if you are pregnant or planning to become pregnant while taking Isotretinoin, breast-feeding, diabetic, or taking a Vitamin A supplement (as a multivitamin or Vitamin A alone), or if you or any family member has a history of high blood-triglyceride levels.

Call your doctor if you develop any severe or unusual side effects, including abdominal pain, bleeding from the rectum, severe diarrhea, headache, nausea or vomiting, any visual difficulty, severe muscle or bone and joint aches or pains, and unusual sensitivity to sunlight or to ultraviolet light.

Your acne may actually get a little worse when Isotretinoin treatment begins, but then it starts to improve. Don't be alarmed if this happens, but your doctor should be informed.

Do not donate blood during Isotretinoin treatment (or for up to 30 days after you have stopped), because of possible risk to a developing fetus of a pregnant woman who might receive the blood.

If you forget to take a dose of Isotretinoin, take it as soon as you remember. If it is almost time for your next dose, skip the one you forgot and continue with your regular schedule. Do not take a double dose.

Special Populations

Pregnancy/Breast-feeding

Pregnant women and those who might become pregnant should NEVER take Isotretinoin, because it is known to cause fetal injury. This drug causes head, brain, eye, ear, and hearing abnormalities. Several cases of spontaneous abortion have been linked to Isotretinoin.

Before taking this drug, women of childbearing age or potential should take a simple urine test to confirm that they are not pregnant. Also, you must be **absolutely certain** that effective birth control is used starting 1 month before beginning Isotretinoin treatment and continuing 1 month after ending treatment. Accidental pregnancy during Isotretinoin therapy is considered possible grounds for a therapeutic abortion. Discuss this with your doctor immediately.

It is not known if Isotretinoin passes into breast milk. However, nursing mothers should not take Isotretinoin, because of the possibility that it will affect the nursing infant.

Seniors

Seniors may take this medication without special restriction. Follow your doctor's directions and report any side effects at once.

Generic Name

Isradipine

Brand Name

DynaCirc

Type of Drug

Calcium channel blocker.

Prescribed for

High blood pressure. It has also been prescribed to treat chronic stable angina pectoris.

General Information

Isradipine is one of many calcium channel blockers available in the United States. It works by blocking the passage of calcium into smooth muscle. Since calcium is an essential factor in muscle contraction, any drug that affects calcium in this way will interfere with the contraction of these muscles. When this happens, several things can result. Blood vessels will dilate (widen) because the muscles that normally keep them narrowed are not contracting, and the amount of oxygen used by heart muscle may also be reduced. Therefore, Isradipine dilates (opens) the arteries that carry blood and prevents spasm of these arteries. Isradipine is also used in the treatment of angina, a type of heart pain related to poor oxygen supply to the heart muscles. Isradipine affects the movement of calcium only into muscle cells. It does not have any effect on calcium in the blood. Other calcium channel blockers are used for abnormal heart rhythms, diseases involving blood vessel spasm (migraine headache, Raynaud's syndrome), heart failure, and cardiomyopathy.

Cautions and Warnings

Do not take this drug if you have had an **allergic** reaction to it. Use Isradipine with caution if you have **heart failure,** since the drug can worsen the condition. **Abruptly stopping** this medication can cause increased chest pain. If you must stop, the **drug dose should be gradually reduced.**

On rare occasions, Isradipine may cause **very low blood pressure** in some people. This may lead to **stimulation of the heart** and **rapid heartbeat** and can worsen **angina pains** in some people.

Isradipine may cause **angina pain** when treatment is first started, when dosage is increased, or if the drug is rapidly withdrawn. This can be avoided by gradual dosage reduction.

Studies have shown that people taking **calcium channel blockers** (usually those taken several times a day, not those taken only once daily) have a greater chance of having a **heart attack** than people taking beta blockers or other medicines for the same purposes. Discuss this with your doctor to be sure you are receiving the best possible treatment.

Isradipine can **slow heart rate,** which increases the possibility of worsening heart failure.

People with **severe liver disease** break down Isradipine much more slowly than people with less severe disease or normal livers. Your doctor should take this factor into account when determining your Isradipine dosage.

Possible Side Effects

Isradipine side effects are generally mild and self-limiting.

▼ Most common: headache.

▼ Less common: low blood pressure, chest pain, swelling of the legs, ankles or feet, rapid heartbeat, dizziness, diarrhea, a feeling of warmth, nausea, light-headedness, fatigue and lethargy, itching, rash, flushing, changes in certain blood-cell components, and headache.

▼ Rare: fainting, heart failure, heart attack, abnormal heart rhythms, stroke, numbness, drowsiness, nervousness, depression, paranoia, memory loss, hallucinations, psychoses, visual disturbances, sleeplessness, tingling in the hands or feet, heart palpitations, constipation, stomach upset and cramps, vomiting, dry mouth, frequent urination (especially at night), sweating, reduced sex drive or poor sexual performance, leg and foot cramps, muscle cramps and inflammation, joint pains, sore throat, and cough. Isradipine can cause increases in certain blood enzyme tests.

Drug Interactions

• Isradipine may interact with beta-blocking drugs to cause heart failure, very low blood pressure, or an increased incidence of angina pain. However, in many cases these drugs have been taken together with no problem.

• Taking Isradipine and Fentanyl (a narcotic pain reliever) together can result in very low blood pressure.

Food Interactions

Taking Isradipine with food has a minor effect on the absorption of the drug. You may take it with food if it upsets your stomach. Avoid drinking grapefruit juice if you are taking this medicine.

Usual Dose

5 to 20 mg per day in 2 doses.

Do not stop taking the drug abruptly. The dosage should be gradually reduced over a period of time.

Overdosage

Overdose of Isradipine can cause nausea, dizziness, weakness, drowsiness, confusion and slurred speech, very low blood pressure, reduced heart efficiency, and unusual heart rhythms. Victims of an Isradipine overdose should be taken to a hospital emergency room for treatment. ALWAYS bring the medicine bottle with you.

Special Information

Call your doctor if you develop swelling in the arms or legs, difficulty breathing, abnormal heartbeat, increased heart pains, dizziness, constipation, nausea, light-headedness, or very low blood pressure.

If you forget to take a dose of Isradipine, take it as soon as you remember. If it is almost time for your next regularly scheduled dose, skip the forgotten dose and continue with your regular schedule. Do not take a double dose.

Special Populations

Pregnancy/Breast-feeding

Laboratory studies found Isradipine to affect the development of animal fetuses in laboratory studies. It has not been found to cause human birth defects. Nevertheless, pregnant women, or those who might become pregnant while taking this drug, should not take Isradipine without their doctor's approval. When the drug is considered essential by your doctor, the potential benefit of taking the medicine must be carefully weighed against its risk.

It is not known if Isradipine passes into breast milk. Women who must take Isradipine should consider the possible effect of the drug on their infants before breast-feeding.

Seniors

Older adults may actually absorb more Isradipine than younger adults and may release the drug more slowly from their bodies. Follow your doctor's directions and report any side effects at once.

Generic Name

Itraconazole

Brand Name

Sporanox

Type of Drug

Antifungal.

Prescribed for

Fungal infections (blastomycosis and histoplasmosis) in normal and immuno-deficient people. Itraconazole is also effective against a number of common superficial fungal infections of the skin that don't respond to other medicines, and against many blood-borne fungal infections.

General Information

Itraconazole is effective against a broad variety of fungal organisms. The broad range of its effectiveness may make it an important therapy for people with AIDS or cancer whose immune systems are compromised. It works by inhibiting important enzyme systems in the organisms it attacks. Drug treatment must be continued for at least 3 months until the fungal infection subsides. This drug is broken down in the liver, but the effect of liver disease on Itraconazole is not known.

Cautions and Warnings

The **combination of Itraconazole and either Astemizole or Terfenadine,** nonsedating antihistamines, can cause severe cardiac side effects and should be avoided.

Do not take Itraconazole if you have had an **allergic** reaction to it. People who are allergic to similar antifungals (**Ketoconazole, Miconazole, and Fluconazole**) may also be allergic to Itraconazole, although cross-reactions are uncommon.

On rare occasions, Itraconazole causes **reversible liver damage.** It should be used with caution by people who already have **liver disease.** In studies with laboratory animals, Itraconazole caused an increase in lung tumors.

Possible Side Effects

▼ Most common: nausea, vomiting, and rash.

▼ Less common: diarrhea, abdominal pain, appetite loss, swelling in the legs or feet, fatigue, fever, feeling sick, itching, headache, dizziness, reduced sex drive, tiredness, high blood pressure, liver or kidney function abnormalities, low blood potassium, and male impotence.

▼ Rare: stomach gas, sleeplessness, depression, ringing or buzzing in the ears, and swollen or painful breasts (both sexes).

Drug Interactions

• People who have taken Terfenadine with Itraconazole have experienced severe cardiac side effects. DO NOT TAKE THIS COMBINATION. This restriction also applies to the combination of Astemizole and Itraconazole.

• Itraconazole increases the effects of Cyclosporine, Digoxin, oral antidiabetes drugs (except Metformin), and Warfarin. Your doctor should evaluate your dosage of these drugs if you start taking Itraconazole. Important dosage adjustments may be needed!

• Cimetidine, Ranitidine, Famotidine, Nizatidine, Isoniazid, Phenytoin, and Rifampin can reduce the amount of Itraconazole in your blood, possibly interfering with its effectiveness.

• Itraconazole may increase the effect of Phenytoin by reducing the rate at which Phenytoin is broken down in the body.

Food Interactions

Itraconazole should be taken with food or meals.

Usual Dose

Adult: 200 to 600 mg once per day.

Child (age 3 to 16 years): 100 mg per day has been used, but the long-term effects of Itraconazole in children are not known.

Overdosage

Symptoms of Itraconazole overdose may include any of the drug's side effects; liver toxicity is especially important. Call your doctor, local poison control center, or hospital emergency room for more information. ALWAYS take the medicine bottle with you.

Special Information

Itraconazole must be taken for at least 3 months to determine its effectiveness. Taking this medicine for less than the prescribed time may lead to recurrence of the original infection.

Call your doctor if you develop unusual fatigue, yellowing of the skin or eyes, nausea or vomiting, loss of appetite, dark urine or pale stools, or unusually bothersome or persistent side effects.

If you forget to take a dose of Itraconazole, take it as soon as you remember. If it is almost time for your next dose, skip the missed one and continue with your regular schedule. Do not take a double dose.

Special Populations

Pregnancy/Breast-feeding

Animal studies have shown that doses of Itraconazole 5 to 20 times the human dose cause damage to the developing fetus. The drug's effect in humans is not known. Pregnant women should not use Itraconazole unless the possible benefits have first been carefully weighed against the risks.

Itraconazole passes into breast milk. Nursing mothers should bottle-feed their babies if they must take this drug.

Seniors

Older adults may use this drug without special restriction. Report any side effects to the doctor at once.

K-Dur

see **Potassium Replacement Products**, page 919

Generic Name

Ketoconazole

Brand Name

Nizoral Cream/Tablets/Shampoo

Type of Drug

Antifungal.

Prescribed for

Thrush and other systemic fungus infections, including candidiasis, histoplasmosis, and blastomycosis. Ketoconazole may also be prescribed for fungus infections of the skin, fingernails, and vagina. High-dose Ketoconazole may be effective in treating fungus infections of the brain. The drug has been studied for the treatment of advanced prostate cancer and Cushing's syndrome. Ketoconazole shampoo is used for dandruff.

General Information

This medicine is effective against a wide variety of fungus organisms. It works by disrupting the fungus cell's membrane, ultimately destroying the cell.

Cautions and Warnings

Ketoconazole has been associated with **liver inflammation and damage:** At least 1 of every 10,000 people who take this drug will develop this condition. In most cases, the inflammation subsides when the drug is discontinued.

Do not take Ketoconazole if you have had an **allergic** reaction to it.

It should not be used to treat **fungus infections of the nervous system** because only small amounts of the drug will enter that part of the body.

In studies of Ketoconazole in **prostate cancer,** 11 people died within 2 weeks of starting high-dose Ketoconazole treatment. The reasons for these deaths are not known but may be related to the fact that the medication can suppress the natural production of adrenal corticosteroid hormones.

Ketoconazole reduces **male testosterone levels** and reduces the amount of **natural corticosteroid hormone** produced by your body.

On rare occasions, people taking Ketoconazole for the first time experience **serious, life-threatening reactions including itching, rash, and breathing difficulty**. Victims of this rare reaction must be given emergency treatment at once.

Possible Side Effects

▼ Common: nausea, vomiting, upset stomach, abdominal pain or discomfort, itching, swelling of male breasts. Most of these side effects are mild, and only a small number of people (1.5 percent) have to stop taking the drug because of severe side effects.

▼ Less common: headache, dizziness, drowsiness or tiredness, fever, chills, unusual sensitivity to bright light, diarrhea, male impotence, and reduced levels of blood platelets. Reduced sperm counts have been associated with Ketoconazole, but only at drug doses above 400 mg a day.

Drug Interactions

• Antacids, histamine H_2 antagonists (including Cimetidine, Ranitidine, and others), and other drugs that reduce the acid in the stomach will counteract the effects of Ketoconazole by preventing it from being absorbed. This drug requires an acid environment to pass into the blood.

• When Ketoconazole is taken together with Rifampin, the effect of both drugs may be reduced.

• The combination of Isoniazid and Ketoconazole causes a neutralization of the Ketoconazole's effect. These interactions occur even when drug doses are separated by 12 hours.

• Ketoconazole increases the amount of Cyclosporine in the bloodstream and the chances for kidney damage caused by Cyclosporine. It also increases the effect of oral anticoagulant (blood-thinning) drugs. Ketoconazole increases the blood levels of Cisapride and of the antihistamines Terfenadine and Astemizole, which leads to an increased chance of developing serious cardiac side effects from those drugs.

• Taking Ketoconazole and Phenytoin can affect the amount of either medicine in your blood, increasing or decreasing either drug's effect.

• Ketoconazole may decrease blood Theophylline levels, possibly precipitating an asthmatic attack. Your doctor can adjust your Theophylline dose.

• Ketoconazole may increase the amount of oral corticosteroid drug absorbed into the bloodstream while slowing its removal from the body, possibly leading to more corticosteroid side effects.

Food Interactions

Food stimulates acid release, and Ketoconazole is absorbed much more efficiently when there is acid in the stomach. Take Ketoconazole with food or meals to improve absorption and avoid stomach upset.

Usual Dose

Tablets
Adult: 200 to 400 mg taken once a day. Dosage may continue for several months, depending on the type of infection being treated.

Child (age 2 and older): 1.5 to 3 mg per pound of body weight once a day.

Child (under age 2): do not use.

Cream
Apply to affected and immediate surrounding areas 1 or 2 times a day for 14 days.

Overdosage

The most likely effects of Ketoconazole overdose are liver damage and exaggerated side effects. Victims of overdose should immediately be given Bicarbonate of Soda or any other antacid to reduce the amount of drug absorbed into the blood. Call your local poison control center for more information. If you take the victim to a hospital emergency room for treatment, ALWAYS bring the prescription bottle with you.

Special Information

If you must take antacids or other ulcer treatments, separate doses of those medicines from Ketoconazole by at least 2 hours. Anything that reduces your stomach-acid levels will reduce the amount of Ketoconazole absorbed into the blood.

This drug can cause headaches, dizziness, and drowsiness. Use caution while doing anything that requires intense concentration, like driving or operating machinery.

Call your doctor if you develop pains in the stomach or abdomen, severe diarrhea, a high fever, unusual tiredness, loss of appetite, nausea, vomiting, yellow discoloration of the skin or whites of the eyes, pale stools, or dark urine.

If you forget to take a dose of Ketoconazole, take it as soon as you remember. If it is almost time for your next regularly scheduled dose, space the missed dose and the next dose 10 to 12 hours apart. Then go back to your regular schedule. **Do not take a double dose.**

Special Populations

Pregnancy/Breast-feeding
Ketoconazole, in doses larger than the maximum human dose, has caused damage to developing animal fetuses. This drug should be avoided by pregnant women or women who may become pregnant unless the potential risk of the drug has been carefully weighed against any possible benefit.

Nursing mothers who must take Ketoconazole should bottle-feed their infants because the drug passes into breast milk.

Seniors
Older adults may take this medication without special restriction. Follow your doctor's directions and report any side effects at once.

Generic Name

Ketoprofen

Brand Names
Actron (available over-the-counter)
Orudis*
Orudis KT (available over-the-counter)
Oruvail Controlled-Release Capsules

(*Also available in generic form)

Type of Drug

Nonsteroidal anti-inflammatory drug (NSAID).

Prescribed for

Rheumatoid arthritis, juvenile rheumatoid arthritis, osteoarthritis, mild to moderate pain, menstrual pain, menstrual headaches, sunburn treatment, and migraine prevention. Controlled-release Ketoprofen is prescribed only for various forms of arthritis.

General Information

Ketoprofen is one of 16 nonsteroidal anti-inflammatory drugs (NSAIDs) that are used to relieve pain and inflammation. We do not know exactly how NSAIDs work, but part of their action may be due to an ability to inhibit the body's production of a hormone called *prostaglandin* and to inhibit the action of other body chemicals, including cyclo-oxygenase, lipoxygenase, leukotrienes, lysosomal enzymes, and a host of other factors. NSAIDs are generally absorbed into the bloodstream fairly quickly. Pain relief generally comes within an hour after taking the first dose, but the NSAIDs' anti-inflammatory effect generally takes a lot longer (several days to 2 weeks) to become apparent, and may take a month or more to reach maximum effect. Controlled-release Ketoprofen is not recommended for acute pain relief, because it can take up to 7 hours to reach its maximum concentration in the blood. Ketoprofen is broken down in the liver and eliminated from the body through the kidneys. Low-dose Ketoprofen is sold without a prescription for fever and pain under the name *Actron*.

Cautions and Warnings

People who are **allergic** to Ketoprofen (or any other NSAID) and those with a history of **asthma attacks** brought on by an NSAID, iodides, or Aspirin should not take Ketoprofen.

Ketoprofen can cause **gastrointestinal (GI) bleeding, ulcers,** and **stomach perforation**. This can occur at any time, with or without warning, in people who take chronic Ketoprofen treatment. People with a **history of active GI bleeding** should be cautious about taking any NSAID. **Minor stomach upset, distress,** or **gas** is common during the first few days of treatment with Ketoprofen. People who develop **bleeding** or

ulcers and continue treatment should be aware of the possibility of developing more serious drug toxicity.

Ketoprofen can affect **platelets** and **blood clotting** at high doses, and should be avoided by people with clotting problems and by those taking Warfarin.

People with **heart problems** who use Ketoprofen may experience swelling in their arms, legs, or feet.

Ketoprofen can cause severe toxic effects to the **kidney**. Report any unusual side effects to your doctor, who may need to periodically test your kidney function.

Ketoprofen can make you **unusually sensitive to the effects of the sun** (photosensitivity).

Possible Side Effects

▼ Most common: diarrhea, nausea, vomiting, constipation, stomach gas, stomach upset or irritation, and loss of appetite.

▼ Less common: stomach ulcers, GI bleeding, hepatitis, gallbladder attacks, painful urination, poor kidney function, kidney inflammation, blood and protein in the urine, dizziness, fainting, nervousness, depression, hallucinations, confusion, disorientation, light-headedness, tingling in the hands or feet, itching, increased sweating, dry nose and mouth, heart palpitations, chest pain, difficulty breathing, and muscle cramps.

▼ Rare: severe allergic reactions, including closing of the throat, fever and chills, changes in liver function, jaundice (yellowing of the skin or eyes), and kidney failure. People who experience such effects must be promptly treated in a hospital emergency room or doctor's office.

NSAIDs have caused severe skin reactions; if this happens to you, see your doctor immediately.

Drug Interactions

• Ketoprofen can increase the effects of oral anticoagulant (blood-thinning) drugs, such as Warfarin. You may take this combination, but your doctor may have to reduce your anticoagulant dose.

• Taking Ketoprofen with Cyclosporine may increase the toxic kidney effects of both drugs. Methotrexate toxicity may be increased in people also taking Ketoprofen.

• Ketoprofen may reduce the blood-pressure-lowering effect of beta blockers and loop diuretic drugs.

• Ketoprofen may increase blood levels of Phenytoin, leading to increased Phenytoin side effects. Blood-Lithium levels may be increased in people taking Ketoprofen.

• Ketoprofen blood levels may be affected by Cimetidine because of that drug's effect on the liver.

• Probenecid may interfere with the elimination of Ketoprofen from the body, increasing the chances for Ketoprofen toxic reactions.

• Aspirin and other salicylates may decrease the amount of Ketoprofen in your blood. These medicines should never be taken at the same time.

Food Interactions

Take Ketoprofen with food or a magnesium/aluminum antacid if it upsets your stomach.

Usual Dose

Capsules

Adult: 50 to 75 mg 3 or 4 times per day. No more than 300 mg per day.

Seniors and those with kidney problems: start with ⅓ to ½ the usual dose.

Controlled-Release Capsules

Adult and Senior: 200 mg once per day.

Overdosage

People have died from NSAID overdoses. The most common signs of overdosage are drowsiness, nausea, vomiting, diarrhea, abdominal pain, rapid breathing, rapid heartbeat, increased sweating, ringing or buzzing in the ears, confusion, disorientation, stupor, and coma.

Take the overdose victim to a hospital emergency room at once. ALWAYS bring the medicine bottle with you.

Special Information

Ketoprofen can make you drowsy and/or tired: Be careful

when driving or operating hazardous equipment. Take each dose with a full glass of water, and don't lie down for 15 to 30 minutes after you take the medicine. Do not take any nonprescription products with Acetaminophen or Aspirin while taking this drug; also, avoid alcoholic beverages.

Contact your doctor if you develop skin rash or itching, visual disturbances, weight gain, breathing difficulty, fluid retention, hallucinations, black or tarry stools, persistent headache, or any unusual or intolerable side effects.

If you miss a Ketoprofen dose, take it as soon as you remember. If you take several doses a day and it is within 4 hours of your next dose, skip the one you forgot and continue with your regular schedule. If you take Ketoprofen once a day and it is within 8 hours of your next dose, skip the missed dose and continue with your regular schedule. Do not take a double dose.

Special Populations

Pregnancy/Breast-feeding

NSAIDs may cross into the fetal blood circulation. They have not been found to cause birth defects, but may affect a developing fetal heart during the second half of pregnancy; animal studies indicate a possible effect. Women who are or might become pregnant should not take Ketoprofen without their doctor's approval; pregnant women should be particularly cautious about using this drug during the last 3 months of their pregnancy. When the drug is considered essential by your doctor, its potential benefits must be carefully weighed against its risks.

NSAIDs may pass into breast milk but have caused no problems among breast-fed infants, except for seizures in a baby whose mother was taking Indomethacin. Other NSAIDs have caused problems in animal studies. There is a possibility that a nursing mother taking Ketoprofen could affect her baby's heart or cardiovascular system. If you must take Ketoprofen, bottle-feed your baby.

Seniors

Older adults may be more susceptible to Ketoprofen side effects, especially ulcer disease.

Generic Name

Ketorolac

Brand Names

Acular Eye Drops
Toradol

Type of Drug

Nonsteroidal anti-inflammatory drug (NSAID).

Prescribed for

Short-term treatment of moderately severe pain that has required narcotic pain relievers. Ketorolac tablets should only be taken by people who have first been treated with Ketorolac injection. Total treatment with injectable and oral Ketorolac should not exceed 5 days. Ketorolac eyedrops are prescribed for eye redness and inflammation caused by seasonal allergies.

General Information

Ketorolac is one of 16 NSAIDs used to relieve pain and inflammation. Unlike the others in this group, Ketorolac is a potent drug with many risks (see *Cautions and Warnings*) that can be serious in some people. Taking more than is prescribed only increases risk; it does not offer the possibility of better results. NSAID eyedrops may be used during eye surgery to prevent movement of the eye muscles. Other NSAID eyedrops (including Diclofenac, Flurbiprofen, and Suprofen) are also prescribed during eye surgery, for inflammation following cataract extraction, and for itching and redness caused by seasonal allergies.

We do not know exactly how NSAIDs work, but part of their action may be due to an ability to inhibit the body's production of a hormone called *prostaglandin* and to inhibit the action of other body chemicals, including cyclo-oxygenase, lipoxygenase, leukotrienes, lysosomal enzymes, and a host of other factors. Ketorolac is absorbed into the bloodstream fairly quickly. Pain relief comes within an hour after taking the first dose.

Cautions and Warnings

People who are **allergic** to Ketorolac (or any other NSAID) and those with a history of **asthma attacks** brought on by another NSAID, Iodides, or Aspirin should not take Ketorolac.

Ketorolac can cause **gastrointestinal (GI) bleeding, ulcers, and stomach perforation.** This can occur at any time, with or without warning, in people who take chronic Ketorolac treatment. People with a **history of active GI bleeding** should be cautious about taking any NSAID. **Minor stomach upset, distress,** or **gas** is common during the first few days of treatment with Ketorolac. People who develop **bleeding** or **ulcers** and continue treatment should be aware of the possibility of developing more serious drug toxicity.

Ketorolac can affect **platelets** and **blood clotting** at high doses, and should be avoided by people with clotting problems and by those taking Warfarin.

People with **heart problems** who use Ketorolac may experience swelling in their arms, legs, or feet.

Ketorolac may actually cause **headaches.** If this happens, you may have to stop taking this medicine or switch to another NSAID.

Ketorolac can cause severe toxic effects to the **kidney.** Report any unusual side effects to your doctor, who may need to periodically test your kidney function.

Ketorolac can make you **unusually sensitive to the effects of the sun** (photosensitivity).

People taking this drug on a regular basis should have their **liver function** checked periodically.

Possible Side Effects

▼ Most common: diarrhea, nausea, vomiting, constipation, stomach gas, stomach upset or irritation, and loss of appetite (injectable and oral); temporary burning, stinging, or other minor eye irritation (eyedrops).

▼ Less common: stomach ulcers, GI bleeding, hepatitis, gallbladder attacks, painful urination, poor kidney function, kidney inflammation, blood and protein in the urine, dizziness, fainting, nervousness, depression, hallucinations, confusion, disorientation, tingling in the hands or feet, light-headedness, itching, increased sweating, dry nose and mouth, heart palpitations, chest pain, difficulty breathing, and muscle cramps (injectable and oral); nau-

Possible Side Effects *(continued)*

sea, vomiting, viral infections, and eye reactions (longer-lasting eye redness, burning, itching, or tearing) (eye-drops).

▼ Rare: severe allergic reactions, including closing of the throat, fever and chills, changes in liver function, jaundice (yellowing of the skin or eyes), and kidney failure. People who experience such effects must be promptly treated in a hospital emergency room or doctor's office.

NSAIDs have caused severe skin reactions; if this happens to you, see your doctor immediately.

The risk of developing bleeding problems or other body-wide side effects with Ketorolac eyedrops is small because only a small amount of this drug is absorbed into the blood.

Drug Interactions

• Ketorolac can increase the effects of oral anticoagulant (blood-thinning) medicines, such as Warfarin. You may take this combination; however, your doctor may have to reduce your anticoagulant dose.

• Taking Ketorolac with Cyclosporine may increase the toxic kidney effects of both drugs. Methotrexate toxicity may be increased in people also taking Ketorolac.

• Ketorolac may reduce the blood-pressure-lowering effect of beta blockers and loop diuretics.

• Ketorolac may increase blood levels of Phenytoin, leading to increased Phenytoin side effects. Blood-Lithium levels may be increased in people taking Ketorolac.

• Ketorolac blood levels may be affected by Cimetidine because of that drug's effect on the liver.

• Probenecid may interfere with the body's elimination of Ketorolac, increasing the chances for Ketorolac toxic reactions.

• Aspirin and other salicylates may decrease the amount of Ketorolac in your blood. These medicines should never be taken at the same time.

• No drug interactions have been reported with Ketorolac eyedrops.

Food Interactions

Take Ketorolac with food or a magnesium/aluminum antacid if it upsets your stomach.

Usual Dose

Tablets
Up to 40 mg per day for no more than 5 days in a row.

Eyedrops
1 drop 4 times per day for itching and irritation caused by seasonal allergies.

Overdosage

People have died from NSAID overdoses. The most common signs of overdosage are drowsiness, nausea, vomiting, diarrhea, abdominal pain, rapid breathing, rapid heartbeat, increased sweating, ringing or buzzing in the ears, confusion, disorientation, stupor, and coma. Take the victim to a hospital emergency room at once. ALWAYS bring the medicine bottle with you.

Special Information

Ketorolac can make you drowsy and/or tired: Be careful when driving or operating hazardous equipment. Take each dose with a full glass of water, and don't lie down for 15 to 30 minutes after you take the medicine. Do not take any nonprescription products with Acetaminophen or Aspirin while taking this drug; also, avoid alcoholic beverages.

Contact your doctor if you develop skin rash or itching, visual disturbances, weight gain, breathing difficulty, fluid retention, hallucinations, black or tarry stools, persistent headache, or any unusual or intolerable side effects.

If you forget to take a dose of Ketorolac tablets, take it as soon as you remember. If you take several doses a day and it is within 4 hours of your next dose, skip the one you forgot and continue with your regular schedule. If you take your medicine once a day and it is within 8 hours of your next dose, skip the missed dose and continue with your regular schedule. Do not take a double dose.

To self-administer the eyedrops, lie down or tilt your head back. Hold the dropper above your eye and drop the medicine inside your lower lid while looking up. To prevent possible infection, don't allow the dropper to touch your fingers, eyelids, or any surface. Release the lower lid and keep your eye open. Don't blink for about 30 seconds. Press gently on the bridge of your nose at the inside corner of your eye for about a minute to help circulate the medicine around your eye. Wait at least 5 minutes before using any other eyedrops.

If you forget a dose of Ketorolac eyedrops, take it as soon as you remember. If it is almost time for your next dose, skip the missed dose and continue with your regular schedule. Do not take a double dose.

Special Populations

Pregnancy/Breast-feeding
Ketorolac should not be taken by women who are pregnant because the drug can affect blood circulation in the fetus and prevent normal labor.

There is a possibility that a nursing mother taking Ketorolac could affect her baby's heart or cardiovascular system. If you must take Ketorolac, bottle-feed your baby.

Seniors
Older adults may be more susceptible to Ketorolac side effects, especially ulcer disease.

Klonopin

see *Clonazepam*, page 235

Generic Name
Labetalol Hydrochloride

Brand Names
Normodyne
Trandate

Type of Drug
Adrenergic blocker; antihypertensive.

Prescribed for

High blood pressure.

General Information

Labetolol, first studied for its effect as a beta blocker, is a unique approach to high-blood-pressure treatment because it selectively blocks both alpha- and beta-adrenergic impulses. This combination of actions contributes to its ability to reduce your blood pressure. It may be better than other beta-blocking drugs because it rarely affects heart rate. Other drugs can increase or decrease heart rate.

Cautions and Warnings

People with **asthma, severe heart failure, reduced heart rate,** and **heart block** should not take Labetalol Hydrochloride. **People with angina** who take Labetalol for high blood pressure should have their dose reduced gradually over a 1- to 2-week period, instead of having it discontinued suddenly, to avoid possible aggravation of the angina. Labetalol should be used with caution if you have **liver disease** because your ability to eliminate the drug from your body may be impaired.

Possible Side Effects

Side effects with Labetalol develop early in the course of treatment and increase with larger doses.

▼ Most common: dizziness, tingling of the scalp, nausea, vomiting, upset stomach, taste distortion, fatigue, sweating, male impotence, urinary difficulty, diarrhea, bile-duct blockage, bronchial spasm, breathing difficulty, muscle weakness, cramps, dry eyes, blurred vision, rash, facial swelling, and hair loss.

▼ Less common: aggravation of lupus erythematosus (a disease of the body's connective tissue), stuffy nose, depression, confusion, disorientation, loss of short-term memory, emotional instability, colitis, drug allergy (fever, sore throat, breathing difficulty), and reduction in the levels of white blood cells and blood platelets.

Drug Interactions

• Labetalol may prevent normal signs of low blood sugar from appearing and can also interfere with the action of oral antidiabetes drugs.

• The combination of Labetalol and a tricyclic antidepressant drug can cause tremor.

• This drug may interfere with the effectiveness of some antiasthma drugs, especially Ephedrine, Isoproterenol, and other beta stimulants.

• Cimetidine increases the amount of Labetalol absorbed into the bloodstream from oral tablets.

• Glutethimide decreases the amount of Labetalol in the blood by increasing the rate at which it is broken down by your liver.

• Labetalol may increase the blood-pressure-lowering effect of Nitroglycerin.

Food Interactions

This medicine may be taken with food if it upsets your stomach. In fact, food increases the amount of Labetalol absorbed into the blood.

Usual Dose

The usual starting dose is 100 mg taken twice per day. The dosage may be increased gradually to as much as 1200 mg twice per day, but the usual maintenance dose is in the range of 200 to 400 mg twice daily.

Overdosage

Labetalol overdose slows your heart rate and causes an excessive blood-pressure drop. The possible consequences of these effects can be treated only in a hospital emergency room. ALWAYS bring the medicine bottle with you.

Special Information

You may experience scalp tingling, especially when you first start taking Labetalol.

This medication is meant to be taken on a continuing basis. Do not stop it unless instructed to do so by your doctor.

Weakness; swelling of your ankles, feet, or legs; breathing difficulty; or other side effects should be reported to your doctor as soon as possible. Most side effects are not serious, but a small number of people (about 7 in 100) have to switch to another medicine because of drug side effects.

If you forget to take a dose of Labetalol, take it as soon as possible. However, if it is within 8 hours of your next dose, skip the forgotten dose and go back to your regular schedule. Do not take a double dose.

Special Populations

Pregnancy/Breast-feeding
This drug crosses into the fetal blood circulation. It has not been found to cause birth defects. However, pregnant women and those who might become pregnant should not take this drug without their doctor's approval. When the drug is considered essential by your doctor, its possible benefits must be carefully weighed against its potential risks.

This drug passes into breast milk but has caused no problems among breast-fed infants. Nursing mothers who must take this medicine may want to bottle-feed their babies.

Seniors
Seniors may be more sensitive to the effects of this medicine. Your dosage of this drug must be adjusted to your individual needs by your doctor, especially if you have liver disease. Seniors may be more likely to suffer from cold hands and feet and reduced body temperature, chest pains, a general feeling of ill health, sudden difficulty in breathing, sweating, or changes in heartbeat because of this medicine.

Generic Name

Lamivudine

Brand Name

Epivir (also known as 3TC)

Type of Drug

Antiviral.

Prescribed for

HIV infection.

General Information

Lamivudine is a nucleoside-type antiviral that works on HIV in the same way as Zalcitabine (ddC), Zidovudine, Stavudine, and other drugs of this type. It is only given in combination with Zidovudine for people who do not respond to that drug alone. Lamivudine is rapidly absorbed into the blood, and most of it passes out of the body in urine.

Cautions and Warnings

Do not take this medicine if you are **sensitive** or **allergic** to Lamivudine. People with **kidney disease** need less Lamivudine than those with normal kidneys.

Possible Side Effects

Since Lamivudine is taken with Zidovudine, the listed side effects are those of the drug combination. The long-term effects of Lamivudine are not known.

▼ Most common: headache, feelings of ill health, fever, chills, skin rash, nausea, vomiting, diarrhea, loss of appetite, abdominal pain or cramps, nervous-system problems (tingling, poor coordination), sleeplessness, dizziness, depression, stuffy or runny nose, cough, and muscle pain.

▼ Common: upset stomach, joint pains, and tingling in the hands or feet (in children). Lamivudine can also affect a variety of blood tests.

▼ Rare: pancreas irritation (children taking Lamivudine develop this side effect much more often than adults).

Drug Interactions

• Lamivudine increases maximum blood levels of Zidovudine by 39 percent. This is helpful in fighting HIV.

• Trimethoprim/Sulfamethoxazole (taken for opportunistic infections of AIDS) increases the amount of Lamivudine in the blood.

Food Interactions

Lamivudine is absorbed more slowly when taken with food,

but not enough to affect the total amount of drug in the blood.

Usual Dose

Adult and adolescent (age 12 and older): 150 mg twice a day in combination with Zidovudine. Adults weighing less than 110 pounds should receive about 1 mg per pound twice a day. Dosage is reduced as kidney function decreases.

Child (3 months to 11 years): about 2 mg per pound twice a day, no more than 150 mg per dose.

Overdosage

There has been only one reported case of Lamivudine overdose; no side effects were noted. Call your local poison center for more information.

Special Information

Lamivudine, like other HIV medicines, does not cure AIDS. People taking this medicine will still develop opportunistic infections and other complications of AIDS. This drug does not reduce the risk of transmitting HIV to others.

It is very important to take this drug exactly as prescribed. If you forget a dose, take it as soon as you remember. If it is almost time for your next dose, skip the forgotten dose and continue with your regular schedule. Call your doctor if you forget 2 or more doses in a row.

Call your doctor at once if your child develops signs of pancreas inflammation while taking Lamivudine, including very severe abdominal pain, tense abdominal muscles, sweating, feeling very ill, shallow and rapid breathing, fever, and possible fainting.

Special Populations

Pregnancy/Breast-feeding

Lamivudine passes into the blood circulation of the developing fetus. Some animal studies of the drug indicated that it may be dangerous to the developing fetus, but others showed no effect. There is no information about the effects of Lamivudine in pregnant women, but it should only be taken during pregnancy if absolutely necessary. The manufacturer has organized a registry to help track what happens to pregnant women who take this medicine.

It is not known if Lamivudine passes into breast milk. Nursing mothers who must take this medicine should bottle-feed their babies.

Seniors

Older adults may require less Lamivudine, according to their kidney function. Otherwise, this medicine may be taken by seniors without special restriction.

Generic Name

Lamotrigine

Brand Name

Lamictal

Type of Drug

Anticonvulsant.

Prescribed for

Lamotrigine is used as add-on therapy for adult epilepsy and partial seizures.

General Information

Much like Phenytoin and Carbamazepine, Lamotrigine works on voltage-dependent channels in the brain to stabilize them and prevent the release of chemicals that can stimulate the nervous system and lead to a seizure. Lamotrigine is one of the first new antiseizure medicines available in more than 10 years.

Lamotrigine is absorbed rapidly into the bloodstream after you take it, reaching maximum blood concentration in 1½ to 5 hours. Lamotrigine is eliminated from the body by the liver, but the process can be affected by other drugs (see *Drug Interactions*).

Cautions and Warnings

During studies leading to the approval of Lamotrigine in the United States, a few people died from acute **liver failure** or **multi-organ failure**. Although all the people affected were taking Lamotrigine, it is not known if the drug played a role in these deaths.

Lamotrigine binds to melanin, a body hormone commonly found in the skin and eyes. The long-term effect of Lamotrigine on the eyes is not known.

Possible Side Effects

Lamotrigine is considered relatively safe, and its potential for producing toxic side effects is considered relatively small. Side effects are most common during the first few weeks of treatment and tend to resolve on their own in a few weeks.

▼ Common: dizziness, blurred or double vision, weakness, nausea, and vomiting. These effects are related to the amount of drug in your system and so are more likely to occur with a larger daily dose.

▼ Other: headache, sleepiness, skin rash, and pain.

Several kinds of skin rash can occur with Lamotrigine. Skin rash is more likely to occur with large doses and rapid dosage increases and may be more common in people taking Lamotrigine together with Valproate Sodium.

Drug Interactions

• Lamotrigine increases the rate at which Sodium Valproate is eliminated from the body.

• People taking both Carbamazepine and Lamotrigine may experience more drug side effects.

• Acetaminophen and Lamotrigine are broken down by the same system in the liver. Taking Acetaminophen at the same time as Lamotrigine can slightly increase the rate at which Lamotrigine is broken down, but occasional use of the two drugs together is not likely to be a problem. Regular users of Acetaminophen may need adjustment of their Lamotrigine dosage.

• Unlike other medicines for seizure control, Lamotrigine does not seem to interact with oral contraceptives.

Food Interactions

Lamotrigine may be taken without regard to food or meals.

You may take it with food or meals to prevent nausea and vomiting.

Usual Dose

Adult and child (over age 12): 25 or 50 mg a day to start, increased gradually to a maximum daily dose of 500 mg. Lamotrigine is usually taken twice a day. Be sure to take your doses 12 hours apart.

Child (age 12 and under): not recommended.

Overdosage

The most likely immediate effects of Lamotrigine overdose are dizziness, blurred or double vision, weakness, nausea, and vomiting. The overdose victim should be taken to a hospital emergency room at once for treatment. ALWAYS bring the medicine bottle with you.

Special Information

Once you start taking Lamotrigine, your liver may actually increase the rate at which it breaks down the drug, possibly increasing your dosage requirement. Your doctor will have to check your drug blood levels periodically to see if any dosage changes are needed.

Call your doctor at once if you develop a skin rash, but do not change your Lamotrigine dosage or stop taking it on your own.

Lamotrigine can cause drowsiness, dizziness, or blurred vision, effects that are increased by alcoholic beverages. Be careful when driving or doing anything else that requires intense concentration, alertness, and physical dexterity.

If you take Acetaminophen while on Lamotrigine (especially for a Lamotrigine-associated headache), do not take more than the amount of Acetaminophen specified in the package directions.

If you take Lamotrigine once a day and forget to take a dose, take it as soon as you remember. If it is within 8 hours of your next dose, skip the one you forgot and continue with your regular schedule. Do not take a double dose.

After the first 2 weeks of treatment, most people take Lamotrigine twice a day. If you take it twice a day, be sure to take your medicine every 12 hours. If you take Lamotrigine twice a day and forget a dose, take it as soon as you remember. If it is within 4 hours of your next dose, take one dose as soon as you remember and another in 5 or 6 hours, then go back to your regular schedule.

Special Populations

Pregnancy/Breast-feeding

Animal studies have shown no evidence of causing birth defects, but the effect of Lamotrigine on the developing human fetus is not known. A higher incidence of birth malformations has generally been noted among women with seizure disorders.

Lamotrigine passes into breast milk, but its effect on a nursing infant is unknown. If you are nursing and taking this medicine, discuss with your doctor the possibility of taking another seizure medicine or bottle-feeding your baby.

Seniors

Older adults handle Lamotrigine in much the same way as younger people. You may take it in the same dosage as younger adults.

Lanoxin

see **Digitalis Glycosides**, page 338

Generic Name

Lansoprazole

Brand Name

Prevacid

Type of Drug

Stomach-acid inhibitor; antiulcer.

Prescribed for

Duodenal ulcer, esophagitis, Zollinger-Ellison syndrome.

General Information

Lansoprazole is only the second drug available in the United States (the first was Omeprazole) that interferes with the so-called "proton-pump" in the mucous lining of the stomach. This is the last stage of acid production and, as a result of this effect, Lansoprazole can turn off stomach acid production within 1 hour after it is taken. Lansoprazole is accepted in the United States for short-term treatment of duodenal ulcers (up to 4 weeks) and corrosive esophagitis (up to 8 weeks), a condition in which stomach contents flow backward into the esophagus (the pipe that connects the throat to the stomach), resulting in erosion of the esophagus by stomach acid. This medicine is also approved for other conditions in which stomach acid plays a key role or in which excess stomach acid is produced as a part of the condition; Zollinger-Ellison syndrome is the most common of these. Lansoprazole has not yet been accepted for treatment of stomach ulcers, although Omeprazole is widely prescribed for that purpose.

Cautions and Warnings

Do not take this drug if you are **sensitive** or **allergic** to it. Animal studies indicate that long-term use of this medicine can be related to an increase in **stomach tumors,** but it is not known if this is also a problem for humans. Lansoprazole relieves symptoms very quickly, but this may not mean that the underlying problem has been solved.

Possible Side Effects

Generally, Lansoprazole causes relatively few side effects.

▼ Most common: diarrhea.

▼ Less common: nausea, abdominal pain, and headache.

▼ Other: other side effects experienced by people taking Lansoprazole affected virtually every body system (cardiovascular, stomach and intestines, endocrine, blood, skin, metabolic, nervous, sensory, urinary, and reproductive), but were found in less than 1 of every 100 people taking the medication.

Drug Interactions

• Lansoprazole affects the absorption of drugs into the bloodstream that depend on having acid present in the stomach. Some drugs that may be affected are Ampicillin, Digoxin, Iron, and Ketoconazole.

• Lansoprazole slightly increases the rate at which Theophylline is released from the body, but this may not affect most people taking Theophylline for their asthma.

• Sucralfate interferes with the absorption of Lansoprazole into the blood. If you take both drugs, take the Lansoprazole at least ½ hour before you take your Sucralfate.

Food Interactions

Lansoprazole should be taken before a meal, preferably breakfast. Taking it after meals seriously interferes with the absorption of Lansoprazole into the blood.

Usual Dose

Adult: 15 to 30 mg a day. In some conditions, daily doses can go as high as 120 mg or more. Reduced dosage may be needed in people with severe liver disease.

Child: not recommended.

Overdosage

In one case of a 600-mg overdose, there were no adverse effects. Call your local poison center or hospital emergency room for information if you suspect a Lansoprazole overdose. If you go to an emergency room for treatment, ALWAYS bring the medicine bottle with you.

Special Information

Lansoprazole capsules should be swallowed whole. Don't open or crush them.

If you forget to take a dose of Lansoprazole, take it as soon as you remember. If it is almost time for your next dose, skip the forgotten dose and continue with your regular schedule.

Special Populations

Pregnancy/Breast-feeding

There is no information about the effect of taking Lansoprazole during pregnancy. This drug should not be taken during pregnancy unless absolutely necessary.

This drug may pass into human breast milk and may affect nursing infants. Nursing mothers who must take Lansoprazole should consider bottle-feeding their babies.

Seniors

Older adults clear this drug from their bodies more slowly than younger adults. Daily doses larger than 30 mg should not be taken unless specifically necessary to control disease symptoms.

Lasix

see **Loop Diuretics**, page 617

Generic Name

Levamisole Hydrochloride

Brand Name

Ergamisol

Type of Drug

Immune-system modulator.

Prescribed for

Duke's stage C colon cancer, together with Fluorouracil. Levamisole is also prescribed for malignant melanoma after surgery in people in whom the disease has not spread.

General Information

Levamisole, used to cure worm infections in animals, was found to restore depressed immune function in people. It can stimulate the formulation of antibodies to various agents, enhance T-cell response by stimulating and activating these important immune-system cells, and stimulate the functions of various white-blood-cell types (including their infection-fighting capability). The exact way that it works in concert with Fluorouracil is not known. In one clinical study of Levamisole, the survival rate of Duke's C colon cancer patients was improved by 27 percent for Levamisole plus Fluorouracil and 28 percent for Levamisole alone. The reduced recurrence rate for the disease was 36 percent for the drug combination, and 28 percent for Levamisole alone. Another study showed 33 percent improved survival and 41 percent reduction in disease recurrence for the 2 medicines. The drug is broken down in the liver and passes out of the body through the kidneys.

Cautions and Warnings

Do not take Levamisole if you are **allergic** to this drug or have had an allergic reaction to it.

People taking Levamisole may develop *agranulocytosis*, a potentially **fatal reduction in white-blood-cell levels**. Common symptoms of agranulocytosis are **fever, chills,** and **flu-like symptoms;** agranulocytosis can develop suddenly and without warning. **Regular blood monitoring** is necessary while you are on Levamisole: Your doctor may suddenly stop treatment if blood tests indicate the development of this problem, which may reverse when you stop the medicine.

Possible Side Effects

Virtually all people taking Fluorouracil and Levamisole experience some side effects. Often, side effects are due to either one or both of the drugs, and the actual source of some side effects may not be distinguishable. In Levamisole studies, the most common reasons for people stopping drug treatment were (in order) rash, joint and muscle aches, fever, white-blood-cell depression, urinary infection, and cough.

▼ Most common: nausea, vomiting, diarrhea, mouth sores, appetite loss, abdominal pains, constipation, a metallic taste, joint and muscle aches, dizziness, headache, tingling in the hands or feet, white-blood-cell reductions, rash, hair loss, fatigue, sleepiness, fever, chills, and infections.

▼ Less common: reduced platelet levels, itching, stom-

Possible Side Effects *(continued)*

ach upset, stomach gas, changes in sense of smell, depression, nervousness, sleeplessness, anxiety, blurred vision, and red eyes.

▼ Rare: peeling rashes, swelling around the eyes, vaginal bleeding, severe allergic reactions (breathing difficulty, skin rash, or itching), confusion, convulsions, hallucinations, loss of concentration, and kidney failure.

Drug Interactions

• People taking Levamisole who drink alcoholic beverages may experience severe reactions. Avoid this combination.

• People taking Phenytoin who also take combined therapy with Fluorouracil and Levamisole may have higher than usual levels of Phenytoin in their blood, increasing the chances for drug side effects.

Food Interactions

None known.

Usual Dose

Colon Cancer
50 mg every 8 hours for 3 days starting 7 to 30 days after surgery; then 50 mg every 8 hours for 3 days every 2 weeks.

Malignant Melanoma
2½ mg once daily for 2 consecutive days each week.

Overdosage

A Levamisole dosage was fatal in a child who took the equivalent of 6.8 mg per pound of body weight. An adult died after taking 14.5 mg per pound (usually adults take about 0.5 to 1 mg per pound). The most likely symptoms of overdose are exaggerated side effects, including those that affect the blood system, stomach, and intestines. Overdose victims should be taken to a hospital emergency room at once. ALWAYS bring the medicine bottle with you.

Special Information

Call your doctor if you develop any side effects, especially fever, chills, or flulike symptoms. Taking more than the recommended dose of Levamisole increases side-effect risk without improving the drug's effectiveness. Carefully follow your doctor's directions.

If you forget a dose of Levamisole, do not take the forgotten medication and do not take a double dose. Call your doctor for more information.

Special Populations

Pregnancy/Breast-feeding

While there is no direct information on pregnancy in humans, animal studies indicate that Levamisole may damage a growing fetus. If you are pregnant, do not take this drug unless you have fully discussed all available options and the possible risks and benefits of Levamisole with your doctor. Use effective contraceptive measures to be sure you don't become pregnant while taking Levamisole and Fluorouracil.

Levamisole may pass into breast milk. Nursing mothers who must take Levamisole should bottle-feed their babies.

Seniors

Seniors may take this medicine without special restriction. Report any side effects to your doctor.

Generic Name

Levobunolol

Brand Name

Betagan Liquifilm

Type of Drug

Beta-adrenergic-blocking agent.

Prescribed for

Glaucoma.

General Information

Levobunolol is one of several beta-adrenergic-blocking drugs, or beta blockers, which interfere with the action of a specific part of the nervous system. Beta receptors are found all over the body and affect many body functions, which accounts for the usefulness of beta blockers against a wide variety of conditions.

When applied to the eye, Levobunolol reduces fluid pressure inside the eye by reducing the production of eye fluids and slightly increasing the rate at which fluids flow through and leave the eye. Beta blockers produce a greater drop in eye pressure than either Pilocarpine or Epinephrine, but may be combined with these or other drugs to produce a more pronounced drop in eye pressure.

Betaxolol may be used by people who cannot use Levobunolol because of the possible effect of Levobunolol on heart or lung function.

Cautions and Warnings

Be cautious about taking Levobunolol eyedrops if you have **asthma, severe heart failure, slow heart rate,** or **heart block** because small amounts of the drug may be absorbed into your bloodstream and can aggravate these conditions.

Beta blockers, including Levobunolol, may mask the signs of an **overactive thyroid, low blood sugar,** or **hypoglycemia.**

Possible Side Effects

Levobunolol side effects are usually mild, relatively uncommon, develop early in the course of treatment, and are rarely a reason to stop taking the medication.

Drug Interactions

• If you take other glaucoma eye medicines, separate them from Levobunolol to avoid physically mixing them. Small amounts of Levobunolol are absorbed into the general circulation and may interact with some of the same drugs as beta blockers taken by mouth, but this is unlikely.

Food Interactions

None known.

Usual Dose

One drop in the affected eye 1 or 2 times per day.

Overdosage

Symptoms of Levobunolol overdose are changes in heartbeat (unusually slow, unusually fast, or irregular), severe dizziness or fainting, difficulty breathing, bluish-colored fingernails or palms of the hands, and seizures. Overdose is highly unlikely. Call your local poison control center or hospital emergency room for more information. ALWAYS bring the medicine bottle with you.

Special Information

Call your doctor about the following side effects only if they persist or are bothersome: anxiety, diarrhea, constipation, sexual impotence, mild dizziness, headache, itching, nausea or vomiting, nightmares or vivid dreams, upset stomach, trouble sleeping, stuffed nose, frequent urination, unusual tiredness, or weakness.

To administer the eyedrops, lie down or tilt your head backward and look at the ceiling. Hold the dropper above your eye and drop the medicine inside your lower lid while looking up. To prevent possible infection, don't allow the dropper to touch your fingers, eyelids, or any surface. Release the lower lid and keep your eye open. Don't blink for about 30 seconds. Press gently on the bridge of your nose at the inside corner of your eye for about 1 minute. This will help circulate the medicine around your eye. Wait at least 5 minutes before using any other eyedrops.

If you forget to take a dose of Levobunolol eyedrops, take it as soon as you remember. If it is almost time for your next dose, skip the one you forgot and continue with your regular schedule. Do not take a double dose.

Special Populations

Pregnancy/Breast-feeding

Levobunolol may cross into the blood circulation of the developing fetus, but the amount of drug that could be absorbed from eyedrops is negligible.

Nursing mothers should watch their infants for any drug-related effects, although the chances of anything happening are small.

Seniors

Seniors may be more likely to suffer drug-related effects, should the eyedrops be absorbed into the bloodstream.

Generic Name

Levocabastine Hydrochloride

Brand Name

Livostin

Type of Drug

Antihistamine.

Prescribed for

Temporary relief of allergic conjunctivitis ("pink-eye").

General Information

Levocabastine is an antihistamine eyedrop that is used to relieve the tearing and itching that accompanies seasonal allergies.

Cautions and Warnings

Soft contact lens wearers should take their lenses out before using this product.

Possible Side Effects

▼ Most common: eye burning (temporary), stinging, discomfort, and headache.

▼ Less common: visual disturbances, eye pain, dry eye(s), swelling of the eyelid, dry mouth, fatigue, sore throat, pink-eye, tearing or other eye discharges, cough, nausea, skin rash or redness, and breathing difficulty.

Drug Interactions

• Do not use other eyedrops together with this drug.

Food Interactions

None known.

Usual Dose

Adult and Child (age 12 and older): 1 drop in the affected eye 4 times per day for up to 2 weeks.

Child (age 11 and under): not recommended.

Overdosage

Levocabastine is an antihistamine and, if swallowed, could produce any of the effects listed under *Possible Side Effects*. Call your local poison control center or emergency room for more information.

Special Information

Shake the eyedrop bottle well before using. Protect the bottle from freezing.

To administer eyedrops, lie down or tilt your head back and look at the ceiling. Hold the dropper above your eye, gently squeeze your lower lid to form a small pouch, and drop the medicine inside while looking up. Release the lower lid, keeping your eye open. Don't blink for about 40 seconds. Press gently on the bridge of your nose at the inside corner of your eye for about a minute to help circulate the medicine around your eye. To avoid infection, don't touch the dropper tip to your finger or eyelid. Wait at least 5 minutes before using another eyedrop or ointment.

Call your doctor at once if your eye stinging, itching, burning, redness, irritation, swelling, or pain gets worse, or if you start having trouble seeing.

If you forget to take a dose of Levocabastine eyedrops, take it as soon as you remember. If it is almost time for your next dose, skip the missed dose and continue with your regular schedule. Do not take a double dose.

Special Populations

Pregnancy/Breast-feeding

Levocabastine caused birth defects in laboratory animals

when huge doses were given, but the relevance of this effect to pregnant women is not known. Considering the broad variety of other available options, pregnant women should use this drug only if absolutely necessary.

Very small amounts of Levocabastine find their way into breast milk after the drug is put into the eye. Nursing mothers who use this eyedrop should watch their babies for anything unusual.

Seniors
Seniors may use this drug without special restriction.

Generic Name

Levodopa (L-dopa)

Brand Names

Dopar
Larodopa

(Also available in generic form)

Type of Drug

Antiparkinsonian.

Prescribed for

Parkinson's disease; restless legs syndrome; pain associated with herpes zoster (shingles).

General Information

Parkinson's disease can develop as a result of changes in the utilization of dopamine in the brain or damage to the central nervous system caused by carbon monoxide poisoning or manganese poisoning. It usually develops in older adults because of hardening of the arteries. In many other cases, the cause is not known. Levodopa works by entering the brain, where it is converted to dopamine, a chemical found in the central nervous system. The new dopamine replaces what is deficient in people with Parkinson's disease. Some people who take Levodopa develop the "on-off" phenomenon, in which they may suddenly lose all drug effect and then regain it within minutes or hours. About 15 to 40 percent of people with Parkinson's disease will develop this phenomenon after 2 to 3 years of Levodopa treatment. The on-off effect becomes more frequent after 5 years, and some people may experience a gradual decline of drug effect.

Cautions and Warnings

People with a history of **heart attacks, severe heart** or **lung disease, glaucoma, asthma,** or **kidney, liver,** or **hormone diseases** should be cautious about using this drug. Do not take it if you have a history of **stomach ulcer.** People with a **psychotic history** must be treated with extreme care; this drug can cause **depression** with **suicidal tendencies.** Levodopa may activate an existing **malignant melanoma:** People with a family history of melanoma or suspicious **skin lesions** should not take this drug.

Possible Side Effects

▼ Most common: muscle spasms or inability to control arms, legs, or facial muscles; loss of appetite; nausea; vomiting (with or without stomach pain); dry mouth; drooling; difficulty eating (due to poor muscle control); tiredness; hand tremors; headache; dizziness; numbness; weakness or a faint feeling; confusion; sleeplessness; grinding of the teeth; nightmares; euphoria (feeling "high"); hallucinations; delusions; agitation; anxiousness; and general feelings of ill health.

▼ Less common: heart irregularities or palpitations, dizziness when standing or rising (particularly in the morning), mental changes (depression, with or without suicidal tendencies; paranoia; loss of some intellectual function), difficulty urinating, muscle twitching, burning of the tongue, bitter taste, diarrhea, constipation, unusual breathing patterns, blurred or double vision, hot flashes, weight gain or loss, darkening of the urine, and increased perspiration.

▼ Rare: stomach bleeding, development of an ulcer, high blood pressure, convulsions, adverse effects on the blood, difficulty controlling the eye muscles, feeling of

---

Possible Side Effects *(continued)*

being stimulated, hiccups, loss of hair, hoarseness, decreasing size of male genitalia, and retention of fluids.

Drug Interactions

• The effect of Levodopa is decreased when it is used together with an anticholinergic drug (such as Trihexyphenidyl). Other drugs that may interfere with Levodopa are benzodiazepine-type tranquilizers and sedatives, phenothiazine antipsychotic medicines, Phenytoin, Methionine, Papaverine, Pyridoxine, and tricyclic antidepressants.

• Antacids can increase the effects of Levodopa.

• Metoclopramide may increase the amount of Levodopa absorbed into the bloodstream and Levodopa may reduce Metoclopramide's effects on your stomach.

• Levodopa can interact with drugs for high blood pressure to cause further reduction of pressure. Dosage adjustments in the high blood pressure medication may be needed. Methyldopa (a drug for high blood pressure) may increase the effects of Levodopa.

• People taking monoamine oxidase (MAO) inhibitor drugs should stop taking them at least 2 weeks before starting to take Levodopa.

Food Interactions

Do not take vitamin preparations that contain vitamin B_6 (Pyridoxine), because this vitamin will decrease the effectiveness of Levodopa.

Since this drug can cause stomach upset, take each dose with food. A low-protein diet may help to minimize fluctuations in response to this drug that occur in some people.

Usual Dose

0.5 to 8 grams per day. Dosage must be individualized to your specific needs.

Overdosage

People taking an overdose of Levodopa must be treated in a

hospital emergency room immediately. ALWAYS bring the medicine bottle with you.

Special Information

Be careful while driving or operating any complex or hazardous equipment.

Call your doctor *immediately* if any of the following occur: fainting, dizziness or light-headedness; abnormal diabetic urine tests for sugar or ketones; uncontrollable movements of the face, eyelids, mouth, tongue, neck, arms, hands, or legs; mood changes; palpitations or irregular heartbeats; difficulty urinating; severe nausea or vomiting.

If you forget to take a dose of Levodopa, take it as soon as possible. However, if it is within 2 hours of your next dose, skip the missed dose and go back to your regular schedule. Do not take a double dose.

Special Populations

Pregnancy/Breast-feeding

Levodopa has not been studied in humans; however, animal studies indicate that Levodopa may interfere with fetal development. Pregnant women should take this drug only if it is absolutely necessary.

Nursing mothers taking this drug should bottle-feed their infants.

Seniors

Older adults may require smaller doses because they are less tolerant to the drug's side effects. Also, the body enzyme that breaks the drug down decreases with age, so a large dose is not needed.

Seniors who respond to Levodopa treatments, especially those with osteoporosis, should resume activity gradually. Sudden increases in mobility may increase the risk for broken bones.

Seniors, especially those with heart disease, are more likely to develop abnormal heart rhythms and other cardiac side effects. Regular monitoring by your doctor is essential.

Levoxyl

*see **Thyroid Hormone Replacements**, page 1099*

Generic Name

Lisinopril

Brand Name

Prinivil
Zestril

Combination Product

Lisinopril + Hydrochlorothiazide

Zestoretic

Type of Drug

Angiotensin-converting-enzyme (ACE) inhibitor.

Prescribed for

High blood pressure and congestive heart failure.

General Information

ACE inhibitors work by preventing the conversion of a hormone called *angiotensin I* to another hormone called *angiotensin II*, a potent blood-vessel constrictor. Preventing this conversion relaxes blood vessels and helps to reduce blood pressure and relieve the symptoms of heart failure by making it easier for a failing heart to pump blood around your body. The production of other hormones and enzymes that participate in the regulation of blood vessel dilation is also affected by the ACE inhibitors and probably plays a role in the effectiveness of these medicines. Lisinopril begins working about 1 hour after you take it and lasts for a full 24 hours.

Some people who start taking an ACE inhibitor after they are already on a diuretic experience a rapid drop in blood pressure after their first dose or when the dose is increased. To prevent this, you may be told to stop taking the diuretic 2 or 3 days before starting the ACE inhibitor or increase your salt intake during that time. The diuretic may then be restarted gradually. Heart failure patients generally have been taking both Digoxin and a diuretic before starting on an ACE Inhibitor.

Cautions and Warnings

Do not take Lisinopril if you have had an **allergic** reaction to it in the past. Occasionally, severe allergic reactions have occurred in people undergoing desensitization treatments or certain kinds of kidney dialysis. Lisinopril causes very **low blood pressure** in rare instances and can affect your **kidneys,** especially if you have **congestive heart failure.** It is advisable for your doctor to check your urine for changes during the first few months of treatment.

People with **kidney disease** who are taking Lisinopril may require a lower dosage because they have more drug in their blood and are more likely to develop drug side effects.

ACE inhibitors can affect **white-blood-cell count,** possibly increasing your susceptibility to infection. Blood counts should be monitored periodically.

Possible Side Effects

▼ Most common: headache, dizziness, fatigue, nausea, diarrhea, and chronic cough. The cough is more common in women than men and usually goes away a few days after you stop taking the medicine.

▼ Less common: chest pain, low blood pressure, vomiting, upset stomach, breathing difficulty, rash, and muscle weakness.

▼ Rare: sweating, flushing, itching, rash, male impotence, reduced sex drive, muscle cramps, muscle and joint aches, arthritis, fainting, anemia, blurred vision, fever, blood vessel irritation, angina, heart attack, stroke, heart palpitations, dizziness when rising from a sitting or lying position, rapid heartbeat, abnormal heart rhythms, swelling in the arms or legs, sleep disturbances, sleepiness, confusion, depression, feelings of ill health, nervousness, tingling in the hands or feet, appetite loss, constipation, reduced urine flow, dry mouth, hepatitis, jaundice, urinary infection, pancreas inflammation, asthma, bronchitis, and sinus inflammation.

Drug Interactions

• The blood-pressure-lowering effect of Lisinopril is additive with diuretic drugs and beta blockers. Any other drug that can reduce blood pressure should be used with caution if you are taking an ACE inhibitor.

• Lisinopril may increase your blood potassium levels, especially when taken with Dyazide or other potassium-sparing diuretics.

• Lisinopril may increase the effects of Lithium; this combination should be used with caution.

• Antacids may reduce the amount of Lisinopril absorbed into the blood. Separate doses of the two medicines by at least 2 hours.

• Capsaicin may cause or aggravate cough associated with Lisinopril.

• Indomethacin may reduce the blood-pressure-lowering effect of Lisinopril.

• Phenothiazine tranquilizers and antiemetics may increase the effects of Lisinopril.

• The combination of Allopurinol and Lisinopril increases the chance of a drug reaction.

• Lisinopril increases blood levels of Digoxin, possibly increasing the chance of Digoxin side effects.

Food Interactions

Lisinopril is unaffected by food in the stomach and may be taken without regard to food or meals.

Usual Dose

5 to 40 mg a day. People with severe kidney disease should begin with 2.5 mg per day and can be increased up to 5 to 20 mg per day.

Overdosage

The principal effect of Lisinopril overdose is a rapid drop in blood pressure, as evidenced by dizziness or fainting. Take the overdose victim to a hospital emergency room immediately. ALWAYS bring the medicine bottle with you.

Special Information

Call your doctor if you develop swelling of the face or throat, if you have sudden difficulty breathing, or if you develop a sore throat, mouth sores, abnormal heartbeat, chest pain, a persistent rash, or loss of taste perception.

Unexplained swelling of the face, lips, hands, and feet can also affect the larynx (throat) and tongue and interfere with breathing. If this happens, the victim should be taken to a hospital emergency room at once for treatment.

You may get dizzy if you rise to your feet quickly from a sitting or lying position.

Avoid strenuous exercise and/or very hot weather because heavy sweating or dehydration can cause a rapid drop in blood pressure.

Avoid nonprescription diet pills, decongestants, and stimulants that can raise blood pressure.

If you forget to take a dose of Lisinopril, take it as soon as you remember. If it is within 8 hours of your next dose, skip the one you forgot and continue with your regular schedule. Do not take a double dose.

Special Populations

Pregnancy/Breast-feeding

ACE inhibitors have caused low blood pressure, kidney failure, slow formation of the skull, and death in developing fetuses when taken during the last 6 months of pregnancy. Women who are pregnant should not take Lisinopril. Women who may become pregnant while taking Lisinopril should use an effective contraceptive method and stop taking the medicine if they do become pregnant.

It is not known if Lisinopril passes into breast milk. However, nursing mothers who must take this drug should consider an alternative feeding method since infants, especially newborns, are more susceptible than adults to the effects of ACE inhibitors.

Seniors

Older adults may be more sensitive to the effects of Lisinopril than younger adults because of the possibility of normal age-related reductions in kidney function. Your Lisinopril dosage must be individualized to your needs.

Accutane 20 mg p. 551	**Accutane** 40 mg p. 551	**Acetaminophen with Codeine** 30/300 p. 877
Acetaminophen with Codeine 60/300 p. 877		**Achromycin V** 250 mg p. 1082	**Actigall** 300 mg p. 1155
Albuterol 2 mg p. 30	**Albuterol** 4 mg p. 30	**Aldactazide** 25/25 p. 380
Aldomet 250 mg p. 701		**Aldomet** 500 mg p. 701	
Altace 2.5 mg p. 980	**Altace** 5 mg p. 980	**Alupent** 10 mg p. 685	**Alupent** 20 mg p. 685

A

Amitriptyline 25 mg p. 52	**Amitriptyline** 50 mg p. 52	**Amitriptyline** 100 mg p. 52	**Amoxicillin** 250 mg p. 868
Amoxicillin 500 mg p. 868	**Amoxil** 250 mg p. 868	**Amoxil** 500 mg p. 868	**Amoxil Chewable** 125 mg p. 868
Anafranil 50 mg p. 231	**Anaprox** 275 mg p. 769	**Anaprox DS** 550 mg p. 769	
Ancobon 500 mg p. 463	**Ansaid** 50 mg p. 477	**Antivert** 12.5 mg p. 346	**Asendin** 25 mg p. 61
Asendin 50 mg p. 61	**Atarax** 25 mg p. 516	**Atarax** 50 mg p. 516	**Atenolol** 50 mg p. 96

B

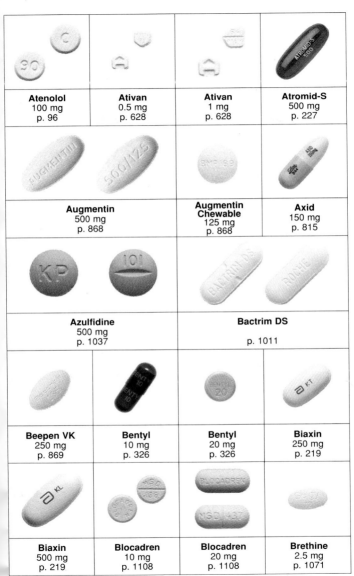

Atenolol 100 mg p. 96	**Ativan** 0.5 mg p. 628	**Ativan** 1 mg p. 628	**Atromid-S** 500 mg p. 227
Augmentin 500 mg p. 868		**Augmentin Chewable** 125 mg p. 868	**Axid** 150 mg p. 815
Azulfidine 500 mg p. 1037		**Bactrim DS** p. 1011	
Beepen VK 250 mg p. 869	**Bentyl** 10 mg p. 326	**Bentyl** 20 mg p. 326	**Biaxin** 250 mg p. 219
Biaxin 500 mg p. 219	**Blocadren** 10 mg p. 1108	**Blocadren** 20 mg p. 1108	**Brethine** 2.5 mg p. 1071

C

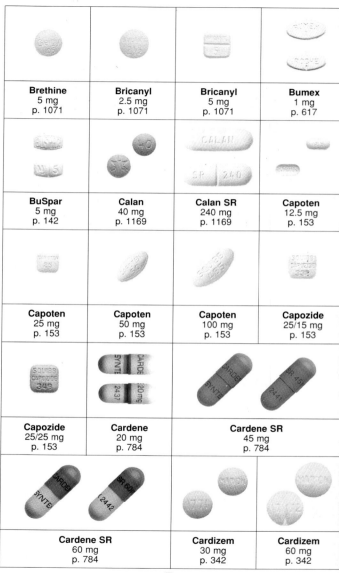

Brethine 5 mg p. 1071	**Bricanyl** 2.5 mg p. 1071	**Bricanyl** 5 mg p. 1071	**Bumex** 1 mg p. 617
BuSpar 5 mg p. 142	**Calan** 40 mg p. 1169	**Calan SR** 240 mg p. 1169	**Capoten** 12.5 mg p. 153
Capoten 25 mg p. 153	**Capoten** 50 mg p. 153	**Capoten** 100 mg p. 153	**Capozide** 25/15 mg p. 153
Capozide 25/25 mg p. 153	**Cardene** 20 mg p. 784	**Cardene SR** 45 mg p. 784	
Cardene SR 60 mg p. 784		**Cardizem** 30 mg p. 342	**Cardizem** 60 mg p. 342

D

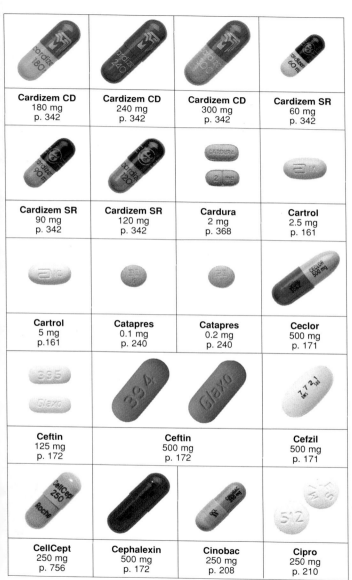

Cardizem CD 180 mg p. 342	**Cardizem CD** 240 mg p. 342	**Cardizem CD** 300 mg p. 342	**Cardizem SR** 60 mg p. 342
Cardizem SR 90 mg p. 342	**Cardizem SR** 120 mg p. 342	**Cardura** 2 mg p. 368	**Cartrol** 2.5 mg p. 161
Cartrol 5 mg p.161	**Catapres** 0.1 mg p. 240	**Catapres** 0.2 mg p. 240	**Ceclor** 500 mg p. 171
Ceftin 125 mg p. 172	**Ceftin** 500 mg p. 172		**Cefzil** 500 mg p. 171
CellCept 250 mg p. 756	**Cephalexin** 500 mg p. 172	**Cinobac** 250 mg p. 208	**Cipro** 250 mg p. 210

E

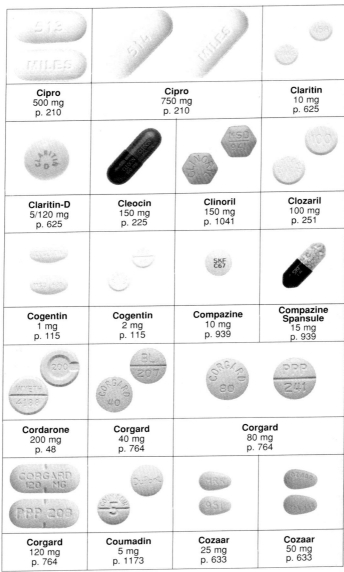

Cipro	Cipro	Claritin
500 mg	750 mg	10 mg
p. 210	p. 210	p. 625

Claritin-D	Cleocin	Clinoril	Clozaril
5/120 mg	150 mg	150 mg	100 mg
p. 625	p. 225	p. 1041	p. 251

Cogentin	Cogentin	Compazine	Compazine Spansule
1 mg	2 mg	10 mg	15 mg
p. 115	p. 115	p. 939	p. 939

Cordarone	Corgard	Corgard
200 mg	40 mg	80 mg
p. 48	p. 764	p. 764

Corgard	Coumadin	Cozaar	Cozaar
120 mg	5 mg	25 mg	50 mg
p. 764	p. 1173	p. 633	p. 633

F

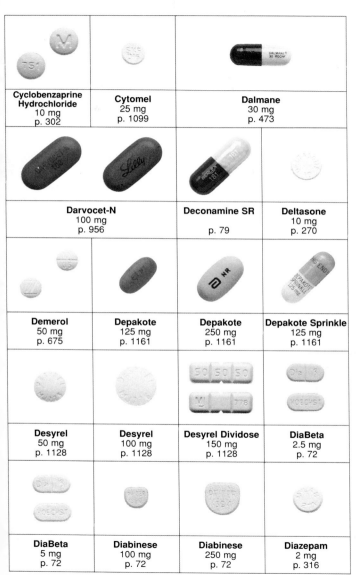

Cyclobenzaprine Hydrochloride 10 mg p. 302	**Cytomel** 25 mg p. 1099	**Dalmane** 30 mg p. 473

Darvocet-N 100 mg p. 956	**Deconamine SR** p. 79	**Deltasone** 10 mg p. 270

Demerol 50 mg p. 675	**Depakote** 125 mg p. 1161	**Depakote** 250 mg p. 1161	**Depakote Sprinkle** 125 mg p. 1161

Desyrel 50 mg p. 1128	**Desyrel** 100 mg p. 1128	**Desyrel Dividose** 150 mg p. 1128	**DiaBeta** 2.5 mg p. 72

DiaBeta 5 mg p. 72	**Diabinese** 100 mg p. 72	**Diabinese** 250 mg p. 72	**Diazepam** 2 mg p. 316

G

Diazepam 5 mg p. 316	**Diazepam** 10 mg p. 316	**Diflucan** 100 mg p. 460	**Diflucan** 150 mg p. 460
Dilantin 100 mg p. 893	**Ditropan** 5 mg p. 849	**Diuril** 500 mg p. 1088	**Dolobid** 250 mg p. 334
Donnatal p. 363	**Donnatal** p. 363	**Doral** 15 mg p.968	**Duricef** 500 mg p. 171
Dyazide p. 380	**Dynabac** 250 mg p. 355	**DynaCirc** 2.5 mg p. 556	**EES** 400 mg p. 406
Effexor 25 mg p. 1165	**Effexor** 37.5 mg p. 1165	**Effexor** 50 mg p. 1165	**Effexor** 75 mg p. 1165

H

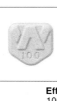		
Effexor 100 mg p. 1165	**E-Mycin** 250 mg p. 406	**E-Mycin** 333 mg p. 406

Elavil 10 mg p. 52	**Elavil** 25 mg p. 52	**Elavil** 150 mg p. 52

Eldepryl 5 mg p. 1007	**Empirin with** **Codeine #3** p. 381	**Empirin with** **Codeine #4** p. 381	**Endep** 10 mg p. 52

Endep 50 mg p. 52	**Entex LA** p. 397

Equagesic p. 401	**EryPed Chewable** 200 mg p. 406

I

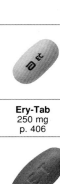		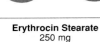	
Ery-Tab 250 mg p. 406	**Ery-Tab** 333 mg p. 406	**Erythrocin Stearate** 250 mg p. 406	

		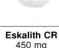	
Erythrocin Stearate 500 mg p. 406		**Erythromycin Base** 250 mg p. 406	**Esgic** p. 446

Esidrix 50 mg p. 1088	**Eskalith** 300 mg p. 603	**Eskalith CR** 450 mg p. 603	**Estrace Oral** 1 mg p. 415

Ethmozine 200 mg p. 745		**Ethmozine** 250 mg p. 745

Ethmozine 300 mg p. 745	**Etrafon 2-10** p. 52

J

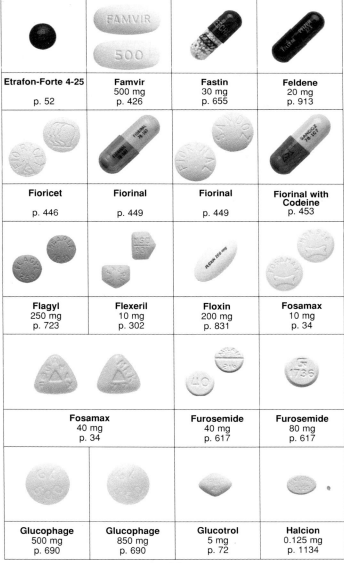

Etrafon-Forte 4-25 p. 52	**Famvir** 500 mg p. 426	**Fastin** 30 mg p. 655	**Feldene** 20 mg p. 913
Fioricet p. 446	**Fiorinal** p. 449	**Fiorinal** p. 449	**Fiorinal with Codeine** p. 453
Flagyl 250 mg p. 723	**Flexeril** 10 mg p. 302	**Floxin** 200 mg p. 831	**Fosamax** 10 mg p. 34
Fosamax 40 mg p. 34		**Furosemide** 40 mg p. 617	**Furosemide** 80 mg p. 617
Glucophage 500 mg p. 690	**Glucophage** 850 mg p. 690	**Glucotrol** 5 mg p. 72	**Halcion** 0.125 mg p. 1134

K

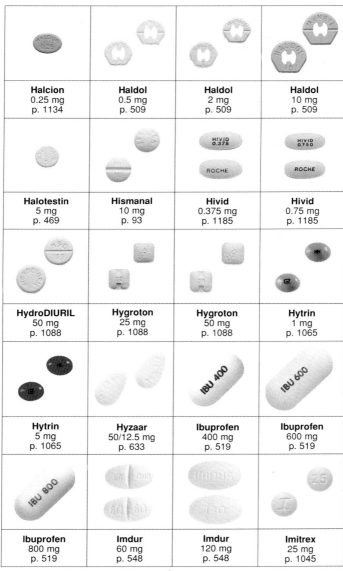

Halcion 0.25 mg p. 1134	**Haldol** 0.5 mg p. 509	**Haldol** 2 mg p. 509	**Haldol** 10 mg p. 509
Halotestin 5 mg p. 469	**Hismanal** 10 mg p. 93	**Hivid** 0.375 mg p. 1185	**Hivid** 0.75 mg p. 1185
HydroDIURIL 50 mg p. 1088	**Hygroton** 25 mg p. 1088	**Hygroton** 50 mg p. 1088	**Hytrin** 1 mg p. 1065
Hytrin 5 mg p. 1065	**Hyzaar** 50/12.5 mg p. 633	**Ibuprofen** 400 mg p. 519	**Ibuprofen** 600 mg p. 519
Ibuprofen 800 mg p. 519	**Imdur** 60 mg p. 548	**Imdur** 120 mg p. 548	**Imitrex** 25 mg p. 1045

L

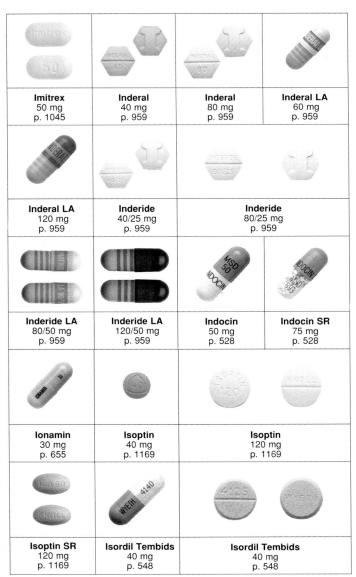

Imitrex 50 mg p. 1045	**Inderal** 40 mg p. 959	**Inderal** 80 mg p. 959	**Inderal LA** 60 mg p. 959
Inderal LA 120 mg p. 959	**Inderide** 40/25 mg p. 959	**Inderide** 80/25 mg p. 959	
Inderide LA 80/50 mg p. 959	**Inderide LA** 120/50 mg p. 959	**Indocin** 50 mg p. 528	**Indocin SR** 75 mg p. 528
Ionamin 30 mg p. 655	**Isoptin** 40 mg p. 1169	**Isoptin** 120 mg p. 1169	
Isoptin SR 120 mg p. 1169	**Isordil Tembids** 40 mg p. 548	**Isordil Tembids** 40 mg p. 548	

M

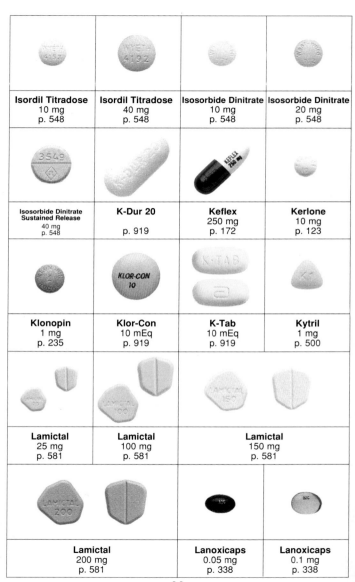

Isordil Titradose 10 mg p. 548	**Isordil Titradose** 40 mg p. 548	**Isosorbide Dinitrate** 10 mg p. 548	**Isosorbide Dinitrate** 20 mg p. 548
Isosorbide Dinitrate Sustained Release 40 mg p. 548	**K-Dur 20** p. 919	**Keflex** 250 mg p. 172	**Kerlone** 10 mg p. 123
Klonopin 1 mg p. 235	**Klor-Con** 10 mEq p. 919	**K-Tab** 10 mEq p. 919	**Kytril** 1 mg p. 500
Lamictal 25 mg p. 581	**Lamictal** 100 mg p. 581	**Lamictal** 150 mg p. 581	
Lamictal 200 mg p. 581		**Lanoxicaps** 0.05 mg p. 338	**Lanoxicaps** 0.1 mg p. 338

N

Lanoxicaps 0.2 mg p. 338	**Lanoxin** 0.125 mg p. 338	**Lanoxin** 0.25 mg p. 338	**Lanoxin** 0.5 mg p. 338
Larodopa 250 mg p. 595	**Lasix** 20 mg p. 617	**Lasix** 40 mg p. 617	**Lasix** 80 mg p. 617
Lescol 20 mg p. 482	**Lescol** 40 mg p. 482	**Levatol** 20 mg p. 864	**Levoxyl** 25 mcg p. 1099
Levoxyl 50 mcg p. 1099	**Levoxyl** 100 mcg p. 1099	**Levoxyl** 125 mcg p. 1099	**Libritabs** 10 mg p. 179
Librium 10 mg p. 179	**Limbitrol** p. 53	**Limbitrol DS** p. 53	**Lithonate** 300 mg p. 603

O

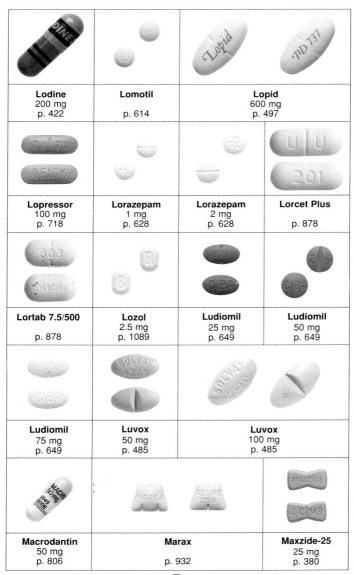

Lodine 200 mg p. 422	**Lomotil** p. 614	**Lopid** 600 mg p. 497	
Lopressor 100 mg p. 718	**Lorazepam** 1 mg p. 628	**Lorazepam** 2 mg p. 628	**Lorcet Plus** p. 878
Lortab 7.5/500 p. 878	**Lozol** 2.5 mg p. 1089	**Ludiomil** 25 mg p. 649	**Ludiomil** 50 mg p. 649
Ludiomil 75 mg p. 649	**Luvox** 50 mg p. 485	**Luvox** 100 mg p. 485	
Macrodantin 50 mg p. 806	**Marax** p. 932		**Maxzide-25** 25 mg p. 380

P

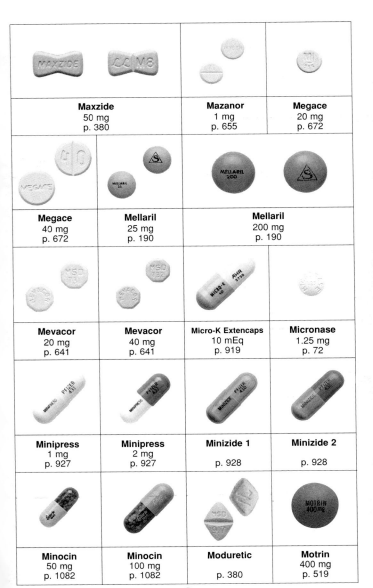

Maxzide 50 mg p. 380	**Mazanor** 1 mg p. 655	**Megace** 20 mg p. 672
Megace 40 mg p. 672	**Mellaril** 25 mg p. 190	**Mellaril** 200 mg p. 190
Mevacor 20 mg p. 641	**Mevacor** 40 mg p. 641	**Micro-K Extencaps** 10 mEq p. 919 · **Micronase** 1.25 mg p. 72
Minipress 1 mg p. 927	**Minipress** 2 mg p. 927	**Minizide 1** p. 928 · **Minizide 2** p. 928
Minocin 50 mg p. 1082	**Minocin** 100 mg p. 1082	**Moduretic** p. 380 · **Motrin** 400 mg p. 519

Q

Motrin 600 mg p. 519	**Motrin** 800 mg p. 519	**Nalfon** 200 mg p. 439	**Nalfon** 300 mg p. 439
Nalfon 600 mg p. 439		**Naprosyn** 250 mg p. 769	**Naprosyn** 375 mg p. 769
Nicorette 2 mg p. 788	**Nizoral** 200 mg p. 563	**Nolvadex** 10 mg p. 1059	**Norgesic Forte** p. 822
Normodyne 200 mg p. 575	**Noroxin** 400 mg p. 818	**Norpace** 100 mg p. 359	**Norpace CR** 100 mg p. 359
Norpramin 50 mg p. 312	**Nortriptyline** 10 mg p. 825	**Nortriptyline** 50 mg p. 825	**Norvasc** 5 mg p. 57

R

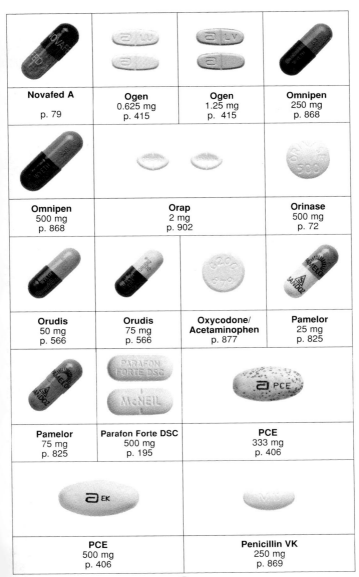

Novafed A p. 79	**Ogen** 0.625 mg p. 415	**Ogen** 1.25 mg p. 415	**Omnipen** 250 mg p. 868
Omnipen 500 mg p. 868	**Orap** 2 mg p. 902		**Orinase** 500 mg p. 72
Orudis 50 mg p. 566	**Orudis** 75 mg p. 566	**Oxycodone/** **Acetaminophen** p. 877	**Pamelor** 25 mg p. 825
Pamelor 75 mg p. 825	**Parafon Forte DSC** 500 mg p. 195	**PCE** 333 mg p. 406	
PCE 500 mg p. 406		**Penicillin VK** 250 mg p. 869	

S

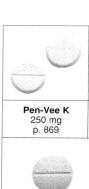			
Pen-Vee K 250 mg p. 869	**Pepcid** 20 mg p. 428	**Percocet** p. 877	

Percodan p. 881		**Permax** 0.05 mg p. 886	**Permax** 0.25 mg p. 886

Phenaphen with Codeine #3 p. 877	**Phenergan** 25 mg p. 943	**Polymox** 500 mg p. 868	**Ponstel** 250 mg p. 668

Potassium Chloride Controlled-Release 8 mEq p. 919	**Pravachol** 20 mg p. 924	

Premarin 0.625 mg p. 415	**Premarin** 1.25 mg p. 415	**Prevacid** 15 mg p. 584	**Prevacid** 30 mg p. 584

T

Prilosec 20 mg p. 837	**Principen** 250 mg p. 868	**Prinivil** 20 mg p. 599	**Procardia** 10 mg p. 794
Procardia 20 mg p. 794	**Procardia XL** 30 mg p. 794	**Procardia XL** 60 mg p. 794	**Procardia XL** 90 mg p. 794
Prograf 1 mg p. 1055	**Prograf** 5 mg p. 1055	**Prolixin** 5 mg p. 190	**Prolixin** 10 mg p. 190
Pronestyl 250 mg p. 934	**Pronestyl SR** 500 mg p. 934	**Propacet 100** p. 956	**Propoxyphene Napsylate and Acetaminophen** 100/650 p. 956
Proventil 4 mg p. 968	**Proventil Repetabs** 4 mg p. 968	**Provera** 2.5 mg p. 665	**Provera** 5 mg p. 665

U

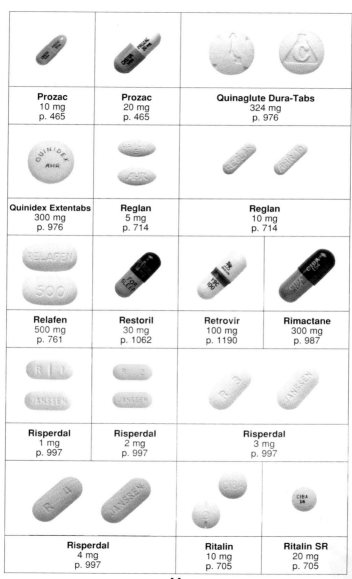

Prozac 10 mg p. 465	**Prozac** 20 mg p. 465	**Quinaglute Dura-Tabs** 324 mg p. 976
Quinidex Extentabs 300 mg p. 976	**Reglan** 5 mg p. 714	**Reglan** 10 mg p. 714

Relafen 500 mg p. 761	**Restoril** 30 mg p. 1062	**Retrovir** 100 mg p. 1190	**Rimactane** 300 mg p. 987

Risperdal 1 mg p. 997	**Risperdal** 2 mg p. 997	**Risperdal** 3 mg p. 997

Risperdal 4 mg p. 997	**Ritalin** 10 mg p. 705	**Ritalin SR** 20 mg p. 705

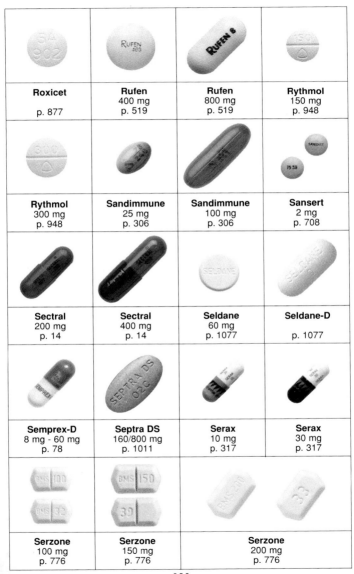

Roxicet p. 877	**Rufen** 400 mg p. 519	**Rufen** 800 mg p. 519	**Rythmol** 150 mg p. 948
Rythmol 300 mg p. 948	**Sandimmune** 25 mg p. 306	**Sandimmune** 100 mg p. 306	**Sansert** 2 mg p. 708
Sectral 200 mg p. 14	**Sectral** 400 mg p. 14	**Seldane** 60 mg p. 1077	**Seldane-D** p. 1077
Semprex-D 8 mg - 60 mg p. 78	**Septra DS** 160/800 mg p. 1011	**Serax** 10 mg p. 317	**Serax** 30 mg p. 317
Serzone 100 mg p. 776	**Serzone** 150 mg p. 776	**Serzone** 200 mg p. 776	

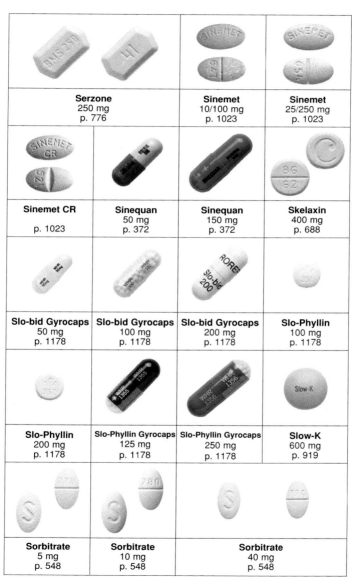

Serzone 250 mg p. 776	**Sinemet** 10/100 mg p. 1023	**Sinemet** 25/250 mg p. 1023
Sinemet CR p. 1023	**Sinequan** 50 mg p. 372	**Sinequan** 150 mg p. 372	**Skelaxin** 400 mg p. 688
Slo-bid Gyrocaps 50 mg p. 1178	**Slo-bid Gyrocaps** 100 mg p. 1178	**Slo-bid Gyrocaps** 200 mg p. 1178	**Slo-Phyllin** 100 mg p. 1178
Slo-Phyllin 200 mg p. 1178	**Slo-Phyllin Gyrocaps** 125 mg p. 1178	**Slo-Phyllin Gyrocaps** 250 mg p. 1178	**Slow-K** 600 mg p. 919
Sorbitrate 5 mg p. 548	**Sorbitrate** 10 mg p. 548	**Sorbitrate** 40 mg p. 548

X

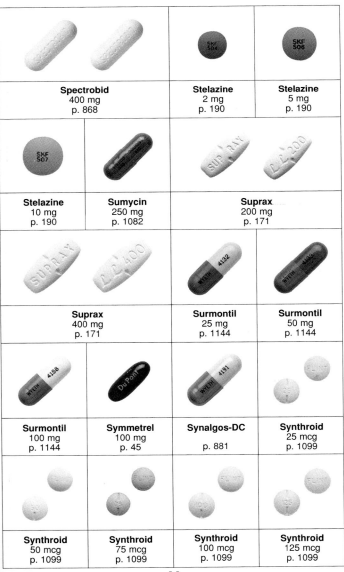

| | Spectrobid
400 mg
p. 868 | Stelazine
2 mg
p. 190 | Stelazine
5 mg
p. 190 |

Spectrobid
400 mg
p. 868

Stelazine
2 mg
p. 190

Stelazine
5 mg
p. 190

Stelazine
10 mg
p. 190

Sumycin
250 mg
p. 1082

Suprax
200 mg
p. 171

Suprax
400 mg
p. 171

Surmontil
25 mg
p. 1144

Surmontil
50 mg
p. 1144

Surmontil
100 mg
p. 1144

Symmetrel
100 mg
p. 45

Synalgos-DC

p. 881

Synthroid
25 mcg
p. 1099

Synthroid
50 mcg
p. 1099

Synthroid
75 mcg
p. 1099

Synthroid
100 mcg
p. 1099

Synthroid
125 mcg
p. 1099

Y

Synthroid 150 mcg p. 1099	**Synthroid** 200 mcg p. 1099	**Synthroid** 300 mcg p. 1099	**Tagamet** 300 mg p. 203
Tagamet 400 mg p. 203	**Tagamet** 800 mg p. 203	**Talwin NX** p. 882	**Tavist** 2.68 mg p. 222
Tavist-1 1.34 mg p. 222	**Tavist-D** p. 81	**Tegopen** 250 mg p. 869	**Tegretol** 200 mg p. 1061
Tegretol Chewable 100 mg p. 157	**Temazepam** 30 mg p. 1062	**Tenex** 1 mg p. 505	**Tenoretic** 50 mg p. 96
Tenoretic 100 mg p. 96	**Tenormin** 50 mg p. 96	**Tenormin** 100 mg p. 96	**Tenuate** 25 mg p. 656

Z

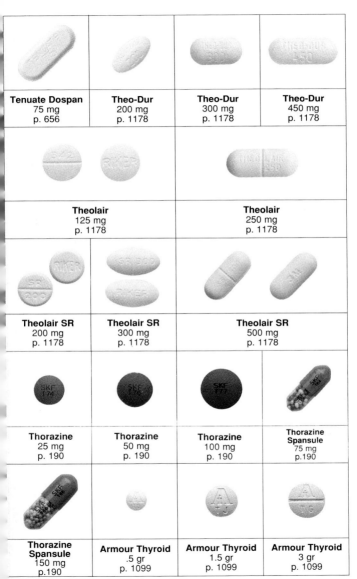

Tenuate Dospan 75 mg p. 656	**Theo-Dur** 200 mg p. 1178	**Theo-Dur** 300 mg p. 1178	**Theo-Dur** 450 mg p. 1178
Theolair 125 mg p. 1178		**Theolair** 250 mg p. 1178	
Theolair SR 200 mg p. 1178	**Theolair SR** 300 mg p. 1178	**Theolair SR** 500 mg p. 1178	
Thorazine 25 mg p. 190	**Thorazine** 50 mg p. 190	**Thorazine** 100 mg p. 190	**Thorazine Spansule** 75 mg p.190
Thorazine Spansule 150 mg p.190	**Armour Thyroid** .5 gr p. 1099	**Armour Thyroid** 1.5 gr p. 1099	**Armour Thyroid** 3 gr p. 1099

AA

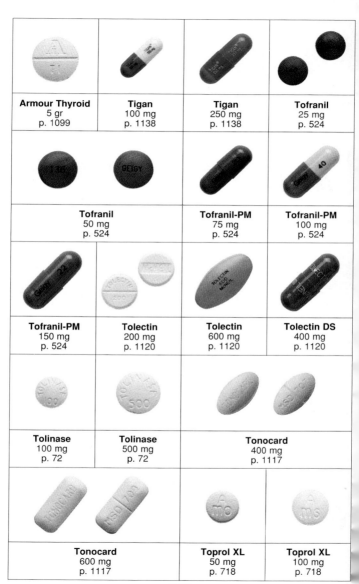

Armour Thyroid 5 gr p. 1099	**Tigan** 100 mg p. 1138	**Tigan** 250 mg p. 1138	**Tofranil** 25 mg p. 524
Tofranil 50 mg p. 524		**Tofranil-PM** 75 mg p. 524	**Tofranil-PM** 100 mg p. 524
Tofranil-PM 150 mg p. 524	**Tolectin** 200 mg p. 1120	**Tolectin** 600 mg p. 1120	**Tolectin DS** 400 mg p. 1120
Tolinase 100 mg p. 72	**Tolinase** 500 mg p. 72	**Tonocard** 400 mg p. 1117	
Tonocard 600 mg p. 1117		**Toprol XL** 50 mg p. 718	**Toprol XL** 100 mg p. 718

BB

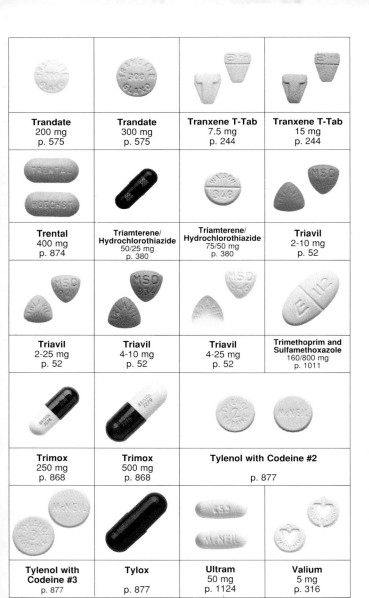

Trandate 200 mg p. 575	**Trandate** 300 mg p. 575	**Tranxene T-Tab** 7.5 mg p. 244	**Tranxene T-Tab** 15 mg p. 244
Trental 400 mg p. 874	**Triamterene/ Hydrochlorothiazide** 50/25 mg p. 380	**Triamterene/ Hydrochlorothiazide** 75/50 mg p. 380	**Triavil** 2-10 mg p. 52
Triavil 2-25 mg p. 52	**Triavil** 4-10 mg p. 52	**Triavil** 4-25 mg p. 52	**Trimethoprim and Sulfamethoxazole** 160/800 mg p. 1011
Trimox 250 mg p. 868	**Trimox** 500 mg p. 868	**Tylenol with Codeine #2** p. 877	
Tylenol with Codeine #3 p. 877	**Tylox** p. 877	**Ultram** 50 mg p. 1124	**Valium** 5 mg p. 316

CC

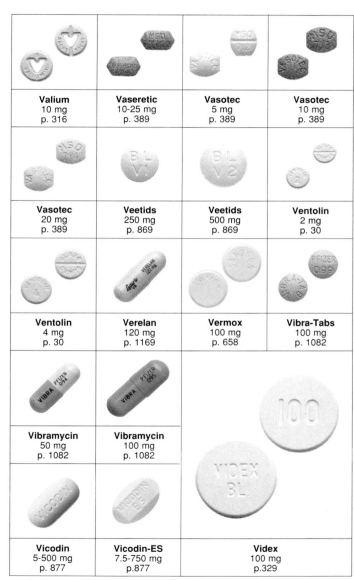

Valium 10 mg p. 316	**Vaseretic** 10-25 mg p. 389	**Vasotec** 5 mg p. 389	**Vasotec** 10 mg p. 389
Vasotec 20 mg p. 389	**Veetids** 250 mg p. 869	**Veetids** 500 mg p. 869	**Ventolin** 2 mg p. 30
Ventolin 4 mg p. 30	**Verelan** 120 mg p. 1169	**Vermox** 100 mg p. 658	**Vibra-Tabs** 100 mg p. 1082
Vibramycin 50 mg p. 1082	**Vibramycin** 100 mg p. 1082		
Vicodin 5-500 mg p. 877	**Vicodin-ES** 7.5-750 mg p.877	**Videx** 100 mg p.329	

DD

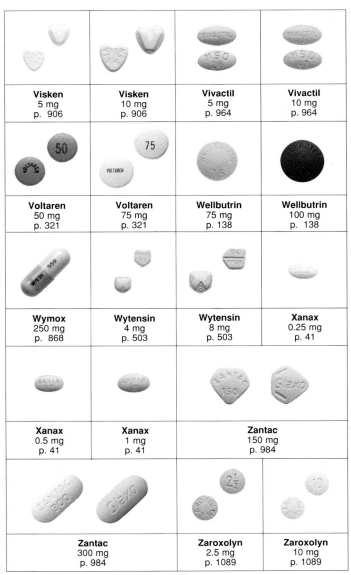

Visken 5 mg p. 906	**Visken** 10 mg p. 906	**Vivactil** 5 mg p. 964	**Vivactil** 10 mg p. 964
Voltaren 50 mg p. 321	**Voltaren** 75 mg p. 321	**Wellbutrin** 75 mg p. 138	**Wellbutrin** 100 mg p. 138
Wymox 250 mg p. 868	**Wytensin** 4 mg p. 503	**Wytensin** 8 mg p. 503	**Xanax** 0.25 mg p. 41
Xanax 0.5 mg p. 41	**Xanax** 1 mg p. 41	**Zantac** 150 mg p. 984	
Zantac 300 mg p. 984		**Zaroxolyn** 2.5 mg p. 1089	**Zaroxolyn** 10 mg p. 1089

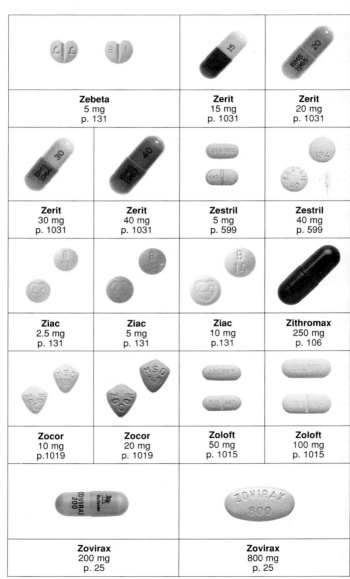

Zebeta 5 mg p. 131	**Zerit** 15 mg p. 1031	**Zerit** 20 mg p. 1031
Zerit 30 mg p. 1031	**Zerit** 40 mg p. 1031	**Zestril** 5 mg p. 599	**Zestril** 40 mg p. 599
Ziac 2.5 mg p. 131	**Ziac** 5 mg p. 131	**Ziac** 10 mg p.131	**Zithromax** 250 mg p. 106
Zocor 10 mg p.1019	**Zocor** 20 mg p. 1019	**Zoloft** 50 mg p. 1015	**Zoloft** 100 mg p. 1015
Zovirax 200 mg p. 25	**Zovirax** 800 mg p. 25		

FF

Generic Name

Lithium

Brand Names

Lithium Carbonate

Eskalith Capsules/Tablets	Lithobid Tablets
Eskalith-CR Controlled	Lithonate
Release Tablets	Lithotabs
Lithane Tablets	

Lithium Citrate

Cibalith-S Syrup   ⑤

(Also available in generic form)

Type of Drug

Antipsychotic; antimanic.

Prescribed for

Treatment of the manic phase of manic-depressive or bipolar illness; suppression and reduction of the number and intensity of manic attacks. Lithium has also been used in cancer and AIDS treatment, in children to improve white blood cell counts; to prevent migraine headaches; to treat premenstrual tension, bulimia, alcoholism (especially in people who are also depressed), postpartum "blues," and overactive thyroid. Lithium lotion has been used for genital herpes and dandruff.

General Information

Lithium is the only medicine that is effective as an antimanic drug. It reduces the level of manic episodes and may produce normal activity within the first 3 weeks of treatment. Typical manic symptoms include rapid speech, elation, hyperactive movements, need for little sleep, grandiose ideas, poor judgment, aggressiveness, and hostility.

Cautions and Warnings

This drug should not be given to anyone with **heart** or **kidney disease, dehydration, low blood sodium,** or to those taking

diuretic drugs. If such people require Lithium they must be very carefully monitored by their doctors, and hospitalization may be needed until the Lithium dose is stabilized.

A few people treated with Lithium and Haloperidol (or another antipsychotic) medicine have developed **encephalo-pathic syndrome.** This is characterized by **weakness, tiredness, fever, confusion,** and **tremulousness** and **uncontrollable muscle spasms.** Also, your doctor may find laboratory indicators of **liver and/or kidney disease.** Rarely, this combination of symptoms is followed by irreversible **brain damage.**

As many as 20 percent of people taking long-term Lithium treatment develop structural changes in their kidneys and **reduced kidney function.** Long-term use of this drug may also lead to **reduced thyroid activity,** enlargement of the thyroid gland, and increased blood levels of thyroid-stimulating hormone. All of these conditions may be treated with thyroid hormone replacement therapy. Overactive thyroid has also occasionally occurred.

Frequent urination and thirst associated with Lithium may be a sign of a condition known as *diabetes insipidus,* in which the kidney stops responding to a hormone called *vasopressin,* which causes the kidney to reabsorb water and make concentrated urine. Lithium may reverse the kidney's ability to perform this function, but things usually go back to normal when Lithium treatment is stopped, Lithium dosage is reduced, or small doses of a thiazide diuretic are taken. Your Lithium dosage may have to be temporarily reduced if you develop an **infection or fever.**

Some Lithium products contain **tartrazine dyes** for product coloring purposes. Tartrazine can stimulate allergic responses in some people, including **asthma.** Ask your pharmacist or doctor for more information.

Possible Side Effects

Side effects of Lithium are directly associated with the amount of this drug in the bloodstream. Few side effects are seen if the blood level is less than 1.5 mEq/L, except in the occasional Lithium-sensitive person. Mild to moderate side effects may occur at blood levels between 1.5 and 2.5 mEq/L. Moderate to severe reactions are seen when Lithium blood levels range from 2 to 2.5 mEq/L.

Possible Side Effects *(continued)*

▼ Most common: fine hand tremor, thirst, and excessive urination when Lithium treatment is first started (these effects may stay throughout treatment); mild nausea and discomfort during the first few days of treatment.

▼ Less common: diarrhea, vomiting, drowsiness, muscle weakness, poor coordination, giddiness, ringing or buzzing in the ears, and blurred vision.

▼ Rare: worsening symptoms in the muscles, nerves, central nervous system (blackouts, seizures, dizziness, incontinence, slurred speech, coma), heart and blood vessels, stomach and intestines (diarrhea, nausea, vomiting), kidney and urinary tract, skin, and thyroid gland. Lithium can also cause changes in tests used to monitor heart-brain function and can cause dry mouth and blurred vision.

Drug Interactions

• When Lithium is combined with Haloperidol, weakness, tiredness, fever, or confusion may result. In some people, these symptoms have been followed by permanent brain damage. Also, Haloperidol may increase the effect of Lithium.

• Lithium and Chlorpromazine may interact to reduce the effect of Chlorpromazine and increase the Lithium effect.

• The effect of Lithium is counteracted by Sodium Bicarbonate, Acetazolamide, Urea, Mannitol, and theophylline drugs, which increase the rate at which Lithium is released from the body. Verapamil may reduce both blood levels of Lithium and the chances of Lithium toxicity.

• The effect of Lithium may be increased by Methyldopa, Fluoxetine, Carbamazepine, thiazide and loop diuretics, and nonsteroidal anti-inflammatory drugs (NSAIDs).

• Lithium may increase the effects of tricyclic antidepressant medications.

Food Interactions

It is essential to maintain a normal diet, including sodium (salt) and fluid intake, because Lithium can cause a natural reduction in body-salt levels. Lithium should be taken immediately after meals or with food or milk.

Usual Dose

Dosage must be individualized to each person's needs. Most people will respond to 1800 mg per day at first. Once the person has responded to Lithium, daily dosage is reduced to the lowest effective level, usually 300 mg 3 to 4 times per day.

Overdosage

Toxic blood levels of Lithium are only slightly above the levels required for treatment. Blood levels should not exceed 2 mEq/L. Early signs of drug toxicity can be diarrhea, vomiting, nausea, tremors, drowsiness, or poor coordination. Later signs of Lithium toxicity include giddiness, weakness, blurred vision, ringing or buzzing in the ears, dizziness, fainting, confusion, muscle twitching or uncontrollable muscle movements, loss of bladder control, worsening of manic symptoms, overactive reflexes, and painful muscles or joints. **If any of these symptoms occur, stop taking the medicine and call your doctor immediately.** ALWAYS bring the medicine bottle with you when you go to a hospital emergency room or to your doctor for treatment.

Special Information

Lithium may cause drowsiness. Be cautious while driving or operating any hazardous machinery.

Lithium causes your body to lose sodium (salt). You must maintain a normal diet and salt intake, and drink 8 to 12 full glasses of water a day while taking Lithium. You may find that excessive sweating (which causes you to lose salt) or diarrhea makes you more sensitive to Lithium side effects.

Call your doctor if you develop diarrhea, vomiting, unsteady walking, tremors, drowsiness, or muscle weakness.

Your tolerance to a particular Lithium dose may be reduced when your manic symptoms decline, causing a need for your doctor to modify your dose.

If you forget to take a dose of Lithium, take it as soon as possible. However, if it is within 2 hours of your next dose (6 hours if you take the long-acting form), skip the missed dose and go back to your regular schedule. Do not take a double dose. Call your doctor if you miss more than 1 dose.

Special Populations

Pregnancy/Breast-feeding

Lithium can cause heart and thyroid birth defects, especially if taken during the first 3 months of pregnancy. It can also affect your newborn baby if the drug is present in your blood during delivery. These effects generally go away in a week or two, when the baby can eliminate the Lithium from his or her system. Talk with your doctor about the risks versus the benefits of taking this drug during your pregnancy.

Lithium passes readily into breast milk and can affect a nursing infant. Signs of these effects are weak muscle tone, low body temperature, bluish discoloration of the skin, and abnormal heart rhythms. You should bottle-feed your baby while taking this medicine.

Seniors

Older adults are more sensitive to the effects of Lithium because they cannot clear it from their bodies via their kidneys as rapidly as younger adults. It is potentially toxic to the central nervous system in older adults, even when Lithium blood levels are in the desired range. Also, seniors taking Lithium are more likely to develop an underactive thyroid.

Lo/Ovral

see Contraceptives, page 262

Lodine

see Etodolac, page 422

Generic Name

Lodoxamide Tromethamine

Brand Name

Alomide

Type of Drug

Cell stabilizer.

Prescribed for

Seasonal "pink-eye" or irritation of the cornea or conjunctiva. Also prescribed for vernal keratoconjunctivitis.

General Information

Lodoxamide stabilizes mast cells in the eye that react to seasonal allergies by releasing histamine and other reactive substances, preventing immediate hypersensitivity reactions. This drug is different from the usual drugs applied to the eye to treat these reactions and is unrelated to the antihistamines, ophthalmic NSAIDs, anti-inflammatory drugs, and vasoconstrictors (nonprescription "pink-eye" drugs).

Cautions and Warnings

Soft contact lens wearers should take their lenses out before using this product.

Possible Side Effects

▼ Most common: temporary eye burning, stinging, and discomfort.

▼ Less common: headache, eye itching or redness, blurred vision, dry eye, tearing or other discharge, crystal deposits in the eye, and a feeling of a foreign object in the eye.

▼ Rare: hot sensation throughout the body, dizziness, tiredness, nausea, upset stomach, sneezing, skin rash, dry nose, corneal abrasions, eye ulcers or erosions, scales forming on the eyelid or eyelash, eye swelling, eye pain or warmth, "tired eyes," allergic reactions, lid irritation, and sticky eyelids.

Drug Interactions

• Do not use other eyedrops together with this drug.

Food Interactions

None known.

Usual Dose

Adult and Child (age 2 and older): 1 or 2 drops in each eye 4 times per day for up to 3 months.

Overdosage

Symptoms that can occur after swallowing up to 10 milliliters (a full bottle) of this product are headache, dizziness, a feeling of warmth or flushing, fatigue, increased sweating, nausea, loose stools, and feelings of urinary urgency or frequent urination. People who have swallowed amounts equal to 12 to 18 bottles of this product experienced temporary warmth, profuse sweating, diarrhea, light-headedness, and stomach upset. No permanent effects were seen. Call your local poison control center or emergency room for more information.

Special Information

To administer eyedrops, lie down or tilt your head back and look at the ceiling. Hold the dropper above your eye, gently squeeze your lower lid to form a small pouch, and drop the medicine inside while looking up. Release the lower lid, keeping your eye open. Don't blink for about 40 seconds. Press gently on the bridge of your nose at the inside corner of your eye for about a minute to help circulate the medicine around your eye. To avoid infection, don't touch the dropper tip to your finger or eyelid. Wait at least 5 minutes before using another eyedrop or ointment.

Call your doctor at once if your eye stinging, itching or burning, redness, irritation, swelling, or pain persists or gets worse, or if you start having trouble seeing.

If you forget to take a dose of Lodoxamide eyedrops, take it as soon as you remember. If it is almost time for your next dose, skip the missed dose and continue with your regular schedule. Do not take a double dose.

Special Populations

Pregnancy/Breast-feeding

There is no information on the effect of Lodoxamide on pregnant women or nursing mothers; it should be used only if absolutely necessary.

Seniors

Seniors may use this drug without special restriction.

Generic Name

Lomefloxacin

Brand Name

Maxaquin

Type of Drug

Fluoroquinolone anti-infective.

Prescribed for

Lower respiratory infections and treating and preventing urinary infections. Lomefloxacin does not work against the common cold, flu, or other viral infections.

General Information

Lomefloxacin works against many organisms that traditional antibiotic treatments have trouble killing. Other fluoroquinolones have been used to treat skin infections, bone and joint infections, infectious diarrhea, lung infections in people with cystic fibrosis, bronchitis, pneumonia, prostate infection, and traveler's diarrhea. It is chemically related to an older antibacterial called *Nalidixic Acid*, but works better than that drug against urinary infections.

Cautions and Warnings

Do not take Lomefloxacin if you have had an **allergic** reaction to it or another fluoroquinolone in the past, or if you have had a reaction to a related medication such as Nalidixic Acid. Severe, **possibly fatal, allergic reactions** can occur even after the very first dose. Some reactions include **cardiovascular collapse, loss of consciousness, tingling, swelling of the face or throat, breathing difficulty, itching,** or **rash.** Stop taking the drug if any of these symptoms occur, and seek medical help at once.

Lomefloxacin dosage must be adjusted in the presence of **kidney failure.**

Lomefloxacin may cause increased pressure on parts of the brain, leading to **convulsions** and **psychotic reactions.**

Other possible adverse effects include **tremors, restlessness, light-headedness, confusion,** and **hallucinations.** Lomefloxacin should be used with caution in people with **seizure disorders** or other **conditions of the nervous system.**

As with any other anti-infective, people taking Lomefoxacin may develop **colitis** that could range from mild to very serious. See your doctor if you develop **diarrhea or cramps** while taking this drug.

Prolonged use of Lomefloxacin can lead to **fungal overgrowth.** Follow your doctor's directions.

People taking Lomefloxacin may experience rash, irritation, and unusual **sensitivity to the sun or to sunlamps,** including exposure through glass, and the risk of **skin cancer** may be increased. Avoid exposure to the sun or to a sunlamp while taking Lomefloxacin. If you experience such a reaction, stop taking the drug and call your doctor.

Possible Side Effects

▼ Most common: nausea, headache, dizziness, unusual sun reactions.

▼ Less common: diarrhea, headache, and rash.

▼ Rare: abdominal pain, vomiting, dry or painful mouth, constipation, gas, colitis, fatigue, drowsiness, not feeling well, depression, seizures, sleeplessness, confusion, tingling in the hands or feet, itching, rash, drug sensitivity, visual disturbances, vaginal irritation, fainting, chills, swelling in the ankles, legs or arms, painful or difficult urination, blood in the urine, kidney failure, vaginal infections, pelvic pains, low blood pressure, rapid heartbeat, abnormal heart rhythms, angina, heart failure, heart attack, pulmonary embolism, vein inflammation, respiratory infection, breathing difficulty, nosebleeds, bronchial spasms, coma, coughing, tremors, fainting, dizziness, anxiety, depersonalization, decreased or increased appetite, stomach inflammation and bleeding, difficulty swallowing, tongue discoloration, taste disturbances, earache, ringing or buzzing in the ears, eye pain, "pink-eye," skin peeling, eczema, flushing, sweating, back or chest pains, facial swelling, muscle and joint pains, leg cramps, low blood sugar, and excessive thirst.

Drug Interactions

- Antacids, Didanosine, Iron and Zinc supplements, and Sucralfate will decrease the amount of Lomefloxacin absorbed into the bloodstream. If you must take any of these products, separate them from your Lomefloxacin dosage by at least 2 hours.
- Anticancer drugs may also reduce the amount of Lomefoxacin in your bloodstream.
- Probenecid cuts the amount of Lomefloxacin released through the kidneys by half, and may increase the chance of drug side effects. Cimetidine also interferes with the release of Lomefloxacin from the body.
- Lomefloxacin may increase the effects of oral anticoagulant (blood-thinning) drugs. Your anticoagulant dose may have to be adjusted.
- Lomefloxacin may increase the toxic effects of Cyclosporine (for organ transplants) on your kidneys.
- Lomefloxacin may reduce the rate at which Theophylline is released from your body, increasing Theophylline blood levels and the chance for related drug side effects.

Food Interactions

Food delays the absorption of Lomefloxacin and reduces the total amount absorbed, but this is not enough to influence the drug's effectiveness. Lomefloxacin may be taken without regard to food or meals.

Usual Dose

400 mg a day. Dosage is adjusted in the presence of kidney failure.

Overdosage

The symptoms of Lomefloxacin overdose are the same as those found under *Possible Side Effects.* One person experienced kidney failure when he took an overdose of Ciprofloxacin, another fluoroquinolone. You may induce vomiting with Syrup of Ipecac (available at any pharmacy) to remove excess medication from the victim's stomach. Consult your local poison control center or hospital emergency room for specific instructions. Overdose victims should be taken to a hospital emergency room for treatment of those symptoms. ALWAYS bring the medicine bottle with you.

Special Information

Take each Lomefloxacin dose with a full glass of water. Be sure to drink at least 8 glasses of water per day while taking this medicine to promote removal of the drug from your system and to help avoid side effects.

If you are taking an antacid or an Iron or Zinc supplement while taking Lomefloxacin, be sure to separate the doses by at least 2 hours to avoid a possible drug interaction.

Drug sensitivity reactions can develop after only one dose of this medicine! Stop taking it and get immediate medical attention if you faint or if you develop itching, rash, facial swelling, difficulty breathing, convulsions, depression, visual disturbances, dizziness, headache, light-headedness, or any sign of a drug reaction.

Colitis can be caused by any anti-infective medication. If diarrhea develops after taking Lomefloxacin, call your doctor at once.

Avoid sun and/or sunlamp exposure.

It is essential that you take Lomefloxacin according to your doctor's directions. Do not stop taking it, even if you begin to feel better in a few days, unless directed to do so by your doctor.

If you forget to take a dose of Lomefloxacin, take it as soon as you remember. If it is almost time for your next dose, skip the forgotten dose and continue with your regular schedule. Do not take a double dose.

Special Populations

Pregnancy/Breast-feeding

Pregnant women should not take Lomefloxacin unless its benefits have been carefully weighed against its risks. Animal studies have shown that Lomefloxacin may reduce your chances for a successful pregnancy or may damage a developing fetus.

It is not known if Lomefloxacin passes into breast milk. Nursing mothers who must take this medication should bottle-feed their babies.

Seniors

Studies in healthy seniors showed that Lomefloxacin is released from their bodies 25 percent more slowly than from the bodies of younger adults because of decreased kidney function. Drug dosage must be reduced according to kidney function.

Brand Name

Lomotil Liquid/Tablets

Ingredients

Atropine Sulfate + Diphenoxylate

Other Brand Names

Logen Tablets
Lomanate Liquid
Lonox Tablets

(Also available in generic form)

Type of Drug

Antidiarrheal.

Prescribed for

Symptomatic relief of diarrhea.

General Information

Lomotil and other antidiarrheal agents should be used only for short periods. They will relieve diarrhea, but not its underlying causes. In some cases, these drugs should not be used even though diarrhea is present: People with certain bowel or stomach diseases may be harmed by taking antidiarrheal drugs. Obviously, the decision to use Lomotil *must* be made by your doctor.

Cautions and Warnings

Do not take Lomotil if you are **allergic** to it or to any other medication containing **Atropine Sulfate**. If you have **jaundice** (yellowing of the eyes and/or skin) or are suffering from **diarrhea caused by antibiotics** such as Clindamycin or Lincomycin, do not take this drug. People with **liver disease** should use this drug with caution.

This medicine may worsen or prolong **diarrhea** associated with *E. Coli*, *Salmonella*, and *Shigella* and with a condition called *pseudomembranous colitis*. You should **stop taking Lomotil if your diarrhea worsens** or if other symptoms develop.

Severe diarrhea can lead to **dehydration** (loss of body fluid and salts), which can cause additional gastric difficulties. This situation can expose some people, especially young children, to a possible delayed drug response or toxic drug effects.

Possible Side Effects

▼ Most common: skin dryness inside the nose or mouth, facial flushing or redness, fever, unusual heart rates, and inability to urinate.

▼ Less common: people taking Lomotil for extended periods may experience abdominal discomfort, swelling of the gums, interference with normal breathing, feeling of numbness in the extremities, drowsiness, restlessness, rashes, nausea, sedation, vomiting, headache, dizziness, depression, feeling unwell, lethargy, loss of appetite, euphoria (feeling "high"), itching, and coma.

Drug Interactions

• Lomotil, a central-nervous-system depressant, may make you tired or unable to concentrate, and may increase the effect of sleeping pills, tranquilizers, and alcohol. Avoid large amounts of alcoholic beverages while taking it.

• Avoid taking Lomotil together with a monamine oxidase (MAO) inhibitor. This combination may cause susceptible people to develop dangerously high blood pressure.

Food Interactions

You may take this drug with food if it upsets your stomach.

Usual Dose

Adult and Adolescent (age 13 and older): 2 tablets 4 times per day until diarrhea has stopped; dose should then be reduced to the lowest level that will control diarrhea (usually 2 tablets per day or less).

Child (age 9 to 12, about 51 to 121 pounds): 3.5 to 5 milliliters 4 times a day.

Child (age 5 to 8, about 35 to 71 pounds): 2.5 to 5 milliliters 4 times a day.

Child (age 4, about 31 to 44 pounds): 2 to 4 milliliters 4 times a day.

Child (age 3, about 26 to 35 pounds): 2 to 3 milliliters 4 times a day.

Child (age 2, about 24 to 31 pounds): 1.5 to 3 milliliters 4 times a day.

Child (under age 2): not recommended.

The liquid form, supplied with a dropper calibrated to deliver medication as desired in milliliters, is used for children age 2 to 12.

Overdosage

Lomotil overdose is generally accidental: some patients, feeling that the prescribed amount has not cured their diarrhea, will take more medication on their own. Symptoms of overdosage (particularly effects on breathing) may not be evident until 12 to 30 hours after the medication has been taken. Symptoms are dryness of skin, mouth, and/or nose; flushing; fever; abnormal heart rates with possible lethargy; coma; or depression of breathing. The victim should be taken to a hospital emergency room immediately. ALWAYS bring the medicine bottle with you.

Special Information

Lomotil may cause drowsiness and difficulty concentrating: Be careful while driving or operating hazardous machinery.

Do not take more Lomotil than is prescribed, and avoid alcohol and other drugs that depress the nervous system.

Notify your doctor if your diarrhea persists or gets worse, if heart palpitations occur, or if you develop any other bothersome or persistent drug side effect.

If you forget to take a dose of Lomotil, take it as soon as you remember. If it is almost time for your next dose, skip the one you forgot and continue with your regular schedule. Do not take a double dose.

Special Populations

Pregnancy/Breast-feeding

Lomotil crosses into the fetal blood circulation, but has not been found to cause birth defects. When the drug is considered essential by your doctor, its potential benefits must be carefully weighed against its risks.

The ingredients in this drug pass into breast milk. You must consider the possible effects of this medicine on a nursing infant.

Seniors

Older adults are more sensitive to the side effects of this drug, especially breathing difficulty. Follow your doctor's directions and report any side effects at once.

Type of Drug

Loop Diuretics

Generic Name	Brand Name
Bumetanide	Bumex*
Ethacrynic Acid	Edecrin
Furosemide	Lasix*
Torsemide	Demadex

(*Also available in generic form)

Prescribed for

Congestive heart failure, cirrhosis of the liver, fluid accumulation in the lungs, kidney dysfunction, high blood pressure, and other conditions where it may be desirable to rid the body of excess fluid. Bumetanide can be used to treat people who urinate frequently at night. It does not work in prostatic hypertrophy.

General Information

Loop diuretics are strong medicines that work similarly to the less potent and more widely used thiazide diuretics. Not only do they affect the same part of the kidney as the thiazide-type diuretics, they also affect the portion of the kidney known as the *loop of Henle*. This double action is what makes the loop diuretics such potent drugs. All 4 loop diuretics can be used for the same purposes, but their doses are quite different.

Cautions and Warnings

Do not take these medicines if you are **sensitive** or **allergic** to them. People **allergic to sulfa drugs** may also be allergic to Furosemide, Torsemide, or Bumetanide.

Loop diuretics are potent medicines and can cause **depletion of water and electrolytes.** They should not be taken without **constant medical supervision.** You should not take these drugs if your **urine production** has been decreased abnormally by some type of **kidney disease.**

Excessive use of loop diuretics will result in **dehydration** or reduction in blood volume, and may cause circulatory collapse or other related problems, particularly in older adults.

Ringing or buzzing in the ears, hearing loss, deafness, fainting, and **fullness in the ears** can occur with these drugs. Hearing usually returns within 24 hours but some loss may be permanent.

These drugs may worsen **systemic lupus erythematosus. Diarrhea** may occur with Ethacrynic Acid or Furosemide solution (because of the sorbitol content). Rarely, people taking Bumetanide have developed **thrombocytopenia** (bleeding caused by very low platelet counts).

Because of the potent effect that these drugs have on blood electrolytes—potassium, sodium, carbon dioxide, and others—frequent laboratory evaluations of these electrolytes should be performed during the few months of therapy and periodically thereafter.

People taking a loop diuretic may develop increased levels of **total cholesterol, LDL cholesterol,** and **triglycerides.**

Possible Side Effects

▼ Common: changes may develop in potassium and other electrolyte concentrations in your body. In the case of hypokalemia (low blood potassium), you may observe dryness of the mouth, excessive thirst, weakness, lethargy, drowsiness, restlessness, muscle pains or cramps, muscular tiredness, low blood pressure, decreased frequency of urination and decreased amount of urine

---

Possible Side Effects *(continued)*

produced, abnormal heart rate, and stomach upset (including nausea and vomiting). To make up for this potassium loss, potassium supplements (tablets, liquids, or powders) and/or potassium-rich foods (bananas, citrus fruits, melons, and tomatoes) are recommended.

Loop diuretics may change sugar metabolism in your body: If you have diabetes mellitus, you may develop high blood sugar or sugar in the urine. To treat this problem, the dosage of your antidiabetes drugs will have to be increased.

▼ Less common: abdominal discomfort, nausea, vomiting, diarrhea, rash, dizziness, light-headedness, headache, blurred vision, fatigue, weakness, jaundice (yellowing of the eyes or skin), acute gout attacks, dermatitis and other skin reactions, tingling in the extremities, dizziness upon rising quickly from a sitting or lying position, and anemias.

▼ Rare: a sweet taste in the mouth, a burning feeling in the stomach and/or mouth, excessive thirst, increased perspiration, and frequent urination.

Drug Interactions

• Loop diuretics increase the action of other blood-pressure-lowering drugs. This is beneficial and is frequently used to help lower blood pressure in patients with hypertension.

• The possibility of developing electrolyte imbalances in body fluids is increased if you take medications such as Digitalis or adrenal corticosteroids while you are taking a loop diuretic. Be aware that the potassium loss caused by loop diuretics will significantly affect the toxicity of Digitalis.

• Loop diuretics may increase the action of oral anticoagulants (blood-thinners); dosage adjustment may be needed if you are taking an anticoagulant.

• If you are taking an oral antidiabetes drug (except Metformin) and begin taking a loop diuretic, the antidiabetes dosage may need to be altered.

• The action of Theophylline may be altered by any loop diuretic. Your doctor should check your Theophylline levels after you have started on a loop diuretic.

- If you are taking Lithium Carbonate, you should probably not take a diuretic, which, by impairing the elimination of Lithium from the blood, adds a high risk of Lithium toxicity.
- People taking Chloral Hydrate (as a nighttime sedative) rarely experience hot flashes, high blood pressure, sweating, abnormal heart rhythms, weakness, and nausea when they also take a loop diuretic.
- Periodic hearing loss or ringing or buzzing in the ears may occur if a loop diuretic is taken with Cisplatin (anticancer drug) or an aminoglycoside antibiotic. Make sure your doctor knows you are taking a loop diuretic before giving you an injection of either of these.
- Clofibrate and thiazide diuretics increase the action of loop diuretics.
- Charcoal tablets, Phenytoin, Probenecid, Aspirin and other salicylate drugs, and nonsteroidal anti-inflammatory drugs (NSAIDs) may decrease the effectiveness of loop diuretics.
- If you are taking a loop diuretic for high blood pressure or congestive heart failure, avoid over-the-counter cough, cold, and allergy products, which often contain stimulant drugs; check with your pharmacist before taking any over-the-counter drug if you're taking a loop diuretic.

Food Interactions

Loop diuretics rob your body of potassium. To counteract this effect, be sure to eat high-potassium foods (including bananas, citrus fruits, melons, and tomatoes).

Furosemide should be taken on an empty stomach, at least 1 hour before or 2 hours after meals. The other loop diuretics (Bumetanide, Torsemide, and Ethacrynic Acid) may be taken without regard to food or meals, and may be taken with food or meals if they upset your stomach.

Usual Dose

Bumetanide
0.5 to 2 mg per day. It may also be taken every other day for 3 or 4 consecutive days followed by 1 or 2 medicine-free days.

Ethacrynic Acid
    Adult: 50 to 200 mg, taken every day or every other day.
    Child: starting dose, 25 mg; increase slowly.

Furosemide

Adult: 20 to 80 mg per day, depending on your response. Doses of 600 mg (or more) per day have been prescribed.

Infant and Child: 0.9 mg per pound of body weight daily in a single dose. If therapy is not successful, the dose may be increased in small steps, but not more than 2.7 mg per pound per day.

Torsemide

Adult: 5 to 20 mg once per day; however, doses up to 200 mg may be prescribed.

Child: not recommended.

Maintenance doses for all of the loop diuretics are adjusted to the minimum effective level to meet the individual's needs.

Overdosage

Symptoms include dehydration, reduced blood volume, passing of tremendous amounts of urine, weakness, dizziness, confusion, loss of appetite, tiredness, vomiting, and cramps. Overdose victims should be taken to an emergency room for treatment. ALWAYS bring the medicine bottle with you.

Special Information

If while taking a loop diuretic the amount of urine you produce each day is dropping or if you suffer from cramps, significant loss of appetite, muscle weakness, tiredness, or nausea, contact your doctor immediately.

Loop diuretics are usually taken once a day after breakfast. If a second dose is needed, it should be taken no later than 2 p.m. to avoid waking up during the night to urinate.

To avoid the dizziness associated with these drugs, rise slowly and carefully when you are getting up from a sitting or lying position.

Loop diuretics can increase blood sugar. Diabetics may have to have their medicine adjusted.

Loop diuretics can make some people very sensitive to the sun or sunlamps. Avoid excess exposure, use sunscreens, and wear protective clothing.

If you forget to take a loop diuretic dose, take it as soon as you remember. If it is almost time for your next dose, skip the one you forgot and continue with your regular schedule. Do not take a double dose.

Special Populations

Pregnancy/Breast-feeding

Loop diuretics have been used to treat specific conditions in pregnancy, but they should be used only when absolutely necessary.

Loop diuretics may pass into breast milk. Bottle-feed your baby if you must take one of these medicines.

Seniors

Seniors are more sensitive to the effects of these drugs. Follow your doctor's directions and report any side effects at once.

Generic Name

Loperamide

Brand Names

Imodium-AD Liquid/Caplets/
   Chewable Tablets
Kaopectate II Caplets
Maalox Anti-Diarrheal
   Caplets

Maalox Anti-Diarrheal
   Caplets
Pepto Diarrhea Control

(Also available in generic form)

Type of Drug

Antidiarrheal.

Prescribed for

Symptomatic treatment of diarrhea, including traveler's diarrhea. Also prescribed to reduce the amount of discharge from ileostomy tubes.

General Information

Loperamide and other antidiarrheal agents should be used only for short periods; they will relieve the diarrhea, but not its underlying causes. Sometimes these drugs should not be used even though diarrhea is present: People with some kinds of bowel, stomach, or other disease may be harmed by taking antidiarrheals. Loperamide can be purchased without a prescription under a variety of brand names. Loperamide is not known to be addictive.

Cautions and Warnings

Do not use Loperamide if you are **allergic** or **sensitive** to it, if you suffer from **diarrhea associated with colitis,** or if you have an intestinal infection of *E. coli*, *Salmonella*, or *Shigella*. Loperamide should not be used together with **Clindamycin**.

If you have **ulcerative colitis** and start taking Loperamide, stop the medicine at once and call your doctor if you develop abdominal problems of any kind.

Possible Side Effects

The incidence of side effects from Loperamide is low. Side effects are most likely to occur when taking Loperamide for longer periods of time to treat chronic diarrhea.

▼ Most common: stomach and abdominal pain, bloating or other discomfort, constipation, dry mouth, dizziness, tiredness, nausea and vomiting, and drug-sensitivity reactions, including rash.

Drug Interactions

• Loperamide, which depresses the central nervous system, may make you tired and unable to concentrate, and may increase the effect of sleeping pills, tranquilizers, and alcohol. Avoid drinking large amounts of alcoholic beverages while taking Loperamide.

Food Interactions

Loperamide should be taken on an empty stomach. However, it is important to maintain a proper diet and to drink plenty of fluids to restore normal bowel function.

Usual Dose

Acute Diarrhea

Adult and Adolescent (age 12 and older): 4 mg to start, followed by 2 mg after each loose stool, up to 16 mg per day maximum. Improvement should be seen in 2 days. People with long-term (chronic) diarrhea usually need 2 to 4 capsules per day. This drug usually is effective within 10 days or not at all.

Child (age 9 to 12): 2 mg 3 times per day to start, then 1 mg for every 22 pounds of body weight after each loose stool, up to 6 mg per day maximum.

Child (age 6 to 8): 2 mg twice per day to start, then 1 mg for every 22 pounds of body weight after each loose stool, up to 4 mg per day maximum.

Child (age 2 to 5): 1 mg, 3 times per day to start, then 1 mg for every 22 pounds of body weight after each loose stool, up to 3 mg per day maximum.

Traveler's Diarrhea

Adult and Adolescent (age 12 and older): 4 mg after the first loose movement, then 2 mg after each following loose movement, up to 8 mg per day for 2 days.

Child (age 9 to 11, or 60 to 95 pounds): 2 mg after the first loose stool and 1 mg after each following loose movement, up to 6 mg per day for 2 days.

Child (age 6 to 8, or 48 to 59 pounds): 1 mg after the first loose stool and 1 mg after each following loose movement, up to 4 mg per day for 2 days.

Overdosage

Symptoms of overdosage are constipation, irritation of the stomach, and tiredness. Large doses usually cause vomiting. The overdose victim should be taken to the emergency room immediately. ALWAYS bring the medicine bottle with you.

Special Information

Loperamide may cause drowsiness and difficulty concentrating: Be careful while driving or operating any appliance or hazardous equipment.

Loperamide may cause dry mouth. Drink plenty of water or other clear fluids to prevent dehydration from the diarrhea. Call your doctor if the diarrhea persists after a few days of Loperamide treatment or if you develop abdominal discomfort or pain, fever, or other drug side effects.

If you forget to take a dose of Loperamide, do not take the

forgotten dose. Skip the dose and go back to your regular schedule. Do not take a double dose.

Special Populations

Pregnancy/Breast-feeding
This drug has not been found to cause birth defects. Pregnant women, or those who might become pregnant while taking this drug, should not take it without their doctors' approval. When the drug is considered essential by your doctor, the risk of taking it must be carefully weighed against the benefits it might produce.

It is not known if Loperamide passes into breast milk. Consider the possible effect on a nursing infant if you are breast-feeding while taking Loperamide.

Seniors
Older adults may be more sensitive to the constipating effects of Loperamide.

Lopressor

see *Metoprolol*, page 718

Lorabid

see *Cephalosporin Antibiotics*, page 171

Generic Name

Loratadine

Brand Name
Claritin

Type of Drug
Antihistamine.

Prescribed for

Seasonal allergy, stuffy and runny nose, itching of the eyes, scratchy throat caused by allergies, and other allergic symptoms such as rash, itching, or hives. Loratadine is also used for asthmatics whose asthma may be triggered by an allergic reaction.

General Information

Loratadine causes less sedation than most other antihistamines available in the United States. It has been widely used and accepted by those who find other antihistamines unacceptable because of the drowsiness and tiredness they cause. Loratadine appears to work in exactly the same way as Chlorpheniramine and other widely used antihistamines.

Cautions and Warnings

Do not take Loratadine if you have had an **allergic** reaction to it in the past.

People with **liver disease** should receive smaller doses of Loratadine than others because they are unable to clear the drug as rapidly from their bodies.

Possible Side Effects

▼ Most common: headache, dry mouth, and drowsiness or fatigue.

▼ Less common: sweating, tearing, male impotence, thirst, flushing, blurred vision, conjunctivitis, earache, eye pain, ringing or buzzing in the ears, weight gain, back pain, leg cramps, chest pain, fever, chills, feelings of ill health, weakness, worsening of allergic symptoms, respiratory infection, breathing difficulty, blood pressure changes, dizziness, fainting, heart palpitations, rapid heartbeat, hyperactivity, tingling in the hands or feet, eye-muscle spasms, migraines, tremors, nausea, vomiting, gas, abdominal distress, stomach irritation or upset, constipation, diarrhea, taste changes, appetite changes, toothache, joint or muscle aches or pains, anxiety, depression, agitation, sleeplessness, memory lapse, loss of concentration, paranoia, confusion, nervousness, loss of

Possible Side Effects *(continued)*

sex drive, breast pain, vaginal irritation, menstrual changes, dry nose, stuffed nose, runny nose, nosebleeds, sore throat, breathing difficulty, coughing, sneezing, vomiting blood, sneezing, bronchitis, bronchial spasm, laryngitis, itching, rash, dry hair or skin, unusual sensitivity to the sun, black-and-blue marks, altered urination, and urine discoloration.

▼ Rare: swelling in the legs, ankles, or feet; yellowing of the skin or eyes; hepatitis; hair loss; seizures; breast enlargement; and erythema multiforme (a very specific skin reaction).

Drug Interactions

• Unlike most other antihistamines, Loratadine is not known to interact with alcohol or other nervous-system depressants to produce drowsiness or loss of coordination.

• Loratadine, like other nonsedating antihistamines, may possibly interact with Ketoconazole, Erythromycin, Cimetidine, Ranitidine, or Theophylline. Conclusive evidence for these interactions has not yet been established due to the small numbers of people taking these drug combinations. If you are taking any of these drugs with Loratadine, be sure to report any problems to your doctor.

Food Interactions

Loratadine should be taken on an empty stomach, 1 hour before or 2 hours after food or meals, although it may be taken with food or milk if it upsets your stomach.

Usual Dose

Adult and Child (over age 12): 10 mg once a day.
People with liver disease should take 10 mg every other day.

Overdosage

Loratadine overdose is likely to cause drowsiness, headache, and rapid heartbeat. Exaggerated drug side effects may also occur. Overdose victims should be given Syrup of Ipecac to make them vomit and be taken to a hospital emergency room for treatment. Call your local poison center or hospital emergency room for instructions. ALWAYS bring the prescription bottle with you.

Special Information

Dizziness or fainting may be the first sign of serious drug side effects. Call your doctor at once if this happens to you.

Report sore throat; unusual bleeding, bruising, tiredness, or weakness; or any other unusual side effects to your doctor.

If you forget to take a dose of Loratadine, take it as soon as you remember. If it is almost time for your next regularly scheduled dose, skip the one you forgot and continue with your regular schedule. Do not take a double dose.

Special Populations

Pregnancy/Breast-feeding

Animal studies of Loratadine have not revealed any adverse effect on the developing fetus. Nevertheless, you should not take any antihistamine without your doctor's knowledge if you are pregnant.

Loratadine passes easily into breast milk and may affect a nursing infant. Nursing mothers should avoid Loratadine or use an alternative feeding method while taking the medicine.

Seniors

Seniors are unlikely to experience nervous-system effects with Loratadine, as opposed to some of the older, more sedating antihistamines. However, older adults, especially those with liver disease, will be more likely to experience drug side effects than their younger counterparts. Report any unusual side effects to your doctor.

Generic Name

Lorazepam

Brand Names

Alzapam
Ativan

(Also available in generic form)

Type of Drug

Benzodiazepine tranquilizer.

Prescribed for

Symptoms of anxiety, tension, fatigue, and agitation. Also prescribed for irritable bowel syndrome, panic attacks, and chronic sleeplessness.

General Information

Lorazepam is a member of a group of drugs known as *benzodiazepines*. All have some activity as antianxiety agents, anticonvulsants, or sedatives. Some are more suited to a specific role because of differences in their chemical makeup that give them greater activity in a certain area or characteristics that make them more desirable for a certain function. Often, individual drugs are limited by the applications for which their research has been sponsored. Benzodiazepines work by a direct effect on the brain. In doing so, they can relax you and make you either more tranquil or sleepier, or slow nervous-system transmissions in such a way as to act as an anticonvulsant, depending on which drug you are taking and how much you take. Many doctors prefer the benzodiazepines to other drugs that can be used for similar effects because they tend to be safer, have fewer side effects, and are usually as, if not more, effective.

Cautions and Warnings

Do not take Lorazepam if you know you are **sensitive** or **allergic** to it or another member of the group, including **Clonazepam,** which is used only as an anticonvulsant.

Lorazepam can aggravate **narrow-angle glaucoma,** but if you have **open-angle glaucoma** you may take it. In any case, check with your doctor. Other conditions where Lorazepam should be avoided are **severe depression, severe lung disease, sleep apnea** (intermittent breathing while sleeping), **liver disease, drunkenness,** and **kidney disease.** In all of these conditions, the depressive effects of Lorazepam may be enhanced and/or could be detrimental to your overall condition.

Lorazepam should not be taken by **psychotic patients**

because it doesn't work for them and can cause unusual excitement, stimulation, and rage.

Lorazepam is not intended to be used for more than **3 to 4 months at a time**. Your doctor should reassess your condition before continuing your prescription beyond that time.

Lorazepam may be **addictive,** and you can experience drug-withdrawal symptoms if you suddenly stop taking it after as little as 4 to 6 weeks of treatment. **Withdrawal symptoms** are more likely with shorter-acting drugs such as Lorazepam taken for long periods. Withdrawal generally begins with increased feelings of **anxiety** and continues with **tingling in the extremities, sensitivity to bright light or the sun, long periods of sleep or sleeplessness,** a **metallic taste, flulike illness, fatigue, difficulty concentrating, restlessness, loss of appetite, nausea, irritability, headache, dizziness, sweating, muscle tension** or **cramps, tremors,** and **feeling uncomfortable or ill at ease.** Other major withdrawal symptoms include confusion, abnormal perception of movement, depersonalization, paranoid delusions, hallucinations, psychotic reactions, muscle twitching, seizures, and memory loss.

Possible Side Effects

▼ Most common: mild drowsiness during the first few days of therapy. Weakness and confusion may also occur, especially in seniors and those who are more sickly. If these effects persist, contact your doctor.

▼ Less common: depression, lethargy, disorientation, headache, inactivity, slurred speech, stupor, dizziness, tremors, constipation, dry mouth, nausea, inability to control urination, sexual difficulties, irregular menstrual cycle, changes in heart rhythm, lowered blood pressure, fluid retention, blurred or double vision, itching, rash, hiccups, nervousness, inability to fall asleep, and occasional liver dysfunction. If you experience any of these symptoms, stop taking the medicine and contact your doctor immediately.

▼ Rare: constipation, diarrhea, dry mouth, coated tongue, sore gums, vomiting, appetite changes, swallowing difficulty, increased salivation, upset stomach, incontinence, changes in sex drive, urinary difficulties, changes

---

Possible Side Effects *(continued)*

in heart rate, palpitations, swelling, stuffed nose, hearing difficulty, hair loss, hairiness, sweating, fever, tingling in the hands or feet, breast pain, muscle disturbances, breathing difficulty, changes in blood components, and joint pain.

Drug Interactions

• Lorazepam is a central-nervous-system depressant. Avoid taking it with alcohol, other tranquilizers, narcotics, barbiturates, monoamine oxidase (MAO) inhibitors, antihistamines, and antidepressants. Taking Lorazepam with these drugs may result in excessive depression, tiredness, sleepiness, difficulty breathing, or similar symptoms.

• Smoking may reduce the effectiveness of Lorazepam by increasing the rate at which it is broken down by the body.

• The effects of Lorazepam may be prolonged when it is taken together with Cimetidine, oral contraceptives, Disulfiram, Fluoxetine, Isoniazid, Ketoconazole, Metoprolol, Probenecid, Propoxyphene, Propranolol, Rifampin, or Valproic Acid. Theophylline may reduce Lorazepam's sedative effects.

• If you take antacids, separate them from your Lorazepam dose by at least 1 hour to prevent them from interfering with the absorption of the Lorazepam into the bloodstream.

• Lorazepam may increase blood levels of Digoxin and the chances for Digoxin toxicity.

• The effect of Levodopa may be decreased if it is taken together with Lorazepam.

• Phenytoin blood concentrations may increase when taken with Lorazepam, resulting in possible Phenytoin toxicity.

Food Interactions

Lorazepam is best taken on an empty stomach but may be taken with food if it upsets your stomach.

Usual Dose

Adult: 2 to 10 mg per day as individualized for maximum benefit, depending on symptoms and response to treatment, which may call for a dose outside the range given. Most people require 2 to 6 mg per day. For sleep, 2 to 4 mg may be taken at bedtime.

Senior: a smaller dose is usually needed to control anxiety and tension.

Child: not recommended.

Overdosage

Symptoms of overdose are confusion, sleepiness, poor coordination, lack of response to pain such as a pin prick, loss of reflexes, shallow breathing, low blood pressure, and coma. The victim should be taken to a hospital emergency room for treatment. ALWAYS bring the medicine bottle with you.

Special Information

Lorazepam can cause tiredness, drowsiness, inability to concentrate, or similar symptoms. Be careful if you are driving, operating machinery, or performing other activities that require concentration.

People taking Lorazepam for more than 3 or 4 months at a time may develop drug withdrawal reactions if the medication is stopped suddenly.

If you forget a dose of Lorazepam, take it as soon as you remember. If it is almost time for your next dose, skip the forgotten pill and continue with your regular schedule. Do not take a double dose.

Special Populations

Pregnancy/Breast-feeding

Lorazepam may cause birth defects if taken during the first 3 months of pregnancy; avoid taking it while pregnant.

Lorazepam passes into breast milk. Because infants break the drug down more slowly than adults, it is possible for the medicine to accumulate and have an undesirable effect on the baby. Bottle-feed your baby while taking this drug.

Seniors

Older adults, especially those with liver or kidney disease, are more sensitive to the effects of Lorazepam and generally require smaller doses to achieve the same effect. Follow your doctor's directions and report any side effects at once.

Generic Name

Losartan Potassium

Brand Name

Cozaar

NOTE: This drug is also available under the brand name Hyzaar in a single-tablet combination that also includes hydrochlorothiazide and potassium.

Type of Drug

Angiotensin-receptor antagonist.

Prescribed for

High blood pressure.

General Information

Losartan is the first of a new class of drug products for high blood pressure called *angiotensin-receptor antagonists*. Losartan works by interfering with the special sites in blood vessels and other tissues where *angiotensin II*, a potent hormone that normally works as part of the body's system for maintaining blood pressure, exerts its effect. Losartan works best when taken with a thiazide-type diuretic. Don't confuse this drug with the many angiotensin-converting-enzyme (ACE) inhibitors that are in use today; they interrupt the body's production of angiotensin II.

After you take Losartan, most of it is transformed in the liver to another, longer-lasting, compound that is actually reponsible for most of the drug's effect. Losartan's effect lasts about 1 day.

Cautions and Warnings

Do not take Losartan if you are **sensitive** or **allergic** to it.

People with serious **liver disease** or **cirrhosis** should receive lower doses of Losartan.

Some people may develop changes in **kidney functioning** while taking Losartan. This effect is similar to that seen in some people who take ACE inhibitor drugs.

Possible Side Effects

In clinical studies of Losartan, the reported chance of having a side effect was about the same for people taking Losartan and those taking a placebo.

▼ Most common: diarrhea, upset stomach, muscle cramps, muscle aches, back and leg pains, dizziness, sleeplessness, stuffy nose, cough, respiratory infection, and sinusitis and other sinus disorders.

▼ Less common: weakness, tiredness, swelling, abdominal pains, chest pains, nausea, headache, and sore throat.

▼ Rare: drug allergy or hypersensitivity and skin peeling. Other rare side effects can affect virtually every body system.

Drug Interactions

• Losartan may interfere with the breakdown of other drugs in the liver. Studies of Losartan have shown no important interactions with Hydrochlorothiazide, Digoxin, Warfarin, and Cimetidine.

• Taking Phenobarbital together with Losartan can reduce the amount of active Losartan in the blood by 20 percent.

• Combining Losartan with another blood-pressure-lowering drug, such as Hydrochlorothiazide, reduces blood pressure more efficiently than either drug taken alone. People already taking a diuretic who start taking Losartan may experience rapid blood pressure lowering at first and should start with a lower Losartan dosage.

Food Interactions

Food slows the absorption of Losartan into the blood, but does not affect overall response to the medicine. You can take Losartan without regard to food or meals.

Usual Dose

Adult: 25 to 50 mg once a day to start, increasing gradually up to 100 mg in one or two doses a day.

Child: Losartan has not been studied in children under age 18 and should not be given to young children.

Overdosage

Animal studies indicate that Losartan could be lethal in massive overdose, but little is known about human overdose. The most likely effects of Losartan overdose are very low blood pressure and rapid heartbeat. Overdose victims should be taken to a hospital emergency room for evaluation and treatment. ALWAYS bring the medicine bottle with you.

Special Information

Studies have shown that Losartan is much less effective in African-Americans than in people of other ethnic backgrounds.

Women tend to absorb twice as much Losartan as men, but the amount of active drug in the blood is about the same; no dosage adjustments are needed.

Avoid strenuous exercise and/or very hot weather because heavy sweating or dehydration can cause a rapid drop in blood pressure.

Avoid nonprescription diet pills, decongestants, and stimulants that can raise blood pressure.

If you take Losartan once a day and forget to take a dose, take it as soon as you remember. If it is within 8 hours of your next dose, skip the one you forgot and continue with your regular schedule. Do not take a double dose.

If you take Losartan twice a day and forget a dose, take it as soon as you remember. If it is within 4 hours of your next dose, take one dose as soon as you remember and another in 5 or 6 hours, then go back to your regular schedule.

Special Populations

Pregnancy/Breast-feeding

Losartan should not be taken during the last 6 months of pregnancy because it can directly affect the developing fetus, possibly causing fetal injury or death. You should take a different medicine for high blood pressure if you are, or may become, pregnant.

Animal studies have shown that Losartan passes into breast milk, but it is not known if this happens in humans. Nursing mothers should avoid Losartan or bottle-feed their babies because of the chance that it will affect the nursing infant.

Seniors

Older adults may take Losartan without special precautions.

Lotensin

see *Benazepril Hydrochloride, page 112*

Brand Name

Lotrel

Ingredients

Amlodipine + Benazepril Hydrochloride

Type of Drug

Antihypertensive.

Prescribed for

High blood pressure.

General Information

This product combines a calcium channel blocker (Amlodipine) and an angiotensin-converting-enzyme (ACE) inhibitor (Benazepril), both of which are often prescribed individually for high blood pressure. Lotrel is not intended for people who are receiving their first treatment for high blood pressure. You should start on this combination only after you have taken an ACE inhibitor or calcium channel blocker and your doctor feels you need another medicine added to control your blood pressure. Both Amlodipine and Benazepril have their own profile in *The Pill Book*. Check them for more information.

Cautions and Warnings

Do not take Lotrel if you are **sensitive** or **allergic** to any of the ingredients in it. People taking any ACE inhibitor drug may experience **severe drug reactions,** including swelling of the face, throat, lips, tongue, hands, and feet. This reaction has occurred in about 5 of every 1000 people who took Benazepril in studies.

In rare instances, people taking a calcium channel blocker

who have severe heart disease have developed increased **angina pain** and/or a **heart attack.**

In people with heart failure, ACE inhibitors can cause **very low blood pressure,** rare kidney failure, and death. It is important to note that ACE inhibitors are currently considered the most beneficial treatment for heart failure. People with heart failure who start taking Lotrel must be under a doctor's care.

Another ACE inhibitor has caused depression of the bone marrow and very low white-blood-cell counts, especially in people with kidney failure. **Fever** and **chills** can be a sign of this problem.

In rare instances, people taking ACE inhibitors have developed **liver failure.** Lotrel should be used with caution by people with **kidney failure.**

All ACE inhibitors can cause a **persistent cough.**

Possible Side Effects

Lotrel side effects are generally considered mild and temporary.

▼ Most common: cough, headache, dizziness, and swelling.

▼ Less common: allergic reactions, weakness and fatigue, dry mouth, nausea, abdominal pains, constipation, diarrhea, upset stomach, throat irritation, low blood-potassium levels, back pain, muscle cramps and pain, sleeplessness, nervousness, anxiety, tremors, reduced sex drive, sore throat, flushing, hot flashes, rashes, impotence, and frequent urination.

▼ Rare: inflammation of the pancreas, hemolytic anemia, chest pain, abnormal heart rhythms, gout, neuritis, ringing or buzzing in the ears.

Drug Interactions

• Mixing a diuretic drug with Lotrel will lower blood pressure, possibly excessively.

• Mixing a potassium-sparing diuretic (Spironolactone, Amiloride, Triamterene) with Benazepril increases the risk of high blood potassium. High blood-potassium levels can lead to abnormal heart rhythms.

• Mixing Lithium with an ACE inhibitor such as Benazepril can increase blood-Lithium levels and lead to Lithium toxicity.

Food Interactions

Food does not affect individual tablets of Amlodipine and Benazepril, but the effects of food on Lotrel have not been studied. Until more information is available, take Lotrel on an empty stomach, 1/2 hour before or 2 hours after meals.

Usual Dose

Adult: Daily dosage ranges from 2.5/10 to 5/20. Daily dosage depends on your needs for each of the two ingredients.

Seniors, small or frail individuals, and people with liver failure: Start with 2.5/10 and increase gradually. You may need to take individual doses of Amlodipine and Benazepril until your daily needs are established.

Overdosage

A few cases of overdose with the individual ingredients in Lotrel have occurred. One person who took 70 mg of Amlodipine and an unknown amount of a Benzodiazepine tranquilizer died. No Lotrel overdoses have been reported. Call your local poison center for more information. Overdose victims should be taken to a hospital emergency room for treatment. ALWAYS bring the medicine bottle with you.

Special Information

Be sure to continue taking your medicine and follow any instructions for diet restriction or other treatments. High blood pressure is a condition with few recognizable symptoms; it may seem to you that you are taking medicine for no good reason. Ask your doctor or pharmacist if you have any questions.

Call your doctor if you develop swelling in the hands or feet, or the face or throat; if you have sudden difficulty breathing; if you develop a sore throat, mouth sores, abnormal heartbeat, increased heart pains, a persistent rash, constipation, nausea, weakness or dizziness, or perceived loss of taste; or if other side effects are particularly bothersome or persistent.

You may get dizzy if you rise to your feet quickly from a sitting or lying position.

Avoid strenuous exercise and/or very hot weather because heavy sweating or dehydration can cause a rapid blood pressure drop.

Avoid nonprescription diet pills, decongestants, and stimulants that can raise blood pressure.

It is important to maintain good dental hygiene while taking Lotrel and to use extra care when using your toothbrush or dental floss because of the chance that the drug will make you more susceptible to some infections.

If you forget to take a dose of Lotrel, take it as soon as you remember. If it is within 8 hours of your next dose, skip the one you forgot and continue with your regular schedule. Do not take a double dose.

Special Populations

Pregnancy/Breast-feeding

This combination product should not be taken by pregnant women, because ACE inhibitors can cause fetal damage or death. If you are taking Lotrel and become pregnant, see your doctor at once about changing medicines.

Small amounts of both active ingredients pass into breast milk. Nursing mothers who must take Lotrel shoud bottle-feed their babies.

Seniors

Older adults may take this product without special restrictions. Older adults should begin with Lotrel 2.5/10.

Brand Name

Lotrisone Cream

Ingredients

Betamethasone + Clotrimazole

Type of Drug

Steroid-antifungal combination.

Prescribed for

Severe fungal infection or rash.

General Information

Lotrisone is one of a number of steroid (Betamethasone)-antifungal (Clotrimazole) combination products available by prescription. All of the other combination products have different ingredients but can be used for the same purpose. Lotrisone Cream is used to relieve the symptoms of itching, rash, or skin inflammation associated with a severe fungal infection. It may treat the underlying cause of the skin problem by killing the fungus and relieving the inflammation that may be associated with the infection.

This combination product should be used only on your doctor's prescription. A combination product such as this may be less effective than applying either Clotrimazole cream or Betamethasone cream alone to the skin, depending on your skin condition.

Improvement usually occurs within the first week of treatment. If you don't see results after 4 weeks, your doctor may need to prescribe a different medicine.

Cautions and Warnings

Do not use Lotrisone if you are **sensitive** or **allergic** to either of its active ingredients.

Do not apply Lotrisone near or in your eyes. Avoid using this product **on the ear** if the **eardrum** is perforated, unless specifically directed to do so by your doctor.

Check with your doctor before using the contents of an old tube of Lotrisone for a new skin problem.

Possible Side Effects

▼ Most common: itching, stinging, burning, skin peeling, and swelling.

Drug and Food Interactions

None known.

Usual Dose

Gently rub a thin film onto affected area(s) and surrounding skin.

Overdosage

Swallowing Lotrisone cream may cause nausea and vomiting. Call your local poison control center for more information.

Special Information

Apply a thin film of Lotrisone to the affected area(s). Washing or soaking the skin before applying the medicine may increase the amount of medicine that penetrates into your skin.

Lotrisone should not be applied to the face, underarms, groin, genitals or genital areas, abdomen, or between the toes for more than a few days. Excessive use on these areas may result in stretch marks.

Do not wear tight clothing after applying Lotrisone, especially when applied to the genitals or genital areas.

Stop using the medicine and call your doctor if Lotrisone causes itching, burning, or skin irritation.

If you forget to apply a dose of Lotrisone, apply it as soon as you remember. If it is almost time for your next application of Lotrisone, skip the missed dose.

Special Populations

Pregnancy/Breast-feeding

Women should not use this product when it is to be applied over large areas of skin during the first 3 months of pregnancy, because Lotrisone can adversely affect fetal development.

Nursing mothers should not apply Lotrisone to the nipple or breast.

Seniors

Seniors may use Lotrisone without special restriction.

Generic Name

Lovastatin

Brand Name

Mevacor

Type of Drug

Cholesterol-lowering agent.

Prescribed for

High blood cholesterol, together with a low-cholesterol diet; slowing the progression of atherosclerosis in people with heart disease. Lovastatin has also been prescribed for lipid problems associated with diabetes, kidney disease, and some inherited blood-lipid problems.

General Information

Lovastatin is one of several HMG-CoA reductase inhibitors. They work by interfering with the natural body process for manufacturing cholesterol, altering that process to produce a harmless by-product. Studies have closely related high blood-fat levels (total cholesterol, LDL cholesterol, and triglycerides) to heart and blood-vessel disease. Drugs that can reduce the amounts of any of these blood-fats and increase HDL cholesterol (the so-called "good" cholesterol) have been assumed to reduce the risk of death and heart attacks. Lovastatin reduces total triglyceride, cholesterol, and LDL-cholesterol counts while raising HDL cholesterol. Lovastatin is also the only one of this group of drugs that has been proven to slow the speed with which blood-vessel plaques (atherosclerosis) develop. This slows the progression of heart disease.

A very small amount of the drug actually reaches the body circulation; most is broken down in the liver. 10 to 20 percent of the drug is released from the body through your kidneys; the rest is eliminated by the liver. A significant blood-fat-lowering response is seen after 1 to 2 weeks of treatment. Blood-fat levels reach their lowest levels within 4 to 6 weeks after you start taking Lovastatin and remain at or close to that level as long as you continue to take the medicine. The effect is known to persist for 4 to 6 weeks after you stop taking it. Lovastatin generally does not benefit anyone under age 30, so it is not usually recommended for children. It may, under special circumstances, be prescribed for teenagers in the same dose as adults.

Cautions and Warnings

Do not take Lovastatin if you are **allergic** to it or to any other member of this group.

People with a history of **liver disease** and those who drink large amounts of **alcohol** should avoid Lovastatin because the drug can aggravate or cause liver disease. Your doctor should take a blood sample to test your liver function every month or so during the first year of treatment to be sure that the drug is not adversely affecting you.

Lovastatin causes **muscle aches** and/or **muscle weakness** in a small number of people that can be a sign of a more serious condition.

At doses between 50 and more than 100 times the maximum human dose, Lovastatin has caused central-nervous-system lesions, liver tumors, and male infertility in lab animals. The importance of this information for people is not known.

Possible Side Effects

Most people who take Lovastatin tolerate it quite well.

▼ Most common: headache, nausea, vomiting, constipation, upset stomach, diarrhea, heartburn, stomach gas, and abdominal pain or cramps.

▼ Less common: muscle aches, dizziness, rash, and itching.

▼ Rare: hepatitis, pancreas inflammation, yellowing of the skin or eyes, appetite loss, muscle cramps and weakness, blurred vision, eye lens changes, changes in taste perception, respiratory infections, common cold symptoms, fatigue, urinary abnormalities, reduced sex drive, male impotence and/or breast pain, anxiety, tingling in the hands or feet, hair loss, swelling in the legs or feet, and blood-cell changes.

Drug Interactions

• The cholesterol-lowering effects of Lovastatin and Colestipol or Cholestyramine are additive when the drugs are taken together.

• Lovastatin may increase Warfarin's anticoagulant (blood-thinning) effect. People taking both drugs should be periodically monitored by their doctor.

• The combination of Cyclosporine, Erythromycin, Gemfibrozil, or Niacin with Lovastatin may cause severe muscle aches, degeneration, or other muscle problems. These combinations should be avoided.

Food Interactions

Take Lovastatin with food to maximize the amount of drug absorbed. Continue your low-cholesterol diet while taking it.

Usual Dose

20 to 80 mg per day, usually with your evening meal. Your daily dosage of these medicines should be adjusted monthly, based on your doctor's assessment of how well the drug is working to reduce your blood cholesterol.

Overdosage

Persons suspected of having taken an overdose of Lovastatin should be taken to a hospital emergency room for evaluation and treatment. The effects of overdose are not well understood, since only a few cases have occurred and all those people recovered.

Special Information

Call your doctor if you develop blurred vision, muscle aches, pain, tenderness, or weakness, especially if you are also feverish or feel sick.

Lovastatin is always prescribed in combination with a low-fat diet. Be sure to follow you doctor's dietary instructions, because both the diet and medicine are necessary to treat your condition.

Do not take more cholesterol-lowering medicine than your doctor has prescribed or stop taking the medicine without your doctor's knowledge.

If you forget to take a dose of Lovastatin, take it as soon as you remember. If it is almost time for your next regularly scheduled dose, skip the one you forgot and continue with your regular schedule. Do not take a double dose.

Special Populations

Pregnancy/Breast-feeding

Pregnant women and those who might become pregnant absolutely must not take Lovastatin. Laboratory studies have shown that daily doses of Lovastatin cause malformations of the skeleton in fetal laboratory animals. Also, cholesterol is essential to the health and development of a fetus. Anything that interferes with that process will cause irreparable damage to the developing brain and nervous system. Because hardening of the arteries is a long-term process, you should be able to stop this medication during pregnancy with no long-term consequences. If you become pregnant while taking Lovastatin, stop the drug immediately and call your doctor.

Lovastatin may pass into breast milk. Women taking Lovastatin should bottle-feed their infants to avoid possible interference with their baby's development.

Seniors
Lovastatin is taken in the same doses for adults of all ages. Be sure to report any side effects to your doctor.

Generic Name

Malathion

Brand Name
Ovide Lotion

Type of Drug
Scabicide.

Prescribed for
Head lice.

General Information
Originally used as an agricultural insecticide, Malathion has been tested and found to be effective against common lice and the eggs they leave behind in the scalp. Malathion works by interfering with the normal breakdown of acetylcholine, a common carrier of nervous-system impulses. The excess acetylcholine produced by Malathion accounts for its toxicity to the lice and eggs.

After it has been applied to the hair, Malathion binds slowly with the hair shaft, providing some protection against future infestations. This binding process, and the protection it carries, takes about 6 hours to develop and reaches its maximum effect in about 12 hours.

Cautions and Warnings

Malathion is an **extremely toxic substance if swallowed** (see *Overdosage* for more information). People with proven **Malathion sensitivity** should not use this product. Normally about 89 percent of the Malathion applied to your skin is absorbed **into the bloodstream, but larger quantities may be absorbed if the lotion is applied to broken skin or open sores.** In rare situations, there is a chance of a toxic reaction if too much Malathion is absorbed through your skin into the blood.

Malathion lotion is flammable. Don't expose the lotion or hair that is still wet with the lotion to an open flame or an electric dryer because of the possibility of fire. Allow hair to dry naturally after application.

Malathion can **severely damage your eyes.** If some of it gets into your eyes, **flush them with water immediately.**

People with any of the following conditions should be cautious when using Malathion because it can precipitate an attack or worsen your condition: **asthma, very slow heartbeat or low blood pressure, stomach spasms or ulcer, recent heart attack, or Parkinson's disease.**

Malathion can worsen the following conditions: **severe anemia, dehydration, insecticide exposure effects, liver disease or cirrhosis, malnutrition, myasthenia or other neuromuscular diseases, and seizure disorders.**

People with **recent brain surgery** should be concerned about using this product because it can initiate toxic nervous-system effects, including **seizures.**

Possible Side Effects

▼ Common: scalp irritation. Malathion is extremely toxic if it is swallowed or gets into your eyes (see *Overdosage* for more information).

▼ Rare: Convulsions and other drug effects can occur if enough drug is absorbed into the blood through the scalp (see *Overdosage* for details).

Drug Interactions

• No drug interactions have been reported. However, unusually large amounts of Malathion could interact with injectable antibiotics (aminoglycosides) to cause breathing problems, with local anesthetics to interfere with their breakdown and cause systemic side effects, and with some eyedrops used to treat glaucoma (Physostigmine, Echothiophate, Demecarium, and Isoflurophate) to cause side effects. Consult your doctor or pharmacist for more information.

Food Interactions

None known.

Usual Dose

Adult and Child (age 2 and older): apply to the hair and scalp and repeat after 7 to 9 days, if necessary.

Overdosage

If swallowed, or absorbed through your skin, Malathion can cause serious problems. Symptoms of Malathion toxicity include abdominal cramps, anxiety, restlessness, clumsiness or unsteadiness, confusion, depression, diarrhea, dizziness, drowsiness, increased sweating, watery eyes or mouth, loss of bowel or bladder control, muscle twitching in the eyelids, face or neck, pinpointed pupils, difficulty breathing, seizures, slow heartbeat, trembling, and weakness.

Malathion overdose is potentially deadly. People who swallow this product may not experience toxic effects for up to 12 hours. However, victims should be made to vomit with Syrup of Ipecac (available at any pharmacy) to remove any remaining drug from the stomach. Anyone who swallows Malathion MUST be taken to a hospital emergency room for treatment. ALWAYS bring the medicine bottle.

If any Malathion gets into your eyes, IMMEDIATELY flush them with water to remove the insecticide and to avoid damage to your vision, then go to a hospital.

Special Information

Follow your prescription exactly, and do not use this product without your doctor's approval.

Sprinkle the lotion onto dry hair and rub in until the hair and scalp are wet. Pay special attention to the back of your head and neck. Avoid contact with the eyes. Wash your hands immediately after applying the lotion to remove any remaining Malathion from your skin. Allow the treated hair to dry naturally; do not cover it or use an electric dryer (or other heat source). Do not shampoo the hair and scalp for 8 to 12 hours to allow the medicine to work. After 8 to 12 hours have passed, shampoo with a plain shampoo. Remove the dead lice and eggs from the scalp with a fine-toothed comb.

Pregnant women should not handle this medication or apply it to others.

Other household members also may have lice and require Malathion treatments. Call your doctor for information.

After head lice have been found, be sure to practice good hygiene to prevent spreading the lice and possible reinfestation of the treated scalp. Wash all clothing, bedding, towels, and washcloths in very hot water or dry-clean them to kill any lice or eggs. Hairbrushes or combs used by people with head lice infestation must be washed in very hot, soapy water to remove any remaining lice or eggs. Do not share brushes and combs because they may spread the lice. Thoroughly clean the entire living area, including furniture and clothing, with a vacuum cleaner to remove any remaining lice or eggs.

Be careful to avoid exposure to other insecticides while being treated with Malathion.

Special Populations

Pregnancy/Breast-feeding
Malathion may be absorbed and can affect a developing fetus. Pregnant women and those who might be pregnant should not use it or apply it to others.

It is not known if Malathion passes into breast milk. There is a chance that some of the insecticide will be absorbed into the bloodstream and possibly passed on to the nursing infant. Nursing mothers should bottle-feed their babies if using this medicine.

Seniors
Seniors may use this product without special restriction.

Generic Name

Maprotiline

Brand Name

Ludiomil Tablets

(Also available in generic form)

Type of Drug

Antidepressant.

Prescribed for

Depression and panic disorder.

General Information

Maprotiline blocks the movement of certain stimulant chemicals in and out of nerve endings, has a sedative effect, and counteracts the effects of a hormone called *acetylcholine* (which makes it anticholinergic). It prevents the reuptake of important neurohormones (norepinephrine or serotonin) at the nerve ending. Theory says that people with depression have a chemical imbalance in their brains and that drugs such as Maprotiline work to reestablish a proper balance. Although Maprotiline and similar antidepressants immediately block neurohormones, it takes about 2 to 4 weeks for their clinical antidepressant effect to come into play. If symptoms are not affected after 6 to 8 weeks, contact your doctor. Maprotiline also elevates mood, increases physical activity and mental alertness, and improves appetite and sleep patterns in a depressed person. Maprotiline is a mild sedative and therefore useful in treating mild forms of depression associated with anxiety. Maprotiline is broken down in the liver.

Cautions and Warnings

Do not take Maprotiline if you are **allergic or sensitive** to it. Don't take Maprotiline if you are recovering from a **heart attack**.

If you have a history of **epilepsy or other convulsive disorders, difficulty in urination, glaucoma, heart disease,**

liver disease, or hyperthyroidism, Maprotiline may be taken, but exercise caution. People who are **schizophrenic or paranoid** may get worse if given a tricyclic antidepressant and manic depressive people may switch phase. This can also happen if you are changing antidepressants or stopping them. **Suicide** is always a possibility in severely depressed people, who should only be allowed to have minimal quantities of medication in their possession at any one time.

Because Maprotiline **lowers the seizure threshold,** seizures can occur at usual doses as well as with overdoses.

Possible Side Effects

▼ Most common: sedation and anticholinergic effects (blurred vision, disorientation, confusion, hallucinations, muscle spasms or tremors, seizures and/or convulsions, dry mouth, constipation [especially in older adults], difficult urination, worsening glaucoma, sensitivity to bright light or sunlight).

▼ Less common: blood-pressure changes, abnormal heart rates, heart attack, anxiety, restlessness, excitement, numbness or tingling in the extremities, poor coordination, rash, itching, retention of fluids, fever, allergy (difficulty breathing, skin rash or itching), changes in blood composition, nausea, vomiting, loss of appetite, stomach upset, diarrhea, enlargement of the breasts in males and females, changes in sex drive, and blood-sugar changes.

▼ Rare: agitation, inability to sleep, nightmares, feelings of panic, a peculiar taste in the mouth, stomach cramps, black discoloration of the tongue, yellowing of the eyes and/or skin, changes in liver function, increased or decreased weight, excessive perspiration, flushing, frequent urination, drowsiness, dizziness, weakness, headache, loss of hair, and feelings of ill health.

Drug Interactions

• Interaction with monoamine oxidase (MAO) inhibitors can cause high fevers, convulsions, and, rarely, death. Don't take MAO inhibitors until at least 2 weeks after Maprotiline has been discontinued. People who take both Maprotiline and an MAO inhibitor require close medical observation.

• Maprotiline interacts with Guanethidine and Clonidine. Tell your doctor if you are taking **any** high-blood-pressure medicine.

• Maprotiline increases the effects of alcohol, barbiturates, tranquilizers, and other sedative drugs. Also, barbiturates may decrease the effectiveness of Maprotiline. Taking Maprotiline and thyroid medicine together will enhance the effects of both medicines, possibly causing abnormal heart rhythms.

• The combination of Maprotiline and Reserpine may cause overstimulation.

• Oral contraceptives can reduce the effect of Maprotiline, as can smoking. Charcoal tablets can prevent Maprotiline's absorption into the bloodstream. Estrogens can increase or decrease the effect of Maprotiline.

• Drugs such as Bicarbonate of Soda, Acetazolamide, Quinidine, and Procainamide will increase the effect of Maprotiline.

• Cimetidine, Methylphenidate, and phenothiazine drugs (such as Thorazine and Compazine) block the liver metabolism of Maprotiline, causing it to stay in the body longer, which can cause severe drug side effects.

Food Interactions

You may take Maprotiline with food if it upsets your stomach.

Usual Dose

Adult: 75 to 225 mg per day. Hospitalized patients may need up to 300 mg per day. The dose of Maprotiline must be tailored to your needs.

Senior: lower doses are recommended for people over 60 years of age, usually 50 to 75 mg per day.

Overdosage

Symptoms are confusion, inability to concentrate, hallucinations, drowsiness, lowered body temperature, abnormal heart rate, heart failure, enlarged pupils of the eyes, seizures or convulsions, very low blood pressure, stupor, and coma. Agitation, stiffening of body muscles, vomiting, and high fever may also develop. The victim should be taken to a hospital emergency room immediately. ALWAYS bring the medicine bottle.

Special Information

Avoid alcohol and other depressants while taking this drug. Do not stop taking this medicine unless your doctor has specifically told you to do so: Abruptly stopping may cause nausea, headache, and a sickly feeling.

This medicine can cause drowsiness, dizziness, and blurred vision. Be careful when driving or operating hazardous machinery. Avoid prolonged exposure to the sun or sun lamps.

Call your doctor at once if you develop seizures, difficult or rapid breathing, fever and sweating, blood-pressure changes, muscle stiffness, loss of bladder control, or unusual tiredness or weakness.

Dry mouth may lead to an increase in dental cavities, gum bleeding, and gum disease. People taking Maprotiline should pay special attention to dental hygiene.

If you forget a dose of Maprotiline, skip it and go back to your regular schedule. Do not take a double dose.

Special Populations

Pregnancy/Breast-feeding

Maprotiline crosses into the fetal circulation, and birth defects have been reported. Avoid taking this medication while pregnant.

Maprotiline passes into breast milk in concentrations equal to those in blood. Nursing mothers taking Maprotiline should consider bottle-feeding.

Seniors

Older adults are more sensitive to the effects of this drug, especially heart-related side effects such as abnormal rhythms. Seniors usually require a lower dose than younger adults to achieve the same result. Follow your doctor's directions and report any side effects at once.

Generic Name

Masoprocol

Brand Name

Actinex

Type of Drug

Antiproliferative.

Prescribed for

Premalignant skin lesions usually associated with excessive exposure to the sun.

General Information

Masoprocol has an antiproliferative (growth-slowing) effect on cell cultures, but how this drug works on the skin is not known. It is prescribed to treat lesions where the horny layer of the skin grows at a much faster rate than the other skin layers. This condition, known as *actinic keratosis*, is thought to be a precursor to the development of skin cancer.

Cautions and Warnings

Do not cover Masoprocol cream with clear plastic wrap or another dressing that occludes (obstructs) the skin.

Masoprocol contains sulfites as preservatives. If you are **allergic to sulfites,** exposure to Masoprocol may cause **hives, itching, wheezing, or anaphylactic shock** (severe allergic reaction).

Possible Side Effects

Skin reactions to Masoprocol are common, but they usually resolve within 2 weeks after you start using the drug.

▼ Most common: skin redness and irritation, itching, dryness, flaking, swelling, burning, and soreness.

▼ Less common: bleeding, crusting, eye irritation, oozing, rash, stinging, tightness, and tingling.

▼ Rare: blistering, eczema, cuts or abrasions in the skin, cracking of the skin, a leathery feeling, wrinkling, and skin roughness.

Drug Interactions

• Do not use other skin products or cosmetics when using Masoprocol.

Food Interactions

None known.

Usual Dose

Adult: wash and dry the areas to which Masoprocol cream is to be applied. Gently massage the cream into the affected areas until it is evenly distributed. Masoprocol should be used morning and night for 28 days.

Overdosage

Animals receiving high doses of Masoprocol developed liver and stomach problems. Anyone who swallows Masoprocol should be made to vomit with Syrup of Ipecac (available at any pharmacy) as soon as possible in order to remove existing material from the stomach. Call your local poison control center for more information and instructions. ALWAYS bring the medicine bottle if you go to a hospital emergency room for treatment.

Special Information

Masoprocol frequently causes allergic contact dermatitis (skin reaction). If this happens to you, stop using the cream and call your doctor.

If you apply Masoprocol directly with your fingers, you must thoroughly wash your hands after each application. Consider using disposable gloves to apply the cream.

You should be careful not to get Masoprocol into your eyes. If Masoprocol cream gets into your eyes, it must be washed out immediately with water.

You should avoid the sun if you are using this product. The lesions being treated are caused by excessive sun exposure and can only be worsened by continuing sun exposure.

Masoprocol cream may stain your skin, clothing, sheets, or furniture.

If you forget to apply a dose of Masoprocol, do so as soon as you remember. If it almost time for your next dose, skip the one you forgot and continue with your regular schedule.

Special Populations

Pregnancy/Breast-feeding

There is no reliable information about the effect of this drug on pregnant women. It should be used during pregnancy only when absolutely necessary.

It is not known if Masoprocol passes into breast milk. Nursing mothers should use this medicine with caution.

Seniors
Seniors may use this medication without special restriction.

Generic Name
Mazindol

Brand Names
Mazanor
Sanorex

Type of Drug
Nonamphetamine appetite suppressant.

A number of other nonamphetamine appetite suppressants are also available for prescription for short-term weight loss, including:

Generic Name
Phentermine Hydrochloride

Brand Names
Adipex-P   Obe-Nix
Fastin   Obephen
Ionamin

Generic Name
Phendimetrazine Tartrate

Brand Names
Anorex   Obalan
Bontril PDM   Weh-less

Sustained-Release Phendimetrazine Products*

Bontril Slow Release	Prelu-2
Dyrexan-OD	Weh-less Timecelles
Melfiat-105	

Generic Name

Diethylpropion Hydrochloride

Brand Names

Tenuate	Tepanil
Tenuate Dospan	Tepanil Ten-Tab

(*Also available in generic form)

Prescribed for

Short-term (2 to 3 months) appetite suppression and obesity. Mazindol may also be prescribed for Duchenne's muscular dystrophy.

General Information

Although this medicine is not an amphetamine, it has many amphetamine-like effects. It suppresses appetite by working on specific areas in the brain, though studies have shown that appetite suppressants are more effective when combined with behavior therapy than when they are taken alone. Each dose of Mazindol works for 8 to 15 hours.

Cautions and Warnings

Do not take Mazindol if you have **heart disease, high blood pressure, thyroid disease, or glaucoma, or if you are sensitive or allergic** to it or any other appetite suppressant. Do not use it if you are **prone to emotional agitation or substance abuse,** since appetite suppressants are inclined to be abused.

Possible Side Effects

▼ Common: a false sense of well-being, nervousness, euphoria (feeling "high"), overstimulation, restlessness, and trouble sleeping.

> **Possible Side Effects** *(continued)*
>
> ▼ Less common: palpitations, high blood pressure, drowsiness or sedation, weakness, dizziness, tremor, headache, dry mouth, nausea, vomiting, diarrhea or other intestinal disturbances, rash, itching, changes in sex drive, hair loss, muscle pains, difficulty urinating, sweating, chills, blurred vision, and fever.

Drug Interactions

- Taking other stimulants (including decongestants, some asthma medicines, nonprescription cold remedies) together with Mazindol may result in excessive stimulation.
- Taking this medicine within 2 weeks of taking any monoamine oxidase (MAO) inhibitor drug may result in very high blood pressure.
- Appetite suppressants may reduce the effects of some medicines used to treat high blood pressure.
- One case of Lithium toxicity occurred in a person taking that drug in combination with Mazindol.

Food Interactions

Do not crush or chew this product. Mazindol may be taken on a full stomach to reduce stomach upset caused by the drug.

Usual Dose

1 mg 3 times a day, 1 hour before meals; or 2 mg once a day, before lunch.

Overdosage

Symptoms of overdosage are restlessness, tremors, shallow breathing, confusion, hallucinations, and fever. These symptoms may be followed by fatigue and depression. Additional symptoms are changes in blood pressure, cold and clammy skin, nausea, vomiting, diarrhea, and stomach cramps. Take the victim to a hospital emergency room immediately, and ALWAYS bring the medicine bottle.

Special Information

Do not take any appetite suppressant for more than 12 weeks

as part of a weight-control program, and take it only under a doctor's supervision. This medicine will not reduce body weight by itself. You must limit or modify your diet and follow your exercise regimen (if applicable).

Appetite suppressants often cause dry mouth, which increases the chances of dental cavities and gum disease. Pay special attention to oral hygiene if you are taking this medicine. The dry mouth usually can be relieved with sugarless candy, gum, or ice chips.

If you forget to take a dose of Mazindol, skip the missed dose and go back to your regular schedule. Do not take a double dose.

Special Populations

Pregnancy/Breast-feeding
Studies have shown that large doses of Mazindol may damage an unborn baby. All appetite suppressants, including Mazindol, should be avoided by women who are or could become pregnant. In cases where this drug is considered essential by your doctor, its potential benefits must be weighed against its possible hazards.

It is not known if Mazindol passes into breast milk. Nursing mothers should not take any appetite suppressant.

Seniors
Older adults should not take this medicine unless prescribed by a doctor. It can aggravate diabetes or high blood pressure, conditions common in older adults.

Generic Name

Mebendazole

Brand Name

Vermox

(Also available in generic form)

Type of Drug

Anthelmintic.

Prescribed for

Whipworm, pinworm, roundworm, hookworm, or mixed-worm infections.

General Information

This drug blocks the mechanism by which susceptible worms get sugar, effectively starving the organism as time passes. This is a slow process; it may take 3 days or more for the worm to be eliminated from your body. Most of the drug passes out of the body unchanged in the feces.

Cautions and Warnings

Do not take this drug if you are **sensitive or allergic** to it.

Possible Side Effects

Side effects are infrequent and passing. Most common are pain and diarrhea in cases of massive infection. Fever has also occurred.

Drug Interactions

• Carbamazepine and Phenytoin-type drugs may reduce blood levels of Mebendazole, possibly interfering with the drug's effect.

Food Interactions

Chew or crush the Mebendazole tablet and mix it with food, especially fatty food, to increase the amount of drug absorbed.

Usual Dose

One tablet morning and night for 3 days in a row. One kind of worm infection may be treated with a single tablet.

Overdosage

Stomach cramps and pain may develop several hours after an overdose. Overdose victims should be given Syrup of Ipecac, available at any pharmacy, to induce vomiting and remove the drug from your system. Call your local poison control center for more information.

Special Information

The same dosage is taken by everyone who takes this product, regardless of age.

Each dose of Mebendazole should be chewed or crushed and taken with food.

In the case of pinworm infection, all family members will have to take 3 days' worth of Mebendazole, even if only 1 member was infected, and a second treatment will be needed 2 or 3 weeks later. Wash (don't shake) all bedclothes after treatment to prevent reinfection.

In the case of hookworm or whipworm, take an Iron supplement every day during treatment and possibly for up to 6 months after treatment is completed if you are anemic.

Call your doctor if you don't start to get better in a few days. If the infection is not cured in 3 weeks, another course of treatment may be needed.

It is essential that you follow the dosage schedule prescribed by your doctor. If you forget a dose, take it as soon as you remember. If it is almost time for your next dose, skip the forgotten dose and continue with your regular schedule. Don't take a double dose.

Special Populations

Pregnancy/Breast-feeding
This drug is toxic to animal fetuses and causes malformations in those animals. It is not recommended for use by women who are pregnant and should be used only if absolutely necessary.

It is not known if Mebendazole passes into breast milk. Nursing mothers should take this drug with caution.

Seniors
Seniors may use this medicine without restriction.

Generic Name

Meclofenamate

Brand Name

Meclomen

(Also available in generic form)

Type of Drug

Nonsteroidal anti-inflammatory drug (NSAID).

Prescribed for

Rheumatoid arthritis, osteoarthritis, mild to moderate pain, sunburn treatment, migraine headaches, menstrual headaches, and discomfort associated with excessive menstrual bleeding.

General Information

Meclofenamate is one of 16 NSAIDs used to relieve pain and inflammation. We do not know exactly how NSAIDs work, but part of their action may be due to an ability to inhibit the body's production of a hormone called *prostaglandin* and to inhibit the action of other body chemicals, including cyclooxygenase, lipoxygenase, leukotrienes, lysosomal enzymes, and a host of other factors. NSAIDs are generally absorbed into the bloodstream fairly quickly. Pain relief comes within an hour after taking the first dose of Meclofenomate, but its anti-inflammatory effect generally takes a lot longer (several days) to become apparent, and may take 2 to 3 weeks to reach its maximum effect. Meclofenamate is broken down in the liver and eliminated through the kidneys.

Cautions and Warnings

People who are **allergic** to this drug (or any other NSAID) and those with a history of **asthma attacks** brought on by other NSAIDs, Iodides, or Aspirin should not take Meclofenamate.

Meclofenamate can cause **gastrointestinal (GI) bleeding, ulcers, and stomach perforation.** This can occur at any time, with or without warning, in people receiving chronic treatment with this drug. People with a history of active GI bleeding should be cautious about taking any NSAID. Minor **stomach upset, distress, or gas** is common during the first few days of treatment with Meclofenamate. People who develop bleeding or ulcers and continue treatment should be aware of the possibility of developing more serious drug toxicity.

Meclofenamate can affect **platelets and blood clotting** at high doses, and should be avoided by people with clotting problems and by those taking Warfarin.

People with **heart problems** who use Meclofenamate may experience swelling in their arms, legs, or feet.

Meclofenamate can cause severe toxic effects to the **kidney.** Report any unusual side effects to your doctor, who may need to periodically test your kidney function.

Meclofenamate can cause **unusual sensitivity to the effects of the sun** (photosensitivity).

Possible Side Effects

▼ Most common: diarrhea, nausea, vomiting, constipation, stomach gas, stomach upset or irritation, and loss of appetite.

▼ Less common: stomach ulcers, GI bleeding, hepatitis, gallbladder attacks, painful urination, poor kidney function, kidney inflammation, blood and protein in the urine, dizziness, fainting, nervousness, depression, hallucinations, confusion, disorientation, tingling in the hands or feet, light-headedness, itching, increased sweating, dry nose and mouth, heart palpitations, chest pain, difficulty breathing, and muscle cramps.

▼ Rare: severe allergic reactions, including closing of the throat, fever and chills, changes in liver function, jaundice (yellowing of the skin or eyes), and kidney failure. People who experience such effects must be promptly treated in a hospital emergency room or doctor's office.

NSAIDs have caused severe skin reactions; if this happens to you, see your doctor immediately.

Drug Interactions

• Meclofenamate can increase the effects of oral anticoagulant (blood-thinning) drugs such as Warfarin. You may take this combination, but your doctor may have to reduce your anticoagulant dose.

• Taking Meclofenamate with Cyclosporine may increase the toxic kidney effects of both drugs. Methotrexate toxicity may be increased in people also taking Meclofenamate.

• Meclofenamate may reduce the blood-pressure-lowering effect of beta blockers and loop diuretic drugs.

• Meclofenamate may increase blood levels of Phenytoin, leading to increased Phenytoin side effects. Blood-Lithium levels may be increased in people taking Meclofenamate.

• Meclofenamate blood levels may be affected by Cimetidine because of that drug's effect on the liver.

• Probenecid may interfere with the elimination of this drug from the body, increasing the risk for Meclofenamate toxic reactions.

• Aspirin and other salicylates may decrease the amount of Meclofenamate in your blood. These medicines should never be taken at the same time.

Food Interactions

Take Meclofenamate with food or a magnesium/aluminum antacid if it upsets your stomach.

Usual Dose

Adult and Adolescent (age 14 and older): 200 to 400 mg per day.

Child (under age 14): not recommended.

Overdosage

People have died from NSAID overdoses. The most common signs of overdosage are drowsiness, nausea, vomiting, diarrhea, abdominal pain, rapid breathing, rapid heartbeat, increased sweating, ringing or buzzing in the ears, confusion, disorientation, stupor, and coma.

Take the victim to a hospital emergency room at once. ALWAYS bring the medicine bottle.

Special Information

Take each dose with a full glass of water and don't lie down for 15 to 30 minutes after you take the medicine.

Meclofenamate can make you drowsy and/or tired: Be careful when driving or operating hazardous equipment. Do not take any nonprescription products with Acetaminophen or Aspirin while taking this drug; also, avoid alcoholic beverages.

Contact your doctor if you develop skin rash or itching, visual disturbances, weight gain, breathing difficulty, fluid retention, hallucinations, black or tarry stools, persistent headache, or any unusual or intolerable side effects.

If you forget to take a dose of Meclofenamate, take it as soon as you remember. If you take several doses a day and it is within 4 hours of your next dose, skip the one you forgot and continue with your regular schedule. If you take your Meclofenamate once a day and it is within 8 hours of your next dose, skip the missed dose and continue with your regular schedule. Do not take a double dose.

Special Populations

Pregnancy/Breast-feeding

NSAIDs may cross into the fetal blood circulation. They have not been found to cause birth defects, but may affect a developing fetal heart during the second half of pregnancy; animal studies indicate a possible effect. Women who are or might become pregnant should not take Meclofenamate without their doctors' approval; pregnant women should be particularly cautious about using this drug during the last 3 months of their pregnancy. When the drug is considered essential by your doctor, its potential benefits must be carefully weighed against its risks.

NSAIDs may pass into breast milk but have caused no problems among breast-fed infants, except for seizures in a baby whose mother was taking Indomethacin. Other NSAIDs have caused problems in animal studies. There is a possibility that a nursing mother taking Meclofenamate could affect her baby's heart or cardiovascular system. If you must take Meclofenamate, bottle-feed your baby.

Seniors

Older adults may be more susceptible to Meclofenamate side effects, especially ulcer disease.

Generic Name

Medroxyprogesterone Acetate

Brand Names

Amen
Curretab

Cycrin
Provera

(Also available in generic form)

Type of Drug

Progestin.

Prescribed for

Oral Medroxyprogesterone is prescribed for irregular menstrual bleeding. Injectable versions of this drug are prescribed to treat endometrial or kidney cancer. Adding Medroxyprogesterone to a cycle of estrogen replacement therapy is helpful in relieving symptoms of menopause. It may also be prescribed to stimulate breathing in people who suffer from sleep apnea and other conditions where breathing rate is abnormally slow or stops completely for short periods of time.

Other progestins have been prescribed for additional medical uses. Rectal or vaginal Progesterone suppositories have been used to treat premenstrual syndrome (PMS), and Progesterone has been used in the late stages of pregnancy to prevent premature labor and earlier in pregnancy to prevent spontaneous abortion. The jury is still out as to whether Progesterone is helpful in preventing abortion.

General Information

Progesterone is the principal hormone involved in the process of pregnancy. It works directly, or indirectly through other hormone systems, on almost every phase of the preparation of the womb for acceptance of the fertilized egg and the maintenance of conditions that allow the growth and development of the fetus.

The decision to take this medication on a regular basis

should be made carefully by you and your doctor because of the possiblity of developing Medroxyprogesterone-related problems. Your continued need for Medroxyprogesterone treatment should be evaluated at least every 6 months.

Cautions and Warnings

Do not take this drug if you have a **history of blood clotting or** similar disorders, or if you have had **convulsions, liver disease,** known or suspected **breast cancer, undiagnosed vaginal bleeding, or a miscarriage.**

Medroxyprogesterone use should be carefully considered if you have had **asthma, cardiac insufficiency, epilepsy, migraine headaches, kidney problems, diabetes, a history of ectopic pregnancy, high blood-fat levels, or depression.**

Possible Side Effects

▼ Common: breakthrough bleeding, spotting, changes in or loss of menstrual flow, water retention, increase or decrease in body weight, breast tenderness, jaundice, acne, skin rash (with or without itching), and mental depression.

▼ Other: changes in libido or sex drive, changes in appetite and mood, headache, nervousness, dizziness, tiredness, backache, loss of scalp hair, growth of hair in unusual quantities or places, itching, symptoms similar to urinary infections, and unusual rashes.

There is a strong relationship between the use of progestin drugs and the development of blood clots in the veins, lungs, or brain.

Drug Interactions

• Medroxyprogesterone may interfere with the effects of Bromocriptine and should not be used at the same time as that drug.

• Rifampin may increase the rate at which Medroxyprogesterone is broken down in the liver, decreasing its effectiveness.

• Diabetics may experience a decrease in glucose tolerance, worsening their condition.

Food Interactions

This medicine is best taken on an empty stomach, but you may take it with food if it upsets your stomach.

Usual Dose

5 to 10 mg per day for 5 to 10 days, beginning on what is assumed to be the 16th to 21st day of the menstrual cycle.

Overdose

Medroxyprogesterone overdose may result in exaggerated side effects. In many cases, small overdoses will result in no unusual symptoms. Call your local poison control center or hospital emergency room for more information.

Special Information

At the first sign of sudden, partial, or complete loss of vision; double vision; sudden falling; calf pain, swelling, and redness; numbness in an arm or leg; leg cramps; water retention; unusual vaginal bleeding; migraine or a sudden and severe headache; or depression; or if you think you have become pregnant, stop the drug immediately and call your doctor.

Medroxyprogesterone may make you unusually sensitive to the sun or bright light. Use extra sunscreen and protective clothing if you must be in the sun and avoid the sun whenever possible.

Medroxyprogesterone may mask the symptoms of menopause.

If you forget to take a dose of Medroxyprogesterone, take it as soon as you remember. If it is almost time for your next regularly scheduled dose, skip the one you forgot and continue with your regular schedule. Do not take a double dose.

Special Populations

Pregnancy/Breast-feeding

Medroxyprogesterone can cause birth defects or interfere with your baby's development; it can double the rate of certain birth defects if used during the first 4 months of your pregnancy. It is not considered safe for use during pregnancy, except under very specific circumstances.

This drug passes into breast milk and does not have an adverse effect on the nursing process. Medroxyprogesterone may increase the volume of milk and length of time you make milk if given after birth.

Seniors

Older adults with severe liver disease are more sensitive to the effects of this drug. Follow your doctor's directions and report any side effects at once.

Generic Name

Mefenamic Acid

Brand Name

Ponstel

Type of Drug

Nonsteroidal anti-inflammatory drug (NSAID).

Prescribed for

Mild to moderate pain (less than 1 week treatment), sunburn treatment, migraine attacks, menstrual pains, menstrual headaches, and premenstrual syndrome (PMS).

General Information

Mefenamic Acid is one of 16 NSAIDs used to relieve pain and inflammation. We do not know exactly how NSAIDs work, but part of their action may be due to an ability to inhibit the body's production of a hormone called *prostaglandin* and to inhibit the action of other body chemicals, including cyclo-oxygenase, lipoxygenase, leukotrienes, lysosomal enzymes, and a host of other factors. NSAIDs are generally absorbed into the bloodstream fairly quickly. Pain relief generally comes within an hour after taking the first dose, but the NSAID's anti-inflammatory effect generally takes a lot longer (several days to 2 weeks) to become apparent, and may take a month or more to reach its maximum effect. Mefenamic Acid is broken down in the liver and eliminated through the kidneys.

Cautions and Warnings

People who are **allergic** to Mefenamic Acid (or any other

NSAID) and those with a history of **asthma attacks** brought on by another NSAID, by Iodides, or by Aspirin should not take Mefenamic Acid.

Mefenamic Acid can cause **gastrointestinal (GI) bleeding, ulcers, and stomach perforation.** This can occur at any time, with or without warning, in people who take chronic Mefenamic Acid treatment. People with a history of **active GI bleeding** should be cautious about taking any NSAID. **Minor stomach upset, distress, or gas is common during the first few days** of treatment with this drug. People who develop bleeding or ulcers and continue treatment should be aware of the possibility of more serious drug toxicity.

Mefenamic Acid can affect **platelets and blood clotting** at high doses, and should be avoided by people with clotting problems and by those taking Warfarin.

People with **heart problems** who use Mefenamic Acid may experience swelling in their arms, legs, or feet.

Mefenamic Acid can cause severe **toxic effects to the kidney.** Report any unusual side effects to your doctor, who may need to periodically test your kidney function.

Mefenamic Acid can cause **unusual sensitivity to the effects of the sun** (photosensitivity).

Possible Side Effects

▼ Most common: diarrhea, nausea, vomiting, constipation, stomach gas, stomach upset or irritation, and appetite loss.

▼ Less common: stomach ulcers, GI bleeding, hepatitis, gallbladder attacks, painful urination, poor kidney function, kidney inflammation, blood and protein in the urine, dizziness, fainting, nervousness, depression, hallucinations, confusion, disorientation, tingling in the hands or feet, light-headedness, itching, increased sweating, dry nose and mouth, heart palpitations, chest pain, difficulty breathing, and muscle cramps.

▼ Rare: severe allergic reactions, including closing of the throat, fever and chills, changes in liver function, jaundice (yellowing of the skin or eyes), and kidney failure. People who experience such effects must be promptly treated in a hospital emergency room or doctor's office.

Possible Side Effects *(continued)*

NSAIDs have caused severe skin reactions; if this happens to you, see your doctor immediately.

Drug Interactions

• Mefenamic Acid can increase the effects of oral anticoagulant (blood-thinning) drugs such as Warfarin. You may take this combination, but your doctor may have to reduce your anticoagulant dose.

• Taking Mefenamic Acid with Cyclosporin may increase the toxic kidney effects of both drugs. Methotrexate toxicity may be increased in people also taking Mefenamic Acid.

• Mefenamic Acid may reduce the blood-pressure-lowering effect of beta blockers and loop diuretic drugs.

• Mefenamic Acid may increase blood levels of Phenytoin, leading to increased Phenytoin side effects. Blood-Lithium levels may be increased in people taking Mefenamic Acid.

• Mefenamic Acid blood levels may be affected by Cimetidine because of that drug's effect on the liver.

• Probenecid may interfere with the elimination of this drug from the body, increasing the risk for Mefenamic Acid toxic reactions.

• Aspirin and other salicylates may decrease the amount of Mefenamic Acid in your blood. These medicines should never be taken at the same time.

Food Interactions

Take Mefenamic Acid with food or a magnesium/aluminum antacid if it upsets your stomach.

Usual Dose

Adult and Adolescent (age 14 and older): 500 mg to start, then 250 mg every 6 hours.

Child (under age 14): not recommended.

Overdosage

People have died from NSAID overdoses. The most common signs of overdosage are drowsiness, nausea, vomiting, diarrhea, abdominal pain, rapid breathing, rapid heartbeat, increased sweating, ringing or buzzing in the ears, confusion, disorientation, stupor, and coma. Take the victim to a hospital emergency room at once. ALWAYS bring the medicine bottle.

Special Information

Take each dose with a full glass of water and don't lie down for 15 to 30 minutes after you take the medicine.

Mefenamic Acid can make you drowsy and/or tired: Be careful when driving or operating hazardous equipment. Do not take any nonprescription products with Acetaminophen or Aspirin while taking this drug; avoid alcoholic beverages.

Contact your doctor if you develop skin rash or itching, visual disturbances, weight gain, breathing difficulty, fluid retention, hallucinations, black or tarry stools, persistent headache, or any unusual or intolerable side effects.

If you forget to take a Mefenamic Acid dose, take it as soon as you remember. If you take several doses a day and it is within 4 hours of your next dose, skip the one you forgot and continue with your regular schedule. If you take it once a day and it is within 8 hours of your next dose, skip the missed dose and continue with your regular schedule. Do not take a double dose.

Special Populations

Pregnancy/Breast-feeding

NSAIDs may cross into the fetal blood circulation. They have not been found to cause birth defects, but may affect a developing fetal heart during the second half of pregnancy; animal studies indicate a possible effect. Women who are or might become pregnant should not take Mefenamic Acid without their doctor's approval; pregnant women should be particularly cautious about using this drug during the last 3 months of their pregnancy. When the drug is considered essential by your doctor, its potential benefits must be carefully weighed against its risks.

NSAIDs may pass into breast milk, but have caused no problems among breast-fed infants, except for seizures in a baby whose mother was taking Indomethacin. Other NSAIDs have caused problems in animal studies. There is a possibility that a nursing mother taking Mefenamic Acid could affect her baby's heart or cardiovascular system. If you must take Mefenamic Acid, bottle-feed your baby.

Seniors
Older adults may be more susceptible to Mefenamic Acid side effects, especially ulcer disease.

Generic Name

Megestrol Acetate

Brand Name
Megace Tablets/Oral Solution

Type of Drug
Progestin.

Prescribed for
Cancer of the breast or endometrium. Megestrol Acetate is also prescribed for decreased appetite and weight loss associated with AIDS.

General Information
Megestrol Acetate has been used quite successfully in the treatment of the cancers cited above. It acts as a hormonal counterbalance in areas rich in estrogen (breast and endometrium). Other progestational hormones, such as Norethindrone (Norlutin or Norlutate), may be used to treat cancer of the endometrium or uterus or to correct hormone imbalance.

Megestrol's action in treating the appetite loss, weight loss, and poor physical condition of AIDS victims is not as well understood; we do know that it stimulates appetite and adds muscle and lean body mass, whereas many other dietary supplements add fat.

Cautions and Warnings
Megestrol should be used only for its two specific indications, and users of this drug should be closely and regularly monitored by their doctors. Megestrol use should be care-

fully considered if you have a history of **blood clots or similar disorders, convulsions, liver disease, undiagnosed vaginal bleeding, asthma, cardiac insufficiency, epilepsy, migraine headaches, kidney problems, diabetes, ectopic pregnancy, high blood-fat levels, or depression.**

Call your doctor at once and stop taking the medicine if you experience a partial or complete loss of vision, double vision, migraine headache, or a sudden fall.

Possible Side Effects

▼ Common: weight gain due to increased appetite. When used for weight gain in AIDS, the major side effect is impotence.

▼ Less common: back or stomach pain, headache, nausea, and vomiting. If any of these symptoms appear, contact your doctor immediately. This drug should be used with caution by those with a history of blood clots in the veins.

▼ Rare: diarrhea, stomach gas, rash, swelling in the legs or feet, and weakness.

Drug Interactions

• Megestrol may interfere with the effects of Bromocriptine; do not combine these drugs.

• Rifampin may increase the rate at which Megestrol is broken down by the liver, possibly decreasing its effects.

Food Interactions

Megestrol is best taken on an empty stomach, but you may take it with food if it upsets your stomach.

Usual Dose

Breast or endometrial cancer
40 to 320 mg per day.

AIDS-related weight loss
800 mg per day to start, reduced to 400 mg per day.

Overdosage

Megestrol overdose may result in exaggerated side effects. In many cases, small overdoses will result in no unusual symptoms. Call your local poison control center or hospital emergency room for more information.

Special Information

Continuous treatment for 2 months is usually required to determine if Megestrol is effective for your condition.

Call your doctor if you develop back or abdominal pain, headache, nausea, vomiting, breast tenderness, or other persistent, severe or bothersome side effects.

Women of childbearing age should use effective contraceptive measures because this drug causes birth defects.

People with AIDS who take Megestrol for weight gain should continue taking it until they reach their desired weight. Then it may be discontinued until needed again.

If you forget to take a dose of Megestrol, take it as soon as you remember. If it is almost time for your next dose, skip the one you forgot and continue with your regular schedule. Do not take a double dose.

Special Populations

Pregnancy/Breast-feeding

This drug is known to cause birth defects and interfere with fetal development. It should not be used during the first 4 months of your pregnancy.

Megestrol passes into breast milk, but has caused no problems among breast-fed infants. However, you must consider possible effects on the nursing infant.

Seniors

Older adults with severe liver disease are more sensitive to the effects of Megestrol. Follow your doctor's directions and report any side effects at once.

Generic Name

Meperidine Hydrochloride

Brand Names

Demerol
Meperidine Hydrochloride
Pethadol

(Also available in generic form)

Type of Drug

Narcotic analgesic.

Prescribed for

Moderate to severe pain.

General Information

Meperidine is a potent narcotic pain reliever and cough
suppressant. It is also used before surgery to reduce anxiety
and help bring the patient into early stages of anesthesia.
Meperidine is probably the most widely used narcotic in
American hospitals. Its effects compare favorably with those
of Morphine Sulfate, the standard for narcotic pain relievers.

It is useful for mild to moderate pain; 25 to 50 mg of
Meperidine are approximately equal in pain-relieving effect
to 2 Aspirin tablets (650 mg). Meperidine may be less active
than Aspirin for pain associated with inflammation because
Aspirin reduces inflammation, whereas Meperidine does not.
Meperidine suppresses the cough reflex but does not cure the
underlying cause of the cough. Sometimes, it may be inappropriate to overly suppress a cough because cough suppression reduces your ability to naturally eliminate excess mucus
produced as a result of respiratory disease.

Cautions and Warnings

Do not take Meperidine if you know you are **allergic** or
sensitive to it. Use this drug with extreme caution if you
suffer from **asthma or other breathing problems**. Long-term
use of Meperidine may cause **drug dependence or addiction**.

Narcotic drug **side effects are exaggerated in the presence of a head injury, brain tumor, or other head problem;** use Meperidine with extreme caution if any of these apply to you. **Narcotics can also hide the symptoms of head injury.**

Possible Side Effects

▼ Most common: light-headedness, dizziness, sleepiness, nausea, vomiting, loss of appetite, and increased sweating. If these occur, consider asking your doctor about lowering your Meperidine dose. These side effects usually will disappear if you simply lie down.

More serious side effects of Meperidine are shallow breathing or difficulty in breathing.

▼ Less common: euphoria (feeling "high"), weakness, headache, agitation, uncoordinated muscle movement, minor hallucinations, disorientation, visual disturbances, dry mouth, constipation, flushing of the face, rapid heartbeat, palpitations, faintness, urinary difficulties or hesitancy, reduced sex drive or potency, itching, skin rashes, anemia, lowered blood-sugar, and a yellowing of the skin or eyes. Narcotic analgesics may aggravate convulsions in those who have had them in the past.

Drug Interactions

• Because of its depressant effect and potential effect on breathing, Meperidine should be taken with extreme care in combination with alcohol, sleeping medicine, tranquilizers, or other depressant drugs.

• People taking Cimetidine and a narcotic pain reliever may experience confusion, disorientation, nervous-system depression, seizures, or breathing difficulty.

• When this drug is taken together with a monamine oxidase (MAO) inhibitor, unusual and possibly fatal reactions may occur. Do not take Meperidine within 2 weeks of your last dose of an MAO inhibitor drug. Some of the symptoms that have occurred are trouble breathing; blood-pressure changes; bluish discoloration of the lips, fingernails, or skin; and coma.

Food Interactions

This drug may be taken with food to reduce stomach upset.

Usual Dose

Adult: 50 to 150 mg every 3 to 4 hours as needed.
Child: 0.5 to 0.8 mg per pound every 3 to 4 hours as needed, up to the adult dose.

Overdosage

Symptoms are slow breathing, extreme tiredness progressing to stupor and then coma, pinpointed pupils, no response to pain stimulation (such as a pin prick), cold or clammy skin, slow heartbeat, low blood pressure, convulsions, and cardiac arrest. The victim should be taken to a hospital emergency room immediately. ALWAYS bring the medicine bottle.

Special Information

If you are taking Meperidine, be extremely careful while driving or operating complicated or hazardous machinery. Avoid alcoholic beverages.

Call your doctor if this drug makes you very nauseous or constipated, if you have trouble breathing, or if any other prominent or persistent side effect occurs.

If you forget to take a dose of Meperidine, take it as soon as you remember. If it is almost time for your next dose, skip the one you forgot and continue with your regular schedule. Do not take a double dose.

Special Populations

Pregnancy/Breast-feeding

Animal studies show that quantities of narcotics can cause problems in a developing fetus. Pregnant women and those who might become pregnant while using this drug should talk to their doctor about the risks of taking this medicine versus the benefits it can provide.

Meperidine passes into breast milk, but no problems in nursing infants have been seen. Bottle-feeding is recommended to avoid possible adverse drug effects in nursing infants.

Large amounts of any narcotic, including Meperidine, taken on a long-term basis during pregnancy and/or breast-feeding may cause the baby to become dependent on the narcotic. Narcotics may also cause breathing problems in the infant during delivery.

Seniors

Seniors are more likely to be sensitive to Meperidine side effects and should take the smallest effective dosages.

Generic Name

Meprobamate

Brand Names

Equanil	Miltown
Meprospan	Neuramate

(Also available in generic form)

Type of Drug

Antianxiety agent.

Prescribed for

Relief of short-term (less than 4 months) anxiety and tension.

General Information

Meprobamate works by directly affecting several areas of the brain. In doing so, it can relax you, relieve anxiety, or act as a muscle relaxant, anticonvulsant, or sleeping pill. This drug should be used only for short-term relief of anxiety and tension.

Cautions and Warnings

Do not take Meprobamate if you are **allergic** to it or to a related drug (Carbromal, Carisoprodol, Felbamate, or Mebutamate). Meprobamate may cause seizures in epileptic patients.

Long-time Meprobamate users have developed severe **physical and psychological drug dependence**. It can produce **chronic intoxication** after prolonged use or if used in greater than recommended doses, leading to slurred speech, dizziness, general sleepiness, or depression. Suddenly stopping Meprobamate after prolonged and excessive use may result in **drug-withdrawal** symptoms, including severe anxiety, vomiting, loss of appetite, sleeplessness, tremors, muscle twitching, severe sleepiness, confusion, hallucinations, and convulsions. Withdrawal symptoms usually begin 12 to 48 hours after Meprobamate has been stopped and may last 1 to 4 days. When stopping treatment with Meprobamate, the drug should be reduced gradually over 1 or 2 weeks.

People with **kidney or liver disease** need to take lower doses of Meprobamate because these conditions will cause the drug to accumulate in your body.

Possible Side Effects

▼ Most common: drowsiness, sleepiness, dizziness, slurred speech, poor muscle coordination, headache, weakness, tingling in the arms and legs, and euphoria (feeling "high").

▼ Less common: nausea, vomiting, diarrhea, abnormal heart rhythms, excitement or overstimulation, low blood pressure, itching, rash, and changes in various blood components.

▼ Rare: people have had allergic reactions to Meprobamate, including high fever, chills, bronchospasm (closing of the throat), and reduced urinary function.

Drug Interactions

• Interactions with nervous-system depressants (including alcohol, other tranquilizers, narcotics, barbiturates, sleeping pills, or antihistamines) can cause excess tranquilization, depression, sleepiness, or fatigue.

Food Interactions

Take this medicine with food if it upsets your stomach.

Usual Dose

Adult and Adolescent (age 13 and older): 1200 to 1600 mg a day in divided doses; maximum daily dose, 2400 mg.
Child (age 6 to 12): 100 to 200 mg 2 to 3 times a day.
Child (under age 6): not recommended.

Overdosage

In attempted suicide or accidental overdose, symptoms are extreme drowsiness, lethargy, stupor, and coma, with possible shock and respiratory collapse (breathing stops). Some people have died after taking only 30 tablets, while others have survived after taking 100. If alcohol or another depressant has also been taken, a much smaller dose of Meprobamate can be fatal. After a large overdose, the victim will go to sleep very quickly, and blood pressure, pulse, and breathing levels will drop rapidly. The overdose victim must be taken to a hospital emergency room immediately, where his or her stomach will be pumped and respiratory assistance and other supportive therapy given. ALWAYS bring the medicine bottle with you.

Special Information

Take this medicine according to your doctor's direction. Do not change your dose without your doctor's approval.

This drug causes drowsiness and poor concentration. Be careful when driving or performing complex activities. Avoid alcohol and other nervous-system depressants, because they increase these effects.

Call your doctor if you develop fever, sore throat, rash, mouth sores, nosebleeds, unexplained black-and-blue marks, or easy bruising or bleeding, or if you become pregnant.

If you forget to take a dose of Meprobamate and you remember within about an hour of your regular time, take it right away. If you do not remember until later, skip the missed dose and go back to your regular schedule. Do not take a double dose.

Special Populations

Pregnancy/Breast-feeding

Meprobamate has been shown to increase the chance of birth defects, particularly during the first 3 months of pregnancy. Inform your doctor immediately if you are, or think you may be, pregnant. There are few good reasons for pregnant women to take Meprobamate.

Meprobamate passes into breast milk in concentrations 2 to 4 times greater than are found in the blood. It may cause tiredness in nursing infants. Nursing mothers who must take this drug should bottle-feed their babies.

Seniors

Older adults are more sensitive to sedative and other effects of this drug, and should take the lowest dose possible. Report any side effects at once.

Generic Name

Mesalamine

Brand Names

Asacol Tablets
Pentasa Capsules
Rowasa Suppositories/Rectal Suspension

Type of Drug

Bowel anti-inflammatory.

Prescribed for

Ulcerative colitis (oral products); distal ulcerative colitis, proctitis, and proctosigmoiditis (rectal products).

General Information

Mesalamine is the breakdown product of Sulfasalazine and Olsalazine, two widely used treatments for ulcerative colitis and other inflammatory conditions, in the body. Mesalamine is the active agent in these drugs in treating symptoms of bowel inflammation. No one knows exactly how Mesalamine, a chemical cousin of Aspirin, produces its effect, but it is thought to have a local effect on the bowel. Mesalamine tablets are coated with an acrylic resin to delay drug release from the tablet until it reaches the colon. Little of the drug is absorbed into the blood; 70 to 90 percent stays in the colon.

Cautions and Warnings

Mesalamine may actually worsen **colitis or cause cramping, sudden abdominal pain, bloody diarrhea, fever, headache,** or a **rash. Call your doctor immediately and stop taking this drug at once if any of these symptoms develop.**

People who are **allergic** to Mesalamine or Aspirin should not use this product. Although people who are **sensitive or allergic to Sulfasalazine** have generally been able to tolerate Mesalamine because so little of the drug is absorbed into the bloodstream, they should be cautious.

Some people taking Mesalamine have developed **kidney problems.** People with a current or past history of kidney disease should be cautious about using this drug. All people taking Mesalamine should have kidney function tests before starting this drug and during the time they are taking it.

Possible Side Effects

Mesalamine is generally well tolerated. Mesalamine tablets have the most side effects, suppositories the least.

▼ Common: abdominal pain, cramps or discomfort, headache, and nausea (all forms); belching, sore throat, and generalized pain (tablets).

▼ Less common: common cold symptoms or flu symptoms, tiredness or weakness, general feelings of ill health, fever, chills, rash, constipation, diarrhea, upset stomach, intestinal gas, joint and leg pains, dizziness, bloating, rectal pain (particularly when inserting the enema tip), hemorrhoids, itching, soreness or burning, acne, hair loss, swelling of the feet or legs, burning sensation upon urinating, urinary infections, weakness, and sleeplessness (all forms); increased sweating, cough or stuffy nose, muscle and joint aches, back pain, painful menstruation, conjunctivitis ("pink-eye"), eye or ear pain, changes in various white blood cells and blood platelets, anxiety, depression, emotional upset, fainting, nervousness, confusion, tremors, tingling in the hands or feet, pancreas inflammation, appetite changes, stomach irritation, gallbladder disease, dry mouth, mouth sores, bloody diarrhea, kidney damage, urges to urinate, blood in the urine, worsening of asthma, psoriasis, dry skin, and other skin reactions (tablets).

▼ Rare: hepatitis, worsening of colitis, and pericarditis (inflammation of the sac surrounding the heart; symptoms include chest pain and breathing difficulty).

Drug Interactions

None known.

Food Interactions

Take this drug with food if it upsets your stomach.

Usual Dose

Capsules
1000 mg 4 times a day for up to 8 weeks.

Tablets
800 mg 3 times a day for 6 weeks.

Rectal Suspension
1 enema (bottle) at bedtime every night for 3 to 6 weeks. The enema liquid should be retained for about 8 hours.

Suppositories
1 suppository 2 times per day for 3 to 6 weeks. Retain the suppository for 1 to 3 hours for maximum benefit.

Overdosage

Symptoms are likely to be similar to an Aspirin overdose: ringing or buzzing in the ears, fainting or dizziness, headache, confusion, drowsiness, sweating, rapid breathing, vomiting, and diarrhea. Overdose victims should be made to vomit with Syrup of Ipecac (available at any pharmacy) to remove the medicine from their stomach and should be taken to a hospital emergency room for treatment. In one case of accidental overdose in a 3-year-old boy who took 2000 mg, treatment with Syrup of Ipecac (available at any pharmacy) and charcoal (to absorb remaining medicine) resulted in no serious consequences. Call your local poison control center before giving the Ipecac. ALWAYS take the medicine bottle with you when you go for treatment.

Special Information

Mesalamine tablets must be swallowed whole. The outer

coating is designed to protect the Mesalamine until it reaches the colon. Call your doctor if you pass whole tablets.

When using suppositories, remove the foil wrapper and insert into the rectum, pointed end first, with as little handling as possible to prevent it from accidentally melting.

When using the rectal suspension, shake the bottle well and remove the protective sheath from the applicator tip. Lie on your left side with your lower leg extended and the upper leg flexed to maintain balance. Gently insert the applicator tip in the rectum pointing toward your navel. Steadily squeeze the bottle to discharge most of the contents into your colon.

Call your doctor if you **develop** chest pains, breathing difficulty, urinary difficulty, **worsening** of your colitis, or any other side effect that is **bothersome** or persistent.

If you forget a dose of Mesalamine, take it as soon as you remember. If you take Mesalamine tablets and it is within 4 hours of your next dose, skip the dose you forgot and continue with your regular schedule.

If you take Mesalamine suppositories or rectal solution and you don't remember until it is almost time for the next dose, skip the one you forgot and continue with your regular schedule. Do not take a double dose of any Mesalamine product.

Special Populations

Pregnancy/Breast-feeding
Mesalamine passes into the developing fetus. As with all drugs, pregnant women should consult their doctor before using Mesalamine.

Small amounts of Mesalamine pass into breast milk, although the importance of this is not known. Nursing mothers taking Mesalamine should exercise caution.

Seniors
Seniors may use this drug without special restriction. Be sure to report any unusual side effects to your doctor.

Generic Name

Metaproterenol

Brand Names

Alupent Inhalation Aerosol/Solution/Syrup/Tablets
Metaprel Inhalation Aerosol/Solution/Syrup/Tablets

(Also available in generic form)

Type of Drug

Bronchodilator.

Prescribed for

Asthma and spasm of the bronchial muscles.

General Information

Metaproterenol can be taken both by mouth as a tablet or
syrup and by inhalation. This drug may be used together with
other drugs to produce the desired relief from asthmatic
symptoms. Oral Metaproterenol begins working 15 to 30
minutes after a dose and its effects may last for up to 4 hours.
Metaproterenol inhalation begins working in 5 to 30 minutes
and lasts for 2 to 6 hours.

Cautions and Warnings

This drug should be used with caution by patients who have
angina, heart disease, high blood pressure, a history of
stroke or **seizures, diabetes, thyroid disease, prostate disease,** or **glaucoma. Excessive use** of Metaproterenol **inhalant**
could lead to **worsening of your condition.**

Using **excessive amounts** of Metaproterenol can lead to
increased difficulty breathing, instead of providing breathing
relief. In the most extreme cases, people have had heart
attacks after using excessive amounts of inhalant.

Possible Side Effects

▼ Common: heart palpitations; rapid heartbeat; tremors;
convulsions; shakiness; nervous tension; dizziness; faint-

Possible Side Effects (continued)

ing; headache; heartburn; upset stomach; nausea and vomiting; cough; sore, dry, or irritated throat; muscle cramps; and urinary difficulties.

▼ Less common: side effects that affect the heart and cardiovascular system, such as high blood pressure, abnormal heart rhythms, and angina. It is less likely to cause these effects than some of the older drugs. Metaproterenol inhalation can also cause diarrhea, bad taste or smell, dry mouth, drowsiness, hoarseness, stuffy nose, worsening of asthma, backache, fatigue, and skin rash.

Drug Interactions

• The effect of this drug may be increased by antidepressant drugs, some antihistamines, Levothyroxine, and monoamine oxidase (MAO) inhibitor drugs.
• The chances of cardiac toxicity may be increased in people taking Metaproterenol and Theophylline.
• Metaproterenol is antagonized by the beta-blocking drugs (Propranolol and others).
• Metaproterenol may antagonize the effects of blood-pressure-lowering drugs, especially Reserpine, Methyldopa, and Guanethidine.

Food Interactions

If the tablets cause an upset stomach, they may be taken with food.

Usual Dose

Oral
Adult and Child (over 60 pounds, or over age 9): 60 to 80 mg a day.

Child (under 60 pounds, or age 6 to 9): 30 to 40 mg a day.

Child (under 6 years): 0.6 to 1.2 mg per pound of body weight a day. Children this age should be treated only with Metaproterenol syrup.

Inhalation
Adult and Adolescent (over age 12): 2 to 3 puffs every 3 to 4 hours.

Child (under age 12): not recommended.

Each canister contains about 300 inhalations. Do not use more than 12 puffs per day.

Overdosage

Symptoms of Metaproterenol overdose are palpitation, abnormal heart rhythms, rapid or slow heartbeat, chest pain, high blood pressure, fever, chills, cold sweat, blanching of the skin, nausea, vomiting, sleeplessness, delirium, tremor, pinpoint pupils, convulsions, coma, and collapse. If you or someone you know has taken an overdose of this drug, call your doctor or bring the patient to a hospital emergency room. ALWAYS remember to bring the prescription bottle or inhaler with you.

Special Information

Be sure to follow your doctor's instructions for this drug. Using more than the amount prescribed can lead to drug tolerance and actually cause your condition to worsen. If your condition worsens instead of improving after using your medicine, stop taking it and call your doctor at once.

Metaproterenol inhalation should be used during the second half of your inward breath, since this allows it to reach more deeply into your lungs.

Call your doctor immediately if you develop chest pain, palpitations, rapid heartbeat, muscle tremors, dizziness, headache, facial flushing, or urinary difficulty, or if you still have trouble breathing after using this medicine.

If you miss a dose of Metaproterenol, take it as soon as possible. Take the rest of that day's dose at regularly spaced time intervals. Go back to your regular schedule the next day.

Special Populations

Pregnancy/Breast-feeding

This drug should be used by women who are pregnant or breast-feeding only when absolutely necessary. The potential hazard to the unborn child or nursing infant is not known at this time. However, Metaproterenol has caused birth defects when given in large amounts to pregnant animals.

It is not known if Metaproterenol passes into breast milk. Nursing mothers must watch for any possible drug effect on their infants while taking Metaproterenol. You may want to consider bottle-feeding.

Seniors
Older adults are more sensitive to the effects of this drug. Closely follow your doctor's directions and report any side effects at once.

Generic Name

Metaxalone

Brand Name

Skelaxin

Type of Drug

Skeletal muscle relaxant.

Prescribed for

Painful muscle spasms.

General Information

Metaxalone is prescribed as a part of a coordinated program of rest, physical therapy, and other measures for the relief of acute (or painful) spasm conditions. It does not directly relax skeletal muscles; exactly how it works is unknown.

Cautions and Warnings

Metaxalone should be taken with caution if you have had a **reaction** to it in the past, if you have a tendency toward **anemia**, or if you have **loss of kidney or liver function**.

Possible Side Effects

▼ Most common: nausea, vomiting, stomach upset or stomach cramps, drowsiness, dizziness, headache, nervousness, and irritability.

▼ Less common: rapid or pounding heartbeat, fainting, convulsions, hallucinations, depression, clumsiness or

---

Possible Side Effects *(continued)*

unsteadiness, constipation, diarrhea, heartburn, hiccups, black or tarry bowel movements, vomiting of "coffee-ground"-like material, agranulocytosis (characterized by fever with or without chills, sore throat, and sores or white spots on the lips or mouth), uncontrolled eye movements, stuffy nose, stinging or burning sensation in the eyes, bloodshot eyes, weakness, unusual tiredness or weakness, chest tightness, swollen glands, unusual bleeding or bruising, and breathing difficulty.

▼ Rare: liver inflammation, yellowing of the eyes or skin, drug-sensitivity reactions (skin rash, hives, itching, changes in facial color, fast or irregular breathing, troubled breathing, wheezing), and allergic skin reactions (itching).

Drug Interactions

• Tranquilizers, alcohol, and other nervous-system depressants may increase the depressant effects of Metaxalone.

Food Interactions

Metaxalone may be taken with food or meals if it upsets your stomach.

Usual Dose

Adult and Adolescent (age 13 and older): 800 mg 3 or 4 times a day.

Child (age 12 and under): not recommended.

Overdosage

Overdose symptoms are likely to be exaggerated side effects but may include some less common reactions as well. Overdose victims should be taken to a hospital emergency room for treatment. ALWAYS bring the medicine bottle.

Special Information

Long-term Metaxalone treatment can cause liver toxicity or damage. If you are using this medicine for an extended period, your doctor should check your liver function about every 1 to 2 months.

People taking Metaxalone must be careful when performing tasks requiring concentration and coordination (such as driving) because of the chance that the drug will make them tired, dizzy, or light-headed.

Call your doctor if you develop trouble breathing, unusual tiredness or weakness, fever, chills, cough or hoarseness, lower back or side pain, painful urination, yellow skin or eyes, skin rash, hives, itching, or redness, or any other particularly bothersome or persistent symptoms.

If you miss a dose of Metaxalone, take it as soon as you remember. If it is almost time for your next dose, take 1 dose as soon as you remember and another in 3 or 4 hours, then go back to your regular schedule. Do not take a double dose.

Special Populations

Pregnancy/Breast-feeding

There are no cases of Metaxalone-related birth defects. As with all drugs, pregnant women should not use Metaxalone unless its benefits have been carefully weighed against its risks.

It is not known if this drug passes into breast milk. Nursing mothers should use this drug with caution.

Seniors

No serious problems have been reported in older adults. However, because seniors are likely to have some loss of some kidney and/or liver function, this factor should be taken into account by your doctor when determining your Metaxalone dosage.

Generic Name

Metformin

Brand Name

Glucophage

Type of Drug

Biguanide antihyperglycemic.

Prescribed for

Diabetes mellitus (sugar in the urine).

General Information

Metformin is chemically different from all other antidiabetes drugs, which belong to the sulfonylurea group. Generally, people are not given Metformin until they have tried one of the sulfonylureas and not gotten a satisfactory response. If neither drug works alone, it is possible that a combination of Metformin and a sulfonylurea may be effective in controlling your diabetes, since the two drugs work by different methods. Metformin can moderately lower blood fats, while sulfonylureas tend to raise blood fat levels; however, the combination of Metformin with a sulfonylurea still lowers blood-fat levels.

Cautions and Warnings

Do not take Metformin if you have had an **allergic reaction** to it. Metformin should not be taken by people with **kidney disease** because the drug is cleared by the kidneys. If you are having **surgery or an x-ray** that requires the injection of an iodine-based contrast material, you should temporarily stop taking Metformin because the combination could result in acute kidney problems.

Metformin is related to an older antidiabetes drug that was moderately popular but was removed from the market because of the possibility of a very rare but serious complication known as **lactic acidosis**. When lactic acidosis does develop, it is fatal approximately half of the time. Lactic acidosis may also occur in association with a number of conditions, including diabetes mellitus. The risk of lactic acidosis increases with age and worsening kidney function. Regular monitoring of kidney function minimizes the chances of developing lactic acidosis, as does the use of the minimum effective dose of Metformin. Metformin should not be taken by people with acidosis, including those with diabetic ketoacidosis. Diabetic ketoacidosis should be treated with Insulin.

People with **liver disease** should not take Metformin because of the increased chance of lactic acidosis.

People taking oral antidiabetes drugs are generally more likely to develop **heart disease,** compared to people taking Insulin or those who can be treated with diet alone.

Possible Side Effects

▼ Most common: diarrhea, nausea, vomiting, abdominal bloating, stomach gas, and appetite loss. These symptoms tend to occur when you first start taking Metformin but are generally transient and resolve on their own. Occasionally, temporary dose reduction may be useful.

People who have been stabilized on Metformin should not consider gastrointestinal (GI) symptoms to be related to the drug unless other causes or lactic acidosis have been excluded.

Metformin can cause about 3 in every 100 people to develop an unpleasant or metallic taste in the mouth. This usually resolves on its own.

About 9 of every 100 people taking Metformin alone developed low blood levels of vitamin B_{12}, without any associated symptoms. This also happened in 6 of every 100 people on combined Metformin-sulfonylurea therapy. Blood folic acid levels did not decrease significantly when vitamin B_{12} was affected. Blood levels of vitamin B_{12} should be periodically checked, or you may take a B_{12} supplement.

Drug Interactions

• Metformin may reduce the effect of Glyburide, a sulfonylurea, but this interaction is highly variable from one person to another.

• Alcohol increases the chance of developing lactic acidosis while taking Metformin.

• Metformin may interfere with Amiloride, Digoxin, Morphine, Procainamide, Quinine, Quinidine, Ranitidine, Triamterene, Trimethoprim, and Vancomycin. Careful monitoring is necessary to avoid any possible problems.

• Cimetidine and Furosemide can cause a large increase in Metformin blood levels and possible side effects. Furosemide levels are reduced by Metformin.

• Nifedipine increases Metformin absorption into the bloodstream, blood levels of Metformin, and the amount of Metformin that is cleared through the kidneys.

Food Interactions

Metformin may be taken with food or meals to reduce upset stomach.

Usual Dose

Adult: 500 mg twice daily, increased gradually to a maximum daily dose of 2550 mg. Starting dosage can be 850 mg in the morning.

Child: not recommended.

Senior: older adults should start with regular doses but generally are not given the maximum daily dose of 2550 mg a day.

Overdosage

Contrary to what you might expect, low blood-sugar is not common with Metformin overdose (it did not even occur in the case of someone swallowing up to 85 grams of Metformin), although lactic acidosis has occurred in cases of Metformin overdose. Overdose victims should be taken to the hospital for treatment at once.

Special Information

Diet and exercise are the mainstays of diabetes treatment. Be sure to follow your doctor's directions in these areas even though you are taking a pill for your disease.

Avoid excessive alcohol intake since alcohol increases the chance of developing lactic acidosis while you are taking Metformin.

Lactic acidosis is a medical emergency that must be treated in a hospital. Metformin treatment must be stopped immediately if you develop lactic acidosis. This disease is often subtle, and accompanied only by nonspecific symptoms such as not feeling well, muscle aches, breathing difficulty, tiredness, and nonspecific upset stomach. Low body temperature, low blood pressure, and slow heartbeat can develop with more severe acidosis. Call your doctor at once if you develop these symptoms while taking Metformin.

Stomach and intestine Metformin side effects may be reduced by gradually increasing your Metformin dose and by taking Metformin with meals.

Metformin should be temporarily stopped if you have

severe diarrhea and/or vomiting because dehydration and reduced kidney function may develop. However, don't stop taking your medicine on your own. Consult your doctor first!

If you forget a dose of Metformin, take it as soon as you remember. If it is almost time for your next dose, skip the forgotten dose and continue with your regular schedule. Do not take a double dose.

Special Populations

Pregnancy/Breast-feeding

Diabetic women who are or who may be pregnant should be taking Insulin injections during their pregnancy. The safety of Metformin during pregnancy is not known.

Metformin passes into breast milk. Nursing mothers who must take Metformin should consider an alternative feeding method.

Seniors

Older adults retain more Metformin than younger adults because of the normal decline in kidney function that accompanies aging and need less medicine to effectively lower their blood sugar levels.

Generic Name

Methenamine Mandelate

Brand Names

Mandelamine

(Also available in generic form)

Information in this profile also applies to:

Generic Name

Methenamine Hippurate

Brand Names

Hiprex
Urex

Type of Drug

Urinary-tract anti-infective.

Prescribed for

Chronic urinary-tract infections.

General Information

The Methenamine anti-infectives work by turning into form-aldehyde and ammonia when the urine is acidic. The formal-dehyde kills bacteria in the urinary tract. These drugs do not break down in the blood. You may need to make your urine more acidic by taking 4 to 12 grams a day of Ascorbic Acid (vitamin C) or Ammonium Chloride.

Cautions and Warnings

People who are **allergic** to any form of Methenamine, and those with **kidney disease, severe dehydration, or severe liver disease** should not use this drug. Methenamine anti-infectives should not be taken together with a **sulfa drug** because sulfa drugs form an insoluble substance in the kidneys when mixed with formaldehyde.

Large doses (8 grams a day and more) of Methenamine can cause **bladder irritation, painful** and **frequent urination,** and **protein and blood in the urine.**

People with gout who take Methenamine may experience some **kidney pain** due to formation of urate crystals in the kidney.

Possible Side Effects

Side effects are relatively rare with Methenamine.

▼ Most common: nausea, vomiting, stomach cramps, diarrhea, appetite loss, and stomach irritation. Large doses over long periods may cause bladder irritation, painful or frequent urination, and protein or blood in the urine. This drug may also cause elevation in liver enzymes.

▼ Less common: headache, breathing difficulty, swelling, lung irritation, and rash (rarely, an itching rash).

Drug Interactions

- Do not take Methenamine with sulfa drugs (see *Cautions and Warnings*).
- Sodium Bicarbonate and Acetazolamide will decrease the effect of Methenamine by making the urine less acidic.

Food Interactions

Take Methenamine with food to minimize stomach upset.

Methenamine's action is decreased by foods that reduce urine acidity, including dairy products. Avoid large amounts of these foods.

Usual Dose

Adult and Adolescent (age 12 and older): 1 gram 2 to 4 times per day.

Child (age 6 to 11): 0.5 to 1 gram 2 to 4 times per day.

Child (under age 6): not recommended.

Overdosage

Upset stomach and exaggerated drug side effects are indicators of Methenamine overdose. Call a poison control center or hospital emergency room for more information. ALWAYS bring the medicine bottle with you if you go for treatment.

Special Information

Make sure you take all the medicine your doctor has prescribed. Stopping too soon can lead to a relapse of your infection.

Take each dose with at least 8 ounces of water.

Call your doctor if you develop pain on urinating, a skin rash, or a severe upset stomach while taking this medicine.

If you miss a dose of Methenamine, take it as soon as possible. Take the rest of that day's doses at regularly spaced time intervals. Go back to your regular schedule the next day.

Special Populations

Pregnancy/Breast-feeding

Methenamine crosses into the fetal blood circulation but has not been found to cause birth defects; it has been used during the last 3 months of pregnancy when many drugs are considered especially dangerous to the fetus, though its safety has never been proven. When the drug is considered essential by your doctor, its potential benefits must be carefully weighed against its risks.

This drug passes into breast milk in concentrations similar to those found in blood, but has caused no problems among breast-fed infants. Nursing mothers taking Methenamine should exercise caution.

Seniors

Older adults without severe kidney or liver disease may take this medication without special restriction. Follow your doctor's directions and report any side effects at once.

Generic Name

Methotrexate

Brand Names

Methotrexate (MTX)
Rheumatrex

(Also available in generic form)

Type of Drug

Antimetabolite; antiarthritic; anti-inflammatory.

Prescribed for

Cancer chemotherapy, psoriasis, psoriatic arthritis, rheumatoid arthritis (adult and juvenile), mycosis fungoides, Reiter's disease, and severe asthma.

General Information

Methotrexate was one of the first drugs found to be effective against certain cancers in the late 1940s. More recent research with smaller doses of this drug has resulted in its acceptance as a treatment for other conditions that respond to immune-system suppressants. Methotrexate doses differ dramatically for each drug use, but you should be aware that Methotrexate can be extremely toxic, even in the relatively low doses prescribed for rheumatoid arthritis. This drug should be considered "last-resort" therapy for all noncancer therapies, to be used only in severe cases that have not responded to other treatments. Methotrexate should be prescribed only by doctors who are familiar with the drug and its potential for producing toxic effects.

Cautions and Warnings

Methotrexate can trigger a unique and dangerous form of **lung disease** at any time during your course of therapy. This reaction can occur at doses as low as 7.5 mg per week (the antiarthritis dose). Symptoms of this condition are **cough, respiratory infection, difficulty breathing, abnormal chest x-ray,** and **low blood-oxygen levels. Report any change** in your **breathing** or **lung status** to your doctor.

Methotrexate can cause **severe liver damage;** this usually occurs only after taking it over a long period. Changes in liver enzymes (measured by a blood test) are common.

Methotrexate should be used with caution, and the dosage should be reduced for people with **kidney disease.**

Methotrexate can cause severe lowering in red- and white-blood-cell and blood-platelet counts.

Your doctor should periodically **test your kidney function, blood components,** and **liver function.**

Methotrexate can cause **severe diarrhea, stomach irritation,** and **mouth or gum sores. Death** can result from intestinal perforation caused by Methotrexate.

Aspirin, nonsteroidal anti-inflammatory drugs **(NSAIDs), and low-dose corticosteroid treatment may be continued** while you are taking Methotrexate for rheumatoid arthritis, although an **increase in drug toxicity** is possible. Previous studies of Methotrexate in rheumatoid arthritis were usually done in people already taking an NSAID.

Possible Side Effects

▼ Most common: liver irritation, loss of kidney function, reduced blood platelet counts, nausea, vomiting, diarrhea, stomach upset and irritation, itching, rash, hair loss, dizziness, and increased susceptibility to infection.

▼ Less common: reduced blood hematocrit (a measure of red-blood-cell count), unusual sensitivity to the

---

Possible Side Effects *(continued)*

sun, acne, headache, drowsiness, blurred vision, respiratory infection and breathing problems, loss of appetite, muscle aches, chest pain, coughing, painful urination, eye discomfort, nosebleeds, fever, infections, blood in the urine, sweating, ringing or buzzing in the ears, defective sperm production, reduced sperm count, menstrual dysfunction, vaginal discharge, convulsions, and slight paralysis.

Drug Interactions

• Fatal reactions have developed in 4 people taking Methotrexate together with some NSAIDs (3 with Ketoprofen, 1 with Naproxen). Do not take another anti-inflammatory or antiarthritic drug (even nonprescription drugs such as Ibuprofen or Naproxen) with Methotrexate unless specifically directed to do so by your doctor.

• Mixing Phenylbutazone and Methotrexate increases the risk of severe white-blood-cell count reductions, but may be medically necessary. In these cases, your doctor will watch especially closely for signs of drug toxicity (see *Cautions and Warnings*).

• Aspirin and other salicylates, some other anticancer drugs, Etretinate, Procarbazine, Probenecid, and sulfa drugs can increase the therapeutic and toxic effects of Methotrexate.

• Folic Acid counteracts the effects of Methotrexate.

• Phenytoin blood levels can be reduced by Methotrexate, possibly reducing Phenytoin's effectiveness.

Food Interactions

Food interferes with Methotrexate absorption into the bloodstream. It is best taken on an empty stomach, at least 1 hour before or 2 hours after meals, but may be taken with food if it upsets your stomach.

Usual Dose

Methotrexate dosage varies with the condition being treated. Some cancers can be treated with 10 to 30 mg per day, while others are treated with hundreds or thousands of mg given by intravenous injection in the hospital.

Rheumatoid Arthritis

Starting dose is 7.5 mg per week by mouth, either as a single dose or in 3 separate doses of 2.5 mg taken every 12 hours. Weekly dosage may be increased gradually up to 20 mg. Doses above 20 mg per week are more likely to cause severe side effects.

Psoriasis

2.5 to 6.5 mg per day by mouth, not to exceed 30 mg per week. In severe cases, dosage may be increased to 50 mg per week.

Overdosage

Methotrexate overdose can be serious and life-threatening. Victims should be taken to a hospital emergency room immediately. A specific antidote to the effects of Methotrexate (called *Calcium Leucovorin*) is available in every hospital. ALWAYS bring the prescription container.

Special Information

If you vomit after taking a dose of Methotrexate, do not take a replacement dose unless instructed to do so by your doctor.

Women taking this drug must use effective birth control.

To avoid possible birth defects, men should not attempt to father a child during treatment or for 3 months after treatment has been completed.

Call your doctor immediately if you develop diarrhea, fever or chills, skin reddening, mouth or lip sores, stomach pain, unusual bleeding or bruising, blurred vision, seizures, cough, or difficulty breathing. The following symptoms are less severe but should still be reported to your doctor: back pain, darkened urine, dizziness, drowsiness, headache, unusual tiredness or sickness, and yellowing of the eyes or skin.

If you forget a dose of Methotrexate, skip the forgotten dose and continue with your regular schedule. Call your doctor at once. Do not take a double dose.

Special Populations

Pregnancy/Breast-feeding

Methotrexate can cause spontaneous abortion or stillbirth, or severe birth defects in a surviving fetus. Do not attempt to become pregnant during Methotrexate treatment or for at least 1 menstrual cycle after the treatment is completed. Use effective birth control while taking this drug.

Men should not attempt to father a child during treatment or for 3 months after treatment has been completed, to avoid possible birth defects. Methotrexate reduces sperm counts and may affect sperm structure.

Nursing mothers who must take Methotrexate should bottle-feed their babies.

Seniors

Older adults may be more susceptible to drug side effects because of their normally reduced kidney and liver function. Seniors may require smaller doses to obtain the same results.

Generic Name

Methyldopa

Brand Name

Aldomet

(Also available in generic form)

Type of Drug

Antihypertensive.

Prescribed for

High blood pressure.

General Information

Methyldopa's mechanism of action in the body is quite complicated and not well understood, but probably has to do with the drug's ability to interfere with body mechanisms involved in making several important neurohormones: serotonin, dopamine, norepinephrine, and epinephrine. People taking Methyldopa have less of these chemicals in their body tissue, reducing blood pressure. It takes about 2 days of treatment for Methyldopa to reach its maximal antihypertensive effect.

Methyldopa is usually prescribed with one or more other

high-blood-pressure medicines or a diuretic. It does not cure high blood pressure, but helps to control it.

Cautions and Warnings

You should not take Methyldopa if you have **hepatitis** or **active cirrhosis** of the liver or if you have ever developed a reaction to Methyldopa. People taking this medicine may develop a **fever with changes in liver function** within the first 3 weeks of treatment. Some people develop yellowing of the eyes or skin (jaundice) during the first 2 or 3 months of treatment. Your doctor should periodically check your liver function during the first 3 months of treatment or if you develop an unexplained fever.

Methyldopa should be used with caution in people with **severe kidney disease.** A reduced dosage is necessary to avoid prolonged and severe lowering of blood pressure.

Possible Side Effects

Most people have little trouble with Methyldopa, but it can cause transient sedation during the first few weeks of therapy or when the dose is increased. Transient headache and weakness are other possible early symptoms.

▼ Less common: dizziness, light-headedness, tingling in the extremities, muscle spasms or weakness, decreased mental acuity, and psychological disturbances, including nightmares, mild psychosis, or depression. Other less common effects are changes in heart rate, increase of pain associated with angina pectoris, water retention (resulting in weight gain), dizziness when rising suddenly from a sitting or lying position, nausea, vomiting, constipation, diarrhea, mild dryness of the mouth, sore and/or black tongue, stuffy nose, male breast enlargement and/or pain, lactation in females, impotence or decreased sex drive in males, mild arthritis symptoms, and skin reactions.

▼ Rare: Methyldopa may affect white blood cells or blood platelets. It may also rarely cause involuntary jerky movements, twitching, restlessness, and slow, continuous, wormlike movements of the fingers, toes, hands, or other body parts.

Drug Interactions

• Methyldopa will increase the effect of other blood-pressure-lowering drugs. This is a desirable interaction for people with high blood pressure. Ironically, the combination of Methyldopa and Propranolol, a beta blocker often prescribed for high blood pressure, has sometimes (although rarely) caused an increase in blood pressure.

• Avoid over-the-counter cough, cold, and allergy preparations containing stimulant drugs that can aggravate your high blood pressure. Information on over-the-counter drugs that are safe for you can be obtained from your pharmacist.

• Methyldopa may increase the blood-sugar-lowering effect of Tolbutamide or other oral antidiabetic drugs.

• If Methyldopa is taken with Phenoxybenzamine, inability to control one's bladder (urinary incontinence) may result.

• The combination of Methyldopa and Lithium may cause symptoms of Lithium overdose, even though blood levels of Lithium do not change.

• Methyldopa, when given together with Haloperidol, may produce irritability, aggressiveness, assaultive behavior, or other psychiatric symptoms.

Food Interactions

This medicine is best taken on an empty stomach, but you may take it with food if it upsets your stomach.

Usual Dose

Adult: starting dose: 250-mg tablet 2 or 3 times per day for the first 2 days. Dosage may then be changed until lower blood pressure is achieved. *Maintenance dose:* 500 to 3,000 mg per day in 2 to 4 divided doses, per patient's needs.

Child: 5 mg per pound of body weight per day in 2 to 4 divided doses per patient's needs. *Maximum dose:* 30 mg per pound of body weight per day or 3000 mg per day.

Overdosage

Symptoms of overdosage are sedation, very low blood pressure, weakness, dizziness, light-headedness, fainting, slow heartbeat, constipation, abdominal gas or bulging, nausea, vomiting, and coma. Overdose victims should be made to vomit if they are still conscious by using Syrup of Ipecac (available at any pharmacy) and then taken to a hospital emergency room for treatment. If some time has passed since the overdose was taken, just take the victim directly to an emergency room. ALWAYS bring the medicine bottle with you.

Special Information

Take this drug exactly as prescribed so that you can maintain maximum control of your high blood pressure.

A mild sedative effect is to be expected from Methyldopa and will resolve within several days.

Your urine may darken if left exposed to air. This is normal and should not be a cause for alarm.

Do not stop taking this medicine unless you are told to do so by your doctor. Call your doctor if you develop fever, prolonged general tiredness, or unusual dizziness.

If you develop involuntary muscle movements, fever, or jaundice, stop taking the drug and contact your physician immediately. If the reactions are due to Methyldopa, your temperature and/or liver abnormalities will reverse toward normal as soon as the drug is discontinued.

If you forget to take a dose of Methyldopa, take it as soon as you remember. If it is almost time for your next dose, skip the one you forgot and continue with your regular schedule. Do not take a double dose.

Special Populations

Pregnancy/Breast-feeding

This drug crosses into the fetal blood circulation, but it has not been found to cause birth defects. Pregnant women and those who might become pregnant should not take this drug without their doctor's approval. When the drug is considered essential by your doctor, its benefits must be carefully weighed against its potential risks.

This drug passes into breast milk in amounts equal to that in the blood. Nursing mothers who must take this medicine should consider bottle-feeding their babies.

Seniors

Older adults are more sensitive to the sedating and blood-pressure-lowering effects of this drug. Follow your doctor's directions, and report any side effects at once.

Generic Name

Methylphenidate

Brand Names

Ritalin
Ritalin-SR (dye free)

(Also available in generic form)

Type of Drug

Central-nervous-system stimulant.

Prescribed for

Attention deficit disorder (ADD) in children; psychological, educational, or social disorders; narcolepsy and mild depression of the elderly. Methylphenidate is also used to treat cancer and to help stroke victims recover.

General Information

Methylphenidate is primarily used for the treatment of minimal brain dysfunction or ADD in children. Common signs of this disease are short attention span, easy distractibility, emotional instability, impulsiveness, and moderate to severe hyperactivity. Children who suffer from ADD will find it difficult to learn. Many professionals feel that Methylphenidate offers only a temporary solution because it does not permanently change behavior patterns. It must be used with other special psychological measures.

Cautions and Warnings

Chronic or abusive use of Methylphenidate can lead to **drug dependence** or **addiction**. This drug can also cause severe psychotic episodes.

Take Methylphenidate with caution if you have **glaucoma or other visual problems, high blood pressure,** or a history of **epilepsy or other seizures,** or if you are extremely **tense** or **agitated,** or are **allergic** to this drug.

Possible Side Effects

▼ Most common: in adults, nervousness and inability to sleep, which are generally controlled by your doctor reducing or eliminating the afternoon or evening dose. The most common side effects in children are loss of appetite, stomach pains, weight loss (especially during prolonged therapy), sleeping difficulty, and abnormal heart rhythms.

▼ Rare: in adults, skin rash, itching, fever, symptoms similar to arthritis, loss of appetite, nausea, dizziness, abnormal heart rhythms, headache, drowsiness, changes in blood pressure or pulse, chest pains, stomach pains, psychotic reactions, effects on components of the blood, loss of some scalp hair.

Drug Interactions

• Methylphenidate will reduce the effectiveness of Guanethidine, a drug used to treat high blood pressure.

• Interaction with monoamine oxidase (MAO) inhibitors may vastly increase the effect of Methylphenidate and cause problems.

• If you take Methylphenidate regularly, avoid alcoholic beverages because this combination will enhance drowsiness.

• Interaction with anticoagulants (blood-thinning drugs), some drugs used to treat epilepsy or other kinds of convulsions, Phenylbutazone and Oxyphenbutazone, and antidepressant drugs will slow the rate at which these drugs are broken down by the body, thereby increasing their levels in the bloodstream. Your doctor may have to lower the dose of these drugs if taken with Methylphenidate.

Food Interactions

This medicine is best taken 30 to 45 minutes before meals.

Usual Dose

Doses should be tailored to individual needs; the doses listed here are only guidelines.

Adult and Adolescent: average doses range from 20 to 30 mg per day but can be prescribed in doses as high as 60 mg per day. The drug is taken in divided doses, 2 to 3 times per day.

Child (over age 6): initial dose, 5 mg before breakfast and lunch; then increase in increments of 5 to 10 mg each week as required, not to exceed 60 mg per day.

Overdosage

Symptoms of overdosage are stimulation of the nervous system, such as vomiting, agitation, tremors (uncontrollable twitching of the muscles), convulsions followed by coma, euphoria (feeling "high"), confusion, hallucinations, delirium, sweating, flushing (redness of the face, hands, and extremities), headache, high fever, abnormal heart rate, high blood pressure, and dryness of the mouth and nose. The victim should be taken to a hospital emergency room immediately. ALWAYS bring the medicine bottle.

Special Information

Methylphenidate is a stimulant that can mask the signs of temporary drowsiness or fatigue: Be careful while driving or operating hazardous machinery. Take your last daily dose no later than 6 p.m. to avoid sleeping problems.

Call your doctor if you develop any unusual, persistent, or bothersome side effects. Do not increase your dose of this drug if the medicine seems to be losing its effect without first talking to your doctor.

If you miss a dose of Methylphenidate, take it as soon as possible. Take the rest of that day's doses at regularly spaced time intervals. Go back to your regular schedule the next day.

Special Populations

Pregnancy/Breast-feeding

Methylphenidate crosses into fetal blood circulation but has not been found to cause birth defects. Pregnant women and those who might become pregnant should not take this drug without their doctor's approval. When the drug is considered essential by your doctor, its potential benefits must be carefully weighed against its risks.

The amount of drug that passes into breast milk is not known, but it has caused no problems among breast-fed

infants. You must consider the potential effect on the nursing
infant if breast-feeding while taking this medicine.

Seniors

Older adults may take this medication without special restriction. Follow your doctor's directions, and report any side
effects at once.

Generic Name

Methysergide Maleate

Brand Name

Sansert

Type of Drug

Migraine-headache preventive.

Prescribed for

Preventing or reducing the intensity of severe migraine headaches.

General Information

Methysergide is prescribed to prevent or reduce the number
and intensity of migraine headache attacks in people who
regularly suffer at least 1 migraine per week or whose
headaches are severe, regardless of how often they occur.
　Methysergide is derived from *ergot*, a natural plant fungus.
The way that Methysergide produces its effects is not known,
but it does block the effects of *serotonin*, a hormone that is
active in many portions of the brain and central nervous
system and in blood vessels that carry blood to the brain.
Serotonin inhibition may be the key to the action of this drug.
　Methysergide must be taken for 1 to 2 days before you feel
the effect of the drug. Its effects will persist for 1 to 2 days
after you stop taking it.

Cautions and Warnings

This medicine should be used only by people whose headaches are **severe** and **uncontrollable** and who are under **close medical supervision.**

People who are **sensitive** or **allergic** to Methysergide or any other ergot-derived medicine should not take this drug. Those with **vascular (blood-vessel) disease, severe hardening of the arteries, very high blood pressure, angina or other signs of coronary artery disease, disease of the heart valves, phlebitis, pulmonary disease, connective tissue disease (lupus and others), liver or kidney disease, or serious infections and those who are severely ill** should be cautious about taking this medication.

People taking Methysergide for long periods of time may develop thickening of tissues surrounding the lung, making it more **difficult to breathe; thickening of the heart valves,** which may interfere with **heart function;** and fibrous tissues in the abdomen. To prevent these effects, you should take a **"drug holiday" (a drug-free period)** of 3 to 4 weeks every 6 months before resuming Methysergide therapy.

Methysergide tablets contain **tartrazine dye,** which should be avoided by asthmatics, people with Aspirin allergy, and those who are allergic to tartrazine. Ask your pharmacist about obtaining tartrazine-free Methysergide.

Possible Side Effects

Side effects are experienced by 30 to 50 percent of people taking Methysergide.

▼ Most common: nausea, vomiting, constipation, diarrhea, heartburn, and abdominal pain usually develop early in drug treatment; they can be avoided by gradually increasing drug dose and taking it with food.

▼ Less common: sleeplessness, drowsiness, mild euphoria (feeling "high"), light-headedness, dizziness, weakness, feelings of disassociation or hallucinations, flushing, raised red spots appearing in the skin, temporary hair loss, swelling, alterations in some blood components, muscle and joint aches, and weight gain.

▼ Rare: lung fibrosis (experienced as chest or abdominal pain, or cold, numb, painful hands or feet with possible tingling and loss of pulse in the arms or legs), visual changes, clumsiness, rash, and depression.

Drug Interactions

• Alcohol, tranquilizers, and other nervous-system depressants will increase the depressant effects of this drug. Also, alcohol worsens migraine headaches.

• Beta blockers and Methysergide may cause reduced blood flow to hands and feet, leading to cold hands or feet and, possibly, gangrene.

Food Interactions

Take this drug with food or milk to avoid stomach upset.

Usual Dose

4 to 8 mg daily, taken with food or meals.

Overdosage

Overdose symptoms include cold and pale hands or feet, severe dizziness, excitement, and convulsions. Overdose victims should be taken to a hospital emergency room for treatment. ALWAYS bring the medicine bottle.

Special Information

Do not take Methysergide for more than 6 months at a time without a 3- to 4-week drug-free period. Do not stop taking it without your doctor's knowledge and approval. Withdrawal headaches can occur if the drug is stopped suddenly. It should be gradually stopped over 2 to 3 weeks.

If Methysergide does not produce an improvement within the first 3 weeks of use, it is unlikely that the drug will be effective for you. Other treatments may be needed.

Heavy smokers experience blood-vessel constriction while taking Methysergide, leading to cold hands or feet, chest and abdominal pains, itching, numbness, and tingling of the toes, fingers, or face. Call your doctor if any of these symptoms develop (especially if you don't smoke) or if you develop visual changes, clumsiness, stimulation, swelling, changes in heart rate, fever, chills, cough, hoarseness, lower back or side pain, urinary difficulty, depression, skin rash, redness or darkening of the face, red spots on the skin, leg cramps, loss of appetite, difficulty breathing, or swelling of the hands, legs, ankles, or feet. Call your doctor if any infection develops because infections can increase your sensitivity to the effects of Methysergide.

People taking Methysergide must be careful when driving or doing things that require concentration and coordination because this drug can cause tiredness, dizziness, or light-headedness.

Exposure to extremely cold weather may worsen feelings of coldness, tingling, or pain caused by Methysergide. Protect yourself from cold winter weather.

If you take Methysergide twice a day and forget a dose, take it as soon as you remember. If it is almost time for your next dose, take one dose as soon as you remember and another in 5 or 6 hours, then go back to your regular schedule. Do not take a double dose.

If you take Methysergide 3 times per day and forget a dose, take it as soon as you remember. If it is almost time for your next dose, take one dose as soon as you remember and another in 3 or 4 hours, then go back to your regular schedule. Do not take a double dose.

Special Populations

Pregnancy/Breast-feeding
Methysergide must not be taken by pregnant women because the drug can cause miscarriage.

Methysergide passes into breast milk and may cause the nursing baby to develop vomiting, diarrhea, or seizures. Nursing mothers who must take Methysergide should bottle-feed their infants.

Seniors
Older adults taking this drug may develop hypothermia (low body temperature) and other drug complications. Seniors are likely to need less Methysergide than younger adults because of natural, age-related losses of kidney function.

Generic Name

Metipranolol

Brand Name

OptiPranolol Ophthalmic Solution

Type of Drug

Beta-adrenergic-blocking agent.

Prescribed for

Glaucoma.

General Information

Metipranolol is one of several beta-adrenergic-blocking drugs, or beta blockers, which interfere with the action of a specific part of the nervous system. Beta receptors are found all over the body and affect many body functions, which accounts for the usefulness of beta blockers against a wide variety of conditions.

Beta-blocker eyedrops generally reduce fluid pressure inside the eye by reducing the production of eye fluids and slightly increasing the rate at which fluids flow through and leave the eye. Metipranolol eyedrops only increase the rate at which fluids leave the eye; they do not affect fluid production in the eye. Beta blockers produce a greater drop in eye pressure than either Pilocarpine or Epinephrine, but may be combined with these or other drugs to produce a more pronounced drop in eye pressure.

People who cannot use Metipranolol because of its possible adverse effects on heart or lung function may be able to use Betaxolol.

Cautions and Warnings

Be cautious about taking a beta-blocker eyedrop if you have **asthma, severe heart failure, very slow heart rate,** or **heart block** because small amounts of the drug may be absorbed into your bloodstream and can aggravate these conditions.

Beta blockers, including Metipranolol, may **mask the signs** of an **overactive thyroid, low blood sugar,** and **hypoglycemia.**

Possible Side Effects

Metipranolol side effects are usually mild, relatively uncommon, develop early in the course of treatment, and are rarely a reason to stop taking the medication.

Drug Interactions

• If you take other glaucoma eye medicines, separate them from Metipranolol to avoid physically mixing them. Small amounts of Metipranolol are absorbed into the general circulation and may interact with some of the same drugs as beta blockers taken by mouth, but this is unlikely.

Food Interactions

None known.

Usual Dose

One drop in the affected eye 1 or 2 times per day.

Overdosage

Symptoms of Metipranolol overdose are changes in heartbeat (unusually slow, unusually fast, or irregular), severe dizziness or fainting, difficulty breathing, bluish-colored fingernails or palms of the hands, and seizures. Overdose is highly unlikely. Call your local poison control center or hospital emergency room for more information.

Special Information

Call your doctor about the following side effects only if they persist or are bothersome: anxiety, diarrhea, constipation, sexual impotence, mild dizziness, headache, itching, nausea or vomiting, nightmares or vivid dreams, upset stomach, trouble sleeping, stuffy nose, frequent urination, unusual tiredness, or weakness.

To administer the eyedrops, lie down or tilt your head backward and look at the ceiling. Hold the dropper above your eye and drop the medicine inside your lower lid while looking up. To prevent possible infection, don't allow the dropper to touch your fingers, eyelids, or any surface. Release the lower lid and keep your eye open. Don't blink for about 30 seconds. Press gently on the bridge of your nose at the inside corner of your eye for about 1 minute. This will help to circulate the medicine around your eye. Wait at least 5 minutes before using any other eyedrops.

If you forget to take a dose, take it as soon as you remember. If it is almost time for your next dose, skip the one you forgot and continue with your regular schedule. Do not take a double dose.

Special Populations

Pregnancy/Breast-feeding

Beta blockers may cross into the blood circulation of the developing fetus, but the amount of drug that could be absorbed from eyedrops is negligible.

Nursing mothers who use these eyedrops should watch their babies for side effects.

Seniors

Seniors may be more likely to suffer drug-related effects if eyedrops are absorbed into the bloodstream.

Generic Name

Metoclopramide

Brand Names

Clopra
Maxolon
Reglan

(Also available in generic form)

Type of Drug

Antiemetic; gastrointestinal stimulant.

Prescribed for

Nausea and vomiting related to cancer chemotherapy, surgery, pregnancy, labor, and other causes. Metoclopramide is also prescribed to treat symptoms of diabetic gastroparesis (stomach paralysis associated with diabetes), including nausea, vomiting, heartburn, fullness after meals, and loss of appetite; gastroesophageal reflux disease (GERD); some cases of stomach ulcers; anorexia nervosa; and bleeding from blood vessels in the esophagus (often associated with severe liver disease). It also helps to facilitate certain diagnostic x-ray procedures, and it can often improve the absorption of antimigraine medicines and narcotic pain relievers. Nursing mothers are occasionally given Metoclopramide to increase milk production.

General Information

Metoclopramide stimulates movement of the upper gastrointestinal (GI) tract but does not stimulate excess stomach acids or other secretions. Its effect against nausea and vomiting may be caused by the drug's direct effect on dopamine receptors in the brain. It also affects the secretion of a variety of hormones in the body and can improve drug absorption into the bloodstream by slowing the movement of the stomach and intestines, keeping the drug in an area where it can be absorbed for a longer time.

Cautions and Warnings

People with **high blood pressure, Parkinson's disease, asthma, liver** or **kidney failure,** or **seizure disorders** should use this drug with caution. Do not take this drug if you are **allergic** to it. Metoclopramide should not be used when a **bleeding ulcer** or another condition is present in which stimulating the GI tract could be dangerous.

Mild to severe depression has occurred in people taking Metoclopramide. People with a history of depression should only use this product if its benefits outweigh the possible dangers.

Uncontrollable motions similar to those that develop in Parkinson's disease have developed as side effects of this drug. These generally occur within 6 months after starting on Metoclopramide and generally subside within 2 to 3 months.

This drug can cause **extrapyramidal side effects** similar to those caused by **phenothiazine drugs.** Do not take the 2 classes of drugs together. Extrapyramidal effects occur in only about 0.2 percent of the people taking the drug; effects include **restlessness and involuntary movements of the arms and legs, face, tongue, lips, or other parts of the body.**

Women taking this drug develop chronic elevations of a hormone called *prolactin.* About one-third of breast tumors are prolactin-dependent, a factor that should be taken into account when this drug is prescribed.

Possible Side Effects

Mild side effects that usually go away when the drug is stopped occur in 20 to 30 percent of people who take Metoclopramide. Side effects are more common as the dose increases or if you take the drug for longer periods of time.

▼ Most common: restlessness, drowsiness, fatigue, sleeplessness, dizziness, anxiety, loss of muscle control, headache, muscle spasm, confusion, severe depression, convulsions, and hallucinations.

▼ Less common: rashes, diarrhea, blood-pressure changes, abnormal heart rhythms, slow heartbeat, oozing fluid from the nipples, tender nipples, loss of regular menstrual periods, breast swelling and tenderness, impotence, reduced white-blood-cell counts, frequent urination, loss of urinary control, visual disturbances, or worsening of bronchial spasms.

▼ Rare: people taking this drug may develop a group of possibly fatal symptoms, collectively called *neuroleptic malignant syndrome* (NMS), that include very high fever, semiconsciousness, rigid muscles, flushing of the face and upper body, and liver toxicity (after high doses).

Drug Interactions

• The effects of Metoclopramide on the stomach are antagonized by narcotics and anticholinergic drugs.

• Metoclopramide may increase the effects of alcoholic beverages and Cyclosporine by increasing the amount absorbed into the bloodstream.

• Metoclopramide may increase the sedative effects of nervous-system depressants, including tranquilizers and sleeping pills.

• Metoclopramide and Levodopa have opposite effects on the same nervous-system receptors and will antagonize each other.

• Metoclopramide may reduce the effects of digitalis drugs and Cimetidine.

• Combining Metoclopramide with a monoamine oxidase (MAO) inhibitor may cause very high blood pressure.

Food Interactions

Take this drug 30 minutes before meals and at bedtime.

Usual Dose

Adult: 5 to 15 mg before meals and at bedtime. Single doses of 10 to 20 mg are used before x-ray diagnostic procedures.

Senior: start at 5 mg.

Child (age 6 to 14): ¼ to ½ the adult dose.

Child (under age 6): 0.05 mg per pound of body weight per dose.

Overdosage

Symptoms of overdose are drowsiness, disorientation, restlessness, or uncontrollable muscle movements; these usually disappear within 24 hours after the drug has been stopped. Anticholinergic drugs will antagonize these symptoms.

Special Information

Call your doctor if you develop chills, fever, sore throat, dizziness, severe or persistent headaches, feelings of ill health, rapid or irregular heartbeat, difficulty speaking or swallowing, loss of balance, stiffness of the arms or legs, a shuffling walk, a masklike face, lip-smacking or puckering, puffing of the cheeks, rapid, wormlike tongue movements, uncontrollable chewing movements, uncontrolled arm and leg movements, or any other persistent or intolerable side effects.

Metoclopramide may cause dizziness, confusion, and drowsiness. Take care while driving or operating hazardous equipment. Avoid alcohol and be cautious about taking tranquilizers or sleeping pills while you are on this drug.

If you forget to take a dose of Metoclopramide, take it as soon as you remember. If it is almost time for your next dose, skip the forgotten dose and continue with your regular schedule. Do not take a double dose.

Special Populations

Pregnancy/Breast-feeding

Metoclopramide crosses into fetal blood circulation, but has not been found to cause birth defects. When the drug is considered essential by your doctor for severe nausea, vomiting, or esophageal irritation, its potential benefits must be carefully weighed against its risks.

Nursing mothers may occasionally be given Metoclopramide to increase milk production. This drug passes into breast milk, but there appears to be no risk for the infant whose nursing mother is taking no more than 45 mg per day. Always consider possible effects on the nursing infant if breast-feeding while taking this medicine.

Seniors

Seniors, especially women, are more sensitive to the side effects of this drug (see *Cautions and Warnings*). Follow your doctor's directions and report any side effects at once.

Generic Name

Metoprolol

Brand Names

Lopressor*
Toprol XL

(*Also available in generic form)

Type of Drug

Beta-adrenergic-blocking agent.

Prescribed for

High blood pressure, angina pectoris, abnormal heart rhythms, preventing second heart attack, migraine headaches, tremors, aggressive behavior, antipsychotic drug side effects, improving cognitive performance, congestive heart failure (in some people), and bleeding from the esophagus.

General Information

Metoprolol is one of 14 beta-adrenergic-blocking drugs that interfere with the action of a specific part of the nervous system. Beta receptors are found all over the body and affect many body functions. This accounts for the usefulness of beta blockers against a wide variety of conditions. The first member of this group, Propranolol, was found to affect the entire beta-adrenergic portion of the nervous system. Newer beta blockers have been refined to affect only a portion of that system, making them more useful in the treatment of cardiovascular disorders and less useful for other purposes. Other beta blockers are mild stimulants to the heart or have other characteristics that make them more useful for a specific purpose or better for certain people. Metoprolol has less of an effect on your pulse and bronchial muscles (asthma), and less of a rebound effect when discontinued. It causes less tiredness, depression, and intolerance to exercise than other beta-blocking drugs. Taking long-acting Metoprolol means you can take the medicine only once a day and still have a steady blood level of the drug for a full 24 hours.

Cautions and Warnings

You should be **cautious about taking Metoprolol** if you have **asthma,** a **very slow heart rate,** or **heart block** because the drug may aggravate these conditions.

People with **angina** who take Metoprolol for high blood pressure should have their **drug dosage reduced gradually** over 1 to 2 weeks rather than suddenly discontinued to avoid possible aggravation of the angina.

Metoprolol should be used with caution if you have **liver or kidney disease** because your ability to eliminate this drug from your body may be impaired.

Metoprolol reduces the amount of blood pumped by the heart with each beat. This reduction in blood flow can aggravate or worsen the condition of people with **poor circulation** or **circulatory disease.**

If you are undergoing **major surgery,** your doctor may want you to stop taking Metoprolol at least 2 days before surgery to permit the heart to respond more acutely to things that happen during the surgery. This is still controversial and may not hold true for all people preparing for surgery.

Possible Side Effects

Metoprolol side effects are usually mild and relatively uncommon, develop early in the course of treatment, and are rarely a reason to stop taking this medication.

▼ Most common: male impotence.

Possible Side Effects *(continued)*

▼ Less common: unusual tiredness or weakness, slow
heartbeat, heart failure (swelling of the legs, ankles, or feet),
dizziness, breathing difficulty, bronchospasm, mental depression, confusion, anxiety, nervousness, sleeplessness,
disorientation, short-term memory loss, emotional instability, cold hands and feet, constipation, diarrhea, nausea,
vomiting, upset stomach, increased sweating, urinary difficulty, cramps, blurred vision, skin rash, hair loss, stuffy
nose, facial swelling, aggravation of lupus erythematosus
(a disease of the body's connective tissues), itching, chest
pains, back or joint pains, colitis, drug allergy (fever, sore
throat), and liver toxicity.

Drug Interactions

• Metoprolol may interact with surgical anesthetics to
increase the risk of heart problems during surgery. Some
anesthesiologists recommend gradually stopping your medicine 2 days before surgery.

• Metoprolol may interfere with the normal signs of low
blood sugar and can interfere with the action of oral antidiabetes medicines.

• Metoprolol enhances the blood-pressure-lowering effects
of other blood-pressure-reducing agents (including Clonidine,
Guanabenz, and Reserpine) and calcium-channel-blocking
drugs (such as Nifedipine).

• Aspirin-containing drugs, Indomethacin, Sulfinpyrazone,
and estrogen drugs can interfere with the blood-pressure-
lowering effect of Metoprolol.

• Cocaine may reduce the effects of all beta-blocking drugs.

• Metoprolol may increase the cold hands and feet associ-
ated with taking ergot alkaloids (for migraine headaches).
Gangrene is a possibility in people taking an ergot and
Metoprolol.

• The effect of benzodiazepine antianxiety drugs may be
increased by Metoprolol.

• Metoprolol will counteract the effects of thyroid-hormone-
replacement medicines.

• Calcium channel blockers, Flecainide, Hydralazine, oral

contraceptives, Propafenone, Haloperidol, phenothiazine tranquilizers (Molindone and others), quinolone antibacterials, and
Quinidine may increase the amount of Metoprolol in the bloodstream and the effect of the drug on the body.
- Metoprolol should not be taken within 2 weeks of taking
a monoamine oxidase (MAO) inhibitor antidepressant drug.
- Cimetidine increases the amount of Metoprolol absorbed
into the bloodstream from oral tablets.
- Metoprolol may interfere with the effectiveness of Theophylline, Aminophylline, and some antiasthma drugs (especially Ephedrine and Isoproterenol).
- The combination of Metoprolol and Phenytoin or digitalis
drugs can result in excessive slowing of the heart, possibly
causing heart block.
- If you stop smoking while taking Metoprolol, your dose
may have to be reduced because your liver will break down
the drug more slowly after you stop.

Food Interactions

Long-acting Metoprolol (Toprol XL) may be taken with food if
it upsets your stomach.
   Food increases the amount of short-acting Metoprolol
(Lopressor) absorbed into the blood, so the drug should be
taken without food.

Usual Dose

100 to 450 mg per day. Metoprolol dosage must be tailored to
your specific needs.

Overdosage

Symptoms of overdosage are changes in heartbeat (unusually slow, unusually fast, or irregular), severe dizziness or
fainting, difficulty breathing, bluish-colored fingernails or
palms, and seizures. The overdose victim should be taken to
a hospital emergency room where proper therapy can be
given. ALWAYS bring the medicine bottle.

Special Information

Metoprolol is meant to be taken continuously. Do not stop
taking it unless directed to do so by your doctor; abrupt
withdrawal may cause chest pain, difficulty breathing, in-

creased sweating, and unusually fast or irregular heartbeat. The dose should be lowered gradually over a period of about 2 weeks.

Call your doctor at once if any of the following symptoms develop: back or joint pains, difficulty breathing, cold hands or feet, depression, skin rash, or changes in heartbeat. This drug may produce an undesirable lowering of blood pressure, leading to dizziness or fainting. Call your doctor if this happens to you. Call your doctor about the following side effects only if they persist or are bothersome: nausea or vomiting, upset stomach, diarrhea, constipation, sexual impotence, headache, itching, anxiety, nightmares or vivid dreams, trouble sleeping, stuffy nose, frequent urination, unusual tiredness, or weakness.

Metoprolol can cause drowsiness, light-headedness, dizziness, or blurred vision. Be careful when driving or performing complex tasks.

It is best to take your medicine at the same time each day. If you forget a dose, take it as soon as you remember. If you take your medicine once a day and it is within 8 hours of your next dose, skip the forgotten tablet and continue with your regular schedule. If you take it twice a day and it is within 4 hours of your next dose, skip the forgotten dose and continue with your regular schedule. Do not take a double dose.

Special Populations

Pregnancy/Breast-feeding
Infants born to women who took a beta blocker weighed less at birth and had low blood pressure and reduced heart rate. Metoprolol should be avoided by pregnant women and those who might become pregnant while taking it. When the drug is considered essential by your doctor, its potential benefits must be carefully weighed against its risks.

Small amounts of Metoprolol pass into breast milk, but problems are rare. Still, nursing mothers taking Metoprolol should bottle-feed their babies.

Seniors
Older adults may absorb and retain more Metoprolol, thus requiring less medicine to achieve the same results. Your doctor will need to adjust your dosage to meet your individual needs. Seniors taking this medicine may be more likely

to suffer from cold hands and feet, reduced body temperature, chest pains, general feelings of ill health, sudden breathing difficulty, increased sweating, or changes in heartbeat.

Generic Name

Metronidazole

Brand Names

Femazole	MetroGel	Protostat
Flagyl	Metryl	Satric
Metizol		

(Also available in generic form)

Type of Drug

Amoebicide; antibiotic.

Prescribed for

Acute amoebic dysentery; infections of the vagina, bone, brain, nervous system, urinary tract, abdomen, and skin caused by bacteria or other micro-organisms that are sensitive to the drug's effects. Metronidazole may also be prescribed for pneumonia, inflammatory bowel disease, colitis caused by other antibiotics, periodontal (gum) infections, and some complications of severe liver disease. Metronidazole gel may be applied to the skin to treat acne. It can also be used for severe decubitus (skin) ulcers and inflammation of the skin around the mouth. Metronidazole given by intravenous injection may be used before, during, and after bowel surgery to prevent infectious complications.

General Information

Metronidazole is effective against a variety of fungi and some bacteria. It may be prescribed for symptomless diseases when the doctor feels that an underlying infection may be involved. For example, asymptomatic women may be treated with this drug when vaginal examination shows evidence of Trichomonas. Because vaginal Trichomonas infection is a venereal disease, asymptomatic sexual partners of treated patients should be treated at the same time if the organism has been found in the woman's genital tract. This is needed to prevent reinfection of the partner. The decision to treat an asymptomatic male partner without evidence of infection must be made by the doctor. Metronidazole kills micro-organisms by disrupting the DNA of the organism after it enters the cell.

Cautions and Warnings

You should not use this drug if you have a history of **blood disease** or if you know that you are **sensitive** or **allergic** to Metronidazole.

People taking this medication have experienced **seizures, numbness,** or **tingling in the hands or feet.** This effect is rare with low doses but may be more common in people taking larger doses for long periods (i.e., in **Crohn's disease**). If this happens to you, stop taking the medicine and **call your doctor at once.** Metronidazole should be taken with caution if you have **active nervous-system disease** (including **epilepsy**) or if you have **severe liver problems.**

Possible Side Effects

▼ Most common: gastrointestinal (GI) tract symptoms, including nausea (sometimes accompanied by head-ache), dizziness, loss of appetite, occasional vomiting, diarrhea, stomach upset, abdominal cramping, and con-stipation. A sharp, unpleasant metallic taste is also asso-ciated with the use of this drug.

▼ Less common: numbness or tingling in the extremi-ties and occasional joint pains, confusion, irritability, depression, difficulty sleeping, and weakness. Itching and a sense of pelvic pressure also have been reported.

▼ Rare: clumsiness or poor coordination, fever, in-creased urination, seizures, incontinence, and reduced sex drive.

Drug Interactions

• Avoid alcoholic beverages: Interaction with Metronida-zole may cause abdominal cramps, nausea, vomiting, headaches, and flushing. Modification of the taste of alcoholic beverages has also been reported. Metronidazole should not be used if you are taking Disulfiram (used to maintain abstinence from alcohol), because the combination can cause confusion and psychotic reactions.

• People taking oral anticoagulant (blood-thinning) drugs such as Warfarin will have to have their dose reduced because Metronidazole increases the effect of anticoagulants.

• Metronidazole raises Lithium blood levels, effects, and toxicity.

• Cimetidine can interfere with the liver's ability to break down Metronidazole, causing increased amounts of Metronidazole in your blood. Your Metronidazole dosage may have to be reduced if you are taking Cimetidine.

• Phenobarbital and other barbiturates can increase the rate at which Metronidazole is broken down, compromising its effectiveness.

• Drugs that cause nervous-system toxicity—such as Mexiletine, Ethambutol, Isoniazid, Lindane, Lincomycin, Lithium, Pemoline, Quinacrine, and long-term high-dose vitamin B_6 (Pyridoxine)—should not be taken with Metronidazole because nervous-system effects may be increased.

• Metronidazole may increase blood levels of Phenytoin by interfering with its breakdown in the liver. This could increase the risk of Phenytoin side effects and might result in the need to adjust your Phenytoin dosage.

Food Interactions

This drug is best taken with food to avoid stomach upset.

Usual Dose

Adult: for the treatment of amoebic dysentery, 500 to 750 mg 3 times per day for 5 to 10 days. For trichomonal infections, 250 mg 3 times per day for 7 days, or 2 grams in 1 dose.

Senior: lower adult doses may be necessary.

Child: for amoebic dysentery, 16 to 23 mg per pound of body weight daily divided in 3 equal doses for 10 days.

Overdosage

Single doses as large as 15,000 mg have been taken in suicide attempts and accidental doses. Overdose symptoms include nausea, vomiting, clumsiness and unsteadiness, seizures, and pain or tingling in the hands or feet. Call your local poison control center for more information. ALWAYS bring the medicine bottle if you go for treatment.

Special Information

Call your doctor if you become dizzy or light-headed while taking this drug, or if you develop numbness, tingling, pain, or weakness in your hands or feet, or seizures (with high doses of Metronidazole). Rare side effects that demand your doctor's attention include clumsiness or unsteadiness; mood changes; unusual vaginal irritation, discharge, or dryness; skin rash, hives, or itching; or severe pain of the back or abdomen accompanied by vomiting, appetite loss, or nausea. Call your doctor if other side effects become particularly bothersome or persistent.

Metronidazole may cause darkening of your urine; this is probably not important, but inform your doctor if this happens.

Follow your doctor's dosage instructions faithfully and don't stop until the full course of therapy has been taken.

Metronidazole may cause dry mouth, which usually can be relieved with ice, hard candy, or gum. Call your doctor or dentist if dry mouth persists for more than 2 weeks.

If you forget to take a dose of Metronidazole, take it as soon as you remember. If it is almost time for your next dose, skip the missed dose and continue with your regular schedule. Do not take a double dose.

Special Populations

Pregnancy/Breast-feeding

Metronidazole passes into the fetal blood circulation soon after it is taken. This drug should not be taken during the first 3 months of pregnancy and should be used with caution during the last 6 months.

About the same amount of Metronidazole passes into breast milk as is in the mother's blood. Breast-feeding while taking this drug may cause side effects in your infant. If you must take Metronidazole, bottle-feed your baby. After you have finished your treatment, express any milk produced while you were taking the drug and discard it plus any pumped breast milk you might have saved. Nursing can be resumed 1 or 2 days after stopping Metronidazole.

Seniors

Seniors, particularly those with advanced liver disease, are more sensitive to the effects of this drug and may require less medicine. Follow your doctor's directions and report any side effects at once.

Generic Name

Mexiletine

Brand Name

Mexitil

(Also available in generic form)

Type of Drug

Antiarrhythmic.

Prescribed for

Abnormal heart rhythms. Mexiletine may be helpful in treating pain, tingling, and loss of the sense of touch that can come with severe diabetes.

General Information

Mexiletine works on the heart in the same way as Lidocaine (a commonly used injectable antiarrhythmic drug). It slows the speed at which nerve impulses are carried through the heart's ventricles, helping the heart to maintain a stable rhythm by making heart muscle cells less easily excited. Mexiletine affects different areas of the heart than many other widely used oral antiarrhythmic drugs. It is usually prescribed for people with life-threatening arrhythmias as a follow-up to intravenous Lidocaine. It should be prescribed only after other drugs have been tried. When Mexiletine is replacing other drug treatments, it may be given 6 to 12 hours after the last dose of Quinidine or Disopyramide, 3 to 6 hours after the last dose of Procainamide, or 12 hours after the last dose of Tocainide.

Cautions and Warnings

Because this drug is broken down by the liver and can cause some **liver problems,** people with severe liver disease must be cautious while taking it. Special considerations also must be made if you have a history of **heart block, heart failure, heart attack, low blood pressure,** or **seizure disorders** (rare) and intend to take Mexiletine.

Like other antiarrhythmic drugs, Mexiletine may occasionally **worsen heart-rhythm problems.** It has **not been proven** to actually help people **live longer.**

Possible Side Effects

▼ Most common: nausea, vomiting, diarrhea, constipation, tremors, dizziness, light-headedness, nervousness, and poor coordination. These can be reversed if drug dose is reduced, if it is taken with food or antacids, or if the drug is stopped.

▼ Less common: heart palpitations, chest pains, angina, changes in appetite, abdominal pains or cramps, stomach ulcers and bleeding, difficulty swallowing, dry mouth, altered taste, changes in the saliva and mucous membranes of the mouth, tingling or numbness in the hands or feet, weakness, fatigue, ringing or buzzing in the ears, depression, speech difficulties, rash, difficulty breathing, and swelling.

▼ Rare: abnormal heart rhythms, memory loss, hallucinations and other psychological problems, fainting, low blood pressure, slow heartbeat, hot flashes, high blood pressure, shock, joint pains, fever, increased sweating, hair loss, impotence, decreased sex drive, feeling sickly, difficulty urinating, hiccups, and dry skin.

Drug Interactions

• Mexiletine's effects are reduced by Aluminum-Magnesium antacids, Atropine, Ammonium Chloride, and vitamin C. Phenytoin, Rifampin, Phenobarbital, narcotics, and other drugs that stimulate the liver to break down drugs more rapidly also reduce this drug's effect.

• Smoking stimulates drug breakdown by the liver, reducing Mexiletine's effectiveness.

• Bicarbonates and Acetazolamide decrease the clearance of Mexiletine through the kidney, thus increasing its effects.

• Cimetidine may raise or lower blood levels of Mexiletine.

• Other drugs for abnormal heart rhythms may produce an additive effect on the heart, although sometimes drug combinations are the only way to control an abnormal rhythm.

• Mexiletine may increase blood levels of Theophylline. Your Theophylline dose may have to lowered if you take this combination.

• Mexiletine may reduce the effects of Caffeine on your body.

Food Interactions

Take this drug with food if it upsets your stomach.

Usual Dose

600 to 1200 mg per day in 2 or 3 divided doses.

Overdosage

Mexiletine overdose can be fatal. The first overdose symptoms are generally dizziness, drowsiness, nausea, low blood pressure, slow pulse, seizures, and tingling in the hands or feet. Coma or respiratory failure can occur after a massive overdose. Overdose victims should be taken to a hospital emergency room immediately. ALWAYS bring the medicine bottle.

Special Information

Call your doctor if you develop chest pain, a fast or irregular heartbeat, breathing problems, seizures, tiredness, yellow skin or eyes, sore throat, fever or chills, unexplained bruising or bleeding, or if any side effect becomes too bothersome.

Avoid diets that can change the acidity of your urine. A high-acid (fruit juice, citrus fruits, etc.) diet will increase the rate at which Mexiletine is removed from your body, and a low-acid diet will cause the drug to be retained in your body. Your doctor or pharmacist can give you more information.

If you miss a dose of Mexiletine, take it as soon as you can. If it is more than 4 hours past your regular dose time, skip the missed dose and continue with your usual dose schedule. Do not take a double dose.

Special Populations

Pregnancy/Breast-feeding

Mexiletine passes into the fetal blood circulation. It is not known to cause human birth defects, but animal experiments have shown some negative effects. When the drug is considered essential by your doctor, its potential benefits must be carefully weighed against its risks.

This drug passes into breast milk in amounts as high or higher than those in the mother's blood. Nursing mothers who must take Mexiletine should bottle-feed their babies.

Seniors

Older adults with severe liver disease are more sensitive to the effects of this drug; others may take it without special restriction. Follow your doctor's directions and report any side effects at once.

Generic Name

Miconazole Nitrate

Brand Names

Micatin Cream/Powder
Monistat 3 Suppositories
Monistat 5 Tampons
Monistat 7 Cream/Suppositories
Monistat-Derm Cream
Monistat 7 Combination Pack
Monistat Dual-Pak

(Also available in generic form)

Type of Drug

Antifungal.

Prescribed for

Treatment of fungal infections of the vagina, skin, and blood.

General Information

Miconazole Nitrate is used to treat a wide variety of fungal infections. Micatin Cream and Powder and Monistat-Derm Cream are applied directly to the skin to treat common fungal infections of the skin, including ringworm, athlete's foot, and jock itch. Monistat 3 and Monistat 7 are used to treat vaginal infections. Hospitalized patients may receive this drug by intravenous injection to ward off serious fungal infections. When used for vaginal or topical infections, it is effective against several nonfungal organisms, as well as fungal-type infections.

Cautions and Warnings

Do not use Miconazole if you are **allergic** to it. Proper diagnosis is essential for effective treatment. **Do not use this product without first consulting your doctor.**

Possible Side Effects

▼ Common: vein irritation, itching, rash, nausea, vomiting, fever, drowsiness, diarrhea, loss of appetite, and flushing (intravenous injection); itching, burning, and irritation (vaginal administration).

▼ Less common: pelvic cramps, hives, rash, and headache (vaginal administration); skin irritation or burning (topical application).

Drug and Food Interactions

None known.

Usual Dose

Vaginal Suppositories and Creams
One applicatorful or suppository into the vagina at bedtime for 3 to 7 days.

Topical Creams, Lotions, and Powders
Apply to affected areas twice a day for up to 1 month.

Overdosage

If accidentally swallowed, little of the drug passes into the bloodstream. Upset stomach may develop. Call your local

poison control center or hospital emergency room for more
information.

Special Information

When using the vaginal cream, insert the whole applicatorful
of cream high into the vagina and be sure to complete the full
course of treatment prescribed for you. Call your doctor if you
develop burning or itching.

If you forget to take a dose of Miconazole, take it as soon as
you remember. If it is almost time for your next dose, skip the
missed dose and continue with your regular schedule. Do not
take a double dose.

Special Populations

Pregnancy/Breast-feeding

Pregnant women should avoid using the vaginal cream
during the first 3 months of pregnancy, and use it during the
next 6 months only if it is absolutely necessary. Your doctor
may want you to avoid using a vaginal applicator during
pregnancy; instead, insert Miconazole vaginal suppositories
by hand.

Miconazole has not been shown to cause problems in
breast-fed infants.

Seniors

Older adults may take this medication without special restriction. Follow your doctor's directions and report any side
effects at once.

Micronase

*see **Antidiabetes Drugs (Oral Sulfonylureas)**, page 72*

Generic Name

Minoxidil

Brand Names

Loniten Tablets
Rogaine Lotion

(Also available in generic form)

Type of Drug

Antihypertensive; hair-growth stimulant.

Prescribed for

Severe high blood pressure not controllable with other drugs. Also prescribed for early male-pattern baldness and for a condition called *alopecia areata*, in which patches of hair fall out all over the body.

General Information

Minoxidil reduces blood pressure by dilating peripheral blood vessels, allowing more blood to flow through arms and legs. This increased blood flow reduces the resistance levels in central vessels (heart, lungs, kidneys, etc.) and therefore reduces blood pressure. Its effect on blood pressure can be seen ½ hour after a dose is taken and lasts up to 3 days. Patients usually take the medicine once or twice a day. Maximum drug effect occurs as early as 3 days after the drug is started, if the dose is large enough (40 mg per day).

Minoxidil stimulates hair growth in men and women with hereditary hair loss. No one knows the exact way that Minoxidil produces this effect, Minoxidil does not work for all people who try it, and you have to continue Minoxidil applications to maintain any new hair growth stimulated by the drug.

The ideal candidate for Minoxidil's hair-restoring effect is a man who has just started to lose his hair. Women may be helped by Minoxidil lotion, too. The drug won't help unless hair in the balding area is at least a half inch long. It takes 4 to

6 months of application before an effect can be expected. This regimen must be followed carefully, because stopping the medication will nullify any benefit you have gained and any hair you have grown will fall out. Some men who used Rogaine continuously for a year found they continued to go bald, but the rate of hair loss was slowed.

Cautions and Warnings

The oral form of Minoxidil can cause severe adverse effects on the heart, including **angina pain** and **fluid around the heart,** which affects cardiac function. Oral Minoxidil should be taken only by people who do not respond to other blood-pressure-lowering treatments. It is usually given together with a beta-blocking antihypertensive drug (Propranolol, Metoprolol, Nadolol, etc.) to prevent rapid heartbeat, and a diuretic to prevent fluid accumulation. Some patients may have to be hospitalized when Minoxidil is started to avoid too rapid a drop in blood pressure.

This drug should not be used by people with **pheochromocytoma,** a rare tumor in which extra body stimulants (catecholamines) are made.

Minoxidil has not been carefully studied in people who have suffered a **heart attack within the previous month;** cardiac side effects can be particularly serious in people with a history of heart disease. People who use Minoxidil for hair growth must have a healthy scalp and no heart disease.

Possible Side Effects

Water and sodium retention can develop, which can worsen heart failure. Also, some patients taking this drug may develop fluid in the sacs surrounding the heart. This is usually treated with diuretic drugs.

▼ Most common: 80 percent of people who start taking Minoxidil by mouth experience thickening, elongation, and darkening of body hair within 3 to 6 weeks, usually first noticed on the temples, between the eyebrows, between the eyebrows and hairline, or on the upper cheek. Later on it often extends to the back, arms, legs, and scalp. This effect stops when the drug is stopped, and

---

Possible Side Effects *(continued)*

symptoms usually disappear in 1 to 6 months. Heart rhythm changes can be detected with electrocardiogram in 60 percent of Minoxidil users but are usually not associated with any symptoms. Some other laboratory tests (blood, liver, kidney) may be affected by Minoxidil.

▼ Less common: bronchitis or other respiratory infections, sinus inflammation, rash, eczema, fungal infection, itching, redness, dry skin or scalp, flaking, worsening of hair loss or hair loss where everything was normal, diarrhea, nausea, vomiting, headache, dizziness, lightheadedness, fainting, back pain, broken bones, tendinitis, aches and pains, swelling of the arms or legs, chest pain, blood-pressure changes, heart palpitations, pulse-rate changes, allergic reactions (such as difficulty breathing, skin rash, or itching), hives, runny nose, facial swelling, conjunctivitis, ear infections, visual disturbances, weight gain, urinary infections, inflammation of the prostate or urethra, vaginal discharge, pain during sex, anxiety, depression, fatigue, menstrual changes, nonspecific breast symptoms, and irritation (pain, inflammation, redness) of the testes, vagina, or vulva.

People using 2% Minoxidil lotion may experience irritation or itching. The amount of Minoxidil absorbed in the scalp is too small to affect blood pressure or cause serious side effects.

Drug Interactions

• Minoxidil may interact with Guanethidine to produce severe dizziness when rising from a sitting or lying position. These drugs should not be taken together.

• Do not take over-the-counter drugs containing stimulants. If you are unsure as to which drugs to avoid, ask your doctor or pharmacist.

Food Interactions

This drug may be taken at any time and is not affected by food or liquid intake.

Usual Dose

Tablets

Adult and Adolescent (age 12 and older): 5 mg to start; may be increased to 40 mg per day. Do not take more than 100 mg per day. The daily dose of Minoxidil must be specifically tailored to your needs. Follow your doctor's directions exactly.

Child (under age 12): 0.1 mg per pound of body weight per day to start; may be increased to 0.5 mg per pound of body weight per day; do not use more than 50 mg per day. The daily dose of Minoxidil must be tailored to the child's specific needs.

Minoxidil is usually taken with a diuretic (Hydrochlorothiazide, 100 mg per day; Chlorthalidone, 50 to 100 mg per day; or Furosemide, 80 mg per day) and a beta-adrenergic blocker (Propranolol, 80 to 160 mg per day, or the equivalent dose of another drug). People who cannot take beta-adrenergic blockers may take Methyldopa, 500 to 1500 mg per day, or 0.2 to 0.4 mg per day of Clonidine.

Lotion

Apply to scalp twice a day.

Overdosage

Symptoms of overdosage may be dizziness, fainting, and rapid heartbeat. Contact your local poison center or hospital emergency room for instructions. ALWAYS bring the medicine bottle if you must go for treatment.

Special Information

Since Minoxidil is usually given with 2 other medications—a beta blocker and a diuretic—do not discontinue any of these drugs unless told to do so by your doctor. Take all medication exactly as prescribed.

The effect of this drug on body hair (see *Possible Side Effects*) is more of a nuisance than a risk and is not a reason to stop taking it.

Call your doctor if you experience an increase in your pulse of 20 or more beats per minute; weight gain of more than 5 pounds; unusual swelling of your arms and/or legs, face, or stomach; chest pain; difficulty in breathing; dizziness; or fainting spells.

If you forget to take a dose of Minoxidil, take it as soon as you remember. If it is almost time for your next regularly scheduled dose, skip the forgotten dose, and continue with your regular schedule. Do not take a double dose.

Special Populations

Pregnancy/Breast-feeding

Minoxidil crosses into the blood circulation of a developing baby but has not been found to cause human birth defects. Pregnant women and those who might become pregnant should not take Minoxidil. When the drug is considered essential by your doctor, its potential benefits must be carefully weighed against its risks.

This drug passes into breast milk and should not be used while nursing. Nursing mothers who must take Minoxidil should bottle-feed their babies.

Seniors

Older adults are usually more sensitive to the blood-pressure-lowering effects of Minoxidil because of a normal loss of some kidney capacity (due to age or other factors) to clear the drug from your body. Follow your doctor's directions, and report any side effects at once.

Generic Name

Misoprostol

Brand Name

Cytotec

Type of Drug

Antiulcer.

Prescribed for

Preventing the stomach ulcers associated with nonsteroidal anti-inflammatory drugs (NSAIDs); treating duodenal ulcers; preventing kidney rejection after organ transplant. Misoprostol has been studied as a vaginal contraceptive.

General Information

Misoprostol is intended to prevent severe stomach irritation or ulcers in people taking a NSAID for arthritis. It helps in treating duodenal ulcers but will not prevent them. Like Cimetidine and some other antiulcer drugs, Misoprostol suppresses stomach acid. It has shown an ability to protect the stomach lining from damage, although the exact way that the drug produces this effect is not known. Misoprostol may stimulate the body to produce more stomach lining; increase the thickness of the protective gel layer that lines the stomach; increase blood flow in the stomach lining, making it repair itself more quickly; or increase the production of bicarbonate, a natural antacid found in the stomach.

Misoprostol is likely to be an effective ulcer treatment for people who have not responded to Cimetidine, Ranitidine, Famotidine, or Nizatidine, or who are unable to take one of these drugs because of side effects or an adverse interaction with another drug.

Misoprostol, which is known to cause the pregnant uterus to contract, has been studied as a vaginal abortion drug. It works in the same way and is as effective as the controversial French abortion drug RU-486. Oral Misoprostol plus one dose of Methotrexate is as effective an abortifacient as vaginal Misoprostol.

This drug is intended for seniors and others with a history of ulcer or stomach disease or those who have been unable to tolerate antiarthritis drugs in the past.

Cautions and Warnings

This drug may make men and women **less fertile**. People who are **allergic** to Misoprostol or any prostaglandin agent should not take this medicine.

People with **kidney disease** routinely have about twice as much medicine in their blood as those with normal kidney function. This is not a problem for most people, but dosage may have to be reduced if side effects become intolerable.

People with **epilepsy** or **blood-vessel disease in the heart or brain** should be cautious about taking this medicine.

Possible Side Effects

▼ Most common: diarrhea and abdominal pain. Most cases of diarrhea are mild, lasting no more than 2 to 3 days.

Possible Side Effects *(continued)*

▼ Less common: headaches, nausea, vomiting, or stomach upset or gas.

▼ Other: spotting, cramps, excessive periodic bleeding, painful menstruation, or other menstrual disorders (in premenopausal women); vaginal bleeding (in postmenopausal women).

Drug Interactions

• Because Misoprostol reduces stomach acid, it may interfere with the absorption of drugs such as Diazepam and Theophylline, which may depend upon the presence of stomach acid for their absorption.

• Antacids reduce the amount of Misoprostol that is absorbed into the bloodstream, but this usually does not interfere with the drug's effectiveness. Magnesium-containing antacids may worsen Misoprostol diarrhea.

Food Interactions

Food interferes with the passage of Misoprostol into your bloodstream; it should be taken with (or after) meals and at bedtime to minimize the drug's gastrointestinal effects.

Usual Dose

800 micrograms per day.

Overdosage

The toxic dose of Misoprostol in humans is not known. Up to 1600 micrograms per day have been taken with only minor discomfort. Overdose symptoms are sedation, tremors, convulsions, breathing difficulty, stomach pain, diarrhea, fever, changes in heart rate (very fast or very slow), and low blood pressure. Overdose victims should be taken to a hospital emergency room for treatment. ALWAYS bring the prescription bottle.

Special Information

Do not stop taking Misoprostol without your doctor's knowledge, keep your follow-up appointments, and don't take it for more than 4 weeks without your doctor's permission. Do not share this drug with anyone else, **especially** a woman of childbearing age.

Call your doctor if drug side effects, especially diarrhea or abdominal or stomach pain, become severe or intolerable. Women who experience Misoprostol-related menstrual problems and postmenopausal women who experience vaginal bleeding should discuss these side effects with their doctors.

If you forget to take a dose of Misoprostol, take it as soon as you remember. If you don't remember until it is almost time to take your next dose, skip the missed dose and continue with your regular schedule. Do not take a double dose.

Special Populations

Pregnancy/Breast-feeding
Misoprostol makes the pregnant uterus contract and will cause a spontaneous miscarriage. Before starting on Misoprostol, you should have had a negative *blood* pregnancy test (an over-the-counter urine test is not sufficient) within 2 weeks before starting the medicine, start the drug on the second or third day of your period, and use effective contraception for the entire time you are taking Misoprostol. Pregnant women should **not** take this drug. Women of childbearing age should take Misoprostol only if they absolutely must take a NSAID and already have, or are at a high risk of developing, stomach ulcers.

Misoprostol is not likely to pass into breast milk because it is broken down rapidly in the body. However, this drug could cause major diarrhea in nursing infants and should be avoided by nursing mothers. If you must take Misoprostol, you should bottle-feed your baby.

Seniors
Older adults absorb more Misoprostol than younger people do, though adverse effects usually do not accompany this phenomenon. The dosage of Misoprostol should be reduced if intolerable side effects develop.

Generic Name

Moexipril

Brand Name

Univasc

Type of Drug

Angiotensin-converting-enzyme (ACE) inhibitor.

Prescribed for

High blood pressure.

General Information

The ACE inhibitors work by preventing the conversion of a hormone called *Angiotensin I* to another hormone called *Angiotensin II*, a potent blood-vessel constrictor. Preventing this conversion relaxes blood vessels and helps to reduce blood pressure and relieve the symptoms of heart failure by making it easier for a failing heart to pump blood around your body. The production of other hormones and enzymes that participate in the regulation of blood vessel dilation are also affected by the ACE inhibitors and probably play a role in the effectiveness of these medicines. Moexipril begins working about 1 hour after you take it and continues its effect for 24 hours.

Some people who start taking an ACE inhibitor after they are already on a diuretic experience a rapid blood-pressure drop after their first dose, or when the dose is increased. To prevent this from happening, you may be told to stop taking the diuretic 2 or 3 days before starting the ACE inhibitor, or to increase your salt intake during that time. The diuretic may then be restarted gradually. Heart failure patients generally will have been on Digoxin and a diuretic before beginning their ACE inhibitor.

Cautions and Warnings

Do not take Moexipril if you have had an **allergic** reaction to it in the past. It can, rarely, cause **very low blood pressure,** and it can affect your **kidneys,** especially if you have **conges-**

tive heart failure. It is advisable for your doctor to check your urine for changes during the first few months of treatment.

Dosage adjustment of Moexipril is necessary if you have **reduced kidney function,** since it is mostly eliminated from the body through the kidneys. ACE inhibitors may cause a decline in kidney function on their own.

Moexipril can occasionally affect **white-blood-cell count,** possibly **increasing** your **susceptibility to infection.** Blood counts should be **monitored** periodically.

Possible Side Effects

▼ Most common: dizziness, tiredness, headache, nausea, low blood pressure, chest pain, and chronic cough. The cough usually goes away in a few days after you stop taking the medicine.

▼ Less common: chest pain, angina, dizziness when rising from a sitting or lying position, fainting, abdominal pain, nausea, vomiting, diarrhea, bronchitis, urinary tract infection, breathing difficulty, weakness, and skin rash.

▼ Infrequent: itching, fever, heart attack, stroke, abnormal heart rhythms, heart palpitations, sleeping difficulty, tingling in the hands or feet, appetite loss, abnormal tastes, upset stomach, hepatitis and jaundice, pancreatitis, blood in the stool, swollen tongue, hair loss, rash, unusual sensitivity to the sun, flushing, anxiety, sleeplessness, nervousness, reduced sex drive, muscle cramps or weakness, impotence, arthritis, muscle aches, asthma, respiratory infection, sinus irritation, confusion, depression, feelings of ill health, sweating, kidney problems, anemia, blurred vision, and swelling of the arms, legs, lips, face, and throat.

Drug Interactions

• The blood-pressure-lowering effect of Moexipril is increased by taking diuretic drugs and beta blockers. Any other drug that causes a rapid blood-pressure drop should be used with caution if you are taking an ACE inhibitor.

• Moexipril may increase potassium levels in your blood, especially when taken with Dyazide or other potassium-sparing diuretics.

• Moexipril may increase the effects of Lithium; this combination should be used with caution.

• Antacids may reduce the amount of Moexipril absorbed into the blood. Separate doses of the two medicines by at least 2 hours.

• Capsaicin may cause or aggravate the cough associated with Moexipril therapy.

• Indomethacin may reduce the blood-pressure-lowering effects of Moexipril.

• Phenothiazine tranquilizers and antiemetics may increase the effects of Moexipril.

• The combination of Allopurinol and Moexipril increases the chance of a drug reaction.

• Moexipril increases the levels of Digoxin in the blood, possibly increasing the chance of Digoxin-related side effects.

Food Interactions

Moexipril should be taken 1 hour before or 2 hours after meals.

Usual Dose

7½ mg to 30 mg once a day. Some people may take their total daily dosage in 2 divided doses. People with poor kidney function should take half the usual dose.

Overdosage

The principal effect of Moexipril overdose is a rapid drop in blood pressure, as evidenced by dizziness or fainting. Take the overdose victim to a hospital emergency room immediately. ALWAYS bring the medicine bottle with you.

Special Information

Call your doctor if you develop swelling of the face or throat, if you have sudden difficulty breathing, or if you develop a sore throat, mouth sores, abnormal heartbeat, chest pain, a persistent rash, or loss of taste perception.

Moexipril can cause unexplained swelling of the face, lips, hands, and feet. This swelling can also affect the larynx (throat) and tongue, and interfere with breathing. If this happens, the victim should be taken to a hospital emergency room at once for treatment.

You may get dizzy if you rise to your feet quickly from a sitting or lying position.

Avoid strenuous exercise and/or very hot weather because heavy sweating or dehydration can cause a rapid blood pressure drop.

Avoid nonprescription diet pills, decongestants, and stimulants that can raise blood pressure.

If you take Moexipril once a day and forget to take a dose, take it as soon as you remember. If it is within 8 hours of your next dose, skip the one you forgot and continue with your regular schedule. Do not take a double dose.

If you take Moexipril twice a day and forget a dose, take it as soon as you remember. If it is within 4 hours of your next dose, take one dose as soon as you remember and another in 5 or 6 hours, then go back to your regular schedule.

Special Populations

Pregnancy/Breast-feeding

ACE inhibitors have caused low blood pressure, kidney failure, slow formation of the skull, and death in developing fetuses when taken during the last 6 months of pregnancy. Women who are pregnant should not take Moexipril. Women who may become pregnant while taking Moexipril should use an effective contraceptive method and stop the medicine if they do become pregnant.

Relatively small amounts of Moexipril pass into breast milk, and the effect on a nursing infant is likely to be minimal. However, nursing mothers who must take this drug should consider an alternative feeding method since infants, especially newborns, are more susceptible to the effects of these medicines than adults.

Seniors

Older adults may be more sensitive to the effects of Moexipril than younger adults because of the possibility of kidney impairment. Your dosage must be individualized to your needs.

Generic Name

Moricizine

Brand Name

Ethmozine

Type of Drug

Antiarrhythmic.

Prescribed for

Life-threatening cardiac arrhythmias.

General Information

Moricizine treatment should always be started in a hospital because of the close cardiac monitoring that is required during the first phase of drug treatment. It should not be prescribed for minor arrhythmias or those that do not cause symptoms of their own. Moricizine works by stabilizing heart tissues and making them less sensitive to excessive stimulation. Moricizine starts working 2 hours after it is taken and lasts for 10 to 24 hours. People with heart failure are usually able to tolerate this drug but should be closely monitored for any sign of worsening of the condition.

Cautions and Warnings

Ironically, Moricizine can **cause abnormal rhythms** of its own or **worsen existing rhythm problems**. This calls for **close monitoring by your doctor**. It is often impossible to distinguish between a drug-induced arrhythmia and one that occurs naturally, except when the problem occurs soon after drug treatment has been started and the patient is on continuous heart monitoring. **Arrhythmias can be serious and life-threatening**.

Do not take this drug if you are allergic to it. People with heart block should also not use this medicine.

Moricizine should be used with caution in patients with a form of **heart disease** called *sick sinus syndrome*, in which the part of the heart that initiates heart contractions is not working properly.

Moricizine causes **changes in electrocardiograms** and may change the actual conduction of electrical impulses throughout the heart.

People with **pacemakers** who start taking Moricizine may need their **pacemakers reset** because of changes in the sensitivity of heart tissue to electrical impulses caused by Moricizine.

This drug should be used with care by people with **liver or kidney disease**. Because Moricizine is partially broken down by the liver and passes out of the body through the kidneys, these organs are essential to the efficient removal of the drug from the body. People with kidney and/or liver disease should receive lower-than-usual doses of the drug and be monitored more closely for unwanted drug effects.

A few people taking Moricizine may develop **fevers or other drug sensitivity reactions**. If fever develops, it should subside within 2 days after stopping the drug.

As is the case with other antiarrhythmic medicines, people taking Moricizine have not been proven to live longer than those who do not take it.

Possible Side Effects

▼ Most common: dizziness, nausea, vomiting, headache, pain, breathing difficulties, fatigue, and drug-induced abnormal heart rhythms (this is the most dangerous).

▼ Common: heart palpitations, chest pain, heart failure, heart attack, cardiac death, changes in blood pressure, fainting, very slow heart rate, blood clots in the lungs, stroke, muscle weakness, nervousness, tingling in the hands or feet, sleep difficulties, tremors, anxiety, depression, euphoria (feeling "high"), confusion, agitation, seizure, coma, difficulty walking, hallucinations, blurred or double vision, speech difficulties, memory loss, coordination difficulties, and ringing or buzzing in the ears.

▼ Less common: urinary difficulty, loss of urinary control, kidney pain, loss of sex drive, male impotence, hyperventilation, asthma, sore throat, cough, sinus irritation, abdominal pain, upset stomach, diarrhea, loss of appetite, a bitter taste, stomach gas and cramps, difficulty swallowing, sweating, dry mouth, muscle pain, drug fever,

Possible Side Effects (continued)

low body temperature, intolerance to heat or cold, eye pains, rash, itching, dry skin, swelling of the lips or tongue, or swelling around the eyes.

▼ Rare: hepatitis or jaundice (yellowing of the skin or eyes).

Drug Interactions

• Cimetidine, Propranolol, and Digoxin may increase the amount of Moricizine in the blood, increasing the possibility of drug side effects.

• Moricizine may drastically decrease the amount of Theophylline in the blood by increasing the rate at which the latter drug is cleared from the body. Theophylline dosage adjustment may be needed.

Food Interactions

Taking Moricizine 30 minutes after eating delays the absorption of the drug into the blood, but does not affect the total amount of medicine absorbed. You may take Moricizine with food if it upsets your stomach.

Usual Dose

Adult: 600 to 900 mg per day.

Seniors and those with kidney or liver disease: a lower starting dose is recommended; the dose should be gradually increased until the maximum effect is achieved.

Overdosage

Symptoms are vomiting, lethargy, fainting, coma, low blood pressure, abnormal heart rhythms, worsening of heart failure, heart attack, and breathing difficulty. Death has occurred after doses of 2250 mg (17 of the 250-mg tablets) and 10,000 mg (33 of the 300-mg tablets). Victims should be taken to an emergency room immediately. ALWAYS bring the medicine bottle.

Special Information

People switching to Moricizine from another antiarrhythmic

should not take their first dose of Moricizine until several hours after their last dose of the old medicine. This is necessary to allow most of the old medicine to clear from the body. The waiting period varies from 3 to 12 hours, depending on which antiarrhythmic is being discontinued.

Some side effects may be related to the size of an individual dose. Therefore, it is usually better to divide the total daily dose into 3 separate doses, rather than 1 or 2 doses.

Call your doctor if you develop cardiac problems; dizziness; anxiety; drug fever; swelling of the tongue, lips, or the area around the eyes; visual or urinary difficulties; yellow discoloration of the skin or eyes; severe nausea; diarrhea; vomiting; or other persistent or intolerable side effects.

If you take Moricizine twice a day and forget a dose, take it as soon as you remember. If it is almost time for your next dose, take one dose as soon as you remember and another in 5 or 6 hours, then go back to your regular schedule. Do not take a double dose.

If you take Moricizine 3 times a day and forget a dose, take it as soon as you remember. If it is almost time for your next dose, take one dose as soon as you remember and another in 3 or 4 hours, then go back to your regular schedule. Do not take a double dose.

Special Populations

Pregnancy/Breast-feeding
In studies of pregnant animals, Moricizine (in doses almost 7 times larger than the maximum human dose) affected the size and weight of offspring or development of the fetuses. There is no information on the effect of Moricizine on pregnant women. The drug should be taken by a pregnant woman only after the possible benefits of taking it have been weighed against the potential harm it might cause.

Moricizine passes into breast milk. Nursing mothers who must take this medicine should bottle-feed their babies.

Seniors
Seniors generally experience the same side effects as younger adults, although studies of the drug showed that stopping drug treatment because of newly discovered arrhythmias was more common among older adults. Seniors are also

more likely to have some kidney and/or liver problem. Those conditions call for starting Moricizine at a lower dose and increasing the dosage more cautiously.

Brand Name

Motofen

Ingredients

Difenoxin + Atropine Sulfate

Type of Drug

Antidiarrheal.

Prescribed for

Acute and chronic diarrhea that does not respond to other treatments.

General Information

Difenoxin is an antidiarrheal agent related to Meperidine (Demerol), a narcotic pain reliever. Difenoxin works by slowing the rate at which intestinal-wall muscles contract. It is a chemical by-product of Diphenoxylate, another popular antidiarrheal. Atropine is added to prevent drug overdose and product abuse because Difenoxin can be addicting. Atropine causes undesirable effects at small doses, thus deterring users from taking larger Motofen doses.

Motofen and other antidiarrheals should be used only for short periods; they relieve diarrhea, but do nothing for the underlying cause. Some people should not use this drug even if diarrhea is present: People with some types of stomach, bowel, or other conditions may be harmed by antidiarrheal drugs. Do not use Motofen without your doctor's advice.

Cautions and Warnings

Do not take Motofen if you are **allergic** to any of its ingredients (including Atropine) or Lomotil. Avoid Motofen if you have **advanced liver disease**, if you have **jaundice (yellowing of the skin or eyes)**, or if your diarrhea was caused by taking **Clindamycin** or **another antibiotic**.

Possible Side Effects

▼ Most common: nausea, vomiting, dry mouth, dizziness, light-headedness, drowsiness, and headache.

▼ Less common: constipation, upset stomach, confusion, and tiredness or sleeplessness.

▼ Rare: burning eyes, blurred vision, dry skin, rapid heartbeat, elevated temperature, and urinary difficulty.

Drug Interactions

• Motofen may increase the effects of alcohol, tranquilizers, pain relievers, and other nervous-system depressants. Avoid these combinations, if possible.

• Monoamine oxidase (MAO) inhibitor antidepressants may, in theory, produce a high-blood-pressure crisis in combination with Motofen. Do not use Motofen if you are taking an MAO-inhibitor drug unless you are under a doctor's care.

Food Interactions

None known.

Usual Dose

Adult and Adolescent (age 12 and older): 2 tablets to start, then 1 after each loose stool or every 3 to 4 hours, as needed; up to 8 tablets in any day. Treatment for more than 2 consecutive days is usually not needed.

Child (age 11 and under): not recommended.

Overdosage

Overdose symptoms include the following: dry skin, mouth, and nose; flushing; fever; and rapid heartbeat. These symptoms may be followed by loss of natural reflexes, pinpointed pupils, droopy eyelids, breathing difficulty, and lethargy or coma. Take the victim to a hospital emergency room immediately. ALWAYS bring the medicine bottle.

Special Information

Be careful when driving or performing complex tasks because Motofen can make you tired, dizzy, or light-headed.

Alcohol, tranquilizers, or other nervous-system depressants will increase the depressant effects of this drug.

Your doctor may prescribe fluid and salt mixtures to replace the body fluids you lose while taking Motofen.

Call your doctor if you develop heart palpitations or if your symptoms don't clear up in 2 days. You may need a different dose or a different medicine for your problem.

If you forget a dose of Motofen, take it as soon as you remember. If it is almost time for your next dose, skip the one you forgot and continue with your regular schedule. Do not take a double dose.

Special Populations

Pregnancy/Breast-feeding

Animal studies with very large doses of Motofen showed no evidence of birth defects, but showed some effect on still-births. Pregnant women should not use Motofen unless its advantages have been carefully weighed against its possible dangers.

Nursing mothers taking Motofen should bottle-feed their babies.

Seniors

No special problems have been reported in older adults. However, those with severe kidney and/or liver disease need lower doses of Motofen.

Motrin

see *Ibuprofen*, page 519

Generic Name

Mupirocin

Brand Name

Bactroban

Type of Drug

Topical antibiotic.

Prescribed for

Impetigo (streptococcal skin infections), eczema, inflammation of the hair follicles, and minor bacterial skin infections.

General Information

Mupirocin is a unique, nonpenicillin product that works against the common micro-organisms that cause impetigo in children. It is used to supplement other treatments for impetigo, although many doctors prefer to prescribe oral medicine for the condition. It is not known how Mupirocin works, but large amounts of this drug kill bacteria and smaller amounts stop the bacteria from growing. It may work where other products fail because of bacterial-resistance problems.

Cautions and Warnings

Do not use this product if you are **allergic** to any of its components. Mupirocin ointment is **not for use in the eye**.

Possible Side Effects

▼ Less common: burning, itching, rash, stinging or pain where the ointment is applied, nausea, skin redness, dry skin, tenderness, swelling, and increased oozing from impetigo lesions.

Drug and Food Interactions

None known.

Usual Dose

Apply a small amount to the affected areas 3 times per day. Cover with gauze, if desired.

Overdosage

There is little experience with Mupirocin overdose. Call your local poison control center or hospital emergency room for more information.

Special Information

Call your doctor if this medicine does not work within 3 to 5 days or if any of the following symptoms develop: dry skin or redness, rash, itching, stinging, or pain.

If you forget to apply a dose of Mupirocin, do so as soon as you remember. If it is almost time for your next dose, skip the one you forgot and continue with your regular schedule. Do not apply a double dose.

Special Populations

Pregnancy/Breast-feeding
Animal studies have revealed no fetal damage. Still, pregnant women should use this drug only if absolutely necessary.

It is not known if Mupirocin passes into breast milk. Nursing mothers who must take this drug should bottle-feed their babies.

Seniors
Seniors may use Mupirocin without special restriction.

Generic Name

Muromonab-CD3

Brand Name
Orthoclone OKT3

Type of Drug
Immunosuppressant.

Prescribed for
Preventing organ rejection after kidney, heart, and liver transplantation.

General Information
Muromonab-CD3, a product of biotechnology processes, is an important alternative to Cyclosporine in preventing organ transplant rejection. This drug acts against human T-cells, which normally protect the body from foreign bodies. By acting against the T-cells, this drug suppresses the immune system and prevents organ rejection. The drug starts working minutes after it is first given and continues working for as

long as it is used. T-cells rapidly return to normal within 1 week after the medicine is stopped.

Cautions and Warnings

This drug should not be used by people with **untreated heart failure, fluid overload,** or a **history of seizures**.

Muromonab-CD3 is made in cells from mouse tissue and causes the development of antimouse antibodies in humans. People who have received other products made in this way may already have high levels of this kind of antibody in their blood and, if they do, should not be treated with this medicine. Your doctor will test for antibody levels.

People who receive this medicine usually develop **cytokine release syndrome (CRS) from 30 minutes to 2 days** after the first dose is given. CRS symptoms range from **mild, flu-like symptoms** (fever, chills, joint aches, weakness, headaches, etc.) to a less common, **life-threatening shock-like reaction** that involves the heart and nervous system. Some of the more severe symptoms of CRS are **shortness of breath, high fever** (up to 107°F), **wheezing, rapid heartbeat, chest pains, respiratory collapse or failure, heart attack, severe drug reactions, seizures, confusion, hallucinations, stiff neck, brain swelling,** and **headaches**. People who are at risk for more severe forms of CRS include those with a **recent heart attack** or **uncontrolled angina pectoris, heart failure, fluid in the lungs, serious lung disease,** and a history of **seizures or shock**. CRS may be prevented or minimized by giving Methylprednisolone 1 to 4 hours before the first dose of Muromonab-CD3.

People receiving this drug (or other immunosuppressants) are **more likely to develop infections**. Preventive antibiotic therapy is sometimes used to reduce the risk of infection.

Possible Side Effects

More than 90 percent of people receiving this drug experience some form of CRS, though it is usually mild (see *Cautions and Warnings*).

▼ Other: increased infection risk, rash, itching, increased sweating, flushing, diarrhea, nausea and vomiting, abdominal gas and pain, reductions in various blood-cell counts, blood-clotting abnormalities, liver inflammation, muscle

---

Possible Side Effects *(continued)*

---

and joint stiffness and pain, arthritis, blindness, blurred or double vision, hearing loss, middle-ear infection, ringing or buzzing in the ears, dizziness or fainting, conjunctivitis ("pink-eye"), stuffy nose and/or ears, sensitivity to bright light, and kidney damage.

Drug Interactions

• Other immunosuppressants (corticosteroids, Cyclosporine, and Azathioprine) and Indomethacin increase the effect of Muromonab-CD3, increasing the chances for drug (CRS) side effects.

Food Interactions

This drug may be taken without regard to food.

Usual Dose

Adult and Adolescent (age 12 and older): 5 mg intravenously per day for 10 to 14 days.

Child (under age 12): 0.1 mg intravenously for every 2.2 pounds of body weight per day for 10 to 14 days.

Overdosage

Call your poison control center for information.

Special Information

Call your doctor at the first sign of skin rash, itching, rapid heartbeat, difficulty swallowing or breathing, any unusual swelling or allergic reaction, or if you experience any other serious or bothersome side effects. It is essential to maintain close contact with your doctor while taking this medicine.

Mild reactions due to CRS may be treated by taking Acetaminophen or antihistamines. Your body temperature should be no higher than 100° F when each dose is given.

Avoid exposure to bacterial infections and immunizations while you are taking this medicine. If an infection develops, your doctor will have to stop Muromonab-CD3 treatments and treat the infection.

It is important to maintain good dental hygiene while taking Muromonab-CD3 and to use extra care when using your toothbrush or dental floss because of the chance that the drug will make you more susceptible to oral infections. See your dentist regularly while taking this medicine.

This drug may cause confusion or interfere with your alertness, dexterity, or coordination. Take care if you are driving or doing anything that requires close concentration.

It is essential to complete the full course of treatment. This medicine should not be stopped unless an infection or other severe side effect develops. If you miss a dose, take it as soon as you remember and call your doctor.

Special Populations

Pregnancy/Breast-feeding

Muromonab-CD3 may cross into the fetal blood circulation, but its effect is not known. Pregnant women and those who become pregnant while taking this drug should consider the possible risks of Muromonab-CD3 to their pregnancy.

It is not known if this drug passes into breast milk. Nursing mothers who must take it should bottle-feed their infants.

Seniors

Older adults may use this drug without special restriction.

Generic Name

Mycophenolate Mofetil

Brand Name

CellCept

Type of Drug

Immunosuppressant.

Prescribed for

Preventing the rejection of transplanted kidneys, together with corticosteroids and Cyclosporine.

General Information

In animals, Mycophenolate extends the survival of transplanted kidney, heart, liver, intestine, limbs, small bowel, pancreas cells, and bone marrow. The drug is rapidly absorbed into the bloodstream where it is metabolized into MPA, the active form of Mycophenolate. MPA inhibits the ability of T and B lymphocytes, key elements of the immune system, to respond in their usual way. MPA also suppresses antibody formation and may act directly on inflammation sites and organ rejection sites to prevent the tissue rejection process from proceeding. People with moderate to severe losses of kidney function may have to have their daily dosage adjusted.

Cautions and Warnings

As with other immunosuppressants, people taking Mycophenolate have a **better chance of developing a lymphoma** or other **malignancy.** The chance increases with the degree of immune suppression and the length of time that the drug is taken.

Two of every 100 people receiving Mycophenolate developed **severe reductions in some white-blood-cell types. Call your physician** if you develop symptoms of **viral infection** or other **unusual symptoms.**

Bleeding in the stomach or **intestines** occurs in about 3 of every 100 people who take this medicine, though many of these people were also taking other medicines that could affect the gastrointestinal (GI) tract. People with stomach or intestinal disease should take this drug with caution.

People with **kidney disease** should receive lower doses of Mycophenolate. People who experience post-transplant reduction in liver function can develop kidney damage.

Mild to moderate **high blood pressure** is a common side effect of Mycophenolate and can be a sign of kidney damage. People taking this drug should **measure** their blood pressure regularly.

Possible Side Effects

▼ Most common: general pain, abdominal pain, fever, headache, infections, blood infections, weakness, chest pain, back pain, high blood pressure, anemia, reduced white-blood-cell and platelet counts, urinary infection,

Possible Side Effects *(continued)*

blood in the urine, swelling of the arms or legs, diarrhea, constipation, nausea and/or vomiting, upset stomach, oral fungus infections, respiratory infections, cough, breathing difficulty, and tremors.

▼ Common: kidney damage, urinary tract problems, high blood cholesterol, low blood-phosphate levels, fluid retention, changes in blood-potassium levels, high blood sugar, sore throat, pneumonia, bronchitis, acne, rash, sleeplessness, and dizziness.

▼ Less common: painful urination, impotence, frequent urination, pyelonephritis, urinary disorders, angina pain, heart palpitations, low blood pressure, dizziness when rising from a sitting or lying position, other cardiovascular disorders, appetite loss, stomach gas, stomach irritation or bleeding, gum irritation or enlargement, liver irritation, mouth ulcers, asthma, lung disorders, stuffy or runny nose, sinus irritation, hair loss, itching, sweating, skin ulcers, anxiety, depression, stiff muscles, tingling in the hands or feet, joint or muscle pains, leg cramps, double vision, cataracts, conjunctivitis ("pink-eye"), chills and fever, abdominal enlargement, facial swelling, cysts, flu symptoms, bleeding, hernia, feeling sick, pelvic pains, and black-and-blue marks.

▼ Rare: lymphomas, skin cancers (not melanomas) and other malignancies; herpes, chickenpox or shingles, some fungus infections, pneumocystis and other opportunistic infections that usually only develop in people with suppressed immune systems.

Drug Interactions

• When Mycophenolate is taken together with Acyclovir, an antiviral drug, the amount of both drugs in the blood rises.

• Use of Cholestyramine and Aluminum/Magnesium antacids decreases the amount of Mycophenolate absorbed into the blood and should be separated from Mycophenolate use by at least 1 hour.

• Azathioprine, another immune-system suppressant, should not be taken together with Mycophenolate because of the chance of excess immune-system suppression.

• Taking Probenecid with Mycophenolate may double or triple the amount of the immunosuppressant in the blood. Aspirin also increases the amount of Mycophenolate in the blood.

• Mycophenolate may moderately decrease the amount of Phenytoin or Theophylline in the blood.

Food Interactions

Mycophenolate should be taken 1 hour before or 2 hours after meals.

Usual Dose

Adult: 2 to 3 grams a day, divided into two doses.
Child: not recommended.

Overdosage

The largest dose given to one person was 4 or 5 grams a day. This dosage is associated with a larger chance of drug side effects (especially those that affect the stomach and intestines) and, sometimes, blood abnormalities. Any person who takes an accidental overdose of Mycophenolate must be taken to a hospital emergency room for treatment. ALWAYS bring the medicine bottle with you.

Special Information

It is **extremely important for you to take this medicine exactly as prescribed.** If you do forget a dose of Mycophenolate, take it as soon as you remember. If it is almost time for your next dose, skip the forgotten dose and continue with your regular schedule. Do not take a double dose, and call your doctor if you forget two or more doses in a row.

Because this drug has been proven to cause birth defects in animals, take extra caution when handling the capsules. Do not open or crush the capsules. Avoid inhaling the powder or allowing it to touch your skin or the membranes inside your mouth or nose. If such contact does occur, make sure to wash thoroughly with soap and water. If the powder gets into your eyes, rinse them thoroughly with plain water.

People taking Mycophenolate require regular testing to monitor their progress.

Call your doctor at the first sign of fever; sore throat;

tiredness; weakness; nervousness; unusual bleeding or bruising; tender or swollen gums; convulsions; irregular heartbeat; confusion; numbness or tingling of your hands, feet, or lips; difficulty breathing; severe stomach pains with nausea; or bloody urine. Other drug effects are less serious but should be brought to your doctor's attention, particularly if they are unusually bothersome or persistent.

It is important to maintain good dental hygiene while taking Mycophenolate and to use extra care when using your toothbrush or dental floss because of the chance that the drug will make you more susceptible to dental infections. Mycophenolate suppresses the normal body systems that fight infection. See your dentist regularly while taking this medicine.

This medicine should be continued for as long as prescribed by your doctor. Do not stop taking it because of side effects or other problems, unless directed by your doctor to stop.

Special Populations

Pregnancy/Breast-feeding

Animal studies show that this drug can be highly toxic to a developing fetus. Women of childbearing age should have a negative pregnancy test at least 1 week before treatment is started. To ensure no pregnancy, they should either use 2 effective contraceptive methods before treatment is started and continuing until 6 weeks after Mycophenolate is discontinued, or they should remain sexually abstinent during this period. Should you accidentally become pregnant during Mycophenolate treatment, discuss the advisability of continuing the pregnancy with your doctor. This drug should not be used during pregnancy unless the benefit outweighs the potential risk of affecting the developing baby.

Nursing mothers who must take this medicine should bottle-feed their babies.

Seniors

Older adults may take this drug, but their dose may have to be reduced to accommodate normal loss of kidney function.

Generic Name

Nabumetone

Brand Name

Relafen

Type of Drug

Nonsteroidal anti-inflammatory drug (NSAID).

Prescribed for

Rheumatoid arthritis and osteoarthritis.

General Information

Nabumetone is one of 16 nonsteroidal anti-inflammatory drugs (NSAIDs) used to relieve pain and inflammation. We do not know exactly how NSAIDs work, but part of their action may be due to an ability to inhibit the body's production of a hormone called *prostaglandin* and to inhibit the action of other body chemicals, including cyclo-oxygenase, lipoxygenase, leukotrienes, lysosomal enzymes, and a host of other factors. NSAIDs are generally absorbed into the blood fairly quickly. Pain relief generally comes within an hour after taking the first dose, but the NSAID's anti-inflammatory effect generally takes a lot longer (several days to 2 weeks) to become apparent, and may take a month or more to reach its maximum effect. Nabumetone is broken down in the liver; it must be converted to its active form by the liver before it can work for your arthritis.

Cautions and Warnings

People who are **allergic** to Nabumetone (or any other NSAID) and those with a history of **asthma attacks** brought on by other NSAIDs, Iodides, or Aspirin should not take it.

Nabumetone can cause **gastrointestinal (GI) bleeding, ulcers,** and **stomach perforation.** This can occur at any time, with or without warning, in people who take chronic Nabumetone treatment. People with a history of **active GI bleeding** should be cautious about taking any NSAID. **Minor stomach upset, distress,** or **gas** is common during the first few days of treatment with Nabumetone. People who develop **bleeding or ulcers** and continue treatment should be aware of the possibility of developing more **serious drug toxicity**.

Nabumetone can affect platelets and blood clotting at high doses, and should be avoided by people with **clotting problems** and by those taking **Warfarin**.

People with **heart problems** who use Nabumetone may experience swelling in their arms, legs, or feet.

Nabumetone can cause **severe toxic effects to the kidney**. Report any unusual side effects to your doctor, who may need to periodically test your kidney function.

Nabumetone can make you **unusually sensitive to the effects of the sun** (photosensitivity).

Possible Side Effects

▼ Most common: diarrhea, nausea, vomiting, constipation, stomach gas, stomach upset or irritation, and loss of appetite.

▼ Less common: stomach ulcers, GI bleeding, hepatitis, gallbladder attacks, painful urination, poor kidney function, kidney inflammation, blood and protein in the urine, dizziness, fainting, nervousness, depression, hallucinations, confusion, disorientation, tingling in the hands or feet, light-headedness, itching, increased sweating, dry nose and mouth, heart palpitations, chest pain, difficulty breathing, and muscle cramps.

▼ Rare: severe allergic reactions, including closing of the throat, fever and chills, changes in liver function, jaundice (yellowing of the skin or eyes), and kidney failure. People who experience such effects must be promptly treated in a hospital emergency room or doctor's office.

NSAIDs have caused severe skin reactions; if this happens to you, see your doctor immediately.

Drug Interactions

• Nabumetone can increase the effects of oral anticoagulant (blood-thinning) drugs such as Warfarin. You may take this combination, but your doctor may have to reduce your anticoagulant dose.

• Taking Nabumetone with Cyclosporine may increase the toxic kidney effects of both drugs. Methotrexate toxicity may be increased in people also taking Nabumetone.

• Nabumetone may reduce the blood-pressure-lowering effect of beta blockers and loop diuretic drugs.

• Nabumetone may increase blood levels of Phenytoin, leading to increased Phenytoin side effects. Blood-Lithium levels may be increased in people taking Nabumetone.

• Nabumetone blood levels may be affected by Cimetidine because of that drug's effect on the liver.

• Probenecid may interfere with the elimination of Nabumetone from the body, increasing the chances for Nabumetone toxic reactions.

• Aspirin and other salicylates may decrease the amount of Nabumetone in your blood. These medicines should never be taken at the same time.

Food Interactions

Take Nabumetone with food or a magnesium/aluminum antacid if it upsets your stomach.

Usual Dose

1000 to 2000 mg per day, taken in 1 or 2 doses. Take each dose with a full glass of water and don't lie down for 15 to 30 minutes after you take the medicine.

Overdosage

People have died from NSAID overdoses. The most common signs of overdosage are drowsiness, nausea, vomiting, diarrhea, abdominal pain, rapid breathing, rapid heartbeat, increased sweating, ringing or buzzing in the ears, confusion, disorientation, stupor, and coma.

Take the victim to a hospital emergency room at once. ALWAYS bring the medicine bottle.

Special Information

Nabumetone can make you drowsy and/or tired: Be careful when driving or operating hazardous equipment. Do not take any nonprescription products with Acetaminophen or Aspirin while taking this drug; also, avoid alcoholic beverages.

Contact your doctor if you develop skin rash or itching,

visual disturbances, weight gain, breathing difficulty, fluid retention, hallucinations, black or tarry stools, persistent headache, or any unusual or intolerable side effects.

If you forget to take a dose of Nabumetone, take it as soon as you remember. If you take several doses a day and it is within 4 hours of your next dose, skip the one you forgot and continue with your regular schedule. If you take Nabumetone once a day and it is within 8 hours of your next dose, skip the missed dose and continue with your regular schedule. Do not take a double dose.

Special Populations

Pregnancy/Breast-feeding

NSAIDs may cross into the fetal blood circulation. They have not been found to cause birth defects, but may affect a developing fetal heart during the second half of pregnancy; animal studies indicate a possible effect. Women who are or might become pregnant should not take Nabumetone without their doctors' approval; be particularly cautious about using this drug during the last 3 months of your pregnancy. When the drug is considered essential by your doctor, its potential benefits must be carefully weighed against its risks.

NSAIDs may pass into breast milk, but have caused no problems among breast-fed infants, except for seizures in a baby whose mother was taking Indomethacin. Other NSAIDs have caused problems in animal studies. There is a possibility that a nursing mother taking Nabumetone could affect her baby's heart or cardiovascular system. If you must take Nabumetone, bottle-feed your baby.

Seniors

Older adults may be more susceptible to Nabumetone side effects, especially ulcer disease.

Generic Name

Nadolol

Brand Name

Corgard

(Available in generic form)

Type of Drug

Beta-adrenergic-blocking agent.

Prescribed for

High blood pressure, angina pectoris, abnormal heart rhythms, migraine headache prevention, tremors, aggressive behavior, antipsychotic drug side effects, and glaucoma.

General Information

Nadolol is one of 14 beta-adrenergic-blocking drugs that interfere with the action of a specific part of the nervous system. Beta receptors are found all over the body and affect many body functions. This accounts for the usefulness of beta blockers against a wide variety of conditions. The first member of this group, *Propranolol,* was found to affect the entire beta-adrenergic portion of the nervous system. Newer beta blockers have been refined to affect only a portion of that system, making them more useful in the treatment of cardiovascular disorders and less useful for other purposes. Other beta blockers are mild stimulants to the heart or have other characteristics that make them more useful for a specific purpose or better for certain people.

Cautions and Warnings

You should be **cautious about taking Nadolol** if you have **asthma, severe heart failure,** a **very slow heart rate,** or **heart block** because the drug may aggravate these conditions.

People with **angina** who take Nadolol for high blood pressure should have their **drug dosage reduced gradually** over 1 to 2 weeks rather than suddenly discontinued to avoid possible aggravation of the angina.

Nadolol should be used with caution if you have **liver or kidney disease** because your ability to eliminate this drug from your body may be impaired.

Nadolol reduces the amount of blood pumped by the heart with each beat. This reduction in blood flow can aggravate or worsen the condition of people with **poor circulation** or **circulatory disease.**

If you are undergoing **major surgery,** your doctor may want you to stop taking Nadolol at least 2 days before surgery to permit the heart to respond more acutely to things that happen during the surgery. This is still controversial and may not hold true for all people preparing for surgery.

Possible Side Effects

Side effects are usually mild, are relatively uncommon, develop early in the course of treatment, and are rarely a reason to stop taking Nadolol.

▼ Most common: male impotence.

▼ Less common: unusual tiredness or weakness, slow heartbeat, heart failure (swelling of the legs, ankles, or feet), dizziness, breathing difficulty, bronchospasm, mental depression, confusion, anxiety, nervousness, sleeplessness, disorientation, short-term memory loss, emotional instability, cold hands and feet, constipation, diarrhea, nausea, vomiting, upset stomach, increased sweating, urinary difficulty, cramps, blurred vision, skin rash, hair loss, stuffy nose, facial swelling, aggravation of lupus erythematosus (a disease of the body's connective tissues), itching, chest pains, back or joint pains, colitis, drug allergy (fever, sore throat), and liver toxicity.

Drug Interactions

• Nadolol may interact with surgical anesthetics to increase the risk of heart problems during surgery. Some anesthesiologists recommend gradually stopping your medicine 2 days before surgery.

• Nadolol may interfere with the normal signs of low blood sugar and can interfere with the action of oral antidiabetes medicines.

• Nadolol enhances the blood-pressure-lowering effects of other blood-pressure-reducing agents (including Clonidine, Guanabenz, and Reserpine) and calcium-channel-blocking drugs (such as Nifedipine).

• Aspirin-containing drugs, Indomethacin, Sulfinpyrazone, and estrogen drugs can interfere with the blood-pressure-lowering effect of Nadolol.

• Cocaine may reduce the effects of all beta-blocking drugs.

• Nadolol may increase the cold hands and feet associated with taking ergot alkaloids (for migraine headaches). Gangrene is a possibility in people taking an ergot and Nadolol.

- Nadolol will counteract the effects of thyroid-hormone-replacement medicines.
- Calcium channel blockers, Flecainide, Hydralazine, oral contraceptives, Propafenone, Haloperidol, phenothiazine tranquilizers (Molindone and others), quinolone antibacterials, and Quinidine may increase the amount of Nadolol in the bloodstream and the effect of that drug on the body.
- Nadolol should not be taken within 2 weeks of taking a monoamine oxidase (MAO) inhibitor antidepressant drug.
- Cimetidine increases the amount of Nadolol absorbed into the bloodstream from oral tablets.
- Nadolol may interfere with the effectiveness of Theophylline, Aminophylline, and some antiasthma drugs (especially Ephedrine and Isoproterenol).
- The combination of Nadolol and Phenytoin or digitalis drugs can result in excessive slowing of the heart, possibly causing heart block.
- If you stop smoking while taking Nadolol, your dose may have to be reduced because your liver will break down the drug more slowly after you stop.

Food Interactions

Nadolol may be taken without regard to food or meals.

Usual Dose

40 to 240 mg per day. People with kidney damage may take their medication as infrequently as once every 60 hours.

Overdosage

Symptoms of overdosage are changes in heartbeat (unusually slow, unusually fast, or irregular), severe dizziness or fainting, difficulty breathing, bluish-colored fingernails or palms, and seizures. The overdose victim should be taken to a hospital emergency room where proper therapy can be given. ALWAYS bring the medicine bottle.

Special Information

Nadolol is meant to be taken continuously. Do not stop taking it unless directed to do so by your doctor; abrupt withdrawal may cause chest pain, difficulty breathing, increased sweating, and unusually fast or irregular heartbeat. The dose should be lowered gradually over a period of about 2 weeks.

Call your doctor at once if any of the following symptoms develop: back or joint pains, difficulty breathing, cold hands or feet, depression, skin rash, or changes in heartbeat. Nadolol may produce an undesirable lowering of blood pressure, leading to dizziness or fainting. Call your doctor if this happens to you. Call your doctor about the following side effects only if they persist or are bothersome: anxiety, diarrhea, constipation, sexual impotence, headache, itching, nausea or vomiting, nightmares or vivid dreams, upset stomach, trouble sleeping, stuffy nose, frequent urination, unusual tiredness, or weakness.

Nadolol can cause drowsiness, dizziness, light-headedness, or blurred vision. Be careful when driving or performing complex tasks.

It is best to take your medicine at the same time each day. If you forget a dose of Nadolol, take it as soon as you remember. If you take your medicine once a day and it is within 8 hours of your next dose, skip the forgotten tablet and continue with your regular schedule. If you take Nadolol twice a day and it is within 4 hours of your next dose, skip the forgotten dose and continue with your regular schedule. Do not take a double dose.

Special Populations

Pregnancy/Breast-feeding

Infants born to women who took a beta blocker weighed less at birth and had low blood pressure and reduced heart rate. Nadolol should be avoided by pregnant women and those who might become pregnant while taking it. When the drug is considered essential by your doctor, its potential benefits must be carefully weighed against its risks.

Nadolol passes into breast milk, but problems are rare. Still, nursing mothers taking this medicine should bottle-feed their babies.

Seniors

Seniors may absorb and retain more Nadolol in their bodies, thus requiring less medicine to achieve the same results. Your doctor will need to adjust your dosage to meet your needs. Seniors taking this medicine may be more likely to suffer from cold hands and feet, reduced body temperature, chest pains, general feelings of ill health, sudden breathing difficulty, increased sweating, or changes in heartbeat.

Generic Name

Naproxen/Naproxen Sodium

Brand Names

Aleve*	Anaprox DS	Naprosyn Tablets/
Anaprox	EC-Naprosyn	Suspension
		Naprelan [once-a-
		day formula]

(Also available in generic form)
(*Available without a prescription)

Type of Drug

Nonsteroidal anti-inflammatory drug (NSAID).

Prescribed for

Rheumatoid arthritis, juvenile rheumatoid arthritis (Naproxen only), osteoarthritis, ankylosing spondylitis, mild to moderate pain, tendinitis, bursitis, gout, fever, sunburn treatment, migraine attacks (Naproxen Sodium only), migraine prevention, menstrual pain, menstrual headaches, and premenstrual syndrome (PMS) (Naproxen Sodium only). Naproxen Sodium is available in an over-the-counter (nonprescription) dosage.

General Information

Naproxen is one of 16 nonsteroidal anti-inflammatory drugs (NSAIDs), used to relieve pain and inflammation. We do not know exactly how NSAIDs work, but part of their action may be due to an ability to inhibit the body's production of a hormone called *prostaglandin* and to inhibit the action of other body chemicals, including cyclo-oxygenase, lipoxygenase, leukotrienes, lysosomal enzymes, and a host of other factors. NSAIDs are generally absorbed into the bloodstream fairly quickly. Pain relief comes within an hour after taking the first dose of Naproxen and lasts for about 7 hours, but its anti-inflammatory effect takes a lot longer (several days to 2 weeks) to become apparent, and may take 1 month to reach its maximum effect. Naproxen is broken down in the liver and eliminated through the kidneys.

Cautions and Warnings

People who are **allergic** to Naproxen (or any other NSAID) and those with a history of **asthma attacks** brought on by an NSAID, Iodides, or Aspirin should not take Naproxen.

Naproxen can cause **gastrointestinal (GI) bleeding, ulcers, and stomach perforation.** This can occur at any time, with or without warning, in people who take chronic Naproxen treatment. People with a history of **active GI bleeding** should be cautious about taking any NSAID. **Minor stomach upset, distress,** or **gas** is common during the first few days of treatment with Naproxen. People who develop **bleeding or ulcers** and continue treatment should be aware of the possibility of developing more **serious drug toxicity.**

Naproxen can affect platelets and blood clotting at high doses, and should be avoided by people with **clotting problems** and by those taking **Warfarin.**

People with **heart problems** who use Naproxen may experience swelling in their arms, legs, or feet.

Naproxen can cause **severe toxic effects to the kidney.** Report any unusual side effects to your doctor, who may need to periodically test your kidney function.

Naproxen can make you **unusually sensitive to the effects of the sun** (photosensitivity).

Naproxen dosage should be reduced in people with **severe liver disease.**

Possible Side Effects

▼ Most common: diarrhea, nausea, vomiting, constipation, stomach gas, stomach upset or irritation, and loss of appetite.

▼ Less common: stomach ulcers, GI bleeding, hepatitis, gallbladder attacks, painful urination, poor kidney function, kidney inflammation, blood and protein in the urine, dizziness, fainting, nervousness, depression, hallucinations, confusion, disorientation, tingling in the hands

Possible Side Effects *(continued)*

or feet, light-headedness, itching, increased sweating, dry nose and mouth, heart palpitations, chest pain, difficulty breathing, and muscle cramps.

▼ Rare: severe allergic reactions, including closing of the throat, fever and chills, changes in liver function, jaundice (yellowing of the skin or eyes), and kidney failure. People who experience such effects must be promptly treated in a hospital emergency room or doctor's office.

NSAIDs have caused severe skin reactions; if this happens to you, see your doctor immediately.

Drug Interactions

• Naproxen can increase the effects of oral anticoagulant (blood-thinning) drugs such as Warfarin. You may take this combination, but your doctor may have to reduce your anticoagulant dose.

• The combination of Naproxen and a thiazide diuretic affects the amount of diuretic in your blood. Naproxen may reduce the effect of the diuretic.

• Taking Naproxen with Cyclosporine may increase the toxic kidney effects of both drugs. Methotrexate toxicity may be increased in people also taking Naproxen.

• Naproxen may reduce the blood-pressure-lowering effect of beta blockers (except Atenolol) and loop diuretic drugs.

• Naproxen may increase blood levels of Phenytoin, leading to increased Phenytoin side effects. Blood-Lithium levels may be increased in people taking Naproxen.

• Naproxen blood levels may be affected by Cimetidine because of that drug's effect on the liver.

• Probenecid may interfere with the body's elimination of Naproxen, increasing the risk of Naproxen toxic reactions.

• Aspirin and other salicylates may decrease the amount of Naproxen in your blood. These medicines should never be taken at the same time.

Food Interactions

Take Naproxen with food or a magnesium/aluminum antacid if it upsets your stomach.

Usual Dose

Adult: 250 mg to 375 mg morning and night, to start. Dose may be increased to 1250 mg per day, if needed. Mild to moderate pain: 250 to 275 mg every 6 to 8 hours.

Nonprescription dose: 1 tablet (200 mg) every 8 to 12 hours. Or, 2 tablets to start, then 1 in 12 hours, and then 1 every 8 to 12 hours. Do not take more than 3 tablets a day.

Seniors (age 65 and older): Do not take more than 200 mg every 12 hours.

Child (age 2 and older): 4.5 mg per pound of body weight divided into 2 doses per day.

Take each dose with a full glass of water and don't lie down for 15 to 30 minutes after you take the medicine.

Overdosage

People have died from NSAID overdoses. The most common signs of overdosage are drowsiness, nausea, vomiting, diarrhea, abdominal pain, rapid breathing, rapid heartbeat, increased sweating, ringing or buzzing in the ears, confusion, disorientation, stupor, and coma.

Take the victim to a hospital emergency room at once. ALWAYS bring the medicine bottle.

Special Information

Naproxen can make you drowsy and/or tired: Be careful when driving or operating hazardous equipment. Do not take any nonprescription products with Acetaminophen or Aspirin while taking this drug; also, avoid alcoholic beverages.

Contact your doctor if you develop skin rash or itching, visual disturbances, weight gain, breathing difficulty, fluid retention, hallucinations, black or tarry stools, persistent headache, or any unusual or intolerable side effects.

If you forget to take a dose of Naproxen, take it as soon as you remember. If you take several doses a day and it is within 4 hours of your next dose, skip the one you forgot and continue with your regular schedule. If you take Naproxen once a day and it is within 8 hours of your next dose, skip the missed dose and continue with your regular schedule. Do not take a double dose.

Special Populations

Pregnancy/Breast-feeding

NSAIDs may cross into the fetal blood circulation. They have not been found to cause birth defects, but may affect a developing fetal heart during the second half of pregnancy; animal studies indicate a possible effect. Women who are or who might become pregnant should not take Naproxen without their doctors' approval; pregnant women should be particularly cautious about using this drug during the last 3 months of their pregnancy. When the drug is considered essential by your doctor, its potential benefits must be carefully weighed against its risks.

NSAIDs may pass into breast milk, but have caused no problems among breast-fed infants, except for seizures in a baby whose mother was taking Indomethacin. Other NSAIDs have caused problems in animal studies. There is a possibility that a nursing mother taking Naproxen could affect her baby's heart or cardiovascular system. If you must take Naproxen, bottle-feed your baby.

Seniors

Older adults may be more susceptible to Naproxen side effects, especially ulcer disease.

Generic Name

Nedocromil Sodium

Brand Name

Tilade Aerosol

Type of Drug

Antiasthmatic.

Prescribed for

Mild to moderate bronchial asthma.

General Information

Nedocromil is an anti-inflammatory agent that is inhaled as part of the process of preventing bronchial asthma. It prevents the usual response to certain inhaled substances that can trigger asthma. The drug does not have specific effects of its own that would treat or prevent asthma; it strictly works to limit the body's response. Very little of this drug is absorbed into the blood after it has been inhaled into your lungs. Clinical studies have shown that Nedocromil improves asthma symptoms and lung function when used with an inhaled bronchodilator as needed.

Cautions and Warnings

Nedocromil should never be used to treat an **acute asthma attack.** It can be used only to **prevent or reduce** the number of asthma attacks and their intensity.

Do not use this product if you are **allergic to** Nedocromil or any of the ingredients in the aerosol.

People taking **corticosteroids,** either inhaled or by mouth, may still need that medicine after starting on Nedocromil, though the daily corticosteroid dose will likely be reduced.

Cough or **bronchial spasm** may occasionally occur after the inhalation of a Nedocromil dose. If this happens, **stop the drug** and talk to your doctor about using a different medicine.

Possible Side Effects

This drug is generally very well tolerated.

▼ Most common: coughing, sore throat, runny nose, upper respiratory infection, bronchospasm, nausea, headache, chest pain, and unpleasant taste.

▼ Less common: increased sputum production, distressed breathing, bronchitis, vomiting, upset stomach, diarrhea, abdominal pains, dry mouth, dizziness, hearing disturbances, fatigue, and viral infections.

▼ Rare: rash, arthritis, tremors, a feeling of warmth, and liver inflammation.

Drug Interactions

None known.

Food Interactions

Make sure you have nothing in your mouth when you inhale Nedocromil.

Usual Dose

Adult and Child (age 12 and over): 2 puffs, 3 or 4 times per day. Each puff provides 1¾ mg of Nedocromil.

Overdosage

There is little potential for serious effects from an overdose of this medicine. Call your local poison control center or hospital emergency room for more information.

Special Information

Nedocromil is taken to prevent or minimize severe asthma attacks. It is imperative that you take this medicine on a regular basis to maintain the protection it provides. Follow the directions in the how-to-use-this-product leaflet that comes with the aerosol. Store the drug at room temperature.

Call your doctor if you develop wheezing, coughing, or an allergic drug reaction. Other side effects should be reported if they are severe or bothersome. Report any symptoms that do not improve or get worse while you are taking this drug.

The effectiveness of this drug depends on taking it regularly. If you forget a dose of Nedocromil, take it as soon as you remember, and space the remaining doses equally throughout the rest of the day. Do not take a double dose of this drug. Call your doctor if symptoms of your condition return because you have skipped too many doses.

Special Populations

Pregnancy/Breast-feeding

There are no reports of birth defects with Nedocromil. However, pregnant women should not use this medicine unless its advantages have been carefully weighed against possible dangers.

It is not known if Nedocromil passes into breast milk. No drug-related problems have been known to occur, but nursing mothers who use Nedocromil should be cautious.

Seniors

No special problems have been reported.

Generic Name

Nefazodone

Brand Name

Serzone

Type of Drug

Antidepressant.

Prescribed for

Depression.

General Information

Nefazodone is a unique chemical compound, unrelated to older antidepressant groups. This drug interferes with the ability of nerve endings in the brain to take up serotonin and norepinephrine, two key neurohormones. Nefazodone is rapidly absorbed, but about 80 percent of each dose is rapidly broken down during its first pass through the liver. Severe liver disease can increase the amount of Nefazodone in the body by 25 percent. Very little of the drug is released through the kidneys.

Cautions and Warnings

The possibility of **suicide** should always be considered in severely depressed people. High-risk persons taking this drug should be considered possible suicide candidates until they significantly improve and be carefully watched at all times.

People with a history of **seizure disorders** may experience seizures while taking Nefazodone.

Recent heart-attack patients should use this drug with caution because it can substantially reduce your heart rate.

Possible Side Effects

▼ Most common: weakness, dry mouth, nausea, constipation, blurred or abnormal vision, tiredness, dizziness, light-headedness, and confusion.

Possible Side Effects *(continued)*

▼ Less common: upset stomach, increased appetite, cough, memory loss, tingling in the hands or feet, flushing or feelings of warmth, poor muscle coordination, and dizziness when rising from a sitting or standing position.

▼ Infrequent: low blood pressure, fever, chills, flu-like effects, joint pains, stiff neck, itching, rash, diarrhea, nausea and vomiting, thirst, sore throat, taste changes, ringing or buzzing in the ears, unusual dreams, poor coordination, tremors, stiff muscles, reduced sex drive, urinary infection and other problems, vaginitis, and breast pain.

▼ Rare: drug allergy, not feeling well, swelling, sensitivity to the sun, pelvic pains, hernia, bad breath, high blood pressure, dizziness, angina pains, periodontal abscess, gum disease, abnormal liver tests, tongue swelling, difficulty swallowing, stomach bleeding, liver inflammation, arthritis, eye pain, impotence, and breast enlargement.

Drug Interactions

• People taking Nefazodone within 2 weeks after having taken a monoamine oxidase (MAO) inhibitor antidepressant may experience severe reactions, including high fever, muscle rigidity or spasm, mental changes, and fluctuations in pulse, temperature, or breathing rate. People stopping Nefazodone should wait at least 1 week before starting an MAO inhibitor drug.

• Nefazodone increases blood levels of Astemizole and Terfenadine, two nonsedating antihistamines, leading to possible cardiac side effects associated with those drugs. It can also increase blood levels of Alprazolam and Triazolam, two benzodiazepine antianxiety drugs. (Lorazepam, another benzodiazepine drug, is not affected by Nefazodone.) Do not take these drugs together with Nefazodone.

• Blood levels of Digoxin may be substantially increased by Nefazodone. People taking these drugs together should have their Digoxin blood levels checked periodically.

• The clearance of Haloperidol, an antipsychotic drug, was drastically reduced by Nefazodone, but the implications of this are not well known.

• Nefazodone caused substantial reductions in the amount of Propranolol absorbed into the blood. At the same time, Nefazodone blood levels increased substantially. Do not take these drugs in combination.

• Drinking alcohol while taking Nefazodone can make you excessively tired. Avoid this combination.

Food Interactions

Food delays the absorption of this drug and can reduce drug levels by 20 percent. Take it on an empty stomach at least 1 hour before or 2 hours after meals.

Usual Dose

Adult: 100 mg twice a day to start. Each dose may be increased by 100 mg a week to about 600 mg a day.

Child: not recommended for use by children under age 18.

Senior: start at half the regular adult dose and increase as needed up to 600 mg a day, if needed.

Overdosage

Symptoms of overdose include nausea, vomiting, and sleepiness. There are no reports of death due to Nefazodone overdose. Nevertheless, Nefazodone overdose victims should be taken to a hospital emergency room for treatment. ALWAYS bring the medicine bottle with you.

Special Information

Several weeks may be needed to see the effects of Nefazodone treatment. Continue taking your medicine during this time even though you may see no changes, and be sure to continue your medicine once changes have taken place.

Call your doctor at once if you develop hives, rash, or other allergic side effects while taking Nefazodone.

Because this drug can make you tired, you should be careful driving, doing complex tasks, or operating equipment while taking Nefazodone. Avoid alcoholic beverages while taking this medicine.

Check with your pharmacist or doctor before you take any nonprescription medicine because of the possibility of drug interaction with Nefazodone.

Special Populations

Pregnancy/Breast-feeding

Animal studies with large doses of this drug have indicated the possibility of decreased fertility and increased risk to the fetus, but no human data are available. Pregnant women or those who may become pregnant should take this drug only if it is absolutely necessary.

It is not known if Nefazodone or its breakdown products pass into breast milk. Women who must take this drug while nursing should watch their infants for possible drug side effects.

Seniors

Older adults, especially women, have difficulty breaking this drug down and should start treatment at half the usual dosage of Nefazodone. Dosage may be gradually increased as needed to the maximum recommended dosage.

Brand Name

Neosporin Ophthalmic Solution

Ingredients

Gramicidin + Neomycin Sulfate + Polymyxin B Sulfate

Other Brand Name

AK-Spore Solution

(Also available in generic form)

Type of Drug

Ophthalmic-antibiotic combination.

Prescribed for

Superficial eye infections.

General Information

Neosporin Ophthalmic Solution is a combination of antibiotics that are effective against the most common eye infections.

It is most useful when the infecting organism is one known to be sensitive to one of the 3 antibiotics contained in Neosporin Ophthalmic Solution. It may also be useful when the infecting organism is not known because of the drug's broad range of coverage.

Prolonged use of any antibiotic product in the eye should be avoided because of the possibility of developing sensitivity to the antibiotic. Frequent or prolonged use of antibiotics in the eye may result in the growth of other organisms, such as fungi. If the infection does not clear up within a few days, contact your doctor.

Neosporin (or its generic equivalent) is also available as an eye ointment with a minor formula change (Bacitracin is substituted for Gramicidin). Both the eyedrops and eye ointment are used for the same kinds of eye infections.

Cautions and Warnings

Do not use Neosporin Ophthalmic Solution if you are **allergic** or **sensitive** to it or any of its ingredients.

Possible Side Effects

▼ Less common: occasional eye irritation, itching, or burning.

Drug and Food Interactions

None known.

Usual Dose

1 to 2 drops in the affected eye(s) 2 to 4 times per day; more frequently if the infection is severe.

Overdosage

The amount of medicine contained in each bottle of Neosporin Ophthalmic Solution is too small to cause serious problems. Call your doctor, hospital emergency room, or local poison control center for more information.

Special Information

To administer the eyedrops, lie down or tilt your head

backward and look at the ceiling. Hold the dropper above your eye and drop the medicine inside your lower lid while looking up. To prevent possible infection, don't allow the dropper to touch your fingers, eyelids, or any surface. Release the lower lid and keep your eye open. Don't blink for about 30 seconds. Press gently on the bridge of your nose at the inside corner of your eye for about 1 minute. This will help circulate the medicine around your eye. Wait at least 5 minutes before using any other eyedrops.

Call your doctor if the itching or burning does not go away after a few minutes, or if redness, irritation, swelling, visual disturbance or loss, or eye pain persists.

In general, you should not wear contact lenses if you have an eye infection, but your doctor may determine that the use of lenses is acceptable in your situation.

If you forget to take a dose of Neosporin, take it as soon as you remember. If it is almost time for your next dose, skip the forgotten dose and continue with your regular schedule. Do not take a double dose.

Special Populations

Pregnancy/Breast-feeding
This drug has been found to be safe for use during pregnancy and breast-feeding. Remember to check with your doctor before taking any drug if you are pregnant.

Seniors
Seniors may take this drug without special restriction.

Generic Name
Niacin (Nicotinic Acid)

Brand Names

Nia-Bid	Nicobid Tempules	Nicotinex
Niacor	Nicolar	Slo-Niacin
Nico-400		

(Also available in generic form)

Type of Drug

Vitamin.

Prescribed for

Treatment of pellagra (Niacin deficiency). Niacin is also used to help lower high blood levels of lipids (or fats) and to help dilate certain blood vessels. Some experts have suggested using it in the treatment of schizophrenia, although there is no good evidence to support megadoses of this vitamin as a treatment for that disorder.

General Information

Niacin, also known as *vitamin B₃*, is essential to normal body function through the part it plays in enzyme activity. It is effective in lowering blood levels of fats and can help dilate (enlarge) certain blood vessels, but we do not know exactly how it does these things. Normally, individual requirements of Niacin are easily supplied in a balanced diet.

Cautions and Warnings

Do not take this drug if you are **sensitive** or **allergic** to it (or to any related drugs) or if you have **liver disease, stomach ulcer, severely low blood pressure, gout,** or **hemorrhage (bleeding)**.

When you are taking Niacin in therapeutic doses, your doctor should periodically check your **liver function** and **blood-sugar level**. Diabetics may experience an increase in blood sugar.

Blood levels of uric acid may rise; people who are prone to **gout** may experience an attack.

Possible Side Effects

▼ Most common: flushing (redness and warmness in the face and hands), which may occur within 2 hours of taking the first dose of Niacin.

▼ Less common: decreased sugar tolerance in diabetics, activation of stomach ulcers, jaundice (yellowing of the eyes and skin), stomach upset, oily or dry skin, aggravation of some skin conditions (such as acne), itching, high blood levels of uric acid, low blood pressure, temporary

---

> **Possible Side Effects** *(continued)*
>
> headache, tingling feeling in the hands or feet, skin rash, abnormal heartbeats, and dizziness.

Drug Interactions

• Niacin can intensify the effect of blood-pressure-lowering drugs, causing postural hypotension (dizziness when rising quickly from a sitting or lying position).

• Niacin may interfere with Sulfinpyrazone's effect (for gout).

• Lovastatin taken together with Niacin may lead to the destruction of skeletal muscle cells. One case of this interaction has been reported.

Food Interactions

Take Niacin with or after meals to reduce the chances of stomach upset.

Usual Dose

Vitamin Supplement
25 mg per day.

Niacin Deficiency
Up to 100 mg per day.

Pellagra
Up to 500 mg per day.

High Blood-Fat Levels
Initial dose, 1 or 2 grams 3 times per day; take with a glass of cold water to help you swallow. The dose should be increased slowly so you can watch for common side effects.

Overdosage

Overdose victims may be expected to show drug side effects. Take the victim to a hospital emergency room for treatment. ALWAYS bring the medicine bottle.

Special Information

Skin reactions may occur within 2 hours after taking the first

Niacin dose, and may include flushing and warmth (especially in the face, ears, or neck), tingling, and itching. Headache may also occur. Call your doctor if these effects don't disappear as you continue taking Niacin.

If you forget to take a dose of Niacin, take it as soon as you remember. If it is almost time for your next dose, skip the missed dose and continue with your regular schedule. Do not take a double dose.

Special Populations

Pregnancy/Breast-feeding
When used in normal doses, Niacin can and should be taken by pregnant women as part of a prenatal vitamin formulation. But if it is used in high doses (to help lower blood-fat levels), there may be some problems.

Although this drug has not been shown to cause birth defects or problems in breast-fed infants, consult with your doctor about taking doses of Niacin large enough to lower blood fats if you are nursing.

Seniors
Seniors may take this medication without special restriction. Follow your doctor's directions and report any side effects at once.

Generic Name

Nicardipine

Brand Names
Cardene
Cardene SR

Type of Drug
Calcium channel blocker.

Prescribed for
Angina pectoris, high blood pressure, and congestive heart failure.

General Information
Nicardipine is one of many calcium channel blockers avail-

able in the United States; some others are Diltiazem, Nifedipine, and Verapamil. These drugs work by slowing the passage of calcium into muscle cells. This causes the muscles in the blood vessels that supply your heart with blood to open wider, allowing more blood to reach heart tissues. They also decrease muscle spasm in those blood vessels. Nicardipine also reduces the speed at which electrical impulses are carried through heart tissue, adding to its ability to slow the heart and prevent the pain of angina. It can help to reduce high blood pressure by causing blood vessels throughout the body to widen, allowing blood to flow more easily through them, especially when combined with a diuretic, beta blocker, or other blood-pressure-lowering drug. Other calcium channel blockers are used to treat abnormal heart rhythms, Raynaud's syndrome, migraine headache, and cardiomyopathy.

Cautions and Warnings

Nicardipine can slow your **heart rate** and interfere with normal electrical conduction in heart muscle. For some people, this can result in temporary heart stoppage; people whose hearts are otherwise healthy will not develop this effect.

Nicardipine should not be used if you have had a **stroke** or **bleeding in the brain,** or if you have **advanced hardening of the arteries,** (particularly the aorta), because the drug can cause heart failure.

People who take Nicardipine for **congestive heart failure** should be aware that the drug can still aggravate heart failure by reducing the effectiveness of the heart in pumping blood.

If you are also taking a **beta blocker,** its dosage should be reduced gradually rather than abruptly stopped when starting on Nicardipine.

Nicardipine dosage should be adjusted in the presence of **kidney** or **liver disease,** since both can prolong the release of Nicardipine from the body.

Nicardipine may cause **angina pain** when treatment is first started, when dosage is increased, or if the drug is rapidly withdrawn. This can be avoided by gradual dosage reduction.

Studies have shown that people taking calcium channel blockers (usually those taken several times a day and not those that are taken only once daily) have shown a tendency toward a greater chance of having a **heart attack** than people taking beta blockers or other medicines for the same purposes. Discuss this with your doctor to be sure you are receiving the best possible treatment.

Possible Side Effects

Calcium channel blocker side effects are generally mild and rarely cause people to stop taking these drugs.

▼ Most common: dizziness or light-headedness; fluid accumulation in the hands, legs, or feet; headache; weakness or fatigue; heart palpitations; angina pains and facial flushing.

▼ Less common: low blood pressure, abnormal heart rhythms, fainting, changes in heart rate (increase or decrease), heart failure, light-headedness, nausea, skin rash, nervousness, tingling in the hands or feet, hallucinations, temporary memory loss, difficulty sleeping, weakness, diarrhea, vomiting, constipation, upset stomach, itching, unusual sensitivity to the sun, painful or stiff joints, liver inflammation, increased urination (especially at night), infection, allergic reactions, sore throat, and hyperactivity.

Drug Interactions

• Taking Nicardipine with a beta-blocking drug to treat high blood pressure is usually well tolerated, but may lead to heart failure in susceptible people.

• Blood levels of Cyclosporine may be increased by Nicardipine, increasing the chance for Cyclosporine-related kidney damage.

• The effect of Quinidine may be altered by Nicardipine.

• Cimetidine and Ranitidine may increase the amount of Nicardipine in the bloodstream.

• Combining Nicardipine with Fentanyl (a narcotic pain reliever) can cause very low blood pressure.

Food Interactions

Nicardipine is best taken on an empty stomach, at least 1 hour before or 2 hours after meals, but it may be taken with food or milk if it upsets your stomach.

Avoid high-fat meals while on this drug, since such a meal taken up to 3 hours after a dose of Nicardipine can significantly reduce the amount of medicine absorbed into the bloodstream. Don't drink grapefruit juice if you are taking Nicardipine.

Usual Dose

Capsules
20 to 40 mg 3 times a day.

Sustained-Release Capsules
30 to 60 mg twice a day.

Kidney Disease
20 mg 3 times a day, or 30 mg 2 times a day of the sustained-release capsules.

Liver Disease
20 mg twice a day (regular tablets).

Overdosage

The major symptoms of Nicardipine overdose are very low blood pressure and reduced heart rate. Nicardipine can be removed from the stomach by giving the victim Syrup of Ipecac to induce vomiting, but this must be done within 30 minutes of the actual overdose, before the drug can be absorbed into the blood. Once symptoms develop or if more than 30 minutes have passed since the overdose, the victim must be taken to a hospital emergency room for treatment. Always bring the prescription bottle with you.

Special Information

Call your doctor if you develop any of the following symptoms: worsening angina pains; swelling of the hands, legs, or feet; severe dizziness; constipation or nausea; or very low blood pressure.

Some people may experience a slight increase in blood pressure just before their next dose is due. You will be able to see this effect only if you use a home blood pressure monitoring device. If this happens, contact your doctor.

If you take Nicardipine 3 times a day and forget a dose, take it as soon as you remember. If it is almost time for your next dose, take it and space the remaining doses evenly throughout the rest of the day.

If you take Nicardipine 2 times a day and forget a dose, take it as soon as you remember. If it is almost time for your next dose, skip the forgotten dose and continue with your regular schedule.

Special Populations

Pregnancy/Breast-feeding

In animal studies, large doses of Nicardipine have been shown to harm the developing fetus. Nicardipine should be avoided by pregnant women or women who may become pregnant while using it. In situations where it is deemed essential, the potential risk of the drug must be carefully weighed against any benefit it might produce.

Nicardipine passes into breast milk, and nursing mothers should consider bottle-feeding their babies if they must take this medicine.

Seniors

Older adults may be more sensitive to the side effects of Nicardipine. Because of the possibility of reduced kidney and/or liver function in older adults, they should receive smaller doses than younger adults, beginning with 20 mg 2 to 3 times a day and continuing with carefully increased doses.

Generic Name

Nicotine

Brand Names

Habitrol Transdermal Patch   Nicorette DS Chewing Gum [$]
Nicoderm Transdermal Patch   Nicotrol Transdermal Patch
Nicorette Chewing Gum   [$]   ProStep Transdermal Patch

Type of Drug

Smoking deterrent.

Prescribed for

Short-term treatment (up to 3 months) of people addicted to cigarettes who need another source of Nicotine to help break the smoking habit. Nicotine gum has been prescribed (with Haloperidol) for children with Tourette's syndrome.

General Information

Nicotine affects many brain functions: It improves memory, increases one's ability to perform a number of different tasks, reduces hunger, and increases tolerance to pain. Nicotine chewing gum and transdermal patches make cigarette withdrawal much easier for many people. Nicotine gum is being considered by federal authorities for sale without a prescription.

Although these products are designed to fulfill a specific need in those trying to quit smoking, there are a great many other social and psychological needs filled by smoking. These must be dealt with through counseling or other psychological support in order for a program to be successful.

The major advantage of the Nicotine patches over the chewing gum is their convenience and ease of use. Also, Nicotine from the chewing gum is released only if the gum is chewed. It will not be released if you swallow it. The amount of Nicotine that gets in your blood depends on how vigorously and how long you chew; the more you chew, the more gets into your blood. With skin patches, you don't have to worry about any of this. You can count on getting a specific amount of Nicotine delivered through the skin directly into the blood. There are some differences between the various patch products in how much is absorbed, but all of the products are labeled according to the amount of Nicotine actually absorbed into the blood. Obese men absorb significantly less Nicotine into their blood.

You may be addicted to Nicotine if you (1) smoke more than 15 cigarettes per day; (2) prefer unfiltered cigarettes or those with a high nicotine content; (3) usually inhale the smoke; (4) have your first cigarette within 30 minutes of getting up in the morning; (5) find the first morning cigarette the hardest to give up; (6) smoke most frequently in the morning hours; (7) find it hard to obey "no smoking" rules; or (8) smoke even when you are sick in bed.

Cautions and Warnings

Do not use any of these products if you are **sensitive** or **allergic** to Nicotine or to any component of any patch or gum product.

Nicotine products should be used only by **smokers** or others who are **addicted to nicotine**. They should not be used during the period immediately following a **heart attack** or if **severe abnormal heart rhythms** or **angina pains** are present.

People with **severe temporomandibular joint (TMJ) disease** should not chew Nicotine gum.

People with other **heart conditions** must be evaluated by a cardiologist (heart doctor) before starting treatment with Nicotine. **Liver disease** or **severe kidney disease** may affect how the body breaks down or eliminates Nicotine.

This product should be used with caution by **diabetics** being treated with Insulin and by people with an **overactive thyroid, kidney** or **liver disease, pheochromocytoma, high blood pressure, stomach ulcers,** or **chronic dental problems** that might be worsened by Nicotine chewing gum.

It is possible for **Nicotine addiction** to be transferred from cigarettes to the gum or patch or for the addiction to worsen while using the product.

Possible Side Effects

Chewing Gum

▼ Most common: injury to gums, jaw, or teeth; sore mouth or throat; stomach growling due to swallowing air while chewing.

▼ Common: nausea, vomiting, stomach upset, and hiccups.

▼ Less common: excessive salivation, dizziness, light-headedness, irritability, headache, increased bowel movement, diarrhea, constipation, gas pains, dry mouth, hoarseness, flushing, sneezing, coughing, sleeplessness, swelling of arms or legs, high blood pressure, heart palpitations, rapid and abnormal heartbeat, confusion, convulsions, depression, euphoria (feeling "high"), numbness, tingling in the hands or feet, ringing or buzzing in the ears, fainting, weakness, skin redness, itching, and rash.

Transdermal Patch

▼ Most common: tiredness and irritation at the patch site. Transdermal systems may be more irritating to people with eczema or other skin conditions.

▼ Common: weakness, back pain, body aches, diarrhea, upset stomach, headache, sleeplessness, dizziness, ner-

Possible Side Effects *(continued)*

vousness, unusual dreams, increased cough or sore throat, muscle and joint pains, taste changes, and painful menstruation.

▼ Less common: chest pains, allergic reactions (including hives, breathing difficulty, and skin peeling), dry mouth, abdominal pains, vomiting, tiredness, poor concentration, tingling in the hands or feet, sinus irritation or inflammation, increased sweating, and high blood pressure.

Drug Interactions

• Heavy smokers who suddenly stop smoking may experience an increase in the effects of a variety of drugs whose breakdown is known to be stimulated by cigarettes. If you are taking any of the following medications, your dosage may have to be reduced to account for this effect: Acetaminophen, Theophylline, Imipramine, Pentazocine, Furosemide, Oxazepam, Propranolol, and Propoxyphene Hydrochloride.

• Smoking increases the rate at which your body breaks down Caffeine. Stopping Nicotine may make you more sensitive to the effects of Caffeine in coffee or tea.

• Any drug that affects the nervous system (either blockers or stimulants) may be affected by Nicotine because of its effect on levels of certain circulating hormones naturally produced by the body. Your doctor should monitor for any dosage adjustments that may be needed during Nicotine therapy.

• Smoking may reduce the effects of Furosemide, a diuretic, on your body. Once you stop smoking, the drug's effect may increase and your dose may need adjustment.

• The absorption of Glutethimide, a sleeping pill, may be increased when you stop smoking. Also, more Insulin may be absorbed into the blood after each injection. Your doctor may have to recheck your Insulin dose after you stop smoking.

• More Propoxyphene, a pain reliever, may get into your blood from each dose after you stop smoking, increasing the chances for drug side effects.

Food Interactions

Food and drinks such as coffee or colas may interfere with the absorption of Nicotine from the chewing gum product. Do not eat or drink while or immediately after you chew the gum.

Usual Dose

Chewing Gum

1 piece of gum whenever you feel the urge for a cigarette; not more than 30 per day. Gradually reduce the number of pieces you chew and the time you chew each piece every 4 to 7 days. Substituting sugarless gum for Nicotine gum may help in the process of gradual dose reduction. Each piece contains 2 to 4 mg of Nicotine.

Transdermal Patch

Apply the Nicotine patch to the skin as soon as you remove it from the package. Nicotrol patches should be placed when you get up in the morning and removed at bedtime. The other Nicotine patches should be left on for 24 hours at a time. Use a different skin site when you put on a new patch each day. The dosage of the patch will be gradually reduced by your doctor to help wean you away from Nicotine.

Overdosage

Nicotine overdosage can be deadly. Symptoms include excessive salivation, nausea, vomiting, diarrhea, abdominal pains, headache, cold sweats, dizziness, hearing and visual disturbances, weakness, and confusion. If untreated, these symptoms will be followed by fainting; very low blood pressure; a pulse that is weak, rapid, and irregular; convulsions; and death by paralysis of the muscles that control breathing. The lethal dose of Nicotine is about 50 mg.

Nicotine stimulates the brain's vomiting center, making this reaction common, but not automatic. Spontaneous vomiting may be sufficient to remove the poison from the victim's system. If this has not occurred, call your doctor or poison control center for instructions on how to make the victim vomit by giving Syrup of Ipecac (available at any pharmacy). If the victim must be treated in a hospital emergency room, ALWAYS bring the Nicotine package with you.

Special Information

Follow the instructions on the patient-information sheet included in each package. Chew each piece of the gum slowly and intermittently for about 30 minutes to promote slow and even absorption of the Nicotine through the tissues in your mouth. Too-rapid chewing releases the Nicotine too quickly and can lead to side effects of nausea, hiccups, or throat irritation. Follow directions for gradually reducing your chewing time and substituting or reducing the number of pieces of Nicotine gum you chew each day.

You will learn to control your daily dose of Nicotine chewing gum so that your smoking habit is broken and side effects are minimized. Do not chew more than 30 pieces of gum per day. The amount of gum chewed should be gradually reduced and stopped after 3 months of successful treatment.

Be careful to properly dispose of used Nicotine patches to avoid accidental poisoning of children or pets. Do not store Nicotine patches in an area that is warmer than 86°F, because the patches are heat sensitive. Slight discoloration is not a sign of loss of potency, but do not store a patch after you have removed it from its pouch. Nicotine treatments are not recommended for more than 3 months at a time.

Special Populations

Pregnancy/Breast-feeding

This product should not be used by pregnant women or those who might become pregnant; Nicotine is known to cause fetal harm when taken during the last 3 months of pregnancy. Regardless of the source, Nicotine interferes with the newborn baby's ability to breathe properly. Additionally, miscarriages have occurred in women using Nicotine. Be sure to use effective contraceptive measures if there is a chance you will become pregnant while using a Nicotine product.

Mothers should not breast-feed while using this product, because Nicotine passes into breast milk and can be harmful to a growing infant. Bottle-feed your baby if you must use one of these products.

Seniors

Older adults may be more sensitive to the effects of this drug, including weakness, dizziness, and body aches. Follow your doctor's directions and report any side effects at once.

Generic Name

Nifedipine

Brand Names

Adalat
Adalat CC
Procardia
Procardia XL

(Also available in generic form, except Procardia XL)

Type of Drug

Calcium channel blocker.

Prescribed for

Angina pectoris; Prinzmetal's angina. In addition, sustained-release Nifedipine is used for high blood pressure.

Nifedipine has also been prescribed to prevent migraine headaches and to treat asthma, heart failure, Raynaud's disease, disorders of the esophagus, gallbladder and kidney stone attacks, and severe high blood pressure associated with pregnancy (preterm labor).

General Information

Nifedipine was the first of many calcium channel blockers to be marketed in the United States. Calcium channel blockers work by blocking the passage of calcium into heart and smooth muscle. Since calcium is an essential factor in muscle contraction, any drug that affects calcium in this way will interfere with the contraction of these muscles. When this happens, the amount of oxygen used by the muscles is also reduced. Therefore, Nifedipine is used in the treatment of angina, a type of heart pain related to poor oxygen supply to the heart muscles. Also, Nifedipine dilates (opens) the vessels that supply blood to the heart muscles and prevents spasm of these arteries. Nifedipine affects the movement of calcium only into muscle cells; it does not have any effect on calcium in the blood.

Nifedipine capsules contain liquid medicine. In cases where

the drug is needed in the blood as rapidly as possible, the capsules may be punctured and their contents squeezed under the tongue; medicine is rapidly absorbed into the blood in this manner. Thus, Nifedipine capsules are useful in situations where extremely high blood pressure must be rapidly lowered. Some researchers feel that biting the capsule in your mouth and swallowing the contents gets the medicine into your blood even faster than keeping it under the tongue.

Cautions and Warnings

Nifedipine may cause unwanted **low blood pressure** in some people taking it for reasons other than hypertension.

Patients taking a **beta-blocking drug** who begin taking Nifedipine may develop **heart failure** or **increased angina pain**. Angina pain may also increase when your Nifedipine dosage is first started, when it is increased, or if it is abruptly stopped. Studies have shown that people taking calcium channel blockers (usually those taken several times a day and not those that are taken only once daily) have a greater chance of having a **heart attack** than people taking beta blockers or other medicines for the same purposes. Discuss this with your doctor to be sure you are receiving the best possible treatment.

Congestive heart failure has rarely developed in people taking Nifedipine. This happens because the drug can reduce the efficiency of an already compromised heart.

Do not take this drug if you have had an **allergic** reaction to it in the past.

Nifedipine may interfere with one of the mechanisms by which blood clots form, especially if you are also taking Aspirin. Call your doctor if you develop **unusual bruises, bleeding,** or **black-and-blue marks**.

People with **severe liver disease** break down Nifedipine much more slowly than people with less severe disease or normal livers. **Kidney disease** can affect the release of Nifedipine from your body. Your doctor should take these into account when determining your Nifedipine dosage.

Possible Side Effects

Nifedipine side effects are generally mild and rarely cause people to stop taking the drug.

Possible Side Effects *(continued)*

▼ Most common: swelling of the ankles, feet, and legs; dizziness or light-headedness, flushing; a feeling of warmth; and nausea.

▼ Less common: nervousness; headache; weakness, shakiness, or jitteriness; giddiness; muscle cramps, inflammation, and pains; nervousness; mood changes; heart palpitations; heart failure; heart attack; difficulty breathing; coughing; fluid in the lungs; wheezing; stuffy nose; fever and chills; and sore throat.

▼ Rare: low blood pressure, unusual heart rhythms, angina pains, fainting, shortness of breath, diarrhea, cramps, constipation, stomach gas, dry mouth, taste changes, frequent urination (especially at night), stiffness and inflammation of the joints, arthritis, shakiness, jitteriness, psychotic reaction, anxiety, memory loss, paranoia, hallucinations, tingling in the hands or feet, tiredness, muscle weakness, liver inflammation, blurred vision, ringing or buzzing in the ears, difficulty sleeping, unusual dreams, respiratory infections, anemia, bleeding, bruising, nosebleeds, swollen gums, weight gain, reduced white-blood-cell counts, difficulty maintaining balance, itching, rash, hair loss, painful breast inflammation, unusual sensitivity to the sun, severe skin reactions, fever, sweating, chills, and sexual difficulties. Nifedipine can cause increases in certain blood-sugar and some enzyme tests.

Drug Interactions

• Nifedipine may interact with beta-blocking drugs to cause heart failure, very low blood pressure, or an increased incidence of angina pain. However, in many cases these drugs have been taken together with no problem.

• Nifedipine may cause unexpected blood pressure reduction in patients already taking medicine to control their high blood pressure through interaction with other antihypertensive drugs. Low blood pressure can also result from taking Nifedipine with Fentanyl, a narcotic pain reliever.

• Cimetidine and Ranitidine increase the amount of Nifedipine in the blood and may account for a slight increase in Nifedipine's effect.

• The combination of Quinidine (for abnormal heart rhythm) and Nifedipine must be used with caution because it can produce low blood pressure, very slow heart rate, abnormal heart rhythms, and swelling in the arms or legs.

• Nifedipine can, rarely, increase the effects of oral antico-agulant (blood-thinning) drugs.

• Nifedipine can increase the effects of Cyclosporine, Digoxin, and Theophylline products, increasing the chances of side effects with those drugs.

Food Interactions

Nifedipine can be taken without regard to food or meals. Avoid drinking grapefruit juice if you are taking this medicine.

Usual Dose

10 to 30 mg 3 times a day of regular Nifedipine. No patient should take more than 180 mg per day. The usual dose for the sustained-release version of Nifedipine (Procardia XL, Adalat CC) is 30 to 60 mg taken once a day.

Do not stop taking Nifedipine abruptly. The dosage should be gradually reduced over a period of time.

Overdosage

Overdose of Nifedipine can cause low blood pressure. If you think you have taken an overdose of Nifedipine, call your doctor or go to a hospital emergency room. ALWAYS bring the medicine bottle.

Special Information

Call your doctor if you develop constipation, nausea, very low blood pressure, worsening angina pains, swelling in the hands or feet, difficulty breathing, increased heart pains, or dizziness or light-headedness, or if other side effects are particularly bothersome or persistent.

If you are taking Nifedipine for high blood pressure, be sure to continue taking your medicine and follow any instructions for diet restriction or other treatments. High blood pressure is a condition with few recognizable symptoms; it may seem to you that you are taking medicine for no good reason. Call your doctor or pharmacist if you have any questions.

If you take Procardia XL, be sure not to break or crush the tablets. You may notice an empty tablet in your stool. This is not a cause for alarm, because the medicine is normally released from the sustained-release tablet without actually destroying it.

It is important to maintain good dental hygiene while taking Nifedipine and to use extra care when using your toothbrush or dental floss because of the chance that the drug will make you more susceptible to some infections.

If you forget a dose of Nifedipine, and take it 3 or more times a day, take it as soon as you remember. If it is almost time for your next regularly scheduled dose, take the forgotten dose and space the rest evenly throughout the remainder of the day.

If you take Nifedipine twice a day and forget to take a dose, take it as soon as you remember. If it is almost time for your next dose, skip the forgotten dose and continue with your regular schedule. Do not take a double dose of Nifedipine.

Special Populations

Pregnancy/Breast-feeding

Nifedipine crosses into the blood circulation of a developing fetus. It has been used to treat severe high blood pressure associated with pregnancy without causing any unusual effect on the fetus. Nevertheless, pregnant women, or those who might become pregnant while taking this drug, should not take it without their doctor's approval. When the drug is considered essential by your doctor, the potential risk of taking the medicine must be carefully weighed against the benefit it might produce.

Small amounts of Nifedipine may pass into breast milk, but the drug has caused no problems among breast-fed infants. You must consider the potential effect on the nursing infant if breast-feeding while taking this medicine.

Seniors

Older adults are more sensitive to the effects of this drug and may develop low blood pressure because it takes longer to pass out of their bodies. Follow your doctor's directions and report any side effects at once.

Generic Name

Nimodipine

Brand Name

Nimotop

Type of Drug

Calcium channel blocker.

Prescribed for

Functional losses following a stroke. Nimodipine may also be prescribed for migraine and cluster headaches.

General Information

Nimodipine is one of several calcium channel blockers available in the United States. Unlike the other members of this group, Nimodipine has a negligible effect on the heart. It is unique because it is the only calcium channel blocker proven effective as a drug to help improve neurological function after a stroke. Other calcium channel blockers are used for abnormal heart rhythms, high blood pressure, Raynaud's disease, angina pains, heart failure, and cardiomyopathy.

Nimodipine readily dissolves in fatty tissues and reaches very high concentrations in the brain and spinal fluid. Because of this, it has a greater effect on blood vessels in the brain than on those in other parts of the body. Nimodipine relieves stroke symptoms but does not reduce spasms in brain blood vessels. A great deal of research still needs to be done to discover exactly how this drug works.

Cautions and Warnings

Nimodipine should not be taken if you are **sensitive** or **allergic** to it.

Liver disease, including cirrhosis, may slow the breakdown of Nimodipine by the body. This can result in the need to take a lower-than-normal dose of the drug.

Possible Side Effects

Calcium channel blocker side effects are generally mild and rarely cause people to stop taking them.

▼ Most common: diarrhea, low blood pressure, and headache.

▼ Less common: swelling of the arms or legs, high blood pressure, heart failure, rapid heartbeat, changes in the electrocardiogram, depression, memory loss, psychosis, paranoid feelings, hallucinations, nausea, itching, acne, rash, anemia, bleeding or bruising, abnormal blood clotting, flushing, breathing difficulty, stomach bleeding, and muscle cramps.

▼ Rare: dizziness, heart attack, liver inflammation or jaundice, vomiting, and sexual difficulties.

Drug Interactions

• Calcium channel blockers may cause bleeding when taken alone or together with Aspirin.

• Taking Nimodipine together with a beta-blocking drug is usually well tolerated but may lead to heart failure in susceptible people.

• Calcium channel blockers, including Nimodipine, may add to the effects of Digoxin, although this effect is not observed with any consistency and only affects people with a large amount of Digoxin already in their system.

Food Interactions

Nimodipine is best taken at least 1 hour before or 2 hours after meals, but may be taken with food or milk if it upsets your stomach. Avoid drinking grapefruit juice if you are taking this medicine.

Usual Dose

Stroke
60 mg 4 times a day beginning within 96 hours after the stroke and continuing for 21 days.

Migraine Headaches
40 mg 3 times a day.

Overdosage

The major symptoms of Nimodipine overdose are nausea, weakness, dizziness, drowsiness, confusion, and slurred speech. Blood pressure and heart rate may also be affected. Nimodipine can be removed from a victim's stomach by giving Syrup of Ipecac to induce vomiting, but this should be done only under a doctor's supervision or direction. Once symptoms develop, the victim must be taken to a hospital emergency room for treatment. ALWAYS bring the medicine bottle with you.

Special Information

Call your doctor if you develop any of the following symptoms: swelling of the arms or legs, breathing difficulty, severe dizziness, constipation, or nausea.

Patients who are unable to swallow Nimodipine capsules because of their condition may have the liquid withdrawn from the capsule with a syringe and mixed with other liquids to be given orally or through a feeding tube.

If you forget a dose of Nimodipine, it should be taken as soon as you remember. If it is almost time for your next dose, skip the forgotten dose and continue with your regular schedule. Call your doctor if more than two consecutive doses are missed.

Special Populations

Pregnancy/Breast-feeding

Animal studies have shown that Nimodipine may cause malformation of a fetus. Very high doses can cause poor fetal growth, death of the fetus, and fetal bone problems. Nimodipine should be avoided by pregnant women or women who may become pregnant while using it. In situations where the drug is deemed essential by your doctor, the potential risk of the drug must be carefully weighed against any benefit it might produce.

In animal studies, Nimodipine has been shown to pass into breast milk. Nursing mothers who must take Nimodipine should use an alternative feeding method.

Seniors

Older adults, especially those with severe liver disease, may be more sensitive to the side effects of Nimodipine.

Generic Name

Nisoldipine

Brand Name

Sular

Type of Drug

Calcium channel blocker.

Prescribed for

High blood pressure.

General Information

Nisoldipine is one of many calcium channel blockers available in the United States. Chemically, it is closely related to Amlodipine, Isradipine, Felodipine, Nicardipine, Nifedipine, and Nimodipine. Nisoldipine works by blocking the passage of calcium into smooth muscle. Since calcium is an essential factor in muscle contraction, any drug that affects calcium in this way will interfere with the contraction of these muscles. When this happens, several things can result. Blood vessels will dilate (widen) because the muscles that normally keep them narrowed are not contracting, and the amount of oxygen used by heart muscle may also be reduced. Therefore, Nisoldipine opens the arteries that carry blood and prevents spasm of these arteries. Calcium channel blockers are also used in the treatment of *angina*, a type of heart pain related to poor oxygen supply to the heart muscles. Nisoldipine affects the movement of calcium into muscle cells only. It does not have any effect on calcium in the blood. Other calcium channel blockers are used for abnormal heart rhythms, diseases involving blood vessel spasm (migraine headache, Raynaud's syndrome), heart failure, and cardio-myopathy.

Cautions and Warnings

Do not take this drug if you have had an **allergic** reaction to it or a chemically similar calcium channel blocker. Use Nisoldipine with caution if you have **heart failure**, since calcium channel blockers may worsen this condition.

On rare occasions, Nisoldipine may cause **very low blood pressure** in some people. This may lead to stimulation of the heart and rapid heartbeat and can worsen angina pains in some people.

Rarely, Nisoldipine causes **angina pain** when treatment is first started, when dosage is increased, or if the drug is rapidly withdrawn. This can be avoided by gradual dosage reduction.

Studies have shown that people taking calcium channel blockers (usually those taken several times a day and not those that are taken only once daily) have a greater chance of having a **heart attack** than people taking beta blockers or other medicines for the same purposes. Discuss this with your doctor to be sure you are receiving the best possible treatment.

Nisoldipine can slow heart rate. This increases the possibility of worsening **heart failure**.

People with **severe liver disease** break down Nisoldipine much more slowly than people with less severe diseases or normal livers. Blood levels can be 5 times as high in people with cirrhosis as in those with normal livers. Your doctor will take this factor into account when determining your Nisoldipine dosage.

Possible Side Effects

Nisoldipine side effects are generally mild and self-limiting.

▼ Most common: headache and swelling in the arms or legs.

▼ Common: sore throat, flushing, sinus irritation, and heart palpitations.

▼ Less common: chest pain, nausea, and rash.

▼ Rare: chills, generalized inflammation, facial swelling, flu symptoms, not feeling well, heart failure, abnormal heart rhythms, stroke, heart block, blood pressure changes, migraines, heart attacks, dizziness when rising from a lying or sitting position, fainting, electrocardiogram abnormalities, appetite loss, colitis, diarrhea, dry mouth, upset stomach, swallowing difficulty, stomach pain, gas, stomach bleeding, swollen gums, swollen tongue, liver

Possible Side Effects (continued)

enlargement, increased appetite, blood in the stool, mouth sores, diabetes, thyroid inflammation, anemia, tiny blood blisters, black-and-blue marks, gout, low blood potassium (weakness or muscle cramps), weight changes, muscle or joint pains, muscle weakness or irritation, abnormal dreaming or thinking, confusion, memory loss, anxiety, depression, reduced sex drive, unusual muscle contractions, sleeplessness, nervousness, tiredness, tingling in the hands or feet, tremors, asthma, breathing difficulty, wheezing, nosebleeds, cough, laryngitis, sore throat, fluid in the lungs, runny and irritated nose, sinus irritation, acne, hair loss, dry skin, skin rashes, fungus infections of the skin, cold sores, shingles, skin sores or discoloration, sweating, itching, visual changes (including temporary loss of vision), pink-eye, eye irritation, detachment of the retina, ringing or buzzing in the ears, glaucoma, itchy eyes, middle ear infection, watery eyes, taste changes, painful urination, blood in the urine, male impotence, nighttime urination, frequent urination, vaginal irritation or bleeding, kidney damage, increases in liver enzyme tests, and increased sensitivity to pain, heat, or other skin senses.

Drug Interactions

• Nisoldipine may interact with beta-blocking drugs to cause heart failure, very low blood pressure, or an increased incidence of angina pain. However, in most cases these drugs can be taken together with no problem.

• When taken with Cimetidine, blood levels of Nisoldipine increased substantially.

• Quinidine reduces the amount of Nisoldipine in the blood by about 25 percent, but maximum blood levels of Nisoldipine are not affected. The importance of this interaction is not known.

Food Interactions

Avoid eating fatty foods or any grapefruit product with Nisoldipine. Taking Nisoldipine with these foods leads to high drug blood levels.

Usual Dose

Adult: 20 mg per day to start, increased gradually to 40 or 60 mg, as needed.

Child: not recommended.

Senior and people with liver disease: 10 mg per day to start, increased gradually as needed and tolerated to 40 or 60 mg.

Overdosage

These is no experience with Nisoldipine overdose. Overdose of chemically similar calcium channel blockers can cause very low blood pressure. Other possible effects include nausea, dizziness, weakness, drowsiness, confusion and slurred speech, reduced heart efficiency, and unusual heart rhythms. Victims of a Nisoldipine overdose should be taken to a hospital emergency room for treatment. ALWAYS bring the medicine bottle with you.

Special Information

Do not crush, chew, or divide Nisoldipine tablets. They must be swallowed whole.

Call your doctor if you develop swelling in the arms or legs, difficulty breathing, abnormal heartbeat, increased heart pains, dizziness, constipation, nausea, dizziness, light-headedness, or very low blood pressure.

If you forget to take a dose of Nisoldipine, take it as soon as you remember. If it is almost time for your next regular dose, skip the forgotten dose and continue with your regular schedule. Do not take a double dose.

Special Populations

Pregnancy/Breast-feeding

Laboratory studies found Nisoldipine to affect the development of animal fetuses at doses that were also toxic to the mother. It has not been found to cause human birth defects. However, pregnant women, or those who might become pregnant while taking this drug, should not take Nisoldipine without their doctor's approval. When your doctor considers Nisoldipine to be essential, the potential risk of taking it must be carefully weighed against the benefit it might produce.

It is not known if Nisoldipine passes into breast milk.

Women who must take Nisoldipine should consider bottle-feeding their babies.

Seniors

Older adults may have two to three times as much Nisoldipine in their blood as younger adults. Lower starting doses should be used. Headache is less common in older adults than younger people.

Generic Name

Nitrofurantoin

Brand Names

Furadantin
Macrobid

Macrodantin
(Macro Crystals)

(Also available in generic form)

Type of Drug

Urinary anti-infective.

Prescribed for

Preventing and treating urinary tract infections—such as pyelonephritis, pyelitis, and cystitis—caused by organisms susceptible to Nitrofurantoin.

General Information

Nitrofurantoin, like several other urinary anti-infectives (including Nalidixic Acid [NegGram]), is helpful in treating urinary tract infections because large amounts of it pass into your urine. Nitrofurantoin works by interfering with the metabolism of carbohydrates (sugars) in the infecting bacteria. It may also affect the formation of the bacterial cell wall. It should not be used to treat infections in other parts of the body.

Cautions and Warnings

Do not take Nitrofurantoin if you have **kidney disease,** or if you are **allergic** to this agent.

Severe chest pain, difficulty breathing, cough, fever, and

chills may rarely develop within a few hours to 3 weeks after taking Nitrofurantoin. These symptoms usually go away within 1 to 2 days after you stop taking the drug. People who take Nitrofurantoin for prolonged periods of time may develop **cough, breathing problems,** and **feelings of ill health** after 1 to 6 months or more of treatment. **Respiratory failure** and **death** have occurred in a few cases.

Nitrofurantoin may cause a rare reaction called *hemolytic anemia*. People with a deficiency of the enzyme G-6-PD are most susceptible to this reaction and should not take Nitrofurantoin.

Rarely, Nitrofurantoin causes **hepatitis**, which may lead to death. This appears to be a rare drug-sensitivity reaction and is most likely to develop if you are taking long-term Nitrofurantoin treatments.

Possible Side Effects

▼ Most common: loss of appetite, nausea, vomiting, stomach pain, and diarrhea. Some people develop hepatitis symptoms.

Side effects are less prominent when Macrodantin (the large-crystal form of Nitrofurantoin) is used rather than Furadantin (the regular-crystal form).

▼ Less common: fever, chills, cough, chest pain, difficulty in breathing, and development of fluid in the lungs. If these reactions occur in the first week of therapy, they can generally be resolved by stopping the medication. If they develop after a longer time on the medicine, they are considered chronic and may be more serious.

▼ Other: rashes, itching, asthmatic attacks (in patients with history of asthma), drug fever, symptoms similar to arthritis, jaundice (yellowing of the whites of the eyes and/or skin), effects on components of the blood, headache, dizziness, drowsiness, and temporary loss of hair.

This drug is known to cause changes in white and red blood cells. Therefore, it should be used only under strict supervision by your doctor.

Drug Interactions

• Nitrofurantoin may increase the toxic effects of other

drugs on the liver and can increase the chances of hemolytic anemia if you are taking another drug associated with that problem, including the oral antidiabetes drugs, Methyldopa, Primaquine, Procainamide, Quinidine, Quinine, and the sulfa drugs.

• Nitrofurantoin interferes with the effect of Nalidixic Acid. Don't take these drugs together.

• Sulfinpyrazone or Probenecid may interfere with the passage of Nitrofurantoin through the kidneys, increasing blood levels of the drug. This reduces the drug's effectiveness because Nitrofurantoin depends on being present in the urine in very large quantities for its effect. Some drug side effects may also be increased by this interaction.

• Anticholinergic drugs, including Propantheline, may increase the amount of Nitrofurantoin absorbed into the bloodstream. This does not improve its antibacterial effect but may increase the chance of drug side effects.

• Magnesium, found most commonly in antacids, delays or decreases the amount of Nitrofurantoin absorbed into the blood.

• Drugs that cause nervous-system toxicity, including Metronidazole, Mexiletine, Ethambutol, Isoniazid, Lindane, Lincomycin, Lithium, Pemoline, Quinacrine, and long-term high-dose vitamin B_6 (Pyridoxine), should not be taken with Nitrofurantoin, because of the chance that nervous-system effects may be increased.

Food Interactions

Nitrofurantoin should be taken with food to help decrease stomach upset, loss of appetite, nausea, or other gastrointestinal symptoms. Avoid eating citrus fruits or milk products while taking Nitrofurantoin. These can change the acidity of your urine and affect the drug's action.

Usual Dose

Adult: 50 to 100 mg 4 times per day (with meals and at bedtime).

Child (over age 1 month): 2 to 3 mg per pound of body weight in 4 divided doses.

Child (age 1 month and under): not recommended.

Nitrofurantoin may be used in lower doses over a long period by people with chronic urinary infections.

Overdosage

Overdose victims should be made to vomit with Syrup of Ipecac if they have not already done so. Call your local poison control center or hospital emergency department for more information.

Special Information

Call your doctor if you develop chest pains or trouble breathing, sore throat, pale skin, unusual tiredness or weakness, dizziness, drowsiness, headache, skin rash and itching, yellow skin, achy joints, fever and chills, or numbness, tingling, or burning of the face or mouth, or if other side effects are especially persistent or bothersome.

Continue to take this medicine at least 3 days after you stop experiencing symptoms of urinary tract infection.

Nitrofurantoin may give your urine a brownish color: This is usual and not dangerous.

The oral liquid form of Nitrofurantoin can stain your teeth if you don't swallow the medicine rapidly.

If you miss a dose of Nitrofurantoin, take it as soon as possible. If it is almost time for your next dose and you take the medicine 3 or more times a day, space the missed dose and your next dose by 2 to 4 hours, or double your next dose and then continue with your regular schedule.

Special Populations

Pregnancy/Breast-feeding

Nitrofurantoin should be taken by pregnant women only if the benefits of taking the drug outweigh any possible risks. It should never be taken by pregnant women with G-6-PD deficiency and those who are near term, because it can interfere with the developing baby's immature enzyme systems and cause hemolytic anemia. Other urinary anti-infectives are preferred in these circumstances.

This medicine passes into breast milk and may affect some nursing infants, especially those who are G-6-PD deficient. You may want to bottle-feed your baby while taking this medication.

Seniors

Older adults with kidney disease may be more sensitive to some nervous system and lung effects of this drug. Follow your doctor's directions and report any side effects at once.

Also, older adults are likely to have some reduction of kidney function and may require a dosage reduction to account for that loss.

Generic Name

Nitroglycerin

Brand Names

Deponit Patches
Minitran Patches
Nitro-Bid Ointment/Plateau Caps
Nitrocine Timecaps
Nitrodisc Patches
Nitro-Dur Patches
Nitrogard Tablets

Nitroglyn Extended Release Capsules
Nitrol Ointment
Nitrolingual Spray
Nitrong Sustained Release Tablets
Nitrostat Sublingual Tablets
Transderm Nitro Patches

(Also available in generic form)

Type of Drug

Antianginal agent.

Prescribed for

Prevention and treatment of chest pains associated with angina pectoris. Nitroglycerin injection is also used as a treatment after a heart attack, for heart failure, and for high blood pressure.

General Information

Nitroglycerin is available in several dosage forms, including sublingual tablets (which are taken under the tongue and allowed to dissolve), capsules (which are swallowed), transmucosal tablets (which are placed between lip or cheek and gum and allowed to dissolve), oral sprays (sprayed directly onto or under the tongue), patches (which deliver Nitroglycerin through the skin over a 24-hour period), and ointment (which is usually spread over the chest wall, although it can be spread on any area of the body). Frequently, patients may take one or more dosage forms of Nitroglycerin to prevent and/or treat the attack of chest pain associated with angina.

Cautions and Warnings

You should not take Nitroglycerin if you are **allergic** to it or another nitrate product, such as Isosorbide. Also, because Nitroglycerin will increase the pressure of fluid inside your head, it should be taken with great caution if **head trauma** or **bleeding in the head** is present. Other conditions where the use of Nitroglycerin should be carefully weighed are **severe anemia, glaucoma, severe liver disease, overactive thyroid, cardiomyopathy (disease of the heart muscle), low blood pressure, recent heart attack, severe kidney problems,** and an **overactive gastrointestinal tract.**

Possible Side Effects

▼ Most common: flushing and headache (may be severe or persistent).

▼ Less common: Occasionally, episodes of dizziness and weakness have been associated with taking Nitroglycerin. There is a possibility that you will experience blurred vision. If this occurs, stop taking the drug and call your physician.

Some people exhibit a marked sensitivity to the blood-pressure-lowering effect of Nitroglycerin and may experience severe responses of nausea, vomiting, weakness, restlessness, loss of facial color (pallor), increased perspiration, and collapse, even with the usual therapeutic dose. Drug rash may also occur.

Drug Interactions

• Avoid over-the-counter drugs containing stimulants (cough, cold, and allergy remedies; appetite suppressants), which may aggravate your heart disease.

• Interaction with large amounts of alcoholic beverages can cause rapid lowering of blood pressure, resulting in weakness, dizziness, and fainting.

• Aspirin and calcium channel blockers can lead to higher nitrate blood levels and increased drug side effects.

• Nitroglycerin may interfere with the effects of Heparin, an injectable anticoagulant drug.

• Nitrates increase the amount of Dihydroergotamine absorbed into the blood, which can either raise blood pressure or work against the effect of Nitroglycerin.

Food Interactions

Do not use any oral form of Nitroglycerin with food or gum in your mouth. Nitroglycerin pills intended for swallowing (most are not) are best taken on an empty stomach.

Usual Dose

Use only as much as is necessary to control chest pains. Since the sublingual dosage form acts within 10 to 15 seconds of being taken, the drug is taken only when necessary.

Transmucosal Tablets

The tablets are placed between the upper lip and gum or between the cheek and gum and allowed to dissolve over a 3- to 5-hour period. The rate at which the tablet releases its medicine is increased by touching the tablet with your tongue or drinking a hot liquid. While you are awake, insert another tablet after the previous one is dissolved.

Long-Acting (Extended-Release) Capsules and Tablets

Generally, these are used to prevent chest pains associated with angina, with the dose being 1 capsule or tablet every 8 to 12 hours.

Ointment

1 to 2 inches of ointment are squeezed from the tube onto a prepared piece of paper with markings on it (some users may require as much as 4 to 5 inches). The ointment is spread on the skin every 3 to 4 hours as needed for control of chest pains. The medicine is absorbed through the skin. The application sites should be rotated to prevent skin inflammation and rash.

Patches

Patches are placed on a hairless spot not associated with excess movement once a day and left on for 12 to 14 hours. Doses start at 0.2 to 0.4 mg per hour and go to 0.8 mg. Higher doses are preferable for once-daily patch applications.

Aerosol

Nitroglycerin aerosol delivers 0.4 mg per dose. Spray 1 or 2 doses under or on your tongue and repeat as needed to relieve an angina attack.

Overdosage

Nitroglycerin overdose can result in low blood pressure, very rapid heartbeat, flushing, increased perspiration (later on, your skin can become cold, bluish, and clammy), headache, heart palpitations, blurring and other visual disturbances, dizziness, nausea, vomiting, slow and difficult breathing, slow pulse, confusion, moderate fever, and paralysis. Overdose victims should be taken to a hospital emergency room immediately. ALWAYS bring the medicine bottle with you.

Special Information

Do not interchange different brands of Nitroglycerin without your doctor's *and* pharmacist's knowledge. Product differences may mean that a different product cannot control your heart pain without a dosage adjustment.

Sublingual Nitroglycerin should be acquired from your pharmacist only in the original, unopened bottle; the tablets must not be transferred to another bottle or container because the tablets may lose potency. Close the bottle tightly after each use or the drug may evaporate from the tablets.

Sublingual Nitroglycerin should be taken while you are sitting down. Sublingual Nitroglycerin frequently produces a burning sensation under the tongue, which has been taken to indicate that the drug is potent and will produce the desired effect. The lack of this sensation is not an indication that the tablet has lost its potency. The only way you can check if the tablets are working is by seeing if it relieves your symptoms. If it doesn't work in 5 minutes, take another tablet. If that one doesn't work, take a third sublingual Nitroglycerin tablet. If the pain continues or gets worse, call your doctor and/or go to an emergency room for treatment at once.

When applying Nitroglycerin ointment, do not rub or massage it into the skin. Any excess ointment should be washed from hands after application.

People who use the patches for more than 12 hours a day for an extended period can become tolerant to the system and may have to return to other forms of Nitroglycerin to maintain an effect. Nitroglycerin patches contain a significant amount of medicine even after they have been used. They can be a hazard to children and small pets if not disposed of properly.

Orthostatic hypotension can be a problem if you take Nitroglycerin over a long period of time. More blood stays in the extremities and less becomes available to the brain, resulting in light-headedness or faintness if you stand up suddenly. Avoid prolonged standing and be careful to stand up slowly.

If you take Nitroglycerin on a regular schedule and forget a dose, take it as soon as you remember. If you use regular Nitroglycerin tablets, and it is within 2 hours of your next dose, skip the forgotten dose and continue with your regular schedule. If you take extended-release Nitroglycerin tablets or capsules, and it is within 6 hours of your next dose, skip the forgotten dose and continue with your regular schedule.

Special Populations

Pregnancy/Breast-feeding

This drug crosses into the blood circulation of a developing baby. It has not been found to cause birth defects. Pregnant women or those who might become pregnant while taking Nitroglycerin, should not take it without their doctor's approval. When the drug is considered essential by your doctor, the potential risk of taking the medicine must be carefully weighed against the benefit it might produce.

This drug passes into breast milk, but has caused no known problems among breast-fed infants. You must consider the potential effect on the nursing infant if breast-feeding while taking this medicine.

Seniors

Older adults may take Nitroglycerin without special restriction. Be sure to follow your doctor's directions. Because saliva is necessary for the absorption of sublingual Nitroglycerin, older adults with reduced saliva secretions and others with dry mouth may need to use another form of Nitroglycerin or a saliva substitute.

Nitrostat

*see **Nitroglycerin**, page 810*
*see **Nitroglycerin**, page 810*

Generic Name

Nizatidine

Brand Name

Axid

Type of Drug

Antiulcer; histamine H$_2$ antagonist.

Prescribed for

Ulcers of the stomach and upper intestine (duodenum). Nizatidine is also prescribed for gastroesophageal reflux disease (GERD).

General Information

Like the other H$_2$ antagonists, Nizatidine works by essentially turning off the system that produces stomach acid and other secretions.

Nizatidine is effective in treating the symptoms of ulcer and preventing complications of the disease. However, because all histamine H$_2$ antagonists work in exactly the same way, it is doubtful that an ulcer that does not respond to one will be effectively treated by another. These drugs vary only in their potency. Cimetidine is the least potent, with 1000 mg roughly equal to 300 mg of Nizatidine and Ranitidine and 40 mg of Famotidine. The ulcer-healing rates of all of these drugs are roughly equivalent, as is the chance of drug side effects with each.

Cautions and Warnings

Do not take Nizatidine if you have had an **allergic** reaction to it or to another **histamine H$_2$ antagonist** in the past.

Caution must be exercised by people with **kidney** and **liver disease** who take Nizatidine because ⅓ of each dose is broken down in the liver and the rest passes out of the body through the kidneys.

Possible Side Effects

Side effects are infrequent.

Possible Side Effects *(continued)*

▼ Most common: tiredness or fatigue and increased sweating.

▼ Rare: headache, dizziness, confusion, sleeplessness, mild diarrhea and constipation, abdominal discomfort, nausea, vomiting, liver inflammation and jaundice (yellowing of the skin and eyes), reduced blood platelet levels, rashes, itching, abnormal heartbeat and heart attack, painful swelling of the breast, impotence, loss of sex drive, joint pains, fever, and high blood uric acid levels (not associated with symptoms of gout).

Drug Interactions

• Antacids, anticholinergic drugs, and Metoclopramide may slightly reduce the amount of Nizatidine absorbed into the blood, but no precaution is needed.

• Enteric-coated tablets should not be taken with Nizatidine. The change in stomach acidity will cause the tablets to disintegrate prematurely in the stomach.

• Nizatidine may increase blood levels of Aspirin in people taking very large doses of Aspirin.

Food Interactions

Take Nizatidine without regard to food or meals. Food may slightly increase the amount of drug absorbed, but this is of no consequence.

Usual Dose

The usual adult dosage is either 300 mg at bedtime or 150 mg twice per day. Dosage is reduced in people with kidney disease.

Overdosage

There is little information on Nizatidine overdosage. Overdose victims might be expected to show exaggerated side effect symptoms, but little else is known. Your local poison control center may advise giving the victim Syrup of Ipecac (available at any pharmacy) to cause vomiting and remove any remaining drug from the stomach. Victims who have definite symptoms should be taken to a hospital emergency room for observation and possible treatment. ALWAYS bring the medicine bottle with you.

Special Information

You must take this medicine exactly as directed and follow your doctor's instructions for diet and other treatments to get the maximum benefit from this drug. Antacids may be taken together with Nizatidine, if needed. Cigarette smoking is known to be associated with stomach ulcers and may reverse the effect of Nizatidine on stomach acid.

Call your doctor at once if any unusual side effects develop. Especially important are unusual bleeding or bruising, unusual tiredness, diarrhea, dizziness, or rash. Black or tarry stools or vomiting "coffee ground"-like material may indicate your ulcer is bleeding.

If you empty the Nizatidine capsule and mix it with juice before taking it, keep it in the refrigerator, but don't store it for more than 2 days before using it. Keeping it longer than that may cause your medicine to be less potent.

If you forget to take a dose of Nizatidine, take it as soon as you remember. If it is almost time for your next regularly scheduled dose, skip the one you forgot and continue with your regular schedule. Do not take a double dose.

Special Populations

Pregnancy/Breast-feeding

Studies with laboratory animals have revealed no damage to a developing fetus, but it is recommended that Nizatidine be avoided by pregnant women and those who might become pregnant while using it. When usage is essential, Nizatidine's potential benefits must be carefully weighed against its possible risks.

Very small amounts of Nizatidine may pass into breast milk. No problems have been identified in nursing babies, but breast-feeding mothers should consider the risk of possible drug side effects.

Seniors

Older adults respond well to Nizatidine but may need less medication to achieve the desired response, because the drug is eliminated through the kidneys, and kidney function tends to decline with age. Older adults may be more susceptible to some drug side effects.

Generic Name

Norfloxacin

Brand Names

Chibroxin Eye Drops
Noroxin Tablets

Type of Drug

Fluoroquinolone anti-infective.

Prescribed for

Urinary infections, sexually transmitted diseases, and prostatitis. Norfloxacin is also available as eyedrops to treat ocular infections.

General Information

The fluoroquinolone antibacterials are widely used and work against many organisms that traditional antibiotic treatments have trouble killing. In addition to the above uses, fluoroquinolone anti-infectives can also be used for lower respiratory infections, skin infections, bone and joint infections, urinary infections (treatment and prevention), infectious diarrhea, lung infections in people with cystic fibrosis, bronchitis, pneumonia, prostate infection, and traveler's diarrhea. Norfloxacin does not work against the common cold, flu, or other viral infections. Norfloxacin is chemically related to an older antibacterial called *Nalidixic Acid* but works better than that drug against urinary infections.

Cautions and Warnings

Do not take Norfloxacin if you have had an **allergic** reaction to it or another fluoroquinolone in the past, or if you have had a reaction to related medications like **Nalidixic Acid**. Severe, possibly fatal allergic reactions can occur even after the very first dose, including **cardiovascular collapse, loss of consciousness, tingling, swelling of the face or throat, breathing difficulty, itching, or rash**. If any of these occur, **stop taking the drug** and seek medical help at once.

The dosage of Norfloxacin must be adjusted in the presence of **kidney failure.**

Norfloxacin may cause increased pressure on parts of the brain, leading to **convulsions** and **psychotic reactions.** Other possible adverse effects include **tremors, restlessness, lightheadedness, confusion,** and **hallucinations.** Norfloxacin should be used with caution in people with **seizure disorders** or other conditions of the nervous system.

People taking fluoroquinolone medicines can be **unusually sensitive to direct or indirect sunlight** (photosensitivity). **Avoid the sun** while taking this drug and for several days following therapy, *even if you are using a sunscreen!*

As with any other anti-infective, people taking Norfloxacin may develop **colitis** that could range from mild to very serious. See your doctor if you develop **diarrhea** or **cramps** while taking this drug.

Prolonged use of Norfloxacin can lead to **fungal overgrowth.** Follow your doctor's directions.

Possible Side Effects

▼ Most common: nausea, headache, dizziness, liver inflammation, and changes in blood components.

▼ Less common: abdominal pain, heartburn, upset stomach, constipation, gas, fatigue, drowsiness, not feeling well, depression, sleeplessness, rash.

▼ Rare: vomiting, diarrhea, dry or painful mouth, colitis, seizures, confusion, psychotic reactions, tingling in the hands or feet, visual disturbances, hearing loss, fever, hepatitis, inflammation of the pancreas, seizures, drug-sensitivity reactions (e.g., itching, redness, skin peeling), joint pains, and increased sensitivity to the sun.

Drug Interactions

• Antacids, Didanosine, Iron supplements, Sucralfate, and Zinc will decrease the amount of Norfloxacin absorbed into the bloodstream. If you must take any of these products, separate them from your Norfloxacin dosage by at least 2 hours.

• Anticancer drugs may also reduce the amount of Norfloxacin in your bloodstream.

• Probenecid cuts the amount of Norfloxacin released through your kidneys in half and may increase the chance of drug side effects. Cimetidine also increases the amount of Norfloxacin in the blood.

• Norfloxacin may increase the effects of oral anticoagulant (blood-thinning) drugs. Your anticoagulant dose may have to be reduced.

• Norfloxacin decreases the clearance of Caffeine from your body, possibly increasing its effect on your system.

• Norfloxacin may increase the toxic effects of Cyclosporine (for organ transplants) on your kidneys.

• Norfloxacin may reduce the rate at which Theophylline is released from your body, increasing Theophylline blood levels and the chance for Theophylline-related drug side effects.

• Nitrofurantoin may antagonize the antibacterial effect of Norfloxacin.

Food Interactions

Food can interfere with Norfloxacin absorption. Take it on an empty stomach, or at least 1 hour before or 2 hours after meals.

Usual Dose

Tablets
800 mg a day. Daily dosage is reduced in the presence of kidney failure.

Eyedrops
1 or 2 drops in the affected eye several times a day.

Overdosage

Overdose symptoms are the same as those found under *Possible Side Effects*. One person experienced kidney failure when he took an overdose of Ciprofloxacin, another fluoroquinolone. Overdose victims should be taken to a hospital emergency room. ALWAYS bring the medicine bottle with you. You may induce vomiting with Syrup of Ipecac (available at any pharmacy) to remove excess medication from the victim's stomach. Consult your local poison control center or hospital emergency room for specific instructions.

Special Information

Take each dose with a full glass of water. Be sure to drink at least 8 glasses of water a day while taking this medicine to promote removal of the drug from your system and to help avoid side effects.

If you are taking an antacid, Didanosine, Sucralfate, or an Iron or Zinc supplement while taking this drug, be sure to separate the doses by at least 2 hours to avoid an adverse drug interaction.

Drug sensitivity reactions can develop even after only one dose of Norfloxacin! Stop taking it and get immediate medical attention if you faint or if you develop itching, rash, facial swelling, difficulty breathing, convulsions, depression, visual disturbances, dizziness, headache, light-headedness, or any sign of a drug reaction.

Colitis can be caused by any anti-infective medication. If diarrhea develops, call your doctor at once.

Avoid excessive sunlight or exposure to a sunlamp and call your doctor if you become unusually sensitive to the sun while taking Norfloxacin.

You must take Norfloxacin according to your doctor's directions. Do not stop taking it even if you begin to feel better after a few days, unless directed to do so by your doctor.

If you forget to take a dose of Norfloxacin (including the eyedrops), take it as soon as you remember. If it is almost time for your next dose, skip the forgotten dose and continue with your regular schedule. Do not take a double dose.

To administer eyedrops, lie down or tilt your head backward and look at the ceiling. Hold the dropper above your eye, gently squeeze your lower lid to make a small pouch, and drop the medicine inside while looking up. Release the lower lid and keep your eye open. Don't blink for about 40 seconds. Press gently on the bridge of your nose at the inside corner of your eye for about a minute to help circulate the Norfloxacin around your eye. To avoid infection, don't touch the dropper tip to your finger or eyelid. Wait 5 minutes before using another eyedrop or ointment.

Call your doctor at once if your vision declines or if eye stinging, itching or burning, redness, irritation, swelling, or pain gets worse with the medicine.

Special Populations

Pregnancy/Breast-feeding

Animal studies have shown that Norfloxacin may reduce your

chances for a successful pregnancy or damage a developing fetus. Pregnant women should not take Norfloxacin unless its potential benefits clearly outweigh its risks.

Nursing mothers who must take Norfloxacin should bottle-feed their babies. Be sure your doctor knows if you are breast-feeding and taking this drug.

Seniors

Studies in healthy seniors showed that Norfloxacin is released from their bodies more slowly because of age-related reductions in kidney function. Your doctor may need to adjust your dose according to your level of kidney function.

Older adults may use Norfloxacin eyedrops without special restriction. Some seniors may have weak eyelid muscles. This creates a small reservoir for the eyedrops and may actually improve the drug's effect by keeping it in contact with your eye for a longer period. Your doctor may take this into account when determining the proper drug dosage.

Brand Name

Norgesic Forte

Ingredients

Aspirin + Caffeine + Orphenadrine Citrate

Other Brand Names

Norgesic
Orphengesic

(Also available in generic form)

Type of Drug

Analgesic combination.

Prescribed for

Pain of muscle spasms, sprains, strains, or back pain. Orphenadrine has been prescribed for nighttime leg cramps.

General Information

The main ingredient in Norgesic Forte is *Orphenadrine Cit-*

rate, a pain reliever. The Aspirin in Norgesic Forte adds extra pain relief.

Norgesic Forte cannot treat the underlying cause of your muscle spasm: It can only temporarily relieve the pain. You must follow any additional advice from your doctor to help solve the basic problem.

Cautions and Warnings

Norgesic Forte should not be used if you have a history of **glaucoma, stomach ulcer, heart disease, intestinal obstruction, difficulty in passing urine,** or known **sensitivity** or **allergy** to this drug or any of its ingredients.

Orphenadrine can make you **light-headed** or **dizzy.** Be careful doing anything that requires concentration or alertness.

Norgesic Forte **should not be taken by children.**

Possible Side Effects

▼ Most common: dryness of the mouth.

▼ Less common: As the daily dose increases, you may also experience rapid heartbeat, palpitations, difficulty in urination, blurred vision, enlarged pupils, weakness, nausea, vomiting, headache, dizziness, constipation, drowsiness, skin rash or itching, runny or stuffy nose, hallucinations, agitation, tremors, and stomach upset.

Large doses or prolonged therapy with Norgesic Forte may lead to Aspirin poisoning, with symptoms of ringing in the ears, fever, confusion, sweating, thirst, dimness of vision, rapid breathing, increased pulse rate, or diarrhea.

Drug Interactions

• The Aspirin in Norgesic Forte may interact with oral anticoagulant (blood-thinning) drugs, increase the effect of Probenecid, and increase the blood-sugar-lowering effects of oral antidiabetic drugs. Norgesic Forte interaction with Propoxyphene (Darvon) may cause confusion, anxiety, and tremors or shaking.

• Long-term users should avoid excessive alcohol, which may worsen stomach upset and bleeding.

Food Interactions

Take with food or at least half a glass of water to prevent stomach upset.

Usual Dose

½ to 1 tablet 3 to 4 times per day.

Overdosage

A single dose of 40 to 60 Norgesic Forte tablets is lethal to adults. Large overdoses below this level can be rapidly fatal. The victim must be taken to a hospital emergency room for treatment immediately. ALWAYS bring the medicine bottle with you.

Special Information

Norgesic Forte may make you drowsy. Be careful while driving or operating complex or hazardous equipment.

Call your doctor if you develop skin rash or itching, rapid heart rate, palpitations, or confusion, or if side effects are persistent or bothersome.

Avoid alcoholic beverages, which can increase the stomach irritation and depressive effects caused by this drug.

If you forget to take a dose of Norgesic Forte and you remember within about an hour of your regular time, take the dose right away. If you do not remember until later, skip the missed dose and go back to your regular schedule. Do not take a double dose.

Special Populations

Pregnancy/Breast-feeding

Taking too much Aspirin late in pregnancy can decrease a newborn's weight and cause other problems. When Orphenadrine is considered essential by your doctor, its potential benefits must be carefully weighed against its risks.

It is not known if Orphenadrine passes into breast milk. Nursing mothers who must take this medicine should watch their infants for drug-related side effects.

Seniors

Older adults may be more sensitive to the side effects of this medication and should take the lowest effective dose of Norgesic Forte. Seniors may occasionally experience some degree of mental confusion.

Generic Name

Nortriptyline

Brand Names

Pamelor Capsules/Solution
Ventyl Capsules/Solution

(Also available in generic form)

Type of Drug

Tricyclic antidepressant.

Prescribed for

Depression, panic disorder, and premenstrual depression.
Nortriptyline is also prescribed for chronic skin disorders.

General Information

Nortriptyline and other tricyclic antidepressants block the
movement of certain stimulant chemicals in and out of nerve
endings, have a sedative effect, and counteract the effects of
a hormone called *acetylcholine* (which makes them anticholinergic). They prevent the reuptake of important neurohormones (norepinephrine or serotonin) at the nerve ending.
One widely accepted theory of depression says that people
with depression have a chemical imbalance in their brain and
that drugs such as Nortriptyline work to reestablish a proper
balance. Although Nortriptyline and similar antidepressants
immediately block neurohormones, it takes weeks for their
clinical antidepressant effect to come into play. They can also
elevate mood, increase physical activity and mental alertness, and improve appetite and sleep patterns in a depressed
person. These drugs are mild sedatives and therefore useful
in treating mild forms of depression associated with anxiety.
You should not expect instant results; it usually takes 2 to 4
weeks. Call your doctor if symptoms are not better after 6 to
8 weeks. Occasionally, Nortriptyline and other tricyclic antidepressants have been used in treating nighttime bed-
wetting in young children, but they do not produce long-
lasting relief, and their use for this condition is of questionable
value. Tricyclic antidepressants are broken down in the liver.

Cautions and Warnings

Do not take Nortriptyline if you are **allergic** or **sensitive** to it or any other **tricyclic antidepressant:** Clomipramine, Doxepin, Amitriptyline, Trimipramine, Amoxapine, Imipramine, Desipramine, and Protriptyline. The drug should not be used if you are recovering from a **heart attack.**

This drug may be taken with caution if you have a history of **epilepsy** or other **convulsive disorders, difficulty in urination, glaucoma, heart** or **liver disease,** or **hyperthyroidism.** People who are **schizophrenic** or **paranoid** may get worse if given a tricyclic antidepressant, and **manic-depressive** people may switch phase. This can also happen if you are changing antidepressants or stopping them. Suicide is always a possibility in severely depressed people, who should be allowed to have only minimal quantities of medication on hand at any given time.

Possible Side Effects

▼ Most common: sedation and anticholinergic effects (blurred vision, disorientation, confusion, hallucinations, muscle spasms or tremors, seizures and/or convulsions, dry mouth, constipation [especially in older adults], difficult urination, worsening glaucoma, sensitivity to bright light or sunlight).

▼ Less common: blood-pressure changes, abnormal heart rates, heart attack, anxiety, restlessness, excitement, numbness or tingling in the extremities, poor coordination, rash, itching, retention of fluids, fever, allergy, changes in blood composition, nausea, vomiting, loss of appetite, stomach upset, diarrhea, enlargement of the breasts (both sexes), changes in sex drive, and blood-sugar changes.

▼ Rare: agitation, inability to sleep, nightmares, feeling of panic, a peculiar taste in the mouth, stomach cramps, black coloration of the tongue, yellowing eyes or skin, changes in liver function, increased or decreased weight, excessive perspiration, flushing, frequent urination, drowsiness, dizziness, weakness, headache, loss of hair, and feelings of ill health.

Drug Interactions

• Interaction with monoamine oxidase (MAO) inhibitors

can cause high fevers, convulsions, and occasionally death. Don't take MAO inhibitors until at least 2 weeks after Nortriptyline has been discontinued. Patients who must take these drugs together require close medical observation.

• Nortriptyline interacts with Guanethidine and Clonidine. Be sure to discuss this if your doctor prescribes Nortriptyline and you are taking **any** high-blood-pressure medicine.

• Nortriptyline increases the effects of barbiturates, tranquilizers, other sedative drugs, and alcohol. Also, barbiturates may decrease the effectiveness of Nortriptyline.

• Taking Nortriptyline and thyroid medicine together will enhance the effects of both medicines, possibly causing abnormal heart rhythms. The combination of Nortriptyline and Reserpine may cause overstimulation.

• Oral contraceptives can reduce the effect of Nortriptyline, as can smoking. Charcoal tablets can prevent Nortriptyline's absorption into the blood. Estrogens can increase or decrease the effect of Nortriptyline.

• Drugs such as Bicarbonate of Soda, Acetazolamide, Quinidine, or Procainamide will increase the effect of Nortriptyline. Cimetidine, Methylphenidate, and phenothiazine drugs (like Thorazine and Compazine) block the liver metabolism of Nortriptyline, causing it to stay in the body longer. This can cause severe drug side effects.

Food Interactions

Take Nortriptyline with food if it upsets your stomach.

Usual Dose

Adult: 25 mg 3 times per day, increased to 150 mg per day if necessary. This medication must be tailored to your specific needs.

Adolescent and Senior: lower doses are recommended—generally, 30 to 50 mg per day.

Child (age 6 to 17): 10 to 20 mg per day.

Child (up to age 5): not recommended.

Overdosage

Symptoms are confusion, inability to concentrate, hallucinations, drowsiness, lowered body temperature, abnormal heart rate, heart failure, enlarged pupils of the eyes, convulsions, severely lowered blood pressure, stupor, and coma (as well as agitation, stiffening of body muscles, vomiting, and high fever). The victim should be taken to a hospital emergency room immediately. ALWAYS bring the medicine bottle with you.

Special Information

Avoid alcohol and other depressants while taking this drug. Do not stop taking this medicine unless your doctor has specifically told you to do so. Abruptly stopping this medicine may cause nausea, headache, and a sickly feeling.

This medicine can cause drowsiness, dizziness, and blurred vision. Be careful when driving or operating hazardous machinery. Avoid long exposure to the sun or sunlamps.

Call your doctor at once if you develop seizures, difficult or rapid breathing, fever and sweating, blood-pressure changes, muscle stiffness, loss of bladder control, or unusual tiredness or weakness. Dry mouth may lead to an increase in dental cavities, gum bleeding, and gum disease. People taking Nortriptyline should pay close attention to dental hygiene.

If you forget to take a dose of Nortriptyline, take it as soon as you remember. If it is almost time for your next dose, skip the missed dose and go back to your regular schedule. Do not take a double dose.

Special Populations

Pregnancy/Breast-feeding

Nortriptyline, like other antidepressants, crosses into fetal circulation, and birth defects have been reported if this drug is taken during the first 3 months of pregnancy. There have been reports of newborn infants suffering from heart, breathing, and urinary problems after their mothers had taken an antidepressant of this type immediately before delivery. Avoid taking Nortriptyline while pregnant.

Small amounts of tricyclic antidepressants pass into breast milk and can cause sedation in the baby. Nursing mothers should consider bottle-feeding if taking Nortriptyline.

Seniors

Older adults are more sensitive to the effects of this drug, especially abnormal rhythms and other heart side effects; thus, they often require a lower dose to achieve the same results. Follow your doctor's directions and report any side effects at once.

Norvasc

see *Amlodipine*, page 57

Generic Name

Nystatin

Brand Names

Mycostatin Pastilles/Tablets/Vaginal Inserts
Nilstat Cream/Drops (Oral Suspension)/Tablets

(Also available in generic form)

Type of Drug

Antifungal.

Prescribed for

Fungal infections.

General Information

Nystatin is a versatile antifungal agent that is available in a number of different dosage forms. It can be prescribed in any situation where fungus infection is a possible complication of either a disease or a treatment. Generally, Nystatin will relieve your symptoms in 1 to 3 days. Nystatin vaginal tablets effectively control troublesome and unpleasant symptoms such as itching, inflammation, and discharge. In most cases, 2 weeks of therapy is sufficient, but prolonged treatment may be necessary. It is important that you continue using this medicine during menstruation. This drug has been used to prevent thrush or *Candida* infection in the newborn infant by treating the mother for 3 to 6 weeks before her due date.

Before the development of Nystatin pastilles, the vaginal tablet was used as a lozenge to treat *Candida* infections of the mouth.

Cautions and Warnings

Do not take this drug if you know you may be **sensitive** or

allergic to Nystatin. Proper diagnosis is essential for effective treatment. Do not use this product without first **consulting your doctor.**

Possible Side Effects

Nystatin is virtually nontoxic and is generally well tolerated.

▼ Most common: When taken by mouth, nausea, upset stomach, and diarrhea may occur with large doses. The only side effect reported with the vaginal product has been intravaginal irritation; if this occurs, discontinue the drug and contact your doctor.

Drug and Food Interactions

None known.

Usual Dose

Oral Suspension or Pastilles
200,000 to 600,000 units 4 or 5 times a day.

Oral Tablets
500,000 to 1,000,000 units 3 times a day.

Vaginal Tablets
1 tablet inserted high in the vagina daily for 2 weeks.

Overdosage

Nystatin overdose may cause stomach irritation or upset. Call your local poison control center for more information.

Special Information

Do not stop taking Nystatin just because you begin to feel better. You must continue taking the medication as prescribed for at least 2 days after the relief of symptoms.

Some Nystatin brands require storage in the refrigerator. Ask your pharmacist for specific instructions.

If you forget a dose of Nystatin, take it as soon as you remember. If it is almost time for your next dose, skip the one you forgot and continue with your regular schedule. Do not take a double dose.

Special Populations

Pregnancy/Breast-feeding
Pregnant and breast-feeding women may use Nystatin without special restriction.

Seniors
Older adults may use Nystatin without special restriction.

Generic Name

Ofloxacin

Brand Names

Floxin
Ocuflox Eye Drops

Type of Drug

Fluoroquinolone anti-infective.

Prescribed for

Lower respiratory infections, skin infections, bone and joint infections, urinary infections (treatment and prevention), infectious diarrhea, lung infections in people with cystic fibrosis, bronchitis, pneumonia, prostate infection, and traveler's diarrhea. Ofloxacin does not work against the common cold, flu, or other viral infections. It is not effective against syphilis. Ofloxacin is also available as eyedrops to treat ocular infections.

General Information

Ofloxacin works against many organisms that traditional antibiotic treatments have trouble killing. This medication is chemically related to an older antibacterial called *Nalidixic Acid*, but works better than that drug against urinary infections.

Cautions and Warnings

Do not take Ofloxacin if you have had an **allergic reaction** to it or another fluoroquinolone in the past, or if you have had a reaction to related medications like Nalidixic Acid. Severe, possibly fatal allergic reactions can occur even after the very first dose, including cardiovascular collapse, loss of consciousness, tingling, swelling of the face or throat, breathing difficulty, itching, or rash. If any of these occur, stop taking the drug and seek medical help at once.

Ofloxacin dosage must be adjusted in the presence of **kidney failure.**

Ofloxacin may cause increased cranial pressure, leading to **convulsions and psychotic reactions.** Other possible adverse effects include tremors, restlessness, light-headedness, confusion, and hallucinations. Ofloxacin should be used with caution in people with **seizure disorders** or other nervous-system conditions.

People taking fluoroquinolone medicines can be unusually **sensitive to direct or indirect sunlight** (photosensitivity). **Avoid the sun** while taking this drug and for several days following therapy, *even if you are using a sunscreen!*

As with any other anti-infective, people taking Ofloxacin may develop **colitis** that could range from mild to very serious. See your doctor if you develop diarrhea or cramps while taking this drug.

Prolonged use of Ofloxacin, as with any other anti-infective, can lead to **fungal overgrowth.** It should only be taken according to your doctor's direction.

Possible Side Effects

▼ Most common: nausea and sleeplessness.

▼ Less common: vomiting; diarrhea; abdominal pain; dry or painful mouth; headache; rash; fatigue; drowsiness; dizziness; not feeling well; rash; itching; visual disturbances; vaginal irritation, infection, or discharge; fever; genital itching; chest pain; taste disruption; nervousness; and decreased appetite.

▼ Rare: depression; hallucinations; tingling in the hands or feet; unusual sensitivity to sunlight; hearing loss; high blood pressure; heart palpitations; fainting; chills; swollen ankles, legs, or arms; vaginal burning; irritation or pain; painful menstruation; frequent or pain-

Possible Side Effects *(continued)*

ful urination; cough; runny nose; sleep disorders; anxiety; abnormal dreams; euphoria (feeling "high"); weight loss; sweating; joint or muscle aches; and excessive thirst.

Drug Interactions

• Antacids, Didanosine, Iron supplements, Sucralfate, and Zinc will decrease the amount of Ofloxacin absorbed into the bloodstream. If you must take any of these products, separate them from your Ofloxacin dose by at least 2 hours.

• Anticancer drugs may also reduce the amount of Ofloxacin in your blood stream.

• Probenecid cuts the amount of Ofloxacin released through your kidneys by half and may increase the chance of drug side effects. Cimetidine may also interfere with the release of Ofloxacin from your body.

• Ofloxacin may increase the effects of oral anticoagulant (blood-thinning) drugs. Your anticoagulant dose may have to be adjusted.

• Ofloxacin may increase the toxic effects of Cyclosporine (for organ transplants) on your kidneys.

• Ofloxacin may reduce the rate at which Theophylline is released from your body, increasing Theophylline blood levels and the chance for Theophylline-related drug side effects.

Food Interactions

Do not take Ofloxacin with food. Take it at least 1 hour before or 2 hours after a meal.

Usual Dose

Tablets

400 to 800 mg a day. Daily dosage is reduced in the presence of kidney failure.

Eyedrops

1 or 2 drops in the affected eye several times a day as directed by your doctor.

Overdosage

Symptoms of overdosage are the same as those found under *Possible Side Effects*. One person experienced kidney failure when he took an overdose of Ciprofloxacin, another fluoro-quinolone. Overdose victims should be taken to a hospital emergency room. ALWAYS bring the medicine bottle. You may induce vomiting with Syrup of Ipecac (available at any pharmacy) to remove excess medication from the victim's stomach. Consult your local poison control center or hospital emergency room for specific instructions.

Special Information

Take each dose with a full glass of water. Be sure to drink at least 8 glasses of water per day while taking Ofloxacin to promote removal of the drug from your system and to help avoid side effects.

If you are taking an antacid, Didanosine, Sucralfate, or an Iron or Zinc supplement while taking Ofloxacin, be sure to separate the doses by at least 2 hours to avoid a drug interaction.

Drug sensitivity reactions can develop even after only one dose of this medicine! Stop taking it and get immediate medical attention if you faint or if you develop itching, rash, facial swelling, difficulty breathing, convulsions, depression, visual disturbances, dizziness, headache, light-headedness, or any sign of a drug reaction.

Colitis can be caused by any anti-infective medication. If diarrhea develops, call your doctor at once.

Avoid excessive sunlight or exposure to a sunlamp while taking Ofloxacin, and call your doctor if you develop a rash or skin reaction.

It is essential that you take Ofloxacin according to your doctor's directions. Even if you feel better after a few days, do not stop taking it unless directed to do so by your doctor.

To administer eyedrops, lie down or tilt your head back-ward and look up. Hold the dropper above your eye, gently pinch your lower lid to make a small pouch, and drop the medicine inside while looking up. Release the lid and keep your eye open. Don't blink for about 40 seconds. Press gently on the bridge of your nose at the inside corner of your eye for about a minute to help circulate the medicine around your eye. To avoid infection, don't touch the dropper tip to your finger or eyelid. Wait 5 minutes before using another eyedrop or ointment.

Call your doctor at once if eye stinging, itching or burning, redness, irritation, swelling, or pain gets worse or if your vision declines.

If you forget to take a dose of Ofloxacin tablets or eyedrops, take it as soon as you remember. If it is almost time for your next dose, skip the missed dose and continue with your regular schedule. Do not take a double dose.

Special Populations

Pregnancy/Breast-feeding
Animal studies have shown that Ofloxacin may reduce your chances for a successful pregnancy or damage a developing fetus. Pregnant women should not take it unless the possible benefits have been carefully weighed against its risks.

Ofloxacin is found in breast milk at levels that are similar to blood levels of the drug. Use an alternative feeding method if you must take this medicine, and be sure your doctor knows if you are breast-feeding and taking this medicine.

Seniors
Studies in healthy seniors showed that Ofloxacin is released from their bodies more slowly because of normal decreases in kidney function. Drug dosage will be adjusted accordingly.

Older adults may use Ofloxacin eyedrops without special restriction. Some seniors may have weaker eyelid muscles. This creates a small reservoir for the eyedrops and may actually increase the drug's effect by keeping it in contact with your eye for a longer period. Your doctor may take this into account when determining the proper drug dosage.

Generic Name

Olsalazine

Brand Name
Dipentum

Type of Drug
Bowel anti-inflammatory.

Prescribed for

Treating and maintaining ulcerative colitis.

General Information

This drug is broken down to an anti-inflammatory compound, *Mesalamine*, after it enters the colon. Mesalamine acts as an anti-inflammatory agent inside the bowel and is effective for ulcerative colitis. Little (10 to 30 percent) of Mesalamine is absorbed into the blood; 70 to 90 percent of it remains in the colon, where it works on your colitis. People who cannot take Sulfasalazine may be able to take Olsalazine.

Cautions and Warnings

Do not take this product if you are **allergic** to it, Mesalamine, or Aspirin (or Aspirin-related compounds) because the active metabolic product of Olsalazine is closely related to Aspirin.

Possible Side Effects

▼ Most common: diarrhea and stomach cramps or pain.

▼ Less common: muscle aches, headaches, fatigue or drowsiness, depression, nausea, vomiting, upset stomach, bloating, yellowing of the skin or eyes, depression, dizziness, fainting, loss of appetite, respiratory infections, and skin rash or itching.

Many other side effects have been reported, but their link to Olsalazine has not been well established.

Drug Interactions

None known.

Food Interactions

Take this drug with food or meals to reduce stomach upset.

Usual Dose

1000 mg a day divided into 2 doses.

Overdosage

Overdose symptoms are diarrhea, vomiting, and lethargy. Overdose victims should be made to vomit with Syrup of Ipecac (available at any pharmacy) to remove any remaining medicine from their stomach. Call your local poison control center or emergency room before giving the Ipecac. Then take the victim to a hospital emergency room for treatment. ALWAYS take the medicine bottle with you.

Special Information

Call your doctor if you develop fever, pale skin, sore throat, unusual bruising or bleeding, unusual tiredness or weakness, yellow eyes or skin, or if your colitis gets worse. Other symptoms, such as diarrhea, abdominal pains, upset stomach, loss of appetite, nausea, and vomiting, should be reported if they become particularly bothersome or severe.

If you forget a dose of Olsalazine, take it as soon as you remember. If it is almost time for your next dose, take one dose right away and another in 5 or 6 hours, then go back to your regular schedule. Do not take a double dose.

Special Populations

Pregnancy/Breast-feeding

Olsalazine has caused birth defects in lab animals. Olsalazine should not be taken unless its possible benefits have been carefully weighed against its risks.

Olsalazine and Mesalamine pass into breast milk, but the importance of this is not known. Nursing mothers should consult their doctors and exercise caution.

Seniors

Seniors may use this drug without special restriction.

Generic Name

Omeprazole

Brand Name

Prilosec

Type of Drug

Stomach-acid inhibitor; antiulcer.

Prescribed for

Gastroesophageal reflux disease and stomach and duodenal ulcers. Omeprazole is also prescribed for conditions in which there is an excess of stomach acid (including Zollinger-Ellison syndrome).

General Information

Omeprazole is officially accepted in the United States for duodenal ulcers and gastroesophageal reflux disease (GERD), a condition in which some stomach contents flow backward into the esophagus (the pipe connecting the throat and stomach). This can result in erosion of the esophagus caused by the stomach acid. Omeprazole actually stops the production of stomach acid by a method that is different from that of Cimetidine, Ranitidine, and the other H_2 antagonists. It interferes with the so-called "proton-pump," the last stage of acid production within the mucous lining of the stomach. As a result, Omeprazole can turn off stomach acid production within 1 hour after it is taken. This medicine is also approved for several other conditions in which stomach acid plays a key role or in which excess stomach acid is produced as a part of the condition.

Omeprazole has not yet been officially accepted for stomach ulcers, although it is widely prescribed for that purpose.

Cautions and Warnings

Do not take Omeprazole if you have had an **allergic** reaction to it in the past.

In laboratory animal studies, Omeprazole was found to **increase** the numbers of **some tumors**. These studies have raised questions about the long-term safety of Omeprazole and the possible relationship between Omeprazole's effects and human tumors. However, there is no current available information that shows a human-tumor risk with Omeprazole.

Possible Side Effects

Generally, Omeprazole causes few side effects.

▼ Most common: headache, diarrhea, abdominal pain, nausea, sore throat, upper respiratory infections, fever,

---

Possible Side Effects *(continued)*

vomiting, dizziness, rash, constipation, muscle pain, unusual tiredness, cough, and back pain.

▼ Rare: abdominal swelling, a feeling of ill health,
angina pain, appetite loss, stool discoloration, irritable
bowel, fungal infection in the esophagus, dry mouth, low
blood sugar, weight gain, muscle cramps, joint and leg
pains, dizziness, fainting, nervousness, sleeplessness,
apathy, anxiety, unusual dreams, tingling in the hands or
feet, nosebleeds, itching and inflammation of the skin,
dry skin, hair loss, sweating, frequent urination, and
testicle pain.

Drug Interactions

• Omeprazole may increase the effects of Diazepam, Phenytoin, and Warfarin by slowing the breakdown of these drugs
by the liver. It may also interact with other drugs broken down
by the liver.

• Omeprazole may interfere with the absorption from the
stomach of drugs that require stomach acid as part of the
process (e.g., Iron, Ampicillin, and Ketoconazole).

• The use of Omeprazole with drugs that reduce the production of blood cells by the bone marrow may increase their
effect.

Food Interactions

Omeprazole should be taken immediately before a meal,
preferably in the morning.

Usual Dose

20 to 80 mg per day. Up to 120 mg per day has been used for
some conditions. Antacids may be taken with Omeprazole, if
needed.

Overdosage

There is limited experience with Omeprazole overdose, although people with Zollinger-Ellison syndrome have taken
360 mg per day without a problem. Overdose symptoms are

likely to be similar to Omeprazole's side effects. If you suspect an Omeprazole overdose, call your local poison control center or hospital emergency room for additional information.

Special Information

Call your doctor if you develop unusual tiredness or weakness, sore throat, fever, sores in the mouth that don't heal, unusual bleeding or bruising, bloody or cloudy urine, or urinary difficulties, or if side effects are unusually persistent or bothersome.

Continue taking the medication until your doctor tells you to stop, even though your symptoms may improve after 1 or 2 weeks.

If you forget to take a dose of Omeprazole, take it as soon as you remember. If it is almost time for your next dose, skip the one you forgot and continue with your regular schedule. Do not take a double dose.

Special Populations

Pregnancy/Breast-feeding

Animal studies with Omeprazole have shown toxic effects in developing fetuses, but no such problems have been reported in humans. However, as with most drugs, pregnant women, and those who might become pregnant, should not use Omeprazole unless its advantages clearly outweigh its possible dangers.

It is not known if Omeprazole passes into breast milk; no drug-related problems have been known to occur. Nursing mothers who use it should exercise caution and watch their babies for possible drug-related side effects.

Seniors

Seniors exhibit the same side effects seen in younger adults. However, older adults are likely to have age-related reduction in kidney and/or liver function, which could account for increased amounts of drug in the bloodstream. Report any unusual side effects to your doctor.

Generic Name

Ondansetron

Brand Name

Zofran

Type of Drug

Antiemetic.

Prescribed for

Preventing nausea and vomiting that occurs after general anesthetics used during surgery and after certain cancer chemotherapy treatments.

General Information

Ondansetron and Granisetron produce their effect in a unique way. They antagonize the receptor for a special form of the neurohormone *serotonin* ($5HT_3$). Receptors of this type are found in both the part of the brain that controls vomiting (the *chemoreceptor trigger zone*), and the vagus nerve in the stomach and intestines. Women absorb more Ondansetron faster than men and clear the drug more slowly from their bodies. This means that women will have more drug in their blood than men after taking the same dose of Ondansetron, but these differences have not been reflected in any difference in response to the drug.

Ondansetron and Granisetron are extremely effective in preventing nausea and vomiting and work in situations where many older antiemetics are ineffective.

Cautions and Warnings

Don't take Ondansetron if you are **allergic** or **sensitive** to it.

People with **liver failure** must take less Ondansetron since the drug accumulates in their body and less is needed to produce the same effect.

Possible Side Effects

▼ Most common: headache and constipation.

Possible Side Effects *(continued)*

▼ Less common: weakness, fever or chills, dry mouth, liver inflammation, diarrhea, abdominal pains, and rash.

▼ Rare: liver failure, drug allergy, bronchial spasm, unusual tiredness or weakness, dizziness or light-headedness, rapid heartbeat, angina pains, low blood potassium, and grand mal seizures.

Drug Interactions

• Ondansetron is broken down in the liver by the same enzyme system that is responsible for breaking down many other drugs. It may be affected by other drugs that stimulate or inhibit these enzymes, but no important interactions have been discovered to date.

Food Interactions

Food increases the amount of Ondansetron absorbed, but does not affect your Ondansetron dose.

Usual Dose

Adult and Adolescent (age 12 and older): 8 mg 3 times a day. People with liver failure should take no more than 8 mg a day.

Child (age 4-11): 4 mg 3 times a day.

Child (under age 4): not recommended.

Overdosage

Doses up to 145 mg have been taken without important side effects. Call your local poison control center or hospital emergency room for more information. If you go to the hospital for treatment, ALWAYS bring the medicine bottle with you.

Special Information

Call your doctor if you begin to have chest tightness, wheezing, trouble breathing, chest pains, or other unusual or severe side effects.

Ondansetron can cause dry mouth, which can increase

your risk of tooth decay or gum disease. Pay special attention to oral hygiene while you are taking this drug.

If you forget to take a dose of Ondansetron, take it as soon as you remember. If it is almost time for your next dose, skip the dose you forgot and continue with the regular schedule. Skipping more than 1 dose may increase your chances of vomiting.

Special Populations

Pregnancy/Breast-feeding
Studies of Ondansetron have revealed no potential to cause birth defects. Nevertheless, pregnant women should not take this, or any other, drug unless the possible risks and benefits to be gained from taking it have been discussed with their doctors.

Ondansetron may pass into breast milk. Nursing mothers who take this medicine should carefully observe for possible drug side effects in their infants.

Seniors
Seniors may take this medicine without restriction.

Ortho-Cept

see *Contraceptives*, page 262

Ortho-Novum

see *Contraceptives*, page 262

Generic Name

Oxaprozin

Brand Name

Daypro

Type of Drug

Nonsteroidal anti-inflammatory drug (NSAID).

Prescribed for

Rheumatoid arthritis and osteoarthritis.

General Information

Oxaprozin is one of 16 NSAIDs used to relieve pain and inflammation. We do not know exactly how NSAIDs work, but part of their action may be due to an ability to inhibit the body's production of a hormone called *prostaglandin*, as well as inhibiting the action of other body chemicals, including cyclo-oxygenase, lipoxygenase, leukotrienes, lysosomal enzymes, and a host of other factors. NSAIDs are generally absorbed into the bloodstream fairly quickly. Pain relief comes within an hour after taking the first dose of Oxaprozin, but its anti-inflammatory effect takes a lot longer (up to 1 week) to become apparent, and may take a month or more to reach its maximum effect. Oxaprozin is broken down in the liver and eliminated through the kidneys.

Cautions and Warnings

People who are **allergic** to Oxaprozin (or any other NSAID) and those with a history of **asthma** attacks brought on by an NSAID, Iodides, or Aspirin should not take Oxaprozin.

Oxaprozin can cause **gastrointestinal (GI) bleeding, ulcers, and stomach perforation**. This can occur at any time, with or without warning, in people who take chronic Oxaprozin treatment. People with a history of active GI bleeding should be cautious about taking any NSAID. Minor stomach upset, distress, or gas is common during the first few days of treatment with Oxaprozin. People who develop bleeding or ulcers and continue treatment should be aware of the possibility of developing more serious drug toxicity.

Oxaprozin can affect platelets and **blood clotting** at high doses, and should be avoided by people with clotting problems and by those taking Warfarin.

People with **heart problems** who use Oxaprozin may experience swelling in their arms, legs, or feet.

Oxaprozin can cause severe toxic effects to the **kidney.**

Report any unusual side effects to your doctor, who may need to periodically test your kidney function.

Oxaprozin can make you unusually **sensitive to the effects of the sun** (photosensitivity).

Possible Side Effects

▼ Most common: diarrhea, nausea, vomiting, constipation, stomach gas, stomach upset or irritation, and loss of appetite.

▼ Less common: stomach ulcers, GI bleeding, hepatitis, gallbladder attacks, painful urination, poor kidney function, kidney inflammation, blood and protein in the urine, dizziness, fainting, nervousness, depression, hallucinations, confusion, disorientation, tingling in the hands or feet, light-headedness, itching, increased sweating, dry nose and mouth, heart palpitations, chest pain, difficulty breathing, and muscle cramps.

▼ Rare: severe allergic reactions, including closing of the throat; fever and chills; changes in liver function; jaundice (yellowing of the skin or eyes); and kidney failure. People who experience such effects must be promptly treated in a hospital emergency room or doctor's office.

NSAIDs have caused severe skin reactions; if this happens to you, see your doctor immediately.

Drug Interactions

• Oxaprozin can increase the effects of oral anticoagulant (blood-thinning) drugs such as Warfarin. You may take this combination, but your doctor may have to reduce your anticoagulant dose.

• Taking Oxaprozin with Cyclosporine may increase the toxic kidney effects of both drugs. Methotrexate toxicity may be increased in people also taking Oxaprozin.

• Oxaprozin may reduce the blood-pressure-lowering effect of beta blockers and loop diuretic drugs.

• Oxaprozin may increase blood levels of Phenytoin, leading to increased Phenytoin side effects. Blood-Lithium levels may be increased in people taking Oxaprozin.

• Oxaprozin blood levels may be affected by Cimetidine because of that drug's effect on the liver.

• Probenecid may interfere with the elimination of Oxaprozin from the body, increasing the chances for Oxaprozin toxic reactions.

• Aspirin and other salicylates may decrease the amount of Oxaprozin in your blood. These medicines should never be taken at the same time as Oxaprozin.

Food Interactions

Take Oxaprozin with food or a magnesium/aluminum antacid if it upsets your stomach.

Usual Dose

600 to 1800 mg taken once a day. Do not take more than 12 mg per pound of body weight in any day. Take each dose with a full glass of water and don't lie down for 15 to 30 minutes after you take the medicine.

Overdosage

People have died from NSAID overdoses. The most common signs of overdosage are drowsiness, nausea, vomiting, diarrhea, abdominal pain, rapid breathing, rapid heartbeat, increased sweating, ringing or buzzing in the ears, confusion, disorientation, stupor, and coma.

Take the victim to a hospital emergency room at once. ALWAYS bring the medicine bottle with you.

Special Information

Oxaprozin can make you drowsy and/or tired: Be careful when driving or operating hazardous equipment. Do not take any nonprescription products that contain Acetaminophen or Aspirin while taking this drug; also, avoid alcoholic beverages.

Contact your doctor if you develop skin rash or itching, visual disturbances, weight gain, breathing difficulty, fluid retention, hallucinations, black or tarry stools, persistent headache, or any unusual or intolerable side effects.

If you forget to take a dose of Oxaprozin, take it as soon as you remember. If you take your Oxaprozin once a day, and it is within 8 hours of your next dose, skip the missed dose and continue with your regular schedule. Do not take a double dose. If you take more than one Oxaprozin dose a day, and it is within 4 hours of your next dose, skip the one you forgot and continue with your regular schedule.

Special Populations

Pregnancy/Breast-feeding
NSAIDs may cross into the fetal blood circulation. They have not been found to cause birth defects, but animal studies indicate that they may affect a developing fetal heart during the second half of pregnancy. Women who are or might become pregnant should not take Oxaprozin without their doctors' approval; pregnant women should be particularly cautious about using this drug during the last 3 months of their pregnancy. When the drug is considered essential by your doctor, its potential benefits must be carefully weighed against its risks.

NSAIDs may pass into breast milk, but have caused no problems among breast-fed infants, except for seizures in a baby whose mother was taking Indomethacin. Other NSAIDs have caused problems in animal studies. There is a possibility that a nursing mother taking Oxaprozin could affect her baby's heart or cardiovascular system. If you must take Oxaprozin, bottle-feed your baby.

Seniors
Older adults may be more susceptible to Oxaprozin side effects, especially ulcer disease.

Generic Name

Oxiconazole

Brand Name
Oxistat Cream

Type of Drug
Antifungal.

Prescribed for
Fungal infections of the skin.

General Information

Oxiconazole is a general-purpose antifungal product. It works by interfering with the cell membrane of the fungus. Oxiconazole penetrates the skin after application, but little is absorbed into the bloodstream.

Cautions and Warnings

Do not use Oxiconazole if you are **allergic** to it or to any other ingredient in Oxistat Cream.

Large doses of Oxiconazole have caused **reduced fertility** in laboratory animals. This should be taken into account when considering the use of this product, although there is no evidence that Oxiconazole reduces fertility in women.

Possible Side Effects

Oxiconazole side effects are infrequent.
▼ Common: itching and burning.
▼ Rare: stinging, irritation, rash, scaling, tingling, pain, eczema, redness and swelling, and cracked skin.

Drug and Food Interactions

None known.

Usual Dose

Oxiconazole should be applied to affected areas every evening for 2 to 4 weeks, depending on the fungus type.

Overdosage

People who accidentally swallow this medicine should be taken to a hospital emergency room for evaluation and treatment. ALWAYS bring the medicine container.

Special Information

Oxiconazole is meant only for application to the skin. Do not put this product into your eyes or mouth.

Stop using the product and call your doctor if skin irritation or redness develops.

If you forget to apply a dose of Oxiconazole, apply it as soon as you remember. If it is almost time for your next dose, skip the missed dose and continue with your regular schedule.

Special Populations

Pregnancy/Breast-feeding

Oxiconazole is not likely to affect your pregnancy because little is absorbed into the bloodstream. Nevertheless, you should not use this drug without your doctor's knowledge and approval.

Significant amounts of Oxiconazole may pass into breast milk. Nursing mothers who use it should watch their infants for possible drug-related side effects.

Seniors

Seniors may use Oxiconazole without special restriction.

Generic Name

Oxybutynin

Brand Name

Ditropan

Type of Drug

Antispasmodic; anticholinergic.

Prescribed for

Excessive urination caused by bladder conditions.

General Information

Oxybutynin directly affects the smooth muscle that controls the opening and closing of the bladder. This antispasmodic is 4 to 10 times more potent than Atropine, but has only 1/5 the anticholinergic effect of that drug and is much less likely to cause side effects.

Cautions and Warnings

Do not take Oxybutynin if you are **allergic** or **sensitive** to it. Skin rash or itching may be mild signs of drug allergy.

Oxybutynin should be used with caution if you have **glaucoma, intestinal obstruction** or **poor intestinal function, megacolon, severe or ulcerative colitis, myasthenia,** or **unstable heart disease,** including abnormal heart rhythm, heart failure, or recent heart attack. Oxybutynin should be used with caution if you have **liver or kidney disease.** It may worsen symptoms of an **overactive thyroid gland, coronary heart disease, abnormal heart rhythm, rapid heartbeat, high blood pressure, prostate disease,** or **hiatal hernia.**

Possible Side Effects

▼ Most common: dry mouth, decreased sweating, and constipation.

▼ Less common: difficulty urinating, blurred vision, enlarging of the pupils, worsening of glaucoma, palpitations, drowsiness, sleeplessness, weakness, nausea, vomiting, bloating, impotence (male), reduced production of breast milk (women), and skin rash or itching.

Drug Interactions

• Oxybutynin may interact with other phenothiazines, some antihistamines, and other anticholinergic drugs to produce increased drug side effects. Oxybutynin may also increase the effects of nervous-system depressants such as alcohol, tranquilizers, antihistamines, barbiturates, pain medicines, and anticonvulsants.

• Oxybutynin may reduce the effect of Haloperidol and increase the chances for some Haloperidol side effects.

• Oxybutynin may increase the blood levels of Digoxin, increasing the chances for developing Digoxin side effects.

Food Interactions

Take this drug with food or milk if it upsets your stomach.

Usual Dose

Adult and Adolescent: 10 to 20 mg per day in divided doses.

Child (age 6 and older): 10 to 15 mg per day in divided doses.

Overdosage

Oxybutynin overdose symptoms may include restlessness, tremors, irritability, convulsions, hallucinations, flushing, fever, nausea, vomiting, rapid heartbeat, blood-pressure changes, respiratory failure, paralysis, delirium, and coma. Victims should be taken to a hospital emergency room at once. ALWAYS bring the prescription bottle.

Special Information

Oxybutynin may interfere with your vision and your ability to concentrate. Be careful while driving or doing anything that requires concentration and clear vision.

Your eyes may become more sensitive to bright light while taking Oxybutynin; wearing sunglasses or protective lenses should help lessen this problem.

Dry mouth may be treated with sugarless gum, candy, or ice chips. Excessive mouth dryness can lead to tooth decay and should be brought to your dentist's attention if it lasts for more than 2 weeks.

If you forget to take a dose of Oxybutynin, take it as soon as you remember. If it is almost time for your next dose, skip the missed dose and continue with your regular schedule. Do not take a double dose.

Special Populations

Pregnancy/Breast-feeding

The safety of Oxybutynin use by pregnant women is not known. It should only be used when its benefits outweigh the possible damage it might do.

It is not known if Oxybutynin passes into breast milk. Nursing mothers should use this drug with caution.

Seniors

Older adults may be more susceptible to the side effects of Oxybutynin and should take it with caution.

Generic Name

Paclitaxel

Brand Name

Taxol

Type of Drug

Antineoplastic drug.

Prescribed for

Ovarian and breast cancer, after other treatments have failed. This drug is also being studied for cancers of the head and neck, lung, upper gastrointestinal tract, and prostate (that does not respond to hormone treatments) and leukemias.

General Information

Paclitaxel is a natural substance that interferes with the process of cell division in cancerous cells. It is important to remember that this drug is recommended for use only in people who have not responded to other treatments. People who receive this drug will be premedicated with other drugs such as Diphenhydramine and Cimetidine or Ranitidine to minimize some side effects.

Studies in ovarian cancer indicated that 22 to 30 percent of women receiving the drug responded. Of a total of 92 women studied, there were 6 complete and 18 partial responses. The average survival for all people taking the drug was between 8 and 16 months. In breast cancer, studies showed response rates ranging from 26 and 30 percent to 57 percent; survival averaged almost 1 year.

Cautions and Warnings

This drug must be prescribed by a physician who is experienced in the use of cancer chemotherapies. Management of drug complications is possible only when **adequate treatment facilities** are available.

Severe drug sensitivity reactions, including **breathing difficulty; low blood pressure (dizziness or fainting); swelling of the face, hands, feet, genitals,** or **internal organs;** and **generalized itching** and **rashes** have occurred in 2 of every 100 people taking this drug. **People who experience these kinds of reactions *should not* receive this drug again.**

Bone-marrow suppression is the major toxic effect of Paclitaxel. People with **low white-blood-cell counts** should not receive Paclitaxel.

Fewer than 1 of every 100 people who take this drug

develop **severe heart problems** and may require additional cardiac therapy while continuing to receive this drug.

This drug is broken down in the liver and should be used with caution in people with **severe liver disease.**

Possible Side Effects

▼ Most common: reduced blood-cell counts, anemia, infections, drug sensitivity reactions, dizziness or fainting, changes in EKG (electrocardiogram) measurements, muscle or joint pains, nausea and vomiting, diarrhea, mouth sores, liver inflammation, hair loss, numbness, tingling or burning in the hands or feet, and swelling or retention of fluid.

▼ Less common: bleeding, blood in the urine, bruising or black, tarry stool, severe sensitivity reactions, and slow heartbeat.

▼ Rare: severe heart problems and nail changes.

Drug Interactions

• When given together with Cisplatin, another antineoplastic drug, side effects were worse when Paclitaxel was given after Cisplatin than before it.

• Ketoconazole may reduce the rate at which Paclitaxel is broken down in the body, increasing the possibility of drug side effects.

Food Interactions

Paclitaxel can be taken without regard to food or meals.

Usual Dose

Adult: Paclitaxel is given by intravenous injection. Dosage is individualized according to body surface area.

Child: not recommended.

Overdosage

There is little information on Paclitaxel overdose, but exaggerated side effects would be expected.

Special Information

It is important that your care is closely supervised by your doctor while receiving this medicine.

Avoid receiving any immunizations or vaccinations while taking this drug, unless approved by your doctor.

Avoid exposure to people with a bacterial or viral infection, especially when your blood counts are likely to be low. Check with your doctor at the first sign of any cold or infection. Don't touch the inside of your mouth or nose unless you have first washed your hands.

Call your doctor if you experience any unusual bleeding or bruising, black or tarry stools, blood in the urine or stool, or pinpoint red spots on the skin.

Be careful about dental hygiene (brushing or flossing) while on this drug because of the possibility of introducing bacteria into your system. Check with your doctor before you have any dental work done, and make sure your dentist knows you are receiving cancer chemotherapy.

Take care to avoid accidental cuts of your skin with a razor, fingernail, or other sharp objects. Avoid contact sports or other situations where bruising or injury could occur.

Special Populations

Pregnancy/Breast-feeding

Paclitaxel use can harm a developing fetus. Women taking this drug must be sure to use an effective contraceptive during treatment. If you are pregnant and must start taking this drug, discuss the possible hazards with your doctor.

It is not known if Paclitaxel passes into breast milk, but nursing mothers who must take this drug should bottle-feed their babies because of the possibility of toxic drug effects.

Seniors

Older adults may use this drug without special restriction.

Generic Name

Paroxetine

Brand Name

Paxil

Type of Drug

Selective serotonin reuptake inhibitor (SSRI)-type antidepressant.

Prescribed for

Depression.

General Information

Paroxetine and the other SSRIs (Fluvoxamine, Fluoxetine, and Sertraline) are chemically unrelated to the older tricyclic and tetracyclic antidepressant medicines. They work by preventing the movement of a neurohormone, *serotonin*, into nerve endings. This forces the serotonin to remain in the spaces surrounding nerve endings, where it works. Paroxetine is effective in treating common symptoms of depression. It can help improve your mood and mental alertness, increase physical activity, and improve sleep patterns. Tolerance to the effects of Paroxetine may develop over time. The drug takes between 1 and 4 weeks to start working, though you may experience some improvement in sleep patterns within 1 to 2 weeks. It stays in the body for several weeks, even after you stop taking it. This may be important when your doctor starts or stops treatment.

Unlike other SSRIs, Paroxetine does not have any weight-reducing effect.

Cautions and Warnings

Do not take Paroxetine if you are **allergic** to it. Allergies to other antidepressants should not prevent you from taking Paroxetine, because the drug is chemically different from other antidepressants.

A 2-week **drug-free period** should be allowed between Paroxetine and a **monoamine oxidase (MAO) inhibitor antidepressant.**

Paroxetine is broken down by your liver; therefore, people with **severe liver disease** should be cautious about taking this drug and should be treated with doses that are lower than normal.

People with **reduced kidney function** should take this drug with caution.

Studies in animals receiving doses 10 to 20 times the

maximum human dose revealed an increase in certain liver tumors and reduced fertility. The importance of this information to humans is not known.

A small number of **manic** or **hypomanic** patients may experience an activation of their condition while taking Paroxetine.

Paroxetine should be given with caution to patients who suffer from **seizure disorders**.

Paroxetine causes a reduced blood level of uric acid but has not caused kidney failure.

The possibility of **suicide** exists in severely depressed patients and may be present until the condition is significantly improved. Depressed patients should be allowed to carry only small quantities of Paroxetine with them to prevent overdose.

Possible Side Effects

Paroxetine side effects are generally mild, often related to the size of the dose you are taking, and occur mostly during the first week you take this medicine.

▼ Most common: headache, weakness, sleep disturbances, dizziness, and tremors.

▼ Common: nausea, sweating, dry mouth, constipation, decreased sex drive, abnormal ejaculations, blurred vision, and weight gain.

▼ Less common: flushing, pinpoint pupils, increased saliva, cold and clammy skin, dizziness when rising quickly from a sitting or standing position, blood-pressure changes, swelling around the eyes and in the arms or legs, coldness in the hands or feet, fainting and dizziness, rapid heartbeat, weakness, loss of coordination, unusual walk, changes in the general level of activity, migraines, droopy eyelids, acne, hair loss, dry skin, difficulty swallowing, stomach gas, joint pains, muscle pains, cramps and weakness, aggressiveness, abnormal dreaming or thinking, memory loss, apathy, delusions, a feeling of detachment, worsened depression, emotional instability, a "high" feeling, hallucinations, neurosis, paranoia, suicide attempts, teeth grinding, menstrual cramps or pain, bleeding between periods, coughing, bronchospasm,

Possible Side Effects *(continued)*

nosebleeds, breathing difficulty, conjunctivitis, double vision, difficulty accommodating to bright lights, eye pain, earaches, painful urination, facial swelling, frequent urination, nighttime urination, loss of urinary control, generalized swelling, a feeling of ill health, weight changes, and lymph swelling.

▼ Other: many other side effects affecting virtually every body system have been reported by people taking this medicine. They are too numerous to mention here but are considered infrequent or rare and affect only a small number of people.

In studies of Paroxetine before it was released in the United States, 15 percent of people taking it had to stop because of drug side effects. Be sure to report anything unusual to your doctor at once.

Drug Interactions

• Serious, sometimes fatal reactions may occur if Paroxetine and an MAO inhibitor are taken together (see *Cautions and Warnings*).

• People taking Warfarin may experience an increase in that drug's effect if they start taking Paroxetine and can experience a bleeding episode. Your doctor will have to reevaluate and/or adjust your Warfarin dosage.

• Paroxetine may decrease blood levels of Digoxin by 15 percent.

• Cimetidine increases blood levels of Paroxetine by about 50 percent when the drugs are taken together.

• Phenobarbital decreases the amount of Paroxetine in the blood and increases the rate at which it is released from the body.

• When taken together, Paroxetine and Phenytoin (for seizure disorders) can affect each other. The amount of both drugs in the blood can be decreased, and both can be released from the body more quickly than normal. Your doctor will adjust your drug dosage.

• Alcoholic beverages may increase the tiredness and other nervous-system-depressant effects of Paroxetine.

• People taking L-Tryptophan and Paroxetine together may develop agitation, restlessness, and upset stomach.

• People taking Paroxetine and Procyclidine (Kemadrin, for Parkinson's disease) experienced increased Procyclidine side effects. Your doctor may reduce your Procyclidine dosage if needed.

Food Interactions

This drug can be taken without regard to food or meals.

Usual Dose

10 to 50 mg once a day in the morning or at night.

Seniors, people with kidney or liver disease, and those taking several different medicines should remain at the lowest possible dosage for their condition.

Overdosage

In the 18 cases of Paroxetine overdose reported, all recovered completely. Symptoms of overdose are likely to be the most frequent drug side effects. There is no specific antidote for Paroxetine overdose. Any person suspected of having taken a Paroxetine overdose should be taken to a hospital emergency room for treatment at once, or you may call your local poison control center for information and directions. If you go to an emergency room, ALWAYS take the medicine bottle with you.

Special Information

Paroxetine can make you dizzy or drowsy. Take care when driving or doing other tasks that require alertness and concentration.

Do not drink alcoholic beverages if you are taking Paroxetine.

Be sure your doctor knows if you are pregnant, breast-feeding, or taking other prescription and nonprescription (over-the-counter) medications while taking Paroxetine. Notify your doctor of any unusual side effects.

If you forget a dose of Paroxetine, take it as soon as you remember. If it is almost time for your next dose, skip the forgotten dose and continue with your regular schedule. Do not take a double dose of Paroxetine.

Special Populations

Pregnancy/Breast-feeding
There are no good studies of the effect of Paroxetine on pregnant women. Do not take this drug if you are, or might become, pregnant without first seeing your doctor and reviewing the benefits of therapy against the risk of taking Paroxetine.

Paroxetine passes into breast milk in roughly the same concentration as it enters the blood. Nursing mothers should use another feeding method if they must take this medicine.

Seniors
Older adults tend to clear this drug more slowly from their bodies, but side-effect patterns are not affected. Any person with liver or kidney disease—problems that are more common among seniors—should receive a lower dose. Be sure to report any unusual side effects to your doctor.

Paxil

see *Paroxetine*, page 854

Brand Name

Pediazole

Ingredients
Erythromycin Ethylsuccinate + Sulfisoxazole

Other Brand Name
Eryzole

(Also available in generic form)

Type of Drug
Antibiotic/anti-infective combination.

Prescribed for
Middle-ear and sinus infections in children.

General Information

This combination of an antibiotic (Erythromycin) and sulfa drug (Sulfisoxazole) was specially formulated for its effect against *Haemophilus influenzae*, an organism responsible for many cases of difficult-to-treat middle-ear infections in children. Pediazole is also useful for a variety of other infections. Each teaspoonful of the medicine contains 200 mg of Erythromycin and 600 mg of Sulfisoxazole. Although the two drugs work by completely different mechanisms, they complement each other in the ways in which they attack different organisms. Pediazole is especially valuable in cases of *H. influenzae* middle-ear infection that do not respond to Ampicillin, a widely used and generally effective antibiotic.

Cautions and Warnings

Pediazole should not be given to **infants under 2 months** of age, because their body systems are not able to break down the Sulfisoxazole in this product. Children who are **allergic** to any **sulfa drug** or to any form of **Erythromycin** should not be given this product.

Possible Side Effects

It is possible for children given this combination product to develop any side effect known to be caused by either Erythromycin or Sulfisoxazole.

▼ Most common: upset stomach, cramps, drug allergy, and rashes.

▼ Less common: nausea, vomiting, and diarrhea. Pediazole may make your child more sensitive to sunlight, an effect that can last for many months after the medicine has been discontinued.

Drug Interactions

• Pediazole may increase the effects of Digoxin, Tolbutamide, Chlorpropamide, Methotrexate, Theophylline, Warfarin, Aspirin (or other salicylates), Phenylbutazone, Carbamazepine, Phenytoin, and Probenecid. Combining Pediazole with any of these drugs may result in an increase in drug side effects; a dosage adjustment of the interacting drug may be necessary.

Food Interactions

Pediazole is best taken on an empty stomach, at least 1 hour before or 2 hours after meals. However, if it causes stomach upset, have your child take each dose with food or meals. Be sure your child drinks lots of water while using Pediazole.

Usual Dose

The dosage of Pediazole depends on your child's body weight and varies from ½ to 2 teaspoons every 6 hours, usually for 10 days. Follow each dose of Pediazole with a full glass of water.

Overdosage

The strawberry/strawberry-banana flavoring of this product makes it a good candidate for accidental overdose, so be sure it is stored in the area of your refrigerator that is least accessible to your child. Pediazole overdosage is most likely to result in blood in the urine, nausea, vomiting, stomach upset and cramps, dizziness, headache, and drowsiness. Overdosage victims must be made to vomit as soon as possible with Syrup of Ipecac (available at any pharmacy) to remove any remaining drug from the stomach. Call your child's doctor or a poison control center before doing this. If you must go to a hospital emergency room, ALWAYS bring the medicine bottle with you.

Special Information

This product must be stored under refrigeration and discarded after 2 weeks. Be sure it is labeled with an expiration date when you leave the pharmacy.

Do not stop giving your child this medicine when symptoms disappear. It must be taken for the complete course of treatment prescribed by your doctor.

Call your child's doctor if nausea, vomiting, diarrhea, stomach cramps, discomfort (especially after giving the dosage with meals or food), or other symptoms persist. These symptoms may mean that your child is unable to tolerate this antibiotic and will have to receive different therapy. Severe or unusual side effects should be reported to the doctor at once. Especially important are yellow discoloration of the eyes or skin, darkening of the urine, pale stools, or unusual tiredness, which can all be signs of liver irritation.

If your child misses a dose of Pediazole, give it as soon as possible. If it is almost time for the next dose, space the missed dose and the next dose by 2 to 4 hours and then continue with your child's regular schedule.

Generic Name

Pemoline

Brand Names

Cylert
Cylert Chewable

Type of Drug

Psychotherapeutic.

Prescribed for

Children with attention deficit disorder (ADD) who are also in a program of social, psychological, and educational counseling. It may also be prescribed to treat daytime sleepiness.

General Information

This drug stimulates the central nervous system, although its exact action in children with ADD is not known. It should always be used as part of a total therapeutic program and only when prescribed by a qualified physician trained to treat ADD.

Cautions and Warnings

People who are **allergic** or **sensitive** to Pemoline should not use it. **Children under age 6** should not take this medication. Psychotic children may get worse while taking it. People on this drug should have **periodic liver function tests**.

Possible Side Effects

▼ Less common: sleeplessness, appetite loss, stomachache, rash, irritability, depression, nausea, dizziness, headache, drowsiness, and hallucinations.

Possible Side Effects *(continued)*

▼ Rare: drug hypersensitivity, wandering eye, and uncontrolled movements of the lips, face, tongue, and extremities.

Drug Interactions

• Pemoline decreases the seizure threshold and may increase the dosage requirement for anticonvulsant medications.

• Pemoline increases the effects of other nervous-system stimulants, causing nervousness, irritability, sleeplessness, and other effects.

Food Interactions

Take this medicine with food if it causes stomach upset.

Usual Dose

37.5 to 75 mg per day; not more than 112.5 mg per day.

Overdosage

Symptoms of overdosage are rapid heartbeat, hallucinations, agitation, uncontrolled muscle movements, and restlessness. Overdose victims must be taken to a hospital emergency room. ALWAYS bring the medicine bottle.

Special Information

Take your daily dose at the same time each morning. Taking Pemoline too late in the day can result in trouble sleeping. Call your doctor if this happens.

If you forget a dose of Pemoline, take it as soon as possible. If it is time for your next dose, skip the missed dose and continue with your regular schedule. Do not take a double dose.

Special Populations

Pregnancy/Breast-feeding

This drug crosses into the fetal blood circulation. Animal studies have shown that large Pemoline doses can cause stillbirths and reduce newborn survival. When the drug is considered essential by your doctor, its potential benefits must be carefully weighed against its risks.

This drug passes into breast milk but has caused no problems among breast-fed infants. Nursing mothers who take Pemoline should watch their babies for possible drug side effects.

Generic Name

Penbutolol

Brand Name

Levatol

Type of Drug

Beta-adrenergic-blocking agent.

Prescribed for

High blood pressure.

General Information

Penbutolol is one of 14 beta-adrenergic-blocking drugs that interfere with the action of a specific part of the nervous system. Beta receptors are found all over the body and affect many body functions. This accounts for the usefulness of beta blockers against a wide variety of conditions. The first member of this group, *Propranolol,* was found to affect the entire beta-adrenergic portion of the nervous system. Newer beta blockers have been refined to affect only a portion of that system, making them more useful in the treatment of cardio-vascular disorders and less useful for other purposes. Other beta blockers are mild stimulants to the heart or have other characteristics that make them more useful for a specific purpose or better for certain people.

Cautions and Warnings

You should be **cautious about taking Penbutolol** if you have **asthma**, **severe heart failure**, a **very slow heart rate**, or **heart block** because the drug may aggravate these conditions.

People with **angina** who take Penbutolol for high blood pressure should have their **drug dosage reduced gradually** over 1 to 2 weeks rather than suddenly discontinued to avoid possible aggravation of the angina.

Penbutolol should be used with caution if you have **liver or kidney disease**, because your ability to eliminate this drug from your body may be impaired.

Penbutolol reduces the amount of blood pumped by the heart with each beat. This reduction in blood flow can aggravate or worsen the condition of people with **poor circulation** or **circulatory disease**.

If you are undergoing **major surgery**, your doctor may want you to stop taking Penbutolol at least 2 days before surgery to permit the heart to respond more acutely to things that happen during the surgery. This is still controversial and may not hold true for all people preparing for surgery.

Possible Side Effects

Side effects are usually mild, relatively uncommon, develop early in the course of treatment, and are rarely a reason to stop taking Penbutolol.

▼ Most common: male impotence.

▼ Less common: unusual tiredness or weakness, slow heartbeat, heart failure (swelling of the legs, ankles, or feet), dizziness, breathing difficulty, bronchospasm, mental depression, confusion, anxiety, nervousness, sleeplessness, disorientation, short-term memory loss, emotional instability, cold hands and feet, constipation, diarrhea, nausea, vomiting, upset stomach, increased sweating, urinary difficulty, cramps, blurred vision, skin rash, hair loss, stuffy nose, facial swelling, aggravation of lupus erythematosus (a disease of the body's connective tissues), itching, chest pains, back or joint pains, colitis, drug allergy (fever, sore throat), and liver toxicity.

Drug Interactions

• Penbutolol may interact with surgical anesthetics to increase the risk of heart problems during surgery. Some anesthesiologists recommend gradually stopping your medicine 2 days before surgery.

• Penbutolol may interfere with the normal signs of low blood sugar and can interfere with the action of oral antidiabetes medicines.

• Penbutolol enhances the blood-pressure-lowering effects of other blood-pressure-reducing agents (including Clonidine, Guanabenz, and Reserpine) and calcium-channel-blocking drugs (such as Nifedipine).

• Aspirin-containing drugs, Indomethacin, Sulfinpyrazone, and estrogen drugs can interfere with the blood-pressure-lowering effect of Penbutolol.

• Cocaine may reduce the effects of all beta-blocking drugs.

• Penbutolol may increase the cold hands and feet associated with taking ergot alkaloids (for migraine headaches). People taking an ergot and Penbutolol may develop gangrene.

• Penbutolol will counteract the effects of thyroid-hormone-replacement medicines.

• Calcium channel blockers, Flecainide, Hydralazine, oral contraceptives, Propafenone, Haloperidol, phenothiazine tranquilizers (Molindone and others), quinolone antibacterials, and Quinidine may increase the amount of Penbutolol in the bloodstream and the effect of that drug on the body.

• Penbutolol should not be taken within 2 weeks of taking a monoamine oxidase (MAO) inhibitor antidepressant drug.

• Cimetidine increases the amount of Penbutolol absorbed into the bloodstream from oral tablets.

• Penbutolol may interfere with the effectiveness of Theophylline, Aminophylline, and some antiasthma drugs (especially Ephedrine and Isoproterenol).

• The combination of Penbutolol and Phenytoin or digitalis drugs can result in excessive slowing of the heart, possibly causing heart block.

• If you stop smoking while taking Penbutolol, your dose may have to be reduced because your liver will break down the drug more slowly after you stop.

Food Interactions

Penbutolol may be taken without regard to food or meals.

Usual Dose

20 mg once a day. Seniors may require more or less medication and must be carefully monitored by their doctors. Those with liver problems may require less medicine.

Overdosage

Symptoms of overdosage are changes in heartbeat (unusually slow, unusually fast, or irregular), severe dizziness or fainting, difficulty breathing, bluish-colored fingernails or palms, and seizures. The overdose victim should be taken to a hospital emergency room where proper therapy can be given. ALWAYS bring the medicine bottle.

Special Information

Penbutolol is meant to be taken continuously. Do not stop taking it unless directed to do so by your doctor; abrupt withdrawal may cause chest pain, difficulty breathing, increased sweating, and unusually fast or irregular heartbeat. The dose should be lowered gradually over a period of about 2 weeks.

Call your doctor at once if any of the following symptoms develop: back or joint pains, difficulty breathing, cold hands or feet, depression, skin rash, or changes in heartbeat. Penbutolol may produce an undesirable lowering of blood pressure, leading to dizziness or fainting. Call your doctor if this happens to you. Call your doctor about the following side effects only if they persist or are bothersome: anxiety, diarrhea, constipation, sexual impotence, headache, itching, nausea or vomiting, nightmares or vivid dreams, upset stomach, trouble sleeping, stuffy nose, frequent urination, unusual tiredness, or weakness.

Penbutolol can cause drowsiness, light-headedness, dizziness, or blurred vision. Be careful when driving or performing complex tasks.

It is best to take your medicine at the same time each day. If you forget a dose of Penbutolol, take it as soon as you remember. If it is within 8 hours of your next dose, skip the forgotten tablet and continue with your regular schedule. Do not take a double dose.

Special Populations

Pregnancy/Breast-feeding

Infants born to women who took a beta blocker weighed less at birth and had low blood pressure and reduced heart rate. Penbutolol should be avoided by pregnant women and those who might become pregnant while taking it. When the drug is considered essential by your doctor, its potential benefits must be carefully weighed against its risks.

It is not known if Penbutolol passes into breast milk. Therefore, nursing mothers taking this medicine should bottle-feed their babies.

Seniors

Older adults may absorb and retain more Penbutolol in their bodies, thus requiring less medicine. Your doctor will need to adjust your dosage to meet your individual needs. Seniors taking this medicine may be more likely to suffer from cold hands and feet, reduced body temperature, chest pains, general feelings of ill health, sudden breathing difficulty, increased sweating, or changes in heartbeat.

Type of Drug

Penicillin Antibiotics

Brand Names

Generic Name: Amoxicillin*

Amoxil	Biomox	Trimox
Amoxil Chewables	Polymox	Wymox

Generic Name: Amoxicillin and Potassium Clavulanate

Augmentin	Augmentin Chewable

Generic Name: Ampicillin*

D-Amp	Polycillin	Totacillin
Omnipen	Principen	

Generic Name: Ampicillin with Probenecid

Polycillin-PRB	Probampacin

Generic Name: Bacampicillin

Spectrobid

Generic Name: Carbenicillin Indanyl Sodium

Geocillin

Generic Name: Cloxacillin Sodium*

Cloxapen	Tegopen

Generic Name: Dicloxacillin Sodium*

Dycill	Dynapen	Pathocil

Generic Name: Nafcillin

Unipen

Generic Name: Oxacillin*

Bactocill	Prostaphlin

Generic Name: Penicillin G*

Pentids

Generic Name: Penicillin V (Phenoxymethyl Penicillin)*

Beepen-VK	Penicillin VK	Robicillin VK
Betapen-VK	Pen-Vee	V-Cillin K
Ledercillin VK	Pen-Vee K	Veetids

(*Also available in generic form)

Prescribed for

Bacterial and other infections susceptible to the individual antibiotic.

General Information

Penicillin-type antibiotics fight infection by killing bacteria and other micro-organisms. They do this by destroying the cell walls of the invading organisms. Other antibiotics simply prevent the invading organisms from reproducing. Many infections can be treated with almost any kind of Penicillin, but some can be treated only by a specific Penicillin antibiotic.

Penicillin cannot cure a cold, flu, or any other viral infection, and should never be taken unless prescribed by a doctor for a specific illness. Always take your antibiotic exactly according to your doctor's directions, including the number of pills to take every day and the number of days to take the medicine. If you do not follow directions, you will not get the antibiotic's full benefit.

Cautions and Warnings

Serious and sometimes fatal **allergic reactions** have occurred with Penicillin. Although this is more common following injection of the drug, it has occurred with Penicillin taken by mouth and is more common among people with a **history of sensitivity** to this or another **Penicillin antibiotic** or those who suffer from **multiple allergies**. About 5 percent of people who are allergic to a Penicillin antibiotic will also be allergic to the cephalosporins.

Some **Penicillin drug reactions** can be treated with **antihistamines** and other medicines. In a small number of cases where the infection is life threatening and can be treated only with Penicillin, minor reactions may be treated with other medicines while the Penicillin is continued. Generally, though, other drugs can be substituted to treat the infection.

Cystic fibrosis patients are more likely to suffer from drug side effects to some Penicillins.

Possible Side Effects

The most important Penicillin side effect, seen in up to 10 percent of people who take these antibiotics, is drug allergy. These reactions are more common among people who have had a previous reaction to Penicillin and those who have had asthma, hay fever, or other allergies. Some of the allergic symptoms include itching, rash, swelling, breathing difficulty, very low blood pressure, blood vessel collapse, skin peeling, and other severe reactions, including chills, fever, muscle aches, arthritis-like pains, and feelings of ill health.

About 9 percent of Ampicillin users develop an itching rash, which is not a true allergic reaction. This is more common if they are also taking Allopurinol (15 to 20 percent).

▼ Common: upset stomach, abdominal pain, nausea, vomiting, diarrhea, colitis, sore mouth, coated tongue, anemias, bleeding abnormalities, low platelet and white blood cell counts, and oral or rectal fungal infections.

▼ Less common: vaginal irritation, appetite loss, itchy eyes, and feelings of body warmth.

▼ Rare: yellowing of the skin or eyes.

Possible Side Effects *(continued)*

People who receive injectable Penicillin may become lethargic, dizzy, or tired, or may experience hallucinations, seizures, anxiety, depression, confusion, agitation, or hyperactivity.

Drug Interactions

• Penicillin should not be given together with a bacteriostatic antibiotic such as Chloramphenicol, Erythromycin, Tetracycline, or Neomycin, which may diminish the effectiveness of Penicillin.

• Penicillin may interfere with the effectiveness of oral contraceptive drugs.

• Penicillin allergic reactions may be intensified by beta-blocking drugs.

• Ampicillin may reduce the effect of Atenolol by interfering with its absorption into the blood.

• Large doses of injectable Penicillin can increase the effect of anticoagulant (blood-thinning) drugs.

Food Interactions

Do not take Penicillin with fruit juice or carbonated beverages, because the acid in these beverages can destroy the drug.

Most of the Penicillins, including Bacampicillin suspension, are best absorbed on an empty stomach. These medications can be taken 1 hour before or 2 hours after meals, or first thing in the morning and last thing at night with the other doses spaced evenly through the day.

Amoxicillin, Amoxicillin and Potassium Clavulanate, and Bacampicillin tablets can be taken without regard to food.

Usual Dose

Amoxicillin
Adult: 250 to 500 mg every 8 hours.
Child: 10 to 20 mg per pound per day, divided into 3 doses.

Amoxicillin and Potassium Clavulanate
Adult: a "250" or "500" tablet every 8 hours.
Child: 10 to 20 mg per pound per day divided into 3 doses.

Ampicillin
Adult: 1 to 12 grams daily, divided into 4 to 6 doses.
Child: 25 to 100 mg per pound per day, divided into 4 to 6 doses.

Ampicillin with Probenecid
3.5 grams of Ampicillin and 1 gram of Probenecid as a single dose for gonorrhea.

Bacampicillin
Adult: 400 to 800 mg every 12 hours; 1,600 mg plus 1 gram of Probenecid for gonorrhea.
Child: 12 to 25 mg per pound per day, divided into 2 doses.

Carbenicillin Indanyl Sodium
Adult: 382 to 764 mg 4 times per day.
Child: not recommended.

Cloxacillin Sodium
Adult: 250 mg every 6 hours.
Child: 25 mg per pound per day, divided into 4 doses.

Dicloxacillin Sodium
Adult: 125 to 250 mg every 6 hours.
Child: 6 to 12 mg per pound per day, divided into 4 doses.

Nafcillin
Adult: 250 to 1,000 mg every 4 to 6 hours.
Child: 5 to 25 mg per pound every 6 to 8 hours.

Oxacillin
Adult: 500 to 1,000 mg every 4 to 6 hours.
Child: 25 to 50 mg per pound per day, divided into 4 or 6 doses.

Penicillin G
Adult: 200,000 to 800,000 units (125 to 500 mg) every 6 to 8 hours for 10 days.
Child (under age 12): 12,000 to 40,000 units per pound per day, divided into 3 to 6 doses.

Penicillin V
Adult: 125 to 500 mg 4 times per day. People with severe kidney disease should not take more than 250 mg every 6 hours.

Child (under age 12): 12 to 25 mg per pound per day, divided into 3 or 4 doses.

Overdosage

Penicillin overdose is unlikely, but if it occurs, diarrhea and upset stomach are the primary symptoms. Massive overdose can result in seizures or excitability. Call your local poison control center or emergency room for more information. ALWAYS bring the medicine bottle with you if you go for treatment.

Special Information

Oral Penicillin liquids should be refrigerated (the bottle should be labeled to that effect) and must be discarded after 14 days in the refrigerator or 7 days at room temperature.

Call your doctor if you develop black tongue, skin rash, itching, hives, diarrhea, wheezing, breathing difficulty, sore throat, nausea, vomiting, fever, swollen joints, unusual bleeding or bruising, or feelings of ill health.

It takes 7 to 10 days for Penicillin to eradicate most susceptible organisms; be sure to take all the medicine prescribed for the full period prescribed. It is best taken at evenly spaced intervals throughout the entire day.

If you miss a dose of a Penicillin antibiotic, take it as soon as possible. If it is almost time for your next dose, space the missed dose and your next dose by 2 to 4 hours and then continue with your regular schedule.

Special Populations

Pregnancy/Breast-feeding
Penicillin has not caused birth defects and is often prescribed for pregnant women. These drugs cross into fetal blood circulation and should be used only if absolutely necessary. Make sure your doctor knows you are taking a Penicillin antibiotic if you are or might become pregnant.

Penicillin is generally safe during breast-feeding; however, small amounts may pass into breast milk and cause upset stomach, diarrhea, allergic reactions, or other problems in the nursing infant.

Seniors
Seniors may take Penicillin without special restriction.

Generic Name

Pentoxifylline

Brand Name

Trental

Type of Drug

Blood-viscosity reducer.

Prescribed for

Relief of intermittent claudication (blood-vessel spasms and painful leg cramps) caused by poor blood supply associated with arteriosclerotic disease. Pentoxifylline has also been used to treat psychopathological symptoms, cases of inadequate blood flow to the brain, and other blood-vessel disease. It has been studied for treating the complications of diabetes, leg ulcers, transient attacks of low blood supply to the brain, strokes, sickle-cell disease, high-altitude sickness, weak sperm and low sperm counts, hearing disorders, and eye circulation disorders.

General Information

Pentoxifylline reduces blood viscosity (thickness) and improves the ability of red blood cells to modify their shape. In doing so, this medication may help people who experience severe leg pains when they walk by improving blood flow to their leg muscles. Leg cramps occur when muscles are deprived of oxygen. When blood flow is improved, the cramps are less severe or may not occur at all. Studies of Pentoxifylline's effectiveness have yielded mixed results, but the drug may be helpful for people who do not respond to other treatments.

Physical exercise and training is probably a better treatment for intermittent claudication than Pentoxifylline. However, the medicine may help people who cannot follow a training program and who are not candidates for surgery, which is another treatment for this condition.

Cautions and Warnings

People who cannot tolerate **Caffeine, Theophylline,** or **Theo-**

bromine should not use this medicine, since Pentoxifylline is chemically related to those products. The dosage of Pentoxifylline should be reduced in people with **kidney disease.**

Possible Side Effects

Side effects are relatively infrequent.

▼ Most common: mild nausea, upset stomach, dizziness, and headache.

▼ Less common: chest pains, difficulty breathing, arm or leg swelling, low blood pressure, stomach gas, loss of appetite, constipation, dry mouth, excessive thirst, tremors, anxiety, confusion, stuffy nose, nosebleeds, flulike symptoms, sore throat, laryngitis, swollen glands, itching, rash, brittle fingernails, blurred vision, conjunctivitis ("pink-eye"), earache, a bad taste in the mouth, feelings of ill health, and changes in body weight.

▼ Rare: rapid or abnormal heart rhythms, hepatitis (yellow discoloration of the skin or eyes), reduced white-blood-cell count, and small hemorrhages under the skin.

Drug Interactions

• Pentoxifylline may increase the blood-pressure-lowering effects of other medicines. Your doctor may have to change the dosage of your blood-pressure medicines.

• Pentoxifylline may increase the effects of Warfarin.

Food Interactions

You may take this drug with food if it upsets your stomach.

Usual Dose

400 mg 2 to 3 times per day.

Overdosage

The severity of overdose symptoms is directly related to the amount of drug taken. Symptoms usually appear 4 to 5 hours after the medicine was taken and can last for about 12 hours. Some of the reported effects of Pentoxifylline overdose are flushing, low blood pressure, fainting, depression, and convulsions. Overdose victims must be made to vomit with Syrup of Ipecac (available at any pharmacy) as soon as possible to remove any remaining drug from their stomach. Call your doctor or a poison control center before doing this. If you must go to a hospital emergency room, ALWAYS bring the medicine bottle with you.

Special Information

Call your doctor if any side effects develop. Some people may have to stop using this medicine if side effects become intolerable. You may feel better within 2 weeks after starting on Pentoxifylline, but the treatments should be continued for at least 2 months to gain maximum benefit.

If you forget to take a dose of Pentoxifylline, take it as soon as you remember. If it is almost time for your next dose, skip the one you forgot and continue with your regular schedule. Do not take a double dose.

Special Populations

Pregnancy/Breast-feeding

Pentoxifylline crosses into fetal blood circulation but has not been found to cause birth defects. When the drug is considered essential by your doctor, its potential benefits must be carefully weighed against its risks.

Pentoxifylline passes into breast milk and may affect breast-fed infants. Nursing mothers who must take this medicine should bottle-feed their babies.

Seniors

Older adults, especially those with kidney disease, are more sensitive to the effects of this drug because they absorb more and eliminate it more slowly than do younger adults. Follow your doctor's directions, and report any side effects at once.

Pepcid

*see **Famotidine**, page 428*

Brand Name
Percocet

Ingredients

Acetaminophen + Oxycodone Hydrochloride

Other Brand Names

Roxicet	Roxilox	Tylox

(Also available in generic form)

Type of Drug

Narcotic-analgesic combination.

Note: The information in this profile also applies to:

Brand Name

Tylenol with Codeine

Ingredients

Acetaminophen + Codeine Phosphate

Other Brand Names

Aceta with Codeine	Capital with Codeine	Phenaphen with Codeine

(Also available in generic form)

Brand Names

Vicodin	Vicodin-ES

Ingredients

Acetaminophen + Hydrocodone Bitartrate

Other Brand Names

Actagesic ES	Bancap HC	Dolacet
Amacodone	Ceta-Plus	Duocet
Anexsia	Co-Gesic	Duradyne DHC

Hydrogesic	Lorcet Plus	Panacet
Hy-Phen	Lortab	Stagesic
Lorcet	Margesic H	T-Gesic
Lorcet HD	Norcet	Zydone

Prescribed for

Relief of mild to moderate pain.

General Information

Percocet is generally prescribed for those who require a greater analgesic effect than Acetaminophen alone can deliver and/or for those who are allergic to, or cannot take, Aspirin.

Percocet is probably not effective for arthritis or other pain caused by inflammation because it does not reduce inflammation.

Cautions and Warnings

Do not take Percocet if you are **allergic** or **sensitive** to it. Use this drug with extreme caution if you suffer from **asthma** or other **breathing problems** or if you have **kidney** or **liver disease** or **viral infections of the liver**. Long-term use of Percocet may cause **drug dependence** or **addiction**.

Oxycodone is a respiratory depressant and affects the central nervous system, producing **sleepiness, tiredness,** and/or **inability to concentrate**. Be careful if you are driving, operating hazardous or complicated machinery, or performing other functions requiring concentration.

Alcohol may increase the chances of Acetaminophen-related liver toxicity and Oxycodone-related drowsiness.

Possible Side Effects

▼ Most common: light-headedness, dizziness, sleepiness, nausea, vomiting, loss of appetite, and increased sweating. If any of these effects occur, consider asking your doctor to lower your dosage. Most of these side effects will disappear if you simply lie down. More serious side effects are shallow breathing or difficulty in breathing.

Possible Side Effects *(continued)*

▼ Rare: euphoria (feeling "high"), weakness, headache, agitation, uncoordinated muscle movement, minor
hallucinations, disorientation and visual disturbances,
dry mouth, constipation, facial flushing, rapid heartbeat,
palpitations, faintness, urinary difficulties or hesitancy,
reduced sex drive and/or potency, skin rash or itching,
anemia, lowered blood sugar, and yellowing of the skin
or eyes. Narcotic pain relievers may aggravate convulsions in those who have had convulsions in the past.

Drug Interactions

• Because of its depressant effect and potential effect on
breathing, Percocet should be taken with extreme care in
combination with alcohol, sleeping medicine, tranquilizers,
antihistamines, or other drugs producing sedation.

Food Interactions

Percocet is best taken with food or at least half a glass of
water to prevent stomach upset.

Usual Dose

Percocet
Adult: 1 or 2 tablets every 4 hours.
Child: not recommended.

Tylenol with Codeine
Adult and Adolescent (age 13 and older): 1 to 2 tablets
every 4 hours.
Child (age 7 to 12): equivalent to 5 to 10 mg of Codeine
every 4 to 6 hours; not to exceed 60 mg in 24 hours.
Child (age 2 to 6): equivalent to 2.5 to 5 mg of Codeine every
4 to 6 hours; not to exceed 30 mg in 24 hours.

Vicodin
Adult: 1 tablet every 6 hours.
Child: not recommended.

Overdosage

Symptoms are depression of respiration (breathing), extreme

tiredness progressing to stupor and then coma, pinpointed
pupils, no response to pain stimulation (such as a pin stick),
cold and clammy skin, slowing of the heart rate, lowering of
blood pressure, yellowing of the skin or eyes, bluish discoloration of the hands or feet, fever, excitement, delirium,
convulsions, cardiac arrest, and liver toxicity (nausea, vomiting, pain in the abdomen, and diarrhea). The overdose victim
should be made to vomit with Syrup of Ipecac (available at
any pharmacy) and be taken to a hospital emergency room
immediately. ALWAYS bring the medicine bottle with you.

Special Information

Percocet is a respiratory depressant that affects the central
nervous system, producing sleepiness, tiredness, and/or inability to concentrate. Be careful if you are driving, operating
hazardous or complicated machinery, or performing other
functions requiring concentration.

If you forget to take a dose of Percocet, take it as soon as
you remember. If it is almost time for your next dose, skip the
forgotten dose and continue with your regular medication
schedule. Do not take a double dose.

Special Populations

Pregnancy/Breast-feeding

High doses of Acetaminophen, one of the ingredients in
Percocet, have caused some problems when taken during
pregnancy. The regular use of Oxycodone, the other active
ingredient in Percocet, during pregnancy can cause the unborn child to become addicted. If used during labor, it can
cause breathing problems in the infant. If you are pregnant,
or may be pregnant, do not take Percocet.

The ingredients in Percocet may pass into breast milk. If
you must take it, wait 4 to 6 hours after taking the drug before
breast-feeding, or consider bottle-feeding your baby.

Seniors

Seniors may be sensitive to the depressant effects of the
narcotic pain reliever in this combination. Follow your doctor's directions, and report any side effects at once.

Brand Name

Percodan

Ingredients

Aspirin + Oxycodone Hydrochloride + Oxycodone
Terephthalate

Other Brand Names

Oxycodone with Aspirin
Percodan-Demi
Roxiprin

(Also available in generic form)

Note: The information in this profile also applies to:

Brand Name

Empirin with Codeine

(Also available in generic form)

Ingredients

Aspirin + Codeine

Brand Name

Synalgos-DC Capsules

(Also available in generic form)

Ingredients

Aspirin + Caffeine + Dihydrocodeine Bitartrate

Type of Drug

Narcotic-aspirin combination.

Pentazocine, another narcotic pain reliever, may be prescribed
for mild to moderate pain. Pentazocine may be addicting, and
you should observe many of the same warnings with this

drug as with any Codeine-containing medicine. Pentazocine is available in the following combinations:

Brand Names

Talacen (Pentazocine with Acetaminophen)
Talwin Compound (Pentazocine with Aspirin)
Talwin Nx (Pentazocine with Naloxone)

Prescribed for

Relief of mild to moderate pain.

General Information

Percodan is one of many combination products containing both a narcotic and a nonnarcotic analgesic. It is prescribed for people who need the combination of pain relief and inflammation reduction offered by Percodan.

Cautions and Warnings

Do not take Percodan if you know you are **allergic** or **sensitive** to it. Use this medication with extreme caution if you suffer from **asthma** or any other **breathing problems**. Long-term use of this drug may cause **drug dependence** or **addiction**. Percodan is a respiratory depressant and affects the central nervous system, producing **sleepiness, tiredness,** and/or **inability to concentrate.**

Do not take this product if you are **allergic** to any salicylate, including **Aspirin,** or any **nonsteroidal anti-inflammatory drug** (NSAID). Check with your doctor or pharmacist if you are not sure. This and all other Aspirin-containing products should not be taken by **children under age 17.**

People with **liver damage** should avoid Percodan and all products that contain either Aspirin or Oxycodone.

Alcoholic beverages can aggravate the **stomach irritation** caused by Aspirin. The risk of Aspirin-related ulcers is increased by alcohol. Alcohol will also increase the **nervous-system depression** caused by the Oxycodone ingredient in this drug.

Do not use Percodan if you develop **dizziness, hearing loss,** or **ringing or buzzing in your ears.**

Percodan can interfere with normal **blood coagulation** and should be avoided for 1 week before **surgery.** Ask your surgeon and dentist for their recommendation before taking an Aspirin-containing product for pain after surgery.

Possible Side Effects

▼ Most common: light-headedness, dizziness, sleepiness, nausea, vomiting, loss of appetite, and increased sweating. If these occur, consider calling your doctor to ask about lowering your dosage. Usually they will go away if you simply lie down.

▼ Less common: shallow breathing or serious difficulty in breathing, euphoria (feeling "high"), weakness, headache, agitation, uncoordinated muscle movement, minor hallucinations, disorientation, visual disturbances, dry mouth, loss of appetite, constipation, facial flushing, rapid heartbeat, palpitations, faintness, urinary difficulties or hesitancy, reduced sex drive and/or potency, skin rashes or itching, anemia, low blood sugar, and yellowing of the skin or eyes. These drugs may aggravate convulsions in those who have had convulsions.

Drug Interactions

• Interaction with alcohol, tranquilizers, barbiturates, or sleeping pills produces sleepiness or inability to concentrate, and seriously increases the depressive effect of Percodan.

• The Aspirin component of Percodan can affect anticoagulant (blood-thinning) therapy. Discuss this with your doctor so that the proper dosage adjustment can be made.

• Interaction with adrenal corticosteroids, Phenylbutazone, or alcohol can cause severe stomach irritation with possible bleeding.

• The Aspirin component of Percodan will counteract the uric-acid-eliminating effect of Probenecid and Sulfinpyrazone; may counteract the blood-pressure-lowering effect of the angiotensin-converting-enzyme (ACE) inhibitor and beta-blocking drugs and the effects of some diuretics when given to people with severe liver disease; and may increase blood levels of Methotrexate and of Valproic Acid when taken together, leading to increased chances of drug toxicity.

• The Aspirin component of Percodan, when taken with

Nitroglycerin tablets, may lead to an unexpected drop in blood pressure.

• Do not take Percodan together with any NSAID. There is no benefit from the combination, and the chance of side effects, especially stomach irritation, is vastly increased.

• Large doses of Aspirin (2000 mg per day or more) can lower blood sugar, which can be a serious problem in diabetics. Percodan tablets contain 325 mg of Aspirin.

Food Interactions

Take with food or ½ glass of water to prevent stomach upset.

Usual Dose

Percodan
Adult: 1 tablet every 6 hours as needed for relief of pain.
Child: not recommended.

Empirin with Codeine
Adult: 1 to 2 tablets, 3 to 4 times per day.
Child: not recommended.

Synalgos-DC
Adult: 2 capsules every 4 hours.
Child: not recommended.

Overdosage

Symptoms of Oxycodone (a component of Percodan) overdosage are breathing difficulty, extreme tiredness progressing to stupor and then coma, pinpointed pupils, no response to pain stimulation (such as a pin stick), cold and clammy skin, slowing of the heartbeat, dizziness or fainting, convulsions, and cardiac arrest.

Severe Aspirin (a component of Percodan) overdose may cause fever, excitement, confusion, convulsions, liver or kidney failure, or bleeding. Symptoms of mild Aspirin overdosage are rapid and deep breathing, nausea, vomiting, dizziness, ringing or buzzing in the ears, flushing, increased sweating, thirst, headache, drowsiness, diarrhea, and rapid heartbeat.

The overdose victim should be taken to a hospital emergency room immediately. ALWAYS bring the medicine bottle with you.

Special Information

Drowsiness may occur: Be careful when driving or operating complicated or hazardous machinery.

Contact your doctor if you develop continuous stomach pain or a ringing or buzzing in the ears.

Do not use an Aspirin product such as Percodan if it has a strong odor of vinegar. This is an indication that the product has started to break down in the bottle.

If you forget a dose of Percodan, take it as soon as you remember. If it is almost time for your next dose, skip the one you forgot and continue with your regular schedule. Do not take a double dose.

Special Populations

Pregnancy/Breast-feeding

Check with your doctor before taking any Aspirin-containing product during pregnancy, including Percodan. Aspirin can cause bleeding problems in the developing fetus, particularly during the last 2 weeks of pregnancy. Taking Aspirin during the last 3 months of pregnancy may lead to a low-birth-weight infant, prolong labor, and extend the length of pregnancy; it can also cause bleeding in the mother before, during, or after delivery.

Oxycodone, the other ingredient in Percodan, has not been associated with birth defects, but taking too much of any other narcotic during pregnancy can lead to the birth of a drug-dependent infant and drug-withdrawal symptoms in the baby. All narcotics can cause breathing problems in the newborn if taken just before delivery.

The ingredients in these products may pass into breast milk. Consider bottle-feeding your baby if you must take this drug.

Seniors

The Oxycodone in this combination product may have more of a depressant effect on seniors than on younger adults. Other effects that may be more prominent are dizziness, light-headedness, and fainting, particularly upon rising suddenly from a sitting or lying position.

Generic Name

Pergolide Mesylate

Brand Name

Permax

Type of Drug

Antiparkinsonian.

Prescribed for

Parkinson's disease.

General Information

Pergolide is combined with Levodopa or Carbidopa to control Parkinson's disease. It works by stimulating a specific nerve ending in the central nervous system that is normally stimulated by the hormone *dopamine*. Pergolide also inhibits the production of a hormone called *prolactin*, which is involved in the production of breast milk. Pergolide affects growth-hormone levels and the reproductive hormone called *luteinizing hormone* (LH).

Cautions and Warnings

If you have had a **previous reaction** to Pergolide or other drugs derived from the **fungus ergot,** do not take this drug.

Pergolide may cause **hallucinations** in about 14 percent of people who take it. **Report this to your doctor at once.**

People who are prone to **abnormal heart rhythms** should be cautious when taking Pergolide because of possible cardiac side effects.

Female animals given Pergolide develop **tumors of the uterus,** but there is no information on this effect in humans.

Possible Side Effects

Pergolide can affect virtually any body part or system because of its effect on basic body hormones. In studies

---

Possible Side Effects *(continued)*

of the drug, about 1 in 4 people who started on Pergolide stopped because of side effects.

▼ Most common: hallucinations, confusion, abnormal twisting body movements, tiredness, difficulty sleeping, nausea, constipation, diarrhea, upset stomach, and runny nose.

▼ Less common: generalized pain, abdominal pain, neck or back pain, migraine headaches, muscle weakness, chest pain, flu-like illness, chills, facial swelling, infections, dizziness when rising from a sitting or lying position, fainting, heart palpitations, blood-pressure changes, abnormal heart rhythms, heart attack, heart failure, appetite changes, dry mouth, vomiting, stomach gas, yellow discoloration of the skin or eyes, enlarged saliva glands, stomach irritation, intestinal ulcer or obstruction, gum irritation, tooth cavities, colitis, loss of bowel control, blood in the stool, vomiting blood, bursitis, muscle twitching, anxiety, tremors, depression, unusual dreams, personality changes, psychosis, changes in how you walk, loss of coordination, tingling in the hands or feet, speech problems, muscle stiffness, difficulty breathing, hiccups, pneumonia, coughing, sinus irritation, bronchitis, asthma, nosebleeds, rash, skin discoloration, skin ulcers, acne, fungal infections, eczema, hair growth or loss, cold sores, increased sweating, vision abnormalities (double vision, conjunctivitis, cataracts, retinal detachment, blindness, eye pain), earaches, middle-ear infection, ringing or buzzing in the ears, deafness, taste changes, frequent or painful urination, urinary infection, blood in the urine, swelling of the arms or legs, weight gain, anemia, breast pain, painful menstruation, breast oozing, underactive thyroid, thyroid tumor, diabetes, and muscle, bone, and joint pains.

Drug Interactions

• Many drugs will counter the effect of Pergolide, including the phenothiazines, the thioxanthenes, Haloperidol, Droperidol, Loxapine, Methyldopa, Molindone, Papaverine, Reserpine, and Metoclopramide, because they all antagonize the neurohormone dopamine.

- Alcohol, tranquilizers, and other nervous-system depressants will increase the depressant effects of this drug.
- Drugs that cause low blood pressure will exaggerate the blood-pressure-lowering effect of Pergolide.

Food Interactions

Take Pergolide with food or meals if it upsets your stomach.

Usual Dose

Start at 0.05 mg per day and gradually increase by 0.1 to 0.25 mg every third day until an effect is achieved, up to 5 mg per day.

Overdosage

Symptoms of a Pergolide overdosage may include nausea, vomiting, agitation, low blood pressure, hallucinations, involuntary body and muscle movements, tingling in the arms or legs, heart palpitations, abnormal heart rhythms, and nervous-system stimulation. Overdose victims should be taken to a hospital emergency room for treatment. ALWAYS bring the medicine bottle with you.

Special Information

Many people taking Pergolide for the first time experience dizziness and fainting caused by low blood pressure. Your doctor will need to gradually increase your Pergolide dose to reduce this effect. However, any dizziness or fainting should be reported to your doctor at once.

Other Pergolide side effects to report to the doctor include any nervous-system effects (confusion, uncontrolled body movements, hallucinations), pain or burning on urination, high blood pressure, severe headache, seizures, sudden vision changes, severe chest pain, fainting, rapid heartbeat, severe nausea, excessive sweating, nervousness, unexplained shortness of breath, and sudden weakness. In addition, make sure your doctor knows about any side effect that is particularly bothersome or persistent.

Do not stop taking Pergolide or change your dose without your doctor's knowledge. It is important to maintain regular contact with your doctor to allow for observation of the drug effects and side effects.

People taking Pergolide must be careful when performing tasks requiring concentration and coordination (such as driving); this drug can make them tired, dizzy, or light-headed.

Dry mouth usually can be relieved by using sugarless gum, candy, ice, or a saliva substitute. Pay special attention to oral hygiene while you are taking Pergolide because dry mouth increases the chances of oral infections.

If you take Pergolide once a day and forget a dose, take it as soon as you remember. If it is almost time for your next dose, skip the one you forgot and continue with your regular schedule. Do not take a double dose.

If you take Pergolide 2 or 3 times a day and forget a dose, take it as soon as you remember. If it is almost time for your next dose, take one dose as soon as you remember and another in 3 or 4 hours, then go back to your regular schedule. Do not take a double dose.

Special Populations

Pregnancy/Breast-feeding
Pregnant women and those who might become pregnant should not use Pergolide unless its advantages have been carefully weighed against its possible dangers.

Pergolide interferes with milk production. Nursing mothers who must take Pergolide should bottle-feed their babies.

Seniors
Older adults may take Pergolide without special restriction.

Phenergan

see **Promethazine Hydrochloride**, page 943

Generic Name
Phenobarbital

Brand Names

Solfoton

(Also available in generic form)

Type of Drug

Hypnotic; sedative; anticonvulsant.

Prescribed for

Epileptic and other seizures; convulsions; daytime sedation; sleeplessness; eclampsia (toxemia in pregnancy).

General Information

Phenobarbital is a long-acting barbiturate. It takes 30 to 60 minutes to start working, and its effect lasts for 10 to 16 hours. Like other barbiturates, Phenobarbital appears to act by interfering with nerve impulses to the brain. When used as an anticonvulsant, Phenobarbital is not very effective by itself, but when used with anticonvulsant agents such as Phenytoin, the combined action is dramatic. This combination has been used very successfully to control epileptic seizures.

Cautions and Warnings

Phenobarbital may dull your **physical and mental reflexes**, so you must be extremely careful when **driving** or doing anything that requires total concentration.

Phenobarbital can be **addicting** if taken for an extended period of time. It can also cause signs of intoxication, including **slurred speech**, a **wobbly walk**, **rolling of the eyes**, **confusion**, **poor judgment**, **irritability**, and **sleeplessness**. Mixing this drug with **alcohol** worsens the situation.

Barbiturates are broken down in the liver and eliminated through the kidneys. Thus, people with **liver or kidney disease** should be cautious about taking Phenobarbital.

You should not take Phenobarbital if you are **sensitive** or **allergic** to any barbiturate, if you have been addicted to **sedatives** or **hypnotics**, or if you have a **respiratory condition**.

People with **chronic pain** should be careful about taking this drug because it can mask some symptoms or cause stimulation, although using Phenobarbital after surgery and in people with cancer has proven effective.

People abruptly stopping this drug can develop **seizures**. Dosage should be reduced gradually.

Barbiturates can increase your need for **vitamin D**. A standard vitamin supplement will take care of this problem.

Possible Side Effects

▼ Most common: drowsiness, lethargy, dizziness, drug "hangover," breathing difficulty, skin rash, and general allergic reactions (such as runny nose, watery eyes, and scratchy throat).

▼ Less common: nausea, vomiting, constipation and diarrhea, slow heartbeat, low blood pressure, and fainting. More severe adverse reactions may include anemia and yellowing of the skin and eyes.

Drug Interactions

• Alcohol, monoamine oxidase (MAO) inhibitor antidepressants, and Valproic Acid increase the effects of Phenobarbital.

• Charcoal, Chloramphenicol, and Rifampin can counteract the effects of Phenobarbital.

• Phenobarbital interferes with the effects of anticoagulant (blood-thinning) drugs, beta-blocker drugs, Carbamazepine, Chloramphenicol, oral contraceptive pills, Corticosteroids, Clonazepam, Digitoxin, Doxorubicin, Doxycycline, Felodipine, Fenoprofen, Griseofulvin, Metronidazole, Phenylbutazone, Quinidine, Theophylline, and Verapamil.

• Phenobarbital enhances the toxic effects of Acetaminophen and Methoxyflurane (an anesthetic).

• Phenobarbital has a variable effect on Phenytoin and other antiseizure medicines and on narcotic drugs. If you are taking one of these drug combinations, your doctor will have to balance your dosages based on the amount of all drugs in the blood.

Food Interactions

Phenobarbital is best taken on an empty stomach, but may be taken with food if it upsets your stomach.

Usual Dose

Anticonvulsant

Adult: 50 to 100 mg 2 to 3 times per day.

Child: 1.3 to 2.25 mg per pound of body weight divided into 2 or 3 doses a day.

Sleeplessness
100 to 320 mg at bedtime.

Daytime Sedation
30 to 120 mg in 2 to 3 divided doses.

Overdosage

Severe barbiturate overdosage can kill; barbiturates have been used many times in suicide attempts. Overdosage symptoms are difficulty breathing, moderate reduction in pupil size, lowered body temperature progressing to fever as time passes, fluid in the lungs, and, eventually, coma. Anyone suspected of having taken a barbiturate overdose must be taken to a hospital immediately. ALWAYS bring the medicine bottle with you.

Special Information

Avoid alcohol and other drugs that depress the nervous system while taking Phenobarbital.

Be sure to take this medicine exactly as prescribed by your doctor.

This drug causes drowsiness and poor concentration and makes it more difficult to drive a car or perform complicated activities.

Call your doctor at once if you develop fever, sore throat, nosebleeds, mouth sores, unexplainable black-and-blue marks, or easy bruising or bleeding.

If you forget to take a dose of Phenobarbital, take it as soon as you remember. If it is almost time for your next dose, skip the one you forgot and continue with your regular schedule. Do not take a double dose.

Special Populations

Pregnancy/Breast-feeding

Barbiturate use during pregnancy can increase the risk of birth defects. However, Phenobarbital may be necessary to control major seizures in some pregnant women. Regular use of a barbiturate during the last 3 months of pregnancy can cause the baby to be born dependent on the medicine. Also, barbiturate use increases the chance of bleeding problems, brain tumors, and breathing difficulties in the newborn. Talk to your doctor about your need to continue Phenobarbital during your pregnancy.

Barbiturates pass into breast milk and can cause drowsiness, slow heartbeat, and breathing difficulty in nursing infants. Nursing mothers who must take Phenobarbital should consider bottle-feeding their babies.

Seniors

Older adults are more sensitive to the effects of barbiturates and often need less medicine than younger adults. Follow your doctor's directions, and report any side effects at once.

Generic Name

Phenytoin

Brand Names

Extended-Action Products

Dilantin Kapseals
Phenytoin Sodium Extended

Prompt-Acting Products

Dilantin Infatab
Dilantin-30 Pediatric
  Suspension

Dilantin-125 Suspension
Diphenylan Sodium
Phenytoin Sodium

(Also available in generic form)

Type of Drug

Anticonvulsant.

Prescribed for

Control of epileptic seizures. Phenytoin may also be prescribed to prevent seizures following neurosurgery in people who don't usually take it, and to control abnormal heart rhythms, especially those caused by digitalis drugs. Phenytoin injection is used to control preeclampsia (a condition in which pregnant women experience severe increases in blood pressure during the second half of their pregnancy), trigeminal neuralgia (tic douloureux), and severe skin conditions characterized by the formation of large pustules.

General Information

Phenytoin is one of several hydantoin antiseizure drugs used to control certain seizure disorders. These drugs all act by affecting the same area of the brain, where the spread of seizure activity is inhibited. The hydantoins actually reduce the activity of that area of the brain responsible for grand mal seizures. People may respond to some hydantoins and not others, but the reason for this is not understood. Phenytoin is the most widely prescribed member of this group of drugs.

There are 2 kinds of Phenytoin: *prompt*, which must be taken several times a day, and *extended*, which can be taken either once or several times a day. Many people find the extended action more convenient, but the prompt product gives the doctor more flexibility in designing a daily dose schedule.

Phenytoin may or may not be used in combination with other anticonvulsants, like Phenobarbital.

Cautions and Warnings

Do not take Phenytoin if you are **allergic** to it or any other **hydantoin**.

If you have been taking Phenytoin for a long time and no longer need it, the **dosage should be reduced gradually** over a period of about a week. Stopping abruptly may bring on **severe epileptic seizures**.

Phenytoin should not be used if you have **low blood pressure, myocardial insufficiency,** a **very slow heart rate,** or other specific **heart problems.** The use of other hydantoins is not limited by these situations.

People with **liver disease** will eliminate Phenytoin more slowly from their bodies than people without liver disease, increasing the chances for drug side effects.

Your doctor will need to take blood tests periodically to be sure that **red- and white-blood-cell counts** have not been affected by Phenytoin. **Sore throat, feelings of ill health, fever, mucous-membrane bleeding, swollen glands, nosebleeds, black-and-blue marks,** and **easy bruising** may be signs of blood problems.

Skin rash may be a sign of a serious reaction and may be cause for stopping this medicine. **Tell your doctor** at once if this happens.

Possible Side Effects

▼ Most common: rapid or unusual growth of the gums, slurred speech, mental confusion, nystagmus (a rhythmic, uncontrolled movement of the eye), dizziness, insomnia, nervousness, uncontrollable twitching, double vision, tiredness, irritability, depression, tremors, and headaches. These side effects will generally disappear as therapy continues and the dosage is reduced.

▼ Less common: nausea, vomiting, diarrhea, constipation, fever, rashes, balding, weight gain, numbness in the hands or feet, chest pains, retention of water, sensitivity to bright light (especially sunlight), conjunctivitis ("pinkeye"), joint pain and inflammation, and high blood sugar.

▼ Other: Phenytoin can cause coarse facial features, lip enlargement, and Peyronie's disease (a condition where the penis is permanently deformed or misshapen). The skin rash seen with Phenytoin may be accompanied by fever and can be serious or fatal. Some fatal blood-system side effects have occurred with Phenytoin.

▼ Rare: liver damage (including hepatitis) or unusual hair growth over the body.

Drug Interactions

• The following drugs may increase the effects of Phenytoin, necessitating a possible decrease in Phenytoin dosage: alcoholic beverages (small amounts), Allopurinol, Amiodarone, Aspirin and other salicylate drugs, benzodiazepine tranquilizers and sedatives, Chloramphenicol, Chlorphiramine, Cimetidine, Disulfiram, Fluconazole, Ibuprofen, Isoniazid, Metronidazole, Miconazole, Omeprazole, Phenacemide, phenothiazine antipsychotic medicines, Phenylbutazone, succinimide antiseizure medicines, sulfa drugs, tricyclic antidepressants, Trimethoprim, and Valproic Acid.

• The following drugs may interfere with the effects of Phenytoin, necessitating a possible increase in Phenytoin dosage: alcoholic beverages (chronic alcoholism), antacids, anticancer drugs, barbiturates, Carbamazepine, Charcoal tablets, Diazoxide, Folic Acid, Influenza virus vaccine, Loxapine Succinate, Nitrofurantoin, Pyridoxine, Rifampin, Sucralfate, and Theophylline drugs.

• Phenytoin may increase the rate at which the following drugs are removed from the body, indicating a need for a possible increase in their dosage: Amiodarone, Carbamazepine, Digitalis drugs, corticosteroids, Dicumarol, Disopyramide, Doxycycline, Estrogen drugs, Haloperidol, Methadone, Metyrapone, Mexiletine, oral contraceptives, Quinidine, Theophylline drugs, and Valproic Acid.

• Phenytoin may increase the chances for liver toxicity from Acetaminophen, especially if you take Phenytoin regularly for a seizure disorder.

• Phenytoin may affect the following drugs, but the exact way in which these drugs are affected cannot be predicted. If you take Phenytoin and one or more of these medicines, your doctor will have to determine what dosage adjustments, if any, are needed: Cyclosporine, Dopamine, Furosemide, Levodopa, Levonorgestrel, Mebendazole, Phenothiazine antipsychotic medicines, or oral antidiabetes medicines.

• The results of taking Clonazepam and Phenytoin together are unpredictable. The effect of either drug may be reduced, or Phenytoin side effects may occur.

• Corticosteroid drugs may mask the effects of Phenytoin-sensitivity reactions.

• Lithium toxicity may be increased if that drug is taken together with Phenytoin.

• The pain-relieving effect of Meperidine may be decreased by Phenytoin, while the chances for Meperidine side effects may be increased. This combination is not recommended.

• Long-term Phenytoin therapy may result in extreme Folic Acid deficiency, known as *megaloblastic anemia*. This is correctable with Folic Acid supplements.

• The effect of Warfarin may be increased by adding Phenytoin. Warfarin dosage adjustment is necessary.

Food Interactions

Take Phenytoin with food or meals to avoid stomach upset. Avoid taking it with high-calcium foods (milk, cheese, almonds, hazelnuts, sesame seeds, etc); the amount of Phenytoin that is absorbed from the small intestine can be decreased if you eat these foods or take calcium supplements.

Usual Dose

Adult: initial dose, 300 mg per day. If this does not result in satisfactory control, gradually increase to up to 600 mg per day. (The most frequent maintenance dose is 300 to 400 mg per day.) Only the extended form of Phenytoin may be taken once daily; the prompt form must be taken throughout the day.

Child: initial dose, 2.5 mg per pound of body weight per day divided into 2 or 3 equal doses; then adjust according to the child's needs and response (normal maintenance dose, 2 to 4 mg per pound of body weight per day). Dilantin-30 has 30 mg of Phenytoin per teaspoon, and Dilantin-125 has 125 mg of Phenytoin per teaspoon. Children over age 6 may require the same dose as an adult, but no child should be given more than 300 mg per day.

Overdosage

Overdose symptoms are the same as those listed under *Possible Side Effects.* The victim should be taken to a hospital emergency room immediately. ALWAYS bring the medicine bottle with you.

Special Information

Contact your doctor immediately if you don't feel well or you develop a skin rash, severe nausea or vomiting, swollen glands, swollen or tender gums, yellowing of the skin or eyes, joint pain, sore throat, fever, unusual bleeding or bruising, persistent headache, infection, slurred speech, or poor coordination. Tell your doctor if you are pregnant.

Do not stop taking your medicine or change dosage without your doctor's knowledge.

Phenytoin can cause drowsiness, dizziness, or blurred vision, effects that are increased by alcoholic beverages. Be careful while driving or doing anything else that requires intense concentration, alertness, or physical dexterity.

Phenytoin sometimes produces a pink-brown color in the urine, which is normal and not a cause for concern. Diabetic patients who take Phenytoin must monitor their urine regularly and report any changes to their doctor.

Good oral hygiene, including gum massage, frequent brushing, and flossing, is very important because Phenytoin can cause abnormal growth of your gums.

Do not change brands of Phenytoin without notifying your doctor, because different brands may not be equivalent to each other and may not produce the same effect on your body. Dosage adjustment may be required if you do switch.

If you or your child takes Phenytoin suspension, you must vigorously shake the bottle immediately before you pour the medicine out.

Do not use Phenytoin capsules that have become discolored. They should be discarded.

If you take Phenytoin once a day and forget to take a dose, take it as soon as you remember. If it is almost time for your next dose, skip the one you forgot and continue with your regular schedule. Do not take a double dose.

If you take it several times a day and forget to take a dose, and you remember within 4 hours of your regular time, take it right away. If you do not remember until later, skip the forgotten dose and go back to your regular schedule. Do not take a double dose.

Special Populations

Pregnancy/Breast-feeding

Phenytoin crosses into the fetal blood circulation. The great majority of mothers who take Phenytoin deliver healthy, normal babies, but some are born with cleft lip, cleft palate, or heart malformations.

There is a recognized group of deformities, known as *fetal hydantoin syndrome*, that affect children of mothers taking Phenytoin (although it has not been definitely established as the cause of these deformities). Fetal hydantoin syndrome consists of abnormalities in the skull and face, small brain, growth deficiency, deformed fingernails, and mental deficiency. Children born of mothers taking Phenytoin are more likely to have a vitamin K deficiency, which can lead to serious, life-threatening hemorrhage during the first 24 hours of life. Also, the mother may be deficient in vitamin K because of Phenytoin, leading to increased bleeding during delivery.

Phenytoin passes into breast milk and may affect a nursing infant. Nursing mothers taking Phenytoin should bottle-feed their babies.

Seniors

Older adults break down this drug more slowly and are more sensitive to its side effects. Follow your doctor's directions, and report any side effects at once.

Generic Name

Pilocarpine

Brand Names

Adsorbocarpine Solution	Ocusert Pilo Ocular Therapeutic System	Pilopine HS Gel Piloptic Pilostat
Akarpine Solution		
Isopto Carpine Solution	Pilagan	Pilopto-Carpine
Ocu-Carpine	Pilocar Solution	Pilocarpine Nitrate

(Also available in generic form)

Type of Drug

Miotic agent.

Prescribed for

Glaucoma (increased pressure in the eye).

General Information

Pilocarpine ophthalmic solution is the drug of choice in the treatment of open-angle glaucoma. It works on muscles in the eye to open passages so fluid can flow out of the eye chamber, lowering fluid pressure inside the eye. Pilocarpine may also help reduce the amount of fluid produced within the eye.

This drug is usually prescribed for long periods of time, so long as eye pressure does not increase or eyesight does not worsen. The form and concentration of Pilocarpine are determined by the physician based on the severity of the disease. The usual concentration of the eyedrops is 0.5% to 4%. The most often used concentrations are 1% and 2%. Concentrations above 4% are used less often.

This drug is also available as a gel—Pilopine HS—and in a special form called Ocusert Pilo, a thin football-shaped wafer designed to continuously release the drug for 1 week. This eliminates the need for putting drops in your eyes 3 to 4 times per day. The wafer is placed under the eyelid, similar to the way contact lenses are placed. Pilocarpine is also available in many combination products, which may be useful in special circumstances.

Cautions and Warnings

Do not use Pilocarpine if you are **allergic** to it. It should be used **only when prescribed** by an ophthalmologist.

Possible Side Effects

▼ Common: stinging and burning in the eyes, blurred vision, and spasms of the eye muscles (resulting in a headachy feeling). You may also find it hard to focus your eyes. These effects are usually seen in younger people and will disappear with continued use. Some people may have trouble seeing in low light.

▼ Less common: allergy or itching and tearing of the eye may develop after prolonged use.

▼ Rare: detachment of the retina.

Although used as eyedrops, Pilocarpine may affect other parts of the body in rare instances, especially after long-term use. Possible effects are high blood pressure, rapid heartbeat, fluid in the lungs, bronchospasm, excessive sweating or salivation, nausea, vomiting, and diarrhea.

Drug and Food Interactions

None known.

Usual Dose

Eyedrops

Initial dose, 1 to 2 drops in the affected eye up to 6 times per day. Maintenance dose is based on severity of disease.

Gel

Apply a ½-inch ribbon of gel inside your lower eyelid at bedtime. If you use other eye medicines, apply them at least 5 minutes before using the gel.

Ocusert Pilo

Insert into eye sac and replace weekly.

Overdosage

After long-term use, small amounts of drug may be absorbed by the drainage systems of the eye. If symptoms of stomach upset, nausea, vomiting, diarrhea, or cramps appear, contact your doctor immediately. If you go to an emergency room for treatment, ALWAYS bring the medicine bottle with you.

If Pilocarpine is swallowed accidentally, the victim should be made to vomit with Syrup of Ipecac (available in any pharmacy). If toxic symptoms develop (tearing, drooling, nausea, vomiting, or diarrhea), take the victim to a hospital emergency room for treatment. ALWAYS bring the medicine bottle with you.

Special Information

When first prescribed, Pilocarpine is also placed in the healthy eye to keep it from becoming diseased.

If you use Pilocarpine eyedrops, be careful not to touch the eyelids or surrounding area with the dropper tip; otherwise you may contaminate the dropper and cause the medicine to become unsterile. Be sure you recap the bottle tightly in order to preserve the sterility of the medicine.

After placing drops in your eye you may feel a stinging sensation; this is normal with these solutions. You should not close your eyes tightly or blink more than normally; blinking removes the drops from the eye.

If you forget to take a dose of Pilocarpine, take it as soon as you remember. If it is almost time for your next dose, skip the one you forgot and continue with your regular schedule. Do not take a double dose.

Special Populations

Pregnancy/Breast-feeding

Check with your doctor before taking any drug if you are

pregnant. Pilocarpine should be used by a pregnant woman only when it is absolutely necessary.

It is not known if Pilocarpine passes into breast milk. Watch nursing infants for possible drug side effects.

Seniors

Older adults are more likely to develop some Pilocarpine side effects, particularly difficulty seeing in low light. Follow your doctor's directions, and report any side effects at once.

Generic Name

Pimozide

Brand Name

Orap

Type of Drug

Antipsychotic.

Prescribed for

Gilles de la Tourette's syndrome and chronic schizophrenia in people who have not responded to other medicines.

General Information

Pimozide works on very specific brain cells, those stimulated by the hormone *dopamine.* This activity allows Pimozide to be effective in reducing the verbal and physical expressions of Tourette's syndrome, including inappropriate noises, physical movements, and verbal statements. It should be used only by people with severe symptoms who cannot tolerate or do not respond to Haloperidol, the usual treatment for Tourette's syndrome. Pimozide may be prescribed for some cases of chronic schizophrenia, but it should be used only for those who do not also suffer from agitation, excitement, or hyperactivity.

Cautions and Warnings

Pimozide should be used only for the conditions listed above because of the risk for **cardiac** and **nervous-system side**

effects. It should not be used for acute schizophrenia or other psychiatric disorders that can be treated with other drugs. People taking Pimozide (especially older adults) are at risk for developing *tardive dyskinesia,* a group of symptoms that includes **rhythmic and involuntary movements of the tongue, jaw, face, or mouth** (puffing, chewing, puckering, etc). There is no treatment for tardive dyskinesia. The chance that these symptoms will occur and become permanent increases as the dose gets larger. If the drug is stopped at the first sign of involuntary movement, tardive dyskinesia may not develop.

People who are **sensitive** or **allergic** to Pimozide or to other **antipsychotic drugs** should avoid Pimozide. Those who are sensitive to Haloperidol, Loxapine, Molindone, and phenothiazine or thioxanthene antipsychotics may also be sensitive to Pimozide.

People with **heart disease** or **severe toxic depression** should use this drug with caution because of the possibility that Pimozide-related side effects will worsen those conditions.

Sudden **cardiac death** and **seizures** have occurred in Tourette's patients taking Pimozide at doses above 20 mg per day. Your doctor should do an electrocardiogram (EKG) before you start on Pimozide, and periodically thereafter, to monitor for signs that might lead to sudden cardiac problems. Dosage reduction at the first sign of EKG abnormalities can avoid serious problems.

A more serious set of side effects, known as *neuroleptic malignant syndrome* (NMS), has been associated with Pimozide. The symptoms that make up NMS include a **high fever, muscle rigidity, mental changes, irregular pulse or blood pressure, increased sweating,** and **abnormal heart rhythms.** NMS is potentially fatal and requires **immediate medical attention.**

Liver and kidney function are very important because Pimozide is removed from the body by these organs. Any loss of organ function must be compensated for by a smaller dose.

Possible Side Effects

Extrapyramidal effects (unusual body movements, twisting, unusual postures, restlessness, etc) often develop during the first few days of Pimozide treatment and

Possible Side Effects (continued)

generally go away if you stop taking the drug. The chance of developing these effects and their severity increases with increasing drug dosage; your doctor may prescribe additional medicines to counteract these side effects.

A potentially fatal group of symptoms called *neuroleptic malignant syndrome* (NMS) has been associated with Pimozide. See *Cautions and Warnings* for details.

A group of symptoms known as *tardive dyskinesia* can develop and worsen as treatment is continued and the dose is increased. See *Cautions and Warnings* for details.

▼ Other: dry mouth, constipation or diarrhea, excessive thirst, appetite changes, belching, salivation, nausea, vomiting, upset stomach, muscle tightness, cramps, posture changes, rigidity, headache, drowsiness or sedation, sleeplessness, speech and/or handwriting changes, dizziness, tremors, fainting, depression, excitement, nervousness, behavioral changes, visual or taste disturbances, unusual sensitivity to bright light, cataracts, spots before the eyes, swelling around the eyes, changes in urinary habits, male impotence, loss of sex drive, dizziness or fainting when rising suddenly from a sitting or lying position, blood-pressure changes, heart palpitations, chest pains, increased sweating, skin irritations, rash, body weight changes, menstrual disorders, and breast secretions.

Drug Interactions

• Antipsychotic drugs should be used with caution by people taking Pimozide because of the possibility of aggravating or bringing on tardive dyskinesia (see *Cautions and Warnings*).

• Pimozide may increase the medication needs of people with seizure disorders.

• Alcohol, tranquilizers, and other nervous-system depressants can increase Pimozide-related drowsiness or sedation.

• Amphetamines, Methylphenidate, and Pemoline should be stopped before starting Pimozide because they can cause abnormal muscle movements that may be confused with Tourette's syndrome.

• Antihistamines and other medicines with an anticholinergic (drying) effect should not be taken with Pimozide, because such a combination may produce more severe side effects (dry mouth, visual disturbances, urinary difficulty, etc).

• Tricyclic antidepressants, Disopyramide, Maprotiline, Quinidine, phenothiazines, and Procainamide may increase the chance of Pimozide cardiac side effects. These drugs and Pimozide should be used together only under a direct doctor's care. Phenothiazines may increase Pimozide's depressive and anticholinergic effects.

Food Interactions

Low blood-potassium levels may increase the risk of cardiac side effects associated with Pimozide. Be sure to eat enough potassium-rich foods (bananas, tomatoes, etc).

Usual Dose

Adult and Adolescent (age 12 and older): 1 to 2 mg per day to start, increasing gradually up to 10 mg.

Child (under age 12): Low doses with gradual increases are given; children are particularly sensitive to Pimozide.

Overdosage

Symptoms of overdosage are cardiac abnormalities, severe involuntary movements (see *Possible Side Effects*), low blood pressure, breathing difficulty, and coma. Pimozide overdose victims must be taken to a hospital emergency room at once. ALWAYS bring the medicine bottle with you.

Special Information

Pimozide can make you drowsy. Avoid alcohol, tranquilizers, and other drugs that can worsen that effect. Take care while driving or doing anything else that requires concentration.

To avoid dizziness, avoid rising rapidly from a sitting or lying position.

Dry mouth caused by Pimozide may increase the chance for dental cavities, oral infections, and gum disease. Dry mouth usually can be eliminated with sugarless gum, candy, ice, or a saliva substitute. Blood disorders associated with Pimozide may delay healing and cause oral bleeding.

Do not take more Pimozide than your doctor has prescribed. Visit your doctor regularly while taking this drug because of the need to monitor for cardiac or other drug side effects. Call your doctor if dry mouth lasts 2 weeks or more or if you develop any unusual side effect, including fever, dehydration, heart pains or abnormal rhythms, muscle rigidity, restlessness, involuntary movements, posture changes, or mood changes, or if other side effects are bothersome or unusually persistent.

If you forget to take a dose of Pimozide, take the forgotten dose as soon as you remember and divide the remaining doses equally throughout the rest of the day. Do not take a double dose.

Special Populations

Pregnancy/Breast-feeding

Some animal studies did not show an effect of Pimozide on fetal development, while others did. Pregnant women should not take Pimozide unless its advantages clearly outweigh its possible dangers.

Nursing mothers who must take Pimozide should bottle-feed their babies because of possible drug side effects.

Seniors

Older adults should receive lower doses of Pimozide because of increased sensitivity to drug side effects. Older adults, especially women, are more likely to develop tardive dyskinesia (see *Cautions and Warnings*) and Parkinson's disease while taking Pimozide.

Generic Name

Pindolol

Brand Name

Visken

(Also available in generic form)

Type of Drug

Beta-adrenergic-blocking agent.

Prescribed for

High blood pressure; abnormal heart rhythms; treating anti-psychotic drug side effects; stage fright and other anxieties.

General Information

Pindolol is one of 14 beta-adrenergic-blocking drugs that interfere with the action of a specific part of the nervous system. Beta receptors are found all over the body and affect many body functions. This accounts for the usefulness of beta blockers against a wide variety of conditions. The first member of this group, *Propranolol*, was found to affect the entire beta-adrenergic portion of the nervous system. Newer beta blockers have been refined to affect only a portion of that system, making them more useful in the treatment of cardio-vascular disorders and less useful for other purposes. Pindolol is a mild stimulant to the heart, which makes it more useful for certain people.

Cautions and Warnings

People with **angina** who take Pindolol for high blood pressure should have their **drug dosage reduced gradually** over 1 to 2 weeks rather than suddenly discontinued to avoid possible aggravation of the angina.

Pindolol should be used with caution if you have **liver or kidney disease** because your ability to eliminate this drug from your body may be impaired.

Pindolol reduces the amount of blood pumped by the heart with each beat. This reduction in blood flow can aggravate or worsen the condition of people with **poor circulation** or **circulatory disease**.

If you are undergoing **major surgery**, your doctor may want you to stop taking Pindolol at least 2 days before surgery to permit the heart to respond more acutely to things that happen during the surgery. This is still controversial and may not hold true for all people preparing for surgery.

Possible Side Effects

Side effects are usually mild, relatively uncommon, de-velop early in the course of treatment, and are rarely a reason to stop taking Pindolol.

Possible Side Effects *(continued)*

▼ Most common: male impotence.

▼ Less common: unusual tiredness or weakness, slow heartbeat, heart failure (swelling of the legs, ankles, or feet), dizziness, breathing difficulty, bronchospasm, mental depression, confusion, anxiety, nervousness, sleeplessness, disorientation, short-term memory loss, emotional instability, cold hands and feet, constipation, diarrhea, nausea, vomiting, upset stomach, increased sweating, urinary difficulty, cramps, blurred vision, skin rash, hair loss, stuffy nose, facial swelling, aggravation of lupus erythematosus (a disease of the body's connective tissues), itching, chest pains, back or joint pains, colitis, drug allergy (fever, sore throat), and liver toxicity.

Drug Interactions

• Pindolol may interact with surgical anesthetics to increase the risk of heart problems during surgery. Some anesthesiologists recommend gradually stopping your medicine 2 days before surgery.

• Pindolol may interfere with the normal signs of low blood sugar and can interfere with the action of oral antidiabetes medicines.

• Pindolol enhances the blood-pressure-lowering effects of other blood-pressure-reducing agents (including Clonidine, Guanabenz, and Reserpine) and calcium-channel-blocking drugs (such as Nifedipine).

• Aspirin-containing drugs, Indomethacin, Sulfinpyrazone, and estrogen drugs can interfere with the blood-pressure-lowering effect of Pindolol.

• Cocaine may reduce the effects of all beta-blocking drugs.

• Pindolol may increase the cold hands and feet associated with taking ergot alkaloids (for migraine headaches). Gangrene is a possibility in people taking an ergot and Pindolol.

• Pindolol will counteract the effects of thyroid hormone replacement medicines.

• Calcium channel blockers, Flecainide, Hydralazine, oral contraceptives, Propafenone, Haloperidol, phenothiazine tranquilizers (Molindone and others), quinolone antibacterials, and Quinidine may increase the amount of Pindolol in the bloodstream and the effect of that drug on the body.

- Pindolol should not be taken within 2 weeks of taking a monoamine oxidase (MAO) inhibitor antidepressant drug.
- Cimetidine increases the amount of Pindolol absorbed into the bloodstream from oral tablets.
- Pindolol may interfere with the effectiveness of Theophylline, Aminophylline, and some antiasthma drugs (especially Ephedrine and Isoproterenol).
- The combination of Pindolol and Phenytoin or digitalis drugs can result in excessive slowing of the heart, possibly causing heart block.
- If you stop smoking while taking Pindolol, your dose may have to be reduced because your liver will break down the drug more slowly after you stop.

Food Interactions

Pindolol may be taken without regard to food or meals.

Usual Dose

10 to 60 mg per day.

Overdosage

Symptoms of overdosage are changes in heartbeat (unusually slow, unusually fast, or irregular), severe dizziness or fainting, difficulty breathing, bluish-colored fingernails or palms, and seizures. The overdose victim should be taken to a hospital emergency room, where proper therapy can be given. ALWAYS bring the medicine bottle.

Special Information

Pindolol is meant to be taken continuously. Do not stop taking it unless directed to do so by your doctor; abrupt withdrawal may cause chest pain, difficulty breathing, increased sweating, and unusually fast or irregular heartbeat. The dose should be lowered gradually over a period of about 2 weeks.

Call your doctor at once if any of the following symptoms develop: back or joint pains, difficulty breathing, cold hands or feet, depression, skin rash, or changes in heartbeat. Pindolol may produce an undesirable lowering of blood pressure, leading to dizziness or fainting. Call your doctor if this happens to you. Call your doctor about the following side effects only if they persist or are bothersome: anxiety, diarrhea, constipation, sexual impotence, headache, itching, nausea or vomiting, nightmares or vivid dreams, upset stomach, trouble sleeping, stuffy nose, frequent urination, unusual tiredness, or weakness.

Pindolol can cause drowsiness, blurred vision, dizziness, and light-headedness. Be careful when driving or performing complex tasks.

It is best to take your medicine at the same time each day. If you forget a dose of Pindolol, take it as soon as you remember. If you take your medicine once a day, and it is within 8 hours of your next dose, skip the forgotten tablet and continue with your regular schedule. If you take your medicine twice a day, and it is within 4 hours of your next dose, skip the forgotten dose and continue with your regular schedule. Do not take a double dose.

Special Populations

Pregnancy/Breast-feeding

Infants born to women who took a beta blocker weighed less at birth and had low blood pressure and reduced heart rate. Pindolol should be avoided by pregnant women and those who might become pregnant while taking it. When the drug is considered essential by your doctor, its potential benefits must be carefully weighed against its risks.

Pindolol passes into breast milk, but problems are rare. Still, nursing mothers taking it should bottle-feed their babies.

Seniors

Older adults may absorb and retain more Pindolol, thus requiring less medicine to achieve the same results. Your doctor will need to adjust your dosage to meet your individual needs. Seniors taking this medicine may be more likely to suffer from cold hands and feet, reduced body temperature, chest pains, general feelings of ill health, sudden breathing difficulty, increased sweating, or changes in heartbeat.

Generic Name

Pirbuterol Acetate

Brand Name

Maxair Inhaler

Type of Drug

Bronchodilator.

Prescribed for

Asthma and bronchospasm.

General Information

Pirbuterol is available only as an inhalation. It may be taken in combination with other medicines to control your asthma. The drug starts working within 5 minutes after it is taken and continues to work for 5 hours. It can be used when necessary to treat an asthmatic attack or on a regular basis to prevent one.

Cautions and Warnings

Pirbuterol should be used with caution if you have had **angina, heart disease, high blood pressure,** a history of **stroke or seizures, diabetes, prostate disease,** or **glaucoma.**

Using excessive amounts of Pirbuterol can lead to **increased difficulty breathing,** instead of providing breathing relief. In the most extreme cases, people have had **heart attacks** after using excessive amounts of inhalant.

Possible Side Effects

Pirbuterol's side effects are similar to those associated with other bronchodilator drugs.

▼ Most common: shakiness, nervousness and tension, headache.

▼ Less common: restlessness, weakness, anxiety, confusion, depression, fatigue, fainting, abdominal cramps or pains, low blood pressure, numbness in the hands or feet, weight gain, weakness, fear, tension, tremors, sleeplessness, convulsions, dizziness, headache, flushing, loss of appetite, unusual tastes or smells, pallor, sweating, nausea, vomiting, diarrhea, dry mouth, cough, muscle cramps, angina, abnormal heart rhythms, and heart palpitations.

Drug Interactions

• Pirbuterol's effects may be enhanced by monoamine oxidase (MAO) inhibitor drugs, antidepressants, thyroid drugs, other bronchodilators, and some antihistamines.

• Pirbuterol may antagonize the effects of blood-pressure-lowering drugs, especially Reserpine, Methyldopa, and Guanethidine.

• The chances of cardiac toxicity may be increased in people taking Pirbuterol and Theophylline.

• Pirbuterol is antagonized by the beta-blocking drugs (Propranolol and others).

Food Interactions

Pirbuterol does not interact with food, since it is taken only by inhalation into the lungs.

Usual Dose

Adult and Child (over age 12): 1 to 2 inhalations (0.2 mg each) every 4 to 6 hours. Do not take more than 12 inhalations per day.

Overdosage

Pirbuterol overdosage can result in exaggerated side effects, including heart pains and high blood pressure, although the pressure can drop after a short period of elevation. People who inhale too much Pirbuterol should see a doctor, who may prescribe a beta-blocking drug like Atenolol or Metoprolol to counter the bronchodilator's effects.

Special Information

The drug should be inhaled during the second half of your breath. This allows the medicine to reach more deeply into your lungs.

Be sure to follow your doctor's directions for using Pirbuterol, and do not take more than 12 inhalations of Pirbuterol each day. Using more medicine than is prescribed can lead to drug tolerance and actually cause your condition to worsen. If your condition worsens instead of improving after using your medicine, stop taking it and call your doctor at once.

Call your doctor at once if you develop chest pains, rapid heartbeat or heart palpitations, muscle tremors, dizziness,

headache, facial flushing, or urinary difficulty, or if you still
have trouble breathing after using the medicine.

If you forget a dose of Pirbuterol, take it as soon as you
remember and then continue with your regular schedule. Do
not take a double dose or take more than your doctor has
prescribed.

Special Populations

Pregnancy/Breast-feeding
Pirbuterol should be used by a pregnant or breast-feeding
woman only when it is absolutely necessary. The potential
benefit of using this medicine must be weighed against the
potential, but unknown, hazard it can pose to your baby.

It is not known if Pirbuterol passes into breast milk. Nursing
mothers must observe their infants for any possible drug
effect while taking this medication. You may want to consider
using an alternate feeding method.

Seniors
Older adults are more sensitive to the effects of this drug.
Follow your doctor's directions closely, and report any side
effects at once.

Generic Name
Piroxicam

Brand Name
Feldene

(Also available in generic form)

Type of Drug
Nonsteroidal anti-inflammatory drug (NSAID).

Prescribed for
Rheumatoid arthritis, juvenile rheumatoid arthritis, osteoarthritis, menstrual pain, and sunburn treatment.

General Information
Piroxicam is one of 16 nonsteroidal anti-inflammatory drugs
(NSAIDs) used to relieve pain and inflammation. We do not

know exactly how NSAIDs work, but part of their action may be due to an ability to inhibit the body's production of a hormone called *prostaglandin* and to inhibit the action of other body chemicals, including cyclo-oxygenase, lipoxygenase, leukotrienes, lysosomal enzymes, and a host of other factors. NSAIDs are generally absorbed into the bloodstream fairly quickly. Pain relief comes within an hour after taking the first dose of Piroxicam and lasts for 2 to 3 days, but its anti-inflammatory effect takes a lot longer (several days to 2 weeks) to become apparent, and may take 3 weeks to reach its maximum effect. Piroxicam is broken down in the liver and eliminated through the kidneys.

Cautions and Warnings

People who are **allergic** to Piroxicam (or any other NSAID) and those with a history of **asthma** attacks brought on by an NSAID, Iodides, or Aspirin should not take Piroxicam.

Piroxicam can cause **gastrointestinal (GI) bleeding, ulcers, and stomach perforation.** This can occur at any time, with or without warning, in people who take chronic Piroxicam treatment. People with a history of active GI bleeding should be cautious about taking any NSAID. Minor stomach upset, distress, or gas is common during the first few days of treatment with Piroxicam. People who develop bleeding or ulcers and continue treatment should be aware of the possibility of developing more serious drug toxicity.

Piroxicam can affect platelets and **blood clotting** at high doses, and should be avoided by people with clotting problems and by those taking Warfarin.

People with **heart problems** who use Piroxicam may experience **swelling in their arms, legs, or feet.**

Piroxicam can cause severe toxic effects to the **kidney.** Report any unusual side effects to your doctor, who may need to test your kidney function periodically.

Piroxicam can make you unusually **sensitive to the effects of the sun** (photosensitivity).

Possible Side Effects

▼ Most common: diarrhea, nausea, vomiting, constipation, stomach gas, stomach upset or irritation, and loss of appetite.

Possible Side Effects *(continued)*

▼ Less common: stomach ulcers, GI bleeding, hepatitis, gallbladder attacks, painful urination, poor kidney function, kidney inflammation, blood and protein in the urine, dizziness, fainting, nervousness, depression, hallucinations, confusion, disorientation, tingling in the hands or feet, light-headedness, itching, increased sweating, dry nose and mouth, heart palpitations, chest pain, difficulty breathing, and muscle cramps.

▼ Rare: severe allergic reactions, including closing of the throat, fever and chills, changes in liver function, jaundice (yellowing of the skin or eyes), and kidney failure. People who experience such effects must be promptly treated in a hospital emergency room or doctor's office.

NSAIDs have caused severe skin reactions; if this happens to you, see your doctor immediately.

Drug Interactions

• Piroxicam can increase the effects of oral anticoagulant (blood-thinning) drugs such as Warfarin. You may take this combination, but your doctor may have to reduce your anticoagulant dose.

• Taking Piroxicam with Cyclosporine may increase the toxic kidney effects of both drugs. Methotrexate toxicity may be increased in people also taking Piroxicam.

• Piroxicam may reduce the blood-pressure-lowering effect of beta blockers and loop diuretic drugs.

• Piroxicam may increase blood levels of Phenytoin, leading to increased Phenytoin side effects. Blood-Lithium levels may be increased in people taking Piroxicam.

• Piroxicam blood levels may be affected by Cimetidine because of that drug's effect on the liver.

• Probenecid may interfere with the elimination of Piroxicam from the body, increasing the chances for Piroxicam toxic reactions.

• Aspirin and other salicylates may decrease the amount of Piroxicam in your blood. These medicines should never be taken at the same time.

Food Interactions

Take Piroxicam with food or a magnesium/aluminum antacid if it upsets your stomach.

Usual Dose

Adult: 20 mg per day. Take each dose with a full glass of water and don't lie down for 15 to 30 minutes after you take the medicine.

Child: not recommended.

Overdosage

People have died from NSAID overdoses. The most common signs of overdosage are drowsiness, nausea, vomiting, diarrhea, abdominal pain, rapid breathing, rapid heartbeat, increased sweating, ringing or buzzing in the ears, confusion, disorientation, stupor, and coma.

Take the victim to a hospital emergency room at once. ALWAYS bring the medicine bottle.

Special Information

Check with your pharmacist if you are unsure about whether you may or may not crush or chew Piroxicam.

Piroxicam can make you drowsy and/or tired: Be careful when driving or operating hazardous equipment. Do not take any nonprescription products with Acetaminophen or Aspirin while taking this drug; also, avoid alcoholic beverages.

Contact your doctor if you develop skin rash or itching, visual disturbances, weight gain, breathing difficulty, fluid retention, hallucinations, black or tarry stools, persistent headache, or any unusual or intolerable side effects.

If you forget to take a dose of Piroxicam take it as soon as you remember. If you take it once a day and it is within 8 hours of your next dose, skip the missed dose and continue with your regular schedule. Do not take a double dose.

Special Populations

Pregnancy/Breast-feeding

NSAIDs may cross into the fetal blood circulation. They have not been found to cause birth defects, but may affect a developing fetal heart during the second half of pregnancy; animal studies indicate a possible effect. Women who are or who might become pregnant should not take Piroxicam without their doctors' approval; be particularly cautious about using this drug during the last 3 months of your pregnancy. When the drug is considered essential by your doctor, its potential benefits must be carefully weighed against its risks.

NSAIDs may pass into breast milk, but have caused no problems among breast-fed infants, except for seizures in a baby whose mother was taking Indomethacin. Other NSAIDs have caused problems in animal studies. There is a possibility that a nursing mother taking Piroxicam could affect her baby's heart or cardiovascular system. If you must take Piroxicam, bottle-feed your baby.

Seniors
Older adults may be more susceptible to Piroxicam side effects, especially ulcer disease.

Brand Name
Poly-Vi-Flor Chewable Tablets/ Drops

Ingredients

Folic Acid

Sodium Fluoride

Vitamin A

Vitamin B$_1$ (Thiamine)

Vitamin B$_2$ (Riboflavin)

Vitamin B$_3$ (Niacin)

Vitamin B$_6$ (Pyridoxine)

Vitamin B$_{12}$ (Cyanocobalamin)

Vitamin C

Vitamin D

Vitamin E

Other Brand Names

Florvite

Poly-Vitamins with Fluoride

(Also available in generic form)

Type of Drug

Multivitamin supplement with fluoride.

Prescribed for

Vitamin deficiencies and prevention of dental cavities in infants and children.

General Information

Fluoride taken in small daily doses has been effective in preventing cavities in children by strengthening their teeth and making them resistant to cavity formation. Multivitamins with fluoride are also available in preparations with added iron, if iron supplementation is required.

Cautions and Warnings

Too much fluoride can **damage teeth**. Because of this, Poly-Vi-Flor should not be used in areas where the fluoride content in the water supply exceeds 0.7 ppm (parts per million). Your pediatrician or local water company can tell you the fluoride content of your drinking water.

Possible Side Effects

▼ Common: occasional skin rash, itching, stomach upset, headache, and weakness.

Drug and Food Interactions

None known.

Usual Dose

1 tablet/dropperful per day.

Special Information

As with other medicines, it is easiest to remember to take this medicine if it is given at the same time each day.

If you forget to give your child a dose of Poly-Vi-Flor, do so as soon as you remember. If it is almost time for the next regularly scheduled dose, skip the missed dose and continue with the regular schedule. Do not give a double dose.

Type of Drug

Potassium Replacement Products

Brand Names

Potassium Chloride Liquids*

Cena-K	⑤ Kaon-Cl	⑤ Klorvess
Kaochlor	Kay Ciel	⑤ Potasalan Rum-K
Kaochlor S-F ⑤		

Potassium Gluconate Liquids*

Kaon	⑤ Kaylixir	K-G Elixir

Potassium Chloride Salt Combination Liquids*

Kolyum	⑤ Tri-K	Twin-K

Potassium Chloride Powders*

Gen-K	⑤ Kay Ciel	⑤ K-Lyte/Cl
K+ Care	K-Lor	Micro-K LS
Kato	Klor-Con ⑤	

Potassium Salt Combination Powders*

Klorvess Effervescent	Kolyum ⑤
Granules ⑤	

Potassium Effervescent Tablets*

Effer-K	Klor-Con/EF	K-Lyte/Cl
K+ Care ET	Klorvess ⑤	K-Lyte DS
Kaochlor-Eff ⑤	K-Lyte	

Potassium Chloride Controlled-Release Tablets and Capsules*

K+10	Klor-Con 8	Micro-K Extencaps
Kaon-Cl-10	Klor-Con 10	Micro-K 10
K-Dur 10	Klotrix	Extencaps
K-Dur 20	K-Norm	Slow-K
K-Lease	K-Tab	Ten-K

Potassium Gluconate Tablets

(Available only in generic form)

(*Also available in generic form)

Prescribed for

Replacement of potassium in the body. Long-term, moderate-dose potassium supplements may help reduce blood pressure in people with mild hypertension.

General Information

Potassium is a very important component of body fluids and has a major effect in maintaining the proper tone of all body cells. Potassium is also important for the maintenance of normal kidney function; it is required for the passage of electrical impulses throughout the nervous system; and it has a major effect on the heart and all other muscles of the body. Potassium also plays an important role in how the body uses proteins and carbohydrates.

It is important to maintain blood potassium within a specific range to avoid hypokalemia (too little potassium), which is usually caused by extended diuretic treatment, severe diarrhea and/or vomiting, complications of diabetes, or other medical conditions. Symptoms of hypokalemia are weakness, fatigue, muscle twitching and/or easy excitability, severe bowel obstruction (caused by vastly reduced movement of intestinal muscles), and abnormal heart rhythms. Your electrocardiogram's appearance will be affected by low blood potassium.

Potassium supplements are available in many forms, each designed to meet specific needs or preferences. Potassium Chloride is the form most often prescribed by doctors because it contains the most Potassium per unit weight. Another advantage of Potassium Chloride is that it also gives you Chloride ion, another important body-fluid component. Potassium Gluconate provides about one-third as much potassium as the Chloride, so you have to take 3 times as much to get an equal dose of Potassium. However, it is preferable to Potassium Chloride in certain circumstances when Chloride is undesirable.

Foods rich in potassium can provide a natural potassium source and help you avoid the need to take a Potassium supplement; they include apricots, acorn squash, avocados, bananas, beans, beef, broccoli, brussels sprouts, butternut squash, cantaloupe, chicken, collard greens, dates, fish, ham, kidney beans, lentils, milk, orange juice, potatoes (with skin), prunes, raisins, shellfish, spinach, split peas, turkey, veal, yogurt, white navy beans, watermelon, and zucchini.

Cautions and Warnings

Potassium replacement therapy should always be monitored and controlled by your physician. Potassium tablets have caused **ulcers** in some patients with compression of the esophagus. Potassium supplements for these patients should be given in liquid form. Potassium tablets have been reported to cause small bowel ulcers, leading to bleeding, obstruction, and/or perforation (punching an actual hole through the bowel into the abdomen).

People with **kidney disease** may not be able to efficiently eliminate potassium from their bodies. If people with this problem take a Potassium supplement, they can develop hyperkalemia (**too much potassium in their blood**). Hyperkalemia can develop rapidly, without warning or symptoms, and is potentially fatal. Often your doctor discovers hyperkalemia by looking at an electrocardiogram, but you can experience these symptoms: tingling in the hands and feet; a feeling of heaviness or weakness in your muscles; listlessness; confusion; low blood pressure; extreme difficulty moving your arms and legs; abnormal heart rhythms; weak pulse; loss of consciousness; pallor; restlessness; and low urine output.

Do not take Potassium supplements if you are **dehydrated** or experiencing **muscle cramps** due to excessive sun exposure. The drug should be used with caution in patients who have **kidney and/or heart disease.**

Possible Side Effects

▼ Most common: nausea, vomiting, diarrhea, stomach gas, and abdominal discomfort.

▼ Less common: rash, tingling in hands or feet, weakness and heaviness in the legs, listlessness, mental confusion, decreased blood pressure, and/or heart rhythm changes.

Drug Interactions

• Potassium supplements should not be taken with the potassium-sparing diuretics Spironolactone or Triamterene (diuretics that don't cause the body to lose potassium) or combinations of these drugs. Potassium toxicity may occur.

• The combination of an angiotensin-converting-enzyme (ACE) inhibitor drug plus a Potassium supplement may result in high blood-potassium levels.

• People taking digitalis drugs must be careful to keep their blood-potassium levels within acceptable limits. Too little potassium in the blood can accentuate Digitalis side effects and cause toxic reactions.

Food Interactions

Salt substitutes contain large amounts of potassium. Do not use them while taking a Potassium supplement without your doctor's approval. If stomach upset occurs, take this medicine with food.

Usual Dose

16 to 100 milliequivalents of potassium per day.

Overdosage

Potassium overdose is rare, except when accompanied by another condition that interferes with the body's natural processes of maintaining potassium balance. Toxicity can also occur when high doses of Potassium supplements are taken in combination with foods high in potassium.

Large overdoses of Potassium supplements may cause muscle weakness, tingling in the hands or feet, a feeling of heaviness in the legs, listlessness, confusion, breathing difficulty, low blood pressure, shock, abnormal heart rhythms, and heart attack. Call your doctor, local poison control center, or hospital emergency room for more information. ALWAYS take the medicine bottle with you if you go for treatment.

Special Information

Directions for taking and using any Potassium supplement must be followed closely. Effervescent tablets, powders, and liquids should be properly and completely dissolved or diluted in 3 to 8 ounces of cold water or juice and drunk slowly.

Oral tablets or capsules should never be chewed or crushed; they must be swallowed whole.

Many of the controlled-release Potassium supplements are made with the Potassium distributed throughout an indigestible wax core or matrix; you may notice the depleted wax matrix of a tablet in your stool several hours after you swallow the pill. This is normal and should not be a cause for alarm.

Call your doctor at once if you have tingling in your hands or feet, a feeling of heaviness in the legs, unusual tiredness or weakness, nausea, vomiting, continued abdominal pain, or black stool.

If you forget to take a dose of Potassium, take it right away if you remember within 2 hours of your regular time. If you do not remember until later, skip the forgotten dose and go back to your regular schedule. Do not take a double dose.

Special Populations

Pregnancy/Breast-feeding
This drug has been found to be safe for use during pregnancy, but you should check with your doctor before taking any drug if you are pregnant.

Breast-feeding while taking Potassium may cause unwanted side effects in your infant. If you must take Potassium, consider bottle-feeding your baby while you are on this medicine. Nursing can resume 1 to 2 days after stopping Potassium.

Seniors
Seniors may take this medication without special restriction. Follow your doctor's directions and report any side effects at once.

Pravachol

see **Pravastatin**, page 924

Generic Name

Pravastatin

Brand Name

Pravachol

Type of Drug

Cholesterol-lowering agent (HMG-CoA reductase inhibitor).

Prescribed for

Reducing high blood-cholesterol, LDL cholesterol, and triglyceride levels, together with a low-fat diet. Pravastatin has
also been prescribed for lipid problems associated with
diabetes, kidney disease, and some inherited blood lipid
problems.

General Information

Pravastatin is one of several HMG-CoA reductase inhibitors. It
works by interfering with the natural body process for manufacturing cholesterol, altering the process so that a harmless
by-product is produced instead. The value of drugs that
reduce blood cholesterol lies in the assumption that reducing
levels of blood fats reduces the chance of heart disease.
Studies conducted by the National Heart, Lung, and Blood
Institute have closely related high blood-fat levels (total
cholesterol, LDL cholesterol, and triglycerides) to heart and
blood-vessel disease. Drugs that can reduce the amounts of
any of these blood fats and increase HDL cholesterol ("good"
cholesterol) have been thought to lower the risk of heart
attack and death. In fact, studies have shown that people
taking Pravastatin had 67 percent fewer heart attacks (both
fatal and nonfatal).

The drugs in this group (Fluvastatin, Lovastatin, Pravastatin, and Simvastatin) reduce total triglyceride, cholesterol,
and LDL-cholesterol counts, while raising HDL cholesterol.
Only a very small amount of the drug swallowed actually
reaches the body circulation: 10 to 20 percent of the drug is
released from the body through your kidneys; the rest is

eliminated by the liver. A significant blood-fat-lowering response is seen after 1 to 2 weeks of treatment. Blood-fat levels reach their lowest levels within 4 to 6 weeks after you start taking any of these medications and remain at or close to that level as long as you continue to take the medicine.

Pravastatin generally doesn't benefit anyone under age 30, so it is not generally recommended for children, although it may, under special circumstances, be prescribed for teenagers in the same doses as adults.

Cautions and Warnings

Do not take Pravastatin if you are **allergic** to it or to any other member of this group.

People with a history of **liver disease** and those who drink **large amounts of alcohol** should avoid these medications because of the possibility that the drug can aggravate or cause liver disease. Your doctor should take a blood sample to test your liver function every month or so during the first year of treatment.

Pravastatin causes **muscle aches and/or muscle weakness** in a small number of people, which can be a sign of a more serious condition.

At doses between 50 and 100 or more times the maximum human dose, Pravastatin has caused central-nervous-system lesions, liver tumors, and male infertility in laboratory animals. The true importance of this information for humans is not known.

Possible Side Effects

Most people who take Pravastatin tolerate it quite well.

▼ Most common: headache, nausea, vomiting, constipation, upset stomach, diarrhea, heartburn, stomach gas, abdominal pain, and cramps.

▼ Less common: muscle aches, dizziness, rash, and itching.

▼ Rare: hepatitis, pancreas inflammation, yellowing of the skin or eyes, appetite loss, muscle cramps and weakness, blurred vision, changes in taste perception, respiratory infections, common cold symptoms, fatigue, urinary abnormalities, eye lens changes, reduced sex drive,

Possible Side Effects *(continued)*

male impotence and/or breast pain, anxiety, tingling in the hands or feet, hair loss, swelling, and blood cell changes.

Drug Interactions

• The cholesterol-lowering effects of Pravastatin plus Colestipol or Cholestyramine are additive when these drugs are taken together.

• The anticoagulant effect of Warfarin may be increased by Pravastatin. People taking both drugs should be periodically monitored by their doctor for the blood-thinning effect of Warfarin.

• The combination of Cyclosporine, Erythromycin, Gemfibrozil, or Niacin with Pravastatin may cause severe muscle aches, degeneration, or other muscle problems. These drug combinations should be avoided.

Food Interactions

Pravastatin may be taken without regard to food. Continue your low-cholesterol diet while taking this medicine.

Usual Dose

Adult: 10 to 40 mg per day at bedtime.
Senior: 10 mg per day at bedtime. Your daily dosage of Pravastatin should be adjusted monthly, based on how well the drug is working to reduce your blood cholesterol.

Overdosage

Persons suspected of having taken an overdose of Pravastatin should be taken to a hospital emergency room for evaluation and treatment. The effects of overdose are not well understood, since only a few cases have actually occurred; all of those people recovered.

Special Information

Call your doctor if you develop blurred vision, muscle aches, pain, tenderness, or weakness, especially if you are also feverish or feel sick.

Pravastatin is always prescribed in combination with a low-fat diet. Be sure to follow your doctor's dietary instructions precisely, because both the diet and medicine are necessary to treat your condition. Do not take more cholesterol-lowering medicine than your doctor has prescribed. Do not stop taking the medicine without your doctor's knowledge.

If you forget to take a dose of Pravastatin, take it as soon as you remember. If it is almost time for your next regularly scheduled dose, skip the one you forgot and continue with your regular schedule. Do not take a double dose.

Special Populations

Pregnancy/Breast-feeding

Pregnant women, and those who might become pregnant, absolutely must not take Pravastatin. Since hardening of the arteries is a long-term process, you should be able to stop this medication during pregnancy with no serious problems. If you become pregnant while taking Pravastatin, stop the drug immediately and call your doctor.

Pravastatin may pass into breast milk. Women taking the drug should bottle-feed their infants.

Seniors

Seniors may be more sensitive to the effects of Pravastatin and are likely to require less medication than younger adults. Be sure to report any side effects to your doctor.

Generic Name

Prazosin

Brand Name

Minipress

(Also available in generic form)

Type of Drug

Antihypertensive.

Combination Product

Ingredients: Prazosin + Polythiazide

Minizide

(Prasozin, in combination with the diuretic Polythiazide, is used in the treatment of high blood pressure.)

Prescribed for

High blood pressure, benign prostatic hypertrophy (BPH), congestive heart failure, and Raynaud's disease.

General Information

Prazosin is one of several alpha-adrenergic-blocking agents that work by opening blood vessels and reducing pressure in them. Alpha blockers like Prazosin block nerve endings known as *alpha₁ receptors.* Other blood-pressure-lowering drugs block beta receptors, interfere with the movement of calcium in blood-vessel muscle cells, affect salt and electrolyte balance in the body, or interfere with the process for manufacturing norepinephrine in the body. The maximum blood-pressure-lowering effect of Prazosin is seen between 2 and 6 hours after taking a single dose. In BPH, Prazosin works by relaxing smooth muscles in the prostate and neck of the bladder. Here, too, this effect is produced by blockade of alpha receptors in the affected muscles. Despite the fact that Prazosin reduces the symptoms of BPH, the drug's long-term effect on complications of BPH or the need for urinary surgery is not known. Prazosin's effect in congestive heart failure is seen within 1 hour of taking the drug. There is no difference in response between different races or between older and younger adults. Prazosin's effect lasts only between 6 and 10 hours. It is broken down in the liver, and very little passes out of the body via the kidneys.

Cautions and Warnings

Prazosin can cause **dizziness** and **fainting**, especially with the first few doses. This is known as the *first-dose effect.* It can be minimized by limiting the first dose to 1 mg at bedtime. The first-dose effect occurs in about 1 percent of people taking an alpha blocker and can recur if the drug is stopped for a few days and then restarted.

People **allergic** or **sensitive** to any of the alpha blockers should avoid Prazosin.

Prazosin may slightly reduce cholesterol levels and increase the HDL/LDL (important blood fats) ratio, a positive step for people with a blood-cholesterol problem. People with an already **high blood-cholesterol level** should discuss this situation with their doctors.

Possible Side Effects

The incidence of side effects is much lower for Prazosin than it is for other alpha-blocker drugs.

▼ Most common: dizziness, drowsiness, weakness, nausea, and headache.

▼ Less common: low blood pressure, dizziness when rising from a sitting or lying position, rapid heartbeat, vomiting, dry mouth, diarrhea, constipation, abdominal pain or discomfort, breathing difficulty, stuffy nose, nosebleeds, joint or muscle pains, blurry vision, conjunctivitis ("pink-eye"), ringing or buzzing in the ears, depression, nervousness, tingling in the hands or feet, frequent urination, male impotence, poor urinary control, painful erection of the penis, itching, sweating, rash, hair loss, retaining fluid, and fever.

Drug Interactions

• Prazosin may interact with beta-blocking drugs to produce a higher rate of dizziness or fainting after taking the first dose of Prazosin.

• The blood-pressure-lowering effect of Prazosin may be reduced by Indomethacin.

• When taken with other blood-pressure-lowering drugs, Prazosin produces an exaggerated reduction of blood pressure.

• The blood-pressure-lowering effect of Clonidine may be reduced by Prazosin.

Food Interactions

Prazosin may be taken without regard to food or meals.

Usual Dose

1 mg 2 to 3 times per day to start; the dose may be increased to 20 mg a day, and 40 mg has been used in some cases. The total daily dose of Prazosin must be tailored to the patient's individual needs.

Overdosage

Prazosin overdose may produce drowsiness, poor reflexes, and very low blood pressure. Overdose victims should be taken to a hospital emergency room immediately. ALWAYS bring the prescription bottle.

Special Information

Take Prazosin exactly as prescribed. Do not stop taking Prazosin unless directed to do so by your doctor. Avoid nonprescription drugs that contain stimulants because they can increase your blood pressure. Your pharmacist will be able to tell you what you can and cannot take.

Prazosin can cause dizziness, headache, and drowsiness, especially 2 to 6 hours after you take your first drug dose, although these effects can persist after the first few doses.

Call your doctor if you develop severe dizziness, heart palpitations, or other bothersome or persistent side effects.

Before driving or doing anything that requires intense concentration, wait 12 to 24 hours after taking the first dose of Prazosin. You may take your medication at bedtime to minimize this problem.

Taking your medicine at the same time each day will help you remember to take it. If you forget to take a dose of Prazosin and you take it once a day, take it as soon as you remember. If it is almost time for your next dose, skip the forgotten dose and continue with your regular medication schedule. Do not take a double dose.

Special Populations

Pregnancy/Breast-feeding

There have been no studies of Prazosin in pregnant women, and its safety for use during pregnancy is not known.

Small amounts of Prazosin pass into breast milk. Nursing mothers who must take it should bottle-feed their babies.

Seniors
Older adults, especially those with liver disease, may be more sensitive to the effects and side effects of Prazosin. Report any unusual side effects to your doctor.

Prednisone

see ***Corticosteroids***, *page 269*

Premarin

see ***Estrogen***, *page 415*

Prilosec

see ***Omeprazole***, *page 837*

Brand Name
Primatene Tablets

Ingredients

Ephedrine Hydrochloride + Phenobarbital + Theophylline

(Also available in generic form)

The following products have the same ingredients, but in different amounts:
Tedrigen   Theodrine

(Also available in generic form)

The following products substitute Hydroxyzine for Phenobarbital:

Hydrophed   Marax

(Also available in generic form)

The following products have an expectorant added (Guaifenesin or Potassium Iodide) to help loosen thick mucus:

Lufyllin-EPG Tablets (exchanges Dyphylline for Theophylline)
Mudrane Tablets
Mudrane GG Tablets
Quadrinal Tablets

Type of Drug

Antiasthmatic combination.

Prescribed for

Relief of asthma symptoms or other upper respiratory disorders. There is considerable doubt among medical experts that this type of combination drug produces all the effects claimed for it.

General Information

These products combine a drug to help relax the bronchial muscles, a drug to increase the diameter of the breathing passages, and a mild tranquilizer to help relax the patient. Other products in this class may contain similar ingredients along with an additional drug to help eliminate mucus from the breathing passages. Modern asthma therapy has moved away from using these types of combination products. Most doctors today use a combination of different medicines in oral products and inhalers to treat different aspects of asthma. The Food and Drug Administration is currently reviewing these combination products to determine if they should remain on the market.

Cautions and Warnings

Do not take these medicines if you are **sensitive** or **allergic** to any of their ingredients. These drugs should not be taken if you have severe **kidney or liver disease**.

Possible Side Effects

▼ Common: excitation, shakiness, sleeplessness, nervousness, rapid heartbeat, chest pains, irregular heartbeat, dizziness, dryness of the nose and throat, headache, and increased sweating. Occasionally, people have been known to develop hesitation or difficulty in urination.

▼ Less common: excessive urination, heart stimulation, drowsiness, muscle weakness or twitching, and unsteady walk. These effects can usually be controlled by having your doctor reduce the dose.

Drug Interactions

• These medicines may cause sleeplessness and/or drowsiness. Do not take them with alcoholic beverages, which will enhance these effects. Take care while driving or operating hazardous equipment.

• Taking Primatene (or similar medicines) with a monoamine oxidase (MAO) inhibitor can produce a severe interaction. Consult your doctor first.

• Taking these products with Lithium Carbonate will increase the rate at which Lithium passes out of the body. Your doctor may want to adjust your Lithium dosage.

• These medicines may reduce the effectiveness of Propranolol.

Food Interactions

Take these drugs with food to help prevent stomach upset.

Usual Dose

1 to 2 tablets every 4 hours.

Overdosage

Overdosage symptoms may include stimulation, nausea, vomiting, nervousness, loss of appetite, irritability, headache, abnormal heart rhythms, or convulsions or seizures. Overdose victims should be taken to a hospital emergency room at once. ALWAYS bring the medicine bottle with you.

Special Information

Call your doctor if side effects are persistent or bothersome. If you forget to take a dose of Primatene, take it as soon as you remember. If it is almost time for your next dose, skip the one you forgot and continue with your regular schedule. Do not take a double dose.

Special Populations

Pregnancy/Breast-feeding

Some pregnant women may require asthma medicine even though it can increase the chance of birth defects. Regular use of these drugs during the last 3 months of pregnancy may cause drug dependency in the newborn infant. Their use may prolong or delay delivery, or cause breathing problems in the newborn.

The ingredients in these medicines pass into breast milk and may affect a nursing infant. Bottle-feed your baby if you must take one of these drugs.

Seniors

Older adults are more sensitive to the effects of antiasthmatic combination products. Follow your doctor's directions and report any side effects at once.

Prinivil

see **Lisinopril**, page 599

Generic Name

Procainamide Hydrochloride

Brand Name

Pronestyl

(Also available in generic form)

Sustained-Release Products

Procan SR
Pronestyl SR

Type of Drug

Antiarrhythmic.

Prescribed for

Abnormal heart rhythms.

General Information

Procainamide Hydrochloride is often used as treatment for primary arrhythmia (abnormal heart rhythms). It works by slowing the response of heart muscle to nervous-system stimulation. It also slows the rate at which nervous-system impulses are carried through the heart. This drug may be given to patients who do not respond to or cannot tolerate other antiarrhythmic drugs. Procainamide begins working 30 minutes after you take it and continues for 3 or more hours. As with other antiarrhythmic drugs, studies have not proven that people who take Procainamide live longer than people who do not take it.

Short-acting Procainamide generic products may be interchanged for one another. However, sustained-release or long-acting products may not be equivalent to each other and should not be interchanged without your doctor's knowledge.

Cautions and Warnings

About 1 of every 200 people taking Procainamide in the usual dosage range develop **bone marrow depression,** a drastic drop in white-blood-cell count, low platelet count, or other abnormalities of blood components. Physically, these can be represented by **fever, chills, sore throat, mouth sores, bruising,** or **bleeding.** Call your doctor if any of these occur. Because these abnormalities happen most often in the first 3 months on Procainamide, you should be checked with weekly blood counts during your first 3 months taking this medicine.

Procainamide should not be taken by people who have complete **heart block** or the arrhythmia called *Torsade de pointes,* which Procainamide will worsen rather than improve. Long-term Procainamide use often leads to the development of a positive blood test (antinuclear antibody or ANA) for lupus erythematosus (a connective tissue disease), with or without symptoms. Report anything unusual to your doctor.

If you have a condition called ***myasthenia gravis,*** tell your doctor when Procainamide is first prescribed; you should be taking a drug other than Procainamide. You should also tell your doctor if you are **allergic** to Procainamide or to the local anesthetic Procaine. Patients taking Procainamide should be under strict medical supervision.

Procainamide may aggravate **congestive heart failure** by reducing the output of an already compromised heart.

This drug is eliminated from the body through the kidney and liver. If you have either **kidney or liver disease,** your dose of Procainamide may have to be adjusted.

This drug, like other antiarrhythmics, has not been proven to help people with ventricular arrhythmias live longer.

Possible Side Effects

▼ Common: large oral doses of Procainamide Hydro-chloride may cause loss of appetite, nausea, or itching. A group of symptoms resembling the disease lupus erythe-matosus (fever and chills, nausea, vomiting, muscle aches, skin lesions, arthritis, and abdominal pains) has been reported in as many as 30 percent of patients taking the drug for long periods. Your doctor may detect en-largement of your liver and changes in blood tests, indicating a change in the liver. Soreness of the mouth or throat, unusual bleeding, rash, or fever may occur. If any of these symptoms occur while you are taking Procaina-mide, tell your doctor immediately.

▼ Less common: bitter taste in the mouth, vomiting, diarrhea, weakness, dizziness, mental depression, giddi-ness, hallucinations, and drug allergy (such as rash, itching, and drug fever). Liver inflammation has occurred after a single dose of Procainamide.

Drug Interactions

• Procainamide blood levels and the chances of drug side effects are increased by the following: Propranolol and other beta blockers; Cimetidine, Ranitidine, and other H_2 antago-nists; Lidocaine; Quinidine; and Trimethoprim.

• Do not take Procainamide with other antiarrhythmic drugs unless specifically instructed by your doctor. These combinations can unduly depress heart function.

• The interaction between alcohol and Procainamide is variable, and may possibly alter the effects of Procainamide.

• Avoid over-the-counter cough, cold, or allergy remedies containing drugs that have a direct stimulating effect on your heart. Ask your pharmacist about the ingredients in over-the-counter remedies.

Food Interactions

This medicine is best taken on an empty stomach, but you may take it with food if it upsets your stomach.

Usual Dose

Initial dose: 1000 mg to start. *Maintenance dose:* 23 mg per pound per day in divided doses every 3 hours around the clock, adjusted according to individual needs. Seniors and people with kidney or liver disease are treated with lower doses or given the medicine less often.

Taking a sustained-release product allows doses to be spaced 6 hours apart.

Overdosage

Procainamide overdose leads to a progressive blockage of nerve impulses within heart muscle, slowing heart rate and causing low blood pressure and other drug side effects. Overdose symptoms (abnormal heart rhythms, low blood pressure, tremors, nervous-system depression) can follow an overdose of 2000 mg; 3000 mg taken in 1 dose can be dangerous. Overdose victims should be taken to an emergency room immediately. ALWAYS bring the prescription bottle.

Special Information

Call your doctor at once if you develop any sign of infection, including fever, chills, sore throat, or mouth sores, or if you develop joint or muscle pain, dark urine, wheezing, weakness, chest or abdominal pains, heart palpitations, nausea, vomiting, diarrhea, appetite loss, dizziness, depression, hallucinations, or unusual bruising or bleeding.

Be sure you discuss with your doctor any drug sensitivity or reaction, especially to Procaine or other local anesthetics or to Aspirin. Also, be sure your doctor knows if you have heart failure, lupus erythematosus, liver or kidney disease, or myasthenia gravis.

Because Procainamide is taken so frequently during the day, it is essential that you follow your doctor's directions about taking your medicine. Taking more medicine will not necessarily help you, and skipping doses or taking them less often than directed may lead to a loss of control over your heart problem.

If you forget to take a dose of Procainamide, and remember within 2 hours (4 hours for long-acting Procainamide), take it right away. If it is almost time for your next regularly scheduled dose, skip the one you forgot and continue with your regular schedule. Do not take a double dose.

Special Populations

Pregnancy/Breast-feeding

Procainamide passes into the blood circulation of a developing fetus. It has not been found to cause birth defects. Pregnant women or those who might become pregnant while taking this drug should not take it without considering both possible risks and benefits.

This drug passes into breast milk, and could affect a nursing infant. Nursing women who must take Procainamide should bottle-feed their babies.

Seniors

Older adults are more sensitive to the effects of this drug, especially low blood pressure and dizziness. Follow your doctor's directions and report any side effects at once.

Procardia XL

see **Nifedipine**, page 794

Generic Name

Prochlorperazine

Brand Name

Compazine Spansules/Suppositories/Syrup/Tablets

(Also available in generic form)

Type of Drug

Antinauseant; phenothiazine antipsychotic.

Prescribed for

Severe nausea and vomiting. Also prescribed for psychotic disorders (excessive anxiety, tension, and agitation).

General Information

Prochlorperazine is a member of a group of drugs called *phenothiazines*, which act on a portion of the brain called the *hypothalamus*. These drugs affect areas of the hypothalamus that control metabolism, body temperature, alertness, muscle tone, hormone balance, and vomiting, and may be used to treat problems related to any of these functions. The exact way in which they work is not completely understood.

Cautions and Warnings

Prochlorperazine can **depress the cough (gag) reflex.** Some people who have taken this drug have accidentally choked to death because the cough reflex failed to protect them. Prochlorperazine, because of its effect in reducing vomiting, can obscure signs of toxicity due to overdose of other drugs or symptoms of disease.

Do not take Prochlorperazine if you are **allergic** to it or any other phenothiazine drug. Do not take it if you have **very low blood pressure, Parkinson's disease,** or any **blood, liver, kidney, or heart disease.** If you have **glaucoma, epilepsy, ulcers,** or **difficulty passing urine,** Prochlorperazine should be used with caution and under strict supervision of your doctor.

Avoid exposing yourself to **extreme heat,** because Prochlorperazine can upset your body's normal temperature control mechanism.

Possible Side Effects

▼ Most common: drowsiness, especially during the first or second week of therapy. If the drowsiness becomes troublesome, contact your doctor. Prochlorperazine can cause jaundice (yellowing of the whites of the eyes or skin), usually within the first 4 weeks of treatment. The jaundice usually goes away when the drug is discontinued, but there have been cases when it did not. If you notice this effect or if you develop symptoms such as fever or general feelings of ill health, contact your doctor immediately.

▼ Less common: changes in blood components (including anemia), raised or lowered blood pressure, abnormal heart rate, heart attack, and feeling faint or dizzy.

Phenothiazines can produce extrapyramidal effects, such as spasm of the neck muscles, rolling back of the eyes, convulsions, difficulty in swallowing, and symptoms associated with Parkinson's disease. These effects look very serious but disappear after the drug has been withdrawn; however, face, tongue, and jaw symptoms may persist for as long as several years, especially in older adults with a history of brain damage. If you experience extrapyramidal effects, contact your doctor immediately.

▼ Other: Prochlorperazine may cause an unusual increase in psychotic symptoms or may cause paranoid reactions, tiredness, lethargy, restlessness, hyperactivity, confusion at night, bizarre dreams, inability to sleep, depression, and euphoria (feeling 'high'). Other reactions are itching, swelling, unusual sensitivity to bright lights, and red skin or rash. There have been cases of breast enlargement, false-positive pregnancy tests, changes in menstrual flow, impotence or changes in sex drive in males, stuffy nose, headache, nausea, vomiting, loss of appetite, changes in body temperature, pallor, excessive salivation or perspiration, constipation, diarrhea, changes in urine and bowel habits, worsening of glaucoma,

Possible Side Effects *(continued)*

blurred vision, weakening of eyelid muscles, spasms in bronchial or other muscles, increased appetite, fatigue, excessive thirst, and skin discoloration (particularly in areas exposed to sunlight).

Drug Interactions

• Be cautious about taking Prochlorperazine with barbiturates, sleeping pills, narcotics, other tranquilizers, or any other medication that may produce a depressive effect, including alcohol (which should be avoided).

• Aluminum antacids may interfere with the absorption of Prochlorperazine into the bloodstream, reducing its effectiveness. Anticholinergic drugs can reduce the effectiveness of Prochlorperazine and increase the chance of drug side effects.

• Prochlorperazine can reduce the effects of Bromocriptine and appetite suppressants. The blood-pressure-lowering effect of Guanethidine may be counteracted by this drug.

• Taking Lithium together with this or any other phenothiazine drug may lead to disorientation, loss of consciousness, and uncontrolled muscle movements. Mixing Propranolol and Prochlorperazine may lead to unusually low blood pressure.

• Blood concentrations of tricyclic antidepressant drugs may increase if they are taken together with Prochlorperazine. This can lead to antidepressant side effects.

Food Interactions

The antipsychotic effectiveness of Prochlorperazine may be counteracted by foods with caffeine such as coffee, tea, cola drinks, or chocolate.

Usual Dose

Adult: 15 to 150 mg per day, depending on your disease and response. For nausea and vomiting, 15 to 40 mg per day (by mouth); 25 mg twice a day (in rectal suppositories).

Child (40 to 85 pounds): 10 to 15 mg per day (Prochlorperazine syrup contains 5 mg per teaspoon).

Child (30 to 39 pounds): 2.5 mg 2 to 3 times per day.

Child (20 to 29 pounds): 2.5 mg 1 to 2 times per day.

Child (under 2 years or 20 pounds): not recommended, except if your doctor feels the drug would be life-saving. Usually only 1 to 2 days of therapy is needed to relieve nausea and vomiting.

For psychosis, doses of 25 mg or more per day may be required.

Overdosage

Symptoms of overdosage are depression, extreme weakness, tiredness and/or a desire to sleep, lowered blood pressure, uncontrolled muscle spasms, agitation, restlessness, convulsions, fever, dry mouth, abnormal heart rhythms, and coma. The victim should be taken to a hospital emergency room immediately. ALWAYS bring the medicine bottle.

Special Information

This medication is a tranquilizer and can have a depressive effect, especially during the first few days of therapy. Care should be taken when performing activities requiring a high degree of concentration, such as driving.

Call your doctor if you develop sore throat, fever, skin rash, weakness, tremors, visual disturbances, or yellowing of the skin or eyes.

This drug may cause unusual sensitivity to the sun. It can also turn your urine reddish-brown to pink; this is normal and not a cause for concern.

If dizziness occurs, avoid sudden changes in posture and avoid climbing stairs. Use caution in hot weather, because this medicine may make you more prone to heat stroke.

The liquid form of Prochlorperazine can cause skin irritations or rashes. Do not get it on your skin. Liquid Prochlorperazine must be protected from light. Don't take it out of the opaque bottle in which it is dispensed from the pharmacy.

If you miss a dose of Prochlorperazine, take it as soon as you can. If it is almost time for your next dose, skip the missed dose and go back to your regular dose schedule. Do not double any doses.

Special Populations

Pregnancy/Breast-feeding

Infants born to women who have taken this medication have

experienced drug side effects (liver jaundice, nervous-system effects) immediately after birth. Check with your doctor about taking this medicine if you are, or might become, pregnant.

This drug may pass into breast milk and affect a nursing infant. Consider bottle-feeding if you must take this drug.

Seniors
Older adults are more sensitive to the effects of this medication and usually require a lower dosage to achieve the desired results. Also, because seniors are more likely to develop drug side effects, some experts feel that they should be treated with ½ to ¼ the usual adult dose of this drug.

Generic Name

Promethazine Hydrochloride

Brand Name

Phenergan Suppositories/Tablets/Plain Syrup

(Also available in generic form)

Combination Products

Promethazine + Codeine Phosphate*

Pentazine with Codeine Syrup
Phenergan with Codeine Syrup   Ⓐ
Pherazine with Codeine Syrup
Prometh with Codeine Syrup   Ⓐ

Promethazine + Dextromethorphan Hydrobromide

Phenergan with Dextromethorphan Syrup
Phenameth DM Syrup   Ⓐ
Pherazine DM Syrup
Promethazine DM Liquid

Promethazine Phenylephrine Hydrochloride*

Phenergan VC Syrup
Promethazine VC Plain Syrup
Prometh VC Plain Liquid   Ⓐ

Promethazine Codeine Phosphate + Phenylephrine HCl

Para-Hist AT Syrup
Phenergan VC with Codeine Syrup
Pherazine VC with Codeine Syrup
Prometh VC with Codeine Liquid
Promethist with Codeine Syrup

(*Also available in generic form)

Type of Drug

Antihistamine.

Prescribed for

Allergy symptom relief, motion sickness, nausea, vomiting; nighttime sedation; pain relief (when given with narcotic pain relievers); and postoperative nausea and vomiting.

General Information

Promethazine, one of the older members of the phenothiazine antihistamine group, has been used by millions of people both alone and in combination with cough suppressants and decongestants. Many of the newer antihistamines have replaced Promethazine as a routine antihistamine, but it is still widely used for its other effects.

Cautions and Warnings

Promethazine should be used with caution if you are **allergic** to it or if you cannot tolerate any of the other phenothiazine drugs (including Chlorpromazine and Prochlorperazine).

Promethazine should be used with care if you have **very low blood pressure, Parkinson's disease,** or **heart, blood, liver, or kidney disease.** This drug should be used with caution and under your doctor's strict supervision if you have **ulcers, epilepsy, glaucoma,** or **urinary difficulty.**

Children with a history of **apnea** (intermittent breathing while sleeping), a family history of **sudden infant death syndrome** (SIDS), **liver disease,** or **Reye's syndrome** should not take Promethazine.

Possible Side Effects

▼ Most common: drowsiness, mucus thickening, and sedation.

▼ Less common: sore throat and fever; unusual bleeding or bruising; tiredness or weakness; dizziness; feeling faint; clumsiness or unsteadiness; dry mouth, nose, or throat; facial redness; breathing difficulty; hallucinations; confusion; seizures; muscle spasms (especially in the back and neck); restlessness; a shuffling walk; jerky movements of the head and face; shaking and trembling of the hands; blurring or other visual changes; urinary difficulties; rapid heartbeat; sensitivity to the sun; increased sweating; and loss of appetite. Children and older adults are more likely to develop difficulty sleeping, excitement, nervousness, restlessness, and irritability.

The suppositories can cause rectal burning or stinging.

Drug Interactions

• The sedating effects of Promethazine are amplified by any nervous-system depressants, including tranquilizers, alcohol, hypnotics, sedatives, antianxiety drugs, and narcotics. These combinations should be used with extreme caution.

• Use of a monoamine oxidase (MAO) inhibitor drug together with Promethazine may cause low blood pressure and unusual or uncoordinated movements.

• Promethazine will antagonize the effects of amphetamines and other appetite suppressants (diet pills).

• The combination of Promethazine with an oral antithyroid drug may increase the chances for agranulocytosis (severe reductions in white-blood-cell count).

• The combination of Quinidine and Promethazine may increase the cardiac effects of both drugs.

• Promethazine may increase the need for anticonvulsant medicine, Bromocriptine, Guanadrel, Guanethidine, and Levodopa. Dosage adjustments may be needed.

• Riboflavin requirements are increased in people taking Promethazine.

• Promethazine may interfere with some blood-sugar tests and some home pregnancy tests.

Food Interactions

Take Promethazine with food if it upsets your stomach.

Usual Dose

Allergy
Adult: 12.5 mg before meals and 12.5 to 25 mg at bedtime.
Child: 5 to 12.5 mg 3 times per day and 25 mg at bedtime.

Motion Sickness
Adult: 25 mg ½ hour before travel; repeat in 8 to 12 hours if needed. Then take 1 dose upon arising and another before dinner.
Child: 10 to 25 mg given by mouth or as a suppository.

Nausea and Vomiting
Adult: 25 mg when needed; repeat up to 6 times per day, if needed.
Child: 10 to 25 mg twice a day as needed.

Sedation
Adult: 25 to 50 mg at bedtime.
Child: about ½ the adult dose.

Overdosage

Symptoms of overdosage are likely to be drowsiness; confusion; clumsiness; dry mouth, nose, or throat; hallucinations; seizures; and other Promethazine side effects (see *Possible Side Effects*). Overdose victims should be taken to a hospital emergency room for treatment. ALWAYS bring the medicine bottle.

Special Information

People taking Promethazine must be careful when performing tasks requiring concentration and coordination (such as driving) because of the chance that the drug will make them tired, dizzy, or light-headed; avoid alcoholic beverages.

Call your doctor if you develop any of the following: sore throat; very dry mouth, nose, or throat; fever or chills; unusual bleeding or bruising; unusual tiredness or weakness; clumsiness; unsteadiness; hallucinations; seizures; sleeping problems; faintness; facial flushing; breathing difficulty; or any other persistent or intolerable side effects.

It is important to maintain good dental hygiene while taking this drug and to use extra care when using your toothbrush or dental floss because of the chance that the dry mouth it can cause will make you more susceptible to some oral infections. (If the dry mouth caused by Promethazine is not taken care of by gum or hard candies or lasts more than 2 weeks, check with your doctor or dentist.) Any dental work should be completed prior to starting on this drug.

If you take Promethazine twice a day and forget a dose, take it as soon as you remember. If it is almost time for your next dose, take one dose as soon as you remember and another in 5 or 6 hours, then go back to your regular schedule. Do not take a double dose.

If you take Promethazine 3 or more times a day and forget a dose, take it as soon as you remember. If it is almost time for your next dose, take one dose as soon as you remember and another in 3 or 4 hours, then go back to your regular schedule. Do not take a double dose.

Special Populations

Pregnancy/Breast-feeding
Some babies born to women who have taken other phenothiazines have suffered drug side effects at birth (yellowing of the skin and eyes, nervous-system effects). Promethazine taken within 2 weeks before delivery may affect the baby's blood-clotting system. As with all drug products, pregnant women should not use Promethazine unless its advantages have been carefully weighed against its possible dangers, especially during the last 3 months of pregnancy. Newborns and premature infants may exhibit unusual or severe reactions.

Promethazine should not be taken by nursing mothers, especially those with premature or newborn babies, because of the chance that it will affect nursing infants.

Seniors
Seniors are more sensitive to dizziness, sedation, confusion, and low blood pressure and should be careful when taking this drug. Nervous-system side effects, including parkinsonism and unusual or uncoordinated movements, are also more likely to develop in older adults.

Propacet 100

*see **Propoxyphene**, page 955*

Generic Name

Propafenone

Brand Name

Rythmol

Type of Drug

Antiarrhythmic.

Prescribed for

Life-threatening abnormal heart rhythms.

General Information

Propafenone slows the speed at which nerve impulses travel in the heart and reduces the sensitivity of nerves that are present in heart muscle. It also stabilizes the membranes of heart muscle, making them less sensitive to stimulation by cardiac nerves. Propafenone also has a very mild beta-blocking effect, which helps in stabilizing abnormal rhythms. However, this drug can cause abnormal rhythms of its own and, for that reason, is usually recommended only after other drug treatments have failed.

Cautions and Warnings

Propafenone should not be used by people with **severe heart failure, very low blood pressure,** or a **very slow heart rate.** In some cases, Propafenone is not recommended for use unless an artificial pacemaker has been implanted to control basic heart function. **Cardiac pacemakers** may need some programming adjustments because of changes brought about by the drug in the sensitivity of heart muscle to the device.

Propafenone, like some other antiarrhythmic drugs, can

worsen some abnormal rhythms or create abnormalities of its own, including some severe arrhythmias of the ventricle. Overall, about 5 percent of people who take this drug will develop **abnormal rhythms** because of the drug itself.

Most people's bodies break down Propafenone relatively quickly and efficiently, but others handle Propafenone very differently and eliminate it much more slowly. People in the latter group (less than 10 percent of all users) have 1½ to 2 times as much Propafenone in their blood for a given dose and must be treated carefully by their doctors to avoid drug side effects.

People with **heart failure, chronic bronchitis,** or **emphysema** should probably not use Propafenone because the drug's beta-blocking effect may worsen their condition.

Recent heart attack victims should use other agents before Propafenone because the drug may not be beneficial.

People with **kidney or liver disease** may need lower doses to compensate for reduced drug elimination from the body.

Possible Side Effects

▼ Most common: angina pains, heart failure, heart palpitations, abnormal heart rhythms (including rhythm changes in the ventricles), dizziness, headache, nausea or vomiting, constipation, changes in senses of taste and smell, upset stomach, blurred vision, and breathing difficulty. Generally, side effects increase as drug dosage is increased.

▼ Less common: weakness, tremors, rash, joint pain, swelling, increased sweating, stomach gas, dry mouth, diarrhea, constipation, cramps, tiredness, headache, sleeplessness, drowsiness, dizziness, fainting, muscle weakness, loss of appetite, anxiety, low blood pressure, low heart rate, and chest pain.

▼ Rare: hair loss, impotence, increased blood sugar, low blood potassium, kidney failure, pain, itching, lupus, unusual dreams, flushing, hot flashes, psychosis, seizures, ringing or buzzing in the ears, gallbladder problems, anemia, bruising, bleeding, and changes in blood components.

Drug Interactions

- The combination of Propafenone and some beta blockers (such as Metoprolol and Propranolol) has been shown to increase beta-blocker concentrations and decrease their rate of release from the body. Beta-blocker dosage reduction is likely to be required.
- Alcohol, tranquilizers, and other nervous-system depressants will increase the depressant effects of this drug.
- Cimetidine and Quinidine reduce the rate at which this drug is broken down by the liver and may increase Propafenone blood concentrations by 20 percent; dosage adjustment may be necessary.
- Propafenone increases Digoxin levels between 35 and 80 percent, depending on the drug dosage; the higher the Propafenone dose, the greater the effect. Your doctor will need to balance your Digoxin dose if you must take both drugs.
- Propafenone may increase the nervous-system side effects of local anesthetics (often used during minor surgery or dental work).
- Rifampin may increase the rate at which Propafenone is eliminated from the body, resulting in a possible loss of Propafenone effect.
- Propafenone will increase the amount of Warfarin, an anticoagulant (blood thinner), in the blood by about 40 percent. Warfarin dosage adjustment will solve the problem.

Food Interactions

Propafenone may be taken without regard to food or meals.

Usual Dose

150 mg every 8 hours to start. Dosage may be increased in steps up to 900 mg per day, but the dose may also be reduced. Older adults may need less medicine.

Overdosage

Overdose symptoms are usually worst within 3 hours of swallowing Propafenone, and may include weakness, tiredness, fever, low blood pressure, and slow heart rate. Overdose victims should be taken to a hospital emergency room immediately. ALWAYS bring the medicine bottle.

Special Information

See your doctor regularly while you are taking Propafenone, and call the doctor if you feel that your rhythm problem is worsening or not improving, an effect you are most likely to experience at higher drug doses. Other important problems to report to your doctor are chest pain, breathing difficulty, swelling, trembling or shaking, dizziness or fainting, joint pains, a slow heart rate, fever, or chills. Other side effects should be reported if they are persistent or bothersome.

Be careful when driving or performing other complex tasks because of the chance that the drug will make you tired, dizzy, or light-headed; avoid alcoholic beverages.

It is important to take your Propafenone regularly every day and at evenly spaced times around the clock. Maintaining the drug's effect depends on a steady amount of the drug in your body. If you forget a dose, take it as soon as you remember. If 4 hours or more have passed since the forgotten dose should have been taken, skip it and continue with your regular schedule. Do not take a double dose.

Special Populations

Pregnancy/Breast-feeding

Pregnant animals given 10 to 40 times the maximum pre-scribed human dose of Propafenone have shown that the drug can be toxic to the developing fetus. Pregnant women should not use this drug unless its advantages have been carefully weighed against its possible dangers.

It is not known if this drug passes into breast milk. Nursing mothers who must take it should bottle-feed their babies.

Seniors

Older adults are likely to have age-related loss of kidney and/or liver function and may respond to lower dosages. Propafenone is broken down almost completely by the liver and its by-products are eliminated by the kidneys; this should be taken into account by your doctor when determining your Propafenone dosage.

Generic Name

Propantheline Bromide

Brand Name

Pro-Banthine

(Also available in generic form)

Type of Drug

Anticholinergic.

Prescribed for

Relief of stomach upset, spasms, and peptic ulcers. This medication is also prescribed to treat urinary incontinence.

General Information

Propantheline Bromide works by inhibiting the effects of a neurohormone called *acetylcholine* in the stomach and gastrointestinal (GI) tract. This effect directly reduces the mobility of the GI tract and slows the production of enzymes and other secretions. In doing so, it helps relieve some of the uncomfortable symptoms associated with peptic ulcer, irritable bowel and/or colon, spastic colon, other gastrointestinal disorders, and urinary incontinence. This drug only relieves symptoms; it does not cure the underlying disease. It may also slow the production of saliva (causing dry mouth), reduce sweating, and cause dilation of the pupil, making it more difficult for you to become accomodated to sudden bright light.

Cautions and Warnings

Propantheline Bromide should not be used if you are **sensitive** or **allergic** to it or have **heart disease, Down syndrome, reduced mobility of the stomach and lower esophagus, fever, stomach obstruction, glaucoma, acute bleeding, hiatal hernia, intestinal paralysis, myasthenia gravis, kidney or liver dysfunction, rapid heartbeat, high blood pressure,** or **ulcerative colitis.** Because this drug reduces your ability to sweat, its use in **hot weather** may cause heat exhaustion.

Possible Side Effects

▼ Most common: constipation, decreased sweating, and dry skin, eyes, nose, or throat.

▼ Less common: swallowing difficulty or reduced breast milk flow.

▼ Rare: skin rash, hives or other allergy, confusion (especially in older adults), eye pain, dizziness or fainting when rising from a sitting or lying position, feeling bloated, difficult urination, blurred vision or sensitivity to bright light, drowsiness, headache, memory loss, nausea, vomiting, and unusual tiredness or weakness.

Drug Interactions

• Antacids containing Calcium and/or Magnesium, citrates, or Sodium Bicarbonate and carbonic anhydrase inhibitor drugs may slow the rate at which Propantheline is released from the blood, increasing its therapeutic effect and possible side effects.

• Do not mix Propantheline with other anticholinergic drugs, including Atropine, Belladonna, Clidinium, Dicyclomine, Glycopyrrolate, Hyoscyamine, Isopropamide, Scopalamine, and others, because of the possibility of intensifying drug side effects.

• Propantheline can reduce stomach acidity and reduce the amount of Ketoconazole, an antifungal drug, absorbed into the blood after it is taken by mouth.

• Propantheline may counteract the effect of Metoclopramide in reducing nausea and vomiting.

• Taking this drug together with a narcotic pain reliever can increase the chances of severe constipation.

• Taking this or any other drug that slows the movement of stomach and intestinal muscles together with a Potassium Chloride supplement (especially one that comes in a wax-matrix tablet) can lead to excessive irritation of the stomach.

Food Interactions

Propantheline is usually taken 30 to 60 minutes before a meal.

Usual Dose

Adult: 30 mg at bedtime and 7.5 to 15 mg 3 times a day.

Senior: 7.5 mg 3 times a day.
Child (under age 12): do not use.

Overdosage

Propantheline Bromide overdose may lead to blurred vision; clumsiness; confusion; difficulty breathing; dizziness; drowsiness; dry mouth, nose, or throat; rapid heartbeat; fever; hallucinations; weakness; slurred speech; excitement, restlessness, or irritability; warmth; and dry or flushed skin. Take the victim to a hospital emergency room for treatment. ALWAYS bring the medicine bottle with you.

Special Information

Brush and floss your teeth regularly while taking this drug. Because it can cause dry mouth, you may be more likely to develop cavities or other dental problems while you are taking it. Dry mouth can be relieved by chewing gum or sucking hard candy. Constipation associated with Propantheline Bromide can be treated by using a stool-softening laxative.

Propantheline can make you drowsy or tired and can cause blurred vision. Take care while driving or doing other tasks that require concentration and coordination.

Call your doctor if you develop skin rash or flushing or eye pain, or if you develop other side effects (such as dry mouth, urinary difficulty, constipation, or unusual sensitivity to light) that are persistent or bothersome.

If you forget to take a dose of Propantheline Bromide, take it as soon as you remember. If it is almost time for your next regularly scheduled dose, skip the one you forgot and continue with your regular schedule. Do not take a double dose.

Special Populations

Pregnancy/Breast-feeding

This drug crosses into the blood circulation of a developing baby but has not been found to cause birth defects. Pregnant women, or those who might become pregnant while taking this drug, should not take it without their doctors' approval. When the drug is considered essential by your doctor, the potential risk of taking the medicine must be carefully weighed against the benefit it might produce.

This drug passes into breast milk and may reduce the

amount of milk you make, but has caused no problems among breast-fed infants. You must consider the potential effect on the nursing infant if breast-feeding while taking this medicine.

Seniors

Older adults are more likely to become excited, agitated, confused, or drowsy while taking normal doses of Propantheline. Continued use of Propantheline may lead to loss of memory. This medication blocks the hormone acetylcholine in the brain, which is responsible for many memory functions.

Generic Name

Propoxyphene

Generic Name: Propoxyphene Hydrochloride

Darvon
Dolene

(Also available in generic form)

Combination Products

Propoxyphene Hydrochloride + Aspirin + Caffeine*

Darvon Compound-65

Propoxyphene Hydrochloride + Acetaminophen*

E-Lor
Wygesic

Generic Name: Propoxyphene Napsylate

Darvon-N

Combination Products

Propoxyphene Napsylate + Aspirin

Darvon-N with ASA

Propoxyphene Napsylate + Acetaminophen

Darvocet-N 100
Propacet 100

(Also available in generic form)

Type of Drug

Analgesic.

Prescribed for

Pain relief.

General Information

Propoxyphene is a chemical derivative of *Methadone*, a narcotic pain reliever. Methadone is also used to help detoxify narcotics addicts. It is estimated that Propoxyphene is about ½ to ⅔ as strong a pain reliever as Codeine and about as effective as Aspirin. Propoxyphene is widely used for mild pain; it can produce drug dependence when used for extended periods of time.

Propoxyphene is more effective when combined with Aspirin or Acetaminophen than when used alone. The Propoxyphene used in these combinations is in either the Hydrochloride or Napsylate form. Propoxyphene Hydrochloride is about 30 percent more potent than Propoxyphene Napsylate.

Cautions and Warnings

Never take more of this medicine than is prescribed by your doctor. Do not take Propoxyphene if you are **allergic** to it or to similar drugs. This drug can produce **psychological or physical drug dependence** (addiction) when taken in doses larger than those needed for pain relief for long periods of time. The major sign of dependence is anxiety when the drug is suddenly stopped. Occasionally, people have become physically addicted to Propoxyphene. Propoxyphene can be abused to the same degree as Codeine.

Propoxyphene should be considered a dangerous drug, especially when it is in the hands of anyone who is severely depressed or addiction-prone. Excessive doses of Propoxyphene, either by itself or together with alcohol or other nervous-system depressants, are a major cause of drug-related deaths. Many of these deaths have occurred in people with a history of emotional disturbances, ideas of or attempts at suicide, or misuse of tranquilizers, alcohol, and other nervous-system depressants.

Possible Side Effects

▼ Common: dizziness, sedation, nausea, and vomiting. These effects usually disappear if you lie down and relax for a few moments.

▼ Less common: constipation, stomach pain, skin rashes, light-headedness, headache, weakness, euphoria, and minor visual disturbances. Taking Propoxyphene over long periods of time and in very high doses has caused psychotic reactions and convulsions.

Drug Interactions

• Propoxyphene may cause drowsiness when taken with other drugs that cause drowsiness, such as tranquilizers, sedatives, hypnotics, narcotics, alcohol, and possibly antihistamines.

• Carbamazepine levels may be increased by Propoxyphene, resulting in dizziness, nausea, and poor coordination.

• Charcoal tablets decrease the absorption of Propoxyphene into the bloodstream.

• Cigarette smoking increases the rate at which this drug is broken down in the liver. Heavy smokers may need more Propoxyphene to obtain pain relief and will have to take less medicine if they stop smoking.

• Cimetidine may interfere with the breakdown of this drug in the liver, causing confusion, disorientation, difficulty breathing, seizures, and interrupted breathing.

• Propoxyphene may increase the anticoagulant (blood-thinning) effect of Warfarin.

Food Interactions

Take with a full glass of water or with food if this medicine upsets your stomach.

Usual Dose

Propoxyphene Hydrochloride
65 mg every 4 hours as needed.

Propoxyphene Napsylate
100 mg every 4 hours as needed. Seniors and people with poor liver or kidney function may need to take the medicine less often.

Overdosage

Symptoms resemble those of a narcotic overdose and include the following: decrease in respiratory rate (in some people breathing rate is so low that the heart stops), changes in breathing pattern, pinpointed pupils, convulsions, extreme sleepiness leading to stupor or coma, abnormal heart rhythms, and development of fluid in the lungs. The overdose victim should be taken to a hospital emergency room immediately. ALWAYS bring the medicine bottle.

Special Information

Use caution while driving or performing any tasks that require you to be awake and alert. Avoid alcohol and other nervous-system depressants.

Call your doctor if you develop serious nausea or vomiting while taking this drug, or if you develop difficulty breathing.

If you forget to take a dose of Propoxyphene, take it as soon as you remember. If it is almost time for your next regularly scheduled dose, skip the one you forgot and continue with your regular schedule. Do not take a double dose.

Special Populations

Pregnancy/Breast-feeding
No formal studies of this medication have been done in pregnant women, but a survey of almost 3000 pregnant women who took Propoxyphene found that 46 (1.6 percent) had infants with birth defects. Animal studies show that high doses of the drug can cause problems in a developing fetus. Pregnant women who must take a Propoxyphene product should talk to their doctor about the risks of taking this drug.

Small amounts of Propoxyphene pass into breast milk, but no problems have been seen in nursing infants.

Seniors

Seniors, especially those with reduced kidney or liver function, are more likely to be sensitive to the effects of this drug, and should be treated with smaller dosages than younger adults.

Generic Name

Propranolol

Brand Names

Inderal
Inderal LA

(Also available in generic form)

Combination Products

Ingredients: Propranolol + Hydrochlorothiazide

Inderide
Inderide LA

(These combination products are used to treat high blood pressure and are also available in generic form.)

Type of Drug

Beta-adrenergic-blocking agent.

Prescribed for

High blood pressure, angina pectoris, abnormal heart rhythms, second heart attack prevention, migraine headache prevention, tremors, aggressive behavior, antipsychotic drug side effects, acute panic, stage fright and other anxieties, and schizophrenia. Propranolol is also used to treat bleeding from the stomach or esophagus, as well as symptoms of an overactive thyroid.

General Information

Propranolol is one of 14 beta-adrenergic-blocking drugs that interfere with the action of a specific part of the nervous system. Beta receptors are found all over the body and affect many body functions. This accounts for the usefulness of beta blockers against a wide variety of conditions. Propranolol, the first beta blocker, was found to affect the entire beta-adrenergic portion of the nervous system. Newer beta blockers have been refined to affect only a portion of that system, making them more useful in the treatment of cardiovascular disorders and less useful for other purposes. Other beta blockers are mild stimulants to the heart or have other characteristics that make them more useful for a specific purpose or better for certain people.

Cautions and Warnings

You should be **cautious about taking Propranolol** if you have **asthma**, **severe heart failure**, a **very slow heart rate**, or **heart block** because this drug may aggravate these conditions. People with **angina** who take Propranolol for high blood pressure should have their **drug dosage reduced gradually** over 1 to 2 weeks rather than suddenly discontinued to avoid possible aggravation of the angina.

Propranolol should be used with caution if you have **liver** or **kidney disease** because your ability to eliminate this drug from your body may be impaired.

Propranolol reduces the amount of blood pumped by the heart with each beat. This reduction in blood flow can aggravate or worsen the condition of people with **poor circulation** or **circulatory disease**.

If you are undergoing **major surgery**, your doctor may want you to stop taking Propranolol at least 2 days before surgery to permit the heart to respond more acutely to things that happen during the surgery. This is still controversial and may not hold true for all people preparing for surgery.

Possible Side Effects

Side effects are usually mild, relatively uncommon, develop early in the course of treatment, and are rarely a reason to stop taking Propranolol.

▼ Most common: male impotence.

Possible Side Effects *(continued)*

▼ Less common: tiredness or weakness, slow heart-beat, heart failure (swelling of the legs, ankles, or feet), dizziness, breathing difficulty, bronchospasm, mental depression, confusion, anxiety, nervousness, sleeplessness, disorientation, short-term memory loss, emotional instability, cold hands and feet, constipation, diarrhea, nausea, vomiting, upset stomach, increased sweating, urinary difficulty, cramps, blurred vision, skin rash, hair loss, stuffy nose, facial swelling, aggravation of lupus erythematosus (a disease of the body's connective tissues), itching, chest pains, back or joint pains, colitis, drug allergy (fever, sore throat), and liver toxicity.

Drug Interactions

• Propranolol may interact with surgical anesthetics to increase the risk of heart problems during surgery. Some anesthesiologists recommend gradually stopping your medicine 2 days before surgery.

• Propranolol may interfere with the normal signs of low blood sugar and can interfere with the action of oral antidiabetes medicines.

• Propranolol enhances the blood-pressure-lowering effects of other blood-pressure-reducing agents (including Clonidine, Guanabenz, and Reserpine) and calcium-channel-blocking drugs (such as Nifedipine).

• Aspirin-containing drugs, Indomethacin, Sulfinpyrazone, and estrogen drugs can interfere with the blood-pressure-lowering effect of Propranolol.

• Cocaine may reduce the effects of all beta-blocking drugs.

• Propranolol may increase the cold hands and feet associated with taking ergot alkaloids (for migraine headaches). Gangrene can result from taking an ergot and Propranolol.

• The effect of benzodiazepine antianxiety drugs may be increased by Propranolol.

• Propranolol will counteract the effects of thyroid hormone replacement medicines.

• Calcium channel blockers, Flecainide, Hydralazine, oral contraceptives, Propafenone, Haloperidol, phenothiazine tranquilizers (Molindone and others), quinolone antibacterials, and Quinidine may increase the amount of Propranolol in the bloodstream and the effect of that drug on the body.

• Propranolol should not be taken within 2 weeks of taking a monoamine oxidase (MAO) inhibitor antidepressant drug.

• Cimetidine increases the amount of Propranolol absorbed into the bloodstream from oral tablets.

• Propranolol may interfere with the effectiveness of Theophylline, Aminophylline, and some antiasthma drugs (especially Ephedrine and Isoproterenol).

• The combination of Propranolol and Phenytoin or digitalis drugs can result in excessive slowing of the heart, possibly causing heart block.

• Your Propranolol dose may have to be reduced If you stop smoking because your liver will break down the drug more slowly after you stop.

Food Interactions

Food increases the amount of Propranolol absorbed into the bloodstream. You should take it in the same way at all times to produce a consistent effect on the drug, preferably without food or on an empty stomach.

Usual Dose

30 to 700 mg per day. Propranolol should be given in the smallest dose that will produce the desired effect.

Overdosage

Symptoms of overdosage are changes in heartbeat (unusually slow, fast, or irregular), severe dizziness or fainting, difficulty breathing, bluish-colored fingernails or palms, and seizures. The overdose victim should be taken to a hospital emergency room where proper therapy can be given. ALWAYS bring the medicine bottle with you.

Special Information

Propranolol is meant to be taken continuously. Do not stop taking it unless directed to do so by your doctor; abrupt withdrawal may cause chest pain, difficulty breathing, increased sweating, and unusually fast or irregular heartbeat.

The dose should be lowered gradually over a period of about 2 weeks.

Call your doctor at once if any of the following symptoms develop: back or joint pains, difficulty breathing, cold hands or feet, depression, skin rash, or changes in heartbeat. Propranolol may produce an undesirable lowering of blood pressure, leading to dizziness or fainting. Call your doctor if this happens to you. Call your doctor about the following side effects only if they persist or are bothersome: anxiety, diarrhea, constipation, sexual impotence, headache, itching, nausea or vomiting, nightmares or vivid dreams, upset stomach, trouble sleeping, stuffy nose, frequent urination, unusual tiredness, or weakness.

Propranolol can cause drowsiness, light-headedness, dizziness, or blurred vision. Be careful when driving or performing complex tasks.

It is best to take your medicine at the same time each day. If you forget a dose of Propranolol, take it as soon as you remember. If you take your medicine once a day and it is within 8 hours of your next dose, skip the forgotten dose and continue with your regular schedule. If you take Propranolol twice a day and it is within 4 hours of your next dose, skip the forgotten dose and continue with your regular schedule. Do not take a double dose.

Special Populations

Pregnancy/Breast-feeding

Infants born to women who took a beta blocker weighed less at birth and had low blood pressure and reduced heart rate. Propranolol should be avoided by pregnant women and those who might become pregnant while taking it. When the drug is considered essential by your doctor, its potential benefits must be carefully weighed against its risks.

Propranolol passes into breast milk in concentrations too small to have any effect.

Seniors

Older adults may absorb and retain more Propranolol in their bodies, thus requiring less medicine. Your doctor will need to adjust your dosage to meet your individual needs. Seniors taking this medicine may be more likely to suffer from cold hands and feet, reduced body temperature, chest pains, general feelings of ill health, sudden breathing difficulty, increased sweating, or changes in heartbeat.

Propulsid

see *Cisapride,* page 215

Generic Name

Protriptyline Hydrochloride

Brand Name

Vivactil

(Also available in generic form)

Type of Drug

Tricyclic antidepressant.

Prescribed for

Depression, sleep apnea (intermittent breathing while sleeping), and panic disorder.

General Information

Protriptyline and other tricyclic antidepressants block the movement of certain stimulant chemicals (norepinephrine or serotonin) in and out of nerve endings, have a sedative effect, and have an anticholinergic effect (counteract the effects of a hormone called *acetylcholine*).

Theory says that people with depression have a chemical imbalance in their brains and that drugs such as Protriptyline work to reestablish a proper balance. Although Protriptyline and similar antidepressants immediately block neurohormones, it takes about 2 to 4 weeks for their clinical antidepressant effect to come into play. They can also elevate mood, increase physical activity and mental alertness, and improve appetite and sleep patterns in a depressed patient. These drugs are mild sedatives and therefore useful in treating mild forms of depression associated with anxiety. If symptoms are not affected after 6 to 8 weeks, contact your doctor. Protriptyline is broken down in the liver.

Cautions and Warnings

Do not take Protriptyline if you are **allergic** or **sensitive** to it or any other tricyclic antidepressant. Protriptyline should not be used if you are **recovering from a heart attack**.

Protriptyline may be taken with caution if you have a history of **epilepsy** or other seizure disorders, **difficulty in urination, glaucoma, heart disease, liver disease,** or **hyperthyroidism.** People who are **schizophrenic** or **paranoid** may get worse if given a tricyclic antidepressant and manic depressive people may switch phase. This can also happen if they are changing or stopping antidepressants. **Suicide** is always a possibility in severely depressed people, who should be given only small quantities of medication at a time.

Possible Side Effects

▼ Most common: rapid heartbeat, fainting when rising quickly from a sitting or lying position, sedation, and anticholinergic effects such as blurred vision, disorientation, confusion, hallucinations, muscle spasms or tremors, seizures and/or convulsions, dry mouth, constipation (especially in older adults), difficult urination, worsening glaucoma, and sensitivity to bright light or sunlight.

▼ Less common: blood-pressure changes, abnormal heart rates, heart attack, anxiety, restlessness, excitement, numbness and tingling in the extremities, poor coordination, rash, itching, retention of fluids, fever, allergy, changes in composition of blood, nausea, vomiting, loss of appetite, stomach upset, diarrhea, enlargement of the breasts in males and females, changes in sex drive, and blood-sugar changes.

▼ Rare: agitation, inability to sleep, nightmares, feeling of panic, a peculiar taste in the mouth, stomach cramps, black discoloration of the tongue, yellowing eyes and/or skin, changes in liver function, increased or decreased weight, excessive perspiration, flushing, frequent urination, drowsiness, dizziness, weakness, headache, loss of hair, and general feelings of ill health.

Drug Interactions

• Interaction with monoamine oxidase (MAO) inhibitors

can cause high fevers, convulsions, and occasionally death. Do not take MAO inhibitors until at least 2 weeks after this drug has been discontinued. Patients who must take this drug and an MAO inhibitor require close medical observation.

• Protriptyline interacts with Guanethidine and Clonidine. Be sure your doctor knows if you are taking **any** high blood pressure medicine if Protriptyline is being considered.

• Protriptyline increases the effects of barbiturates, tranquilizers, other sedative drugs, and alcohol. Also, barbiturates may decrease the effectiveness of Protriptyline

• Taking Protriptyline and thyroid medicine together will enhance the effects of both medicines, possibly causing abnormal heart rhythms. The combination of Protriptyline and Reserpine may cause overstimulation.

• Oral contraceptives can reduce the effect of Protriptyline, as can smoking. Charcoal tablets can prevent Protriptyline's absorption into the blood. Estrogens can increase or decrease the effect of Protriptyline.

• Drugs such as Bicarbonate of Soda, Acetazolamide, Quinidine, or Procainamide will increase the effect of Protriptyline. Cimetidine, Methylphenidate, and phenothiazine drugs (like Thorazine and Compazine) block the liver metabolism of Protriptyline, causing it to stay in the body longer. This can cause severe drug side effects.

Food Interactions

Take Protriptyline with food if it upsets your stomach.

Usual Dose

Adult: 15 to 60 mg per day in 3 or 4 divided doses. Protriptyline cannot be taken as a single bedtime dose because of its stimulant effect.

Adolescent and Senior: lower doses are recommended, usually up to 20 mg per day. Seniors taking more than 20 mg per day should have regular heart examinations. The dose must be tailored to your needs.

Child: not recommended.

Overdosage

Overdose symptoms are confusion, inability to concentrate, hallucinations, drowsiness, lowered body temperature, abnormal heart rate, heart failure, enlarged pupils of the eyes, convulsions, severely lowered blood pressure, stupor, and coma. Agitation, stiffening of body muscles, vomiting, and high fever may also occur. The victim should be taken to a hospital emergency room immediately. ALWAYS bring the medicine bottle.

Special Information

Avoid alcohol and other depressants while taking this drug. Do not stop taking Protriptyline unless your doctor has specifically told you to do so. Abruptly stopping this medicine may cause nausea, headache, and a sickly feeling.

Protriptyline can cause drowsiness, dizziness, and blurred vision. Be careful when driving or operating hazardous machinery. Avoid prolonged exposure to the sun or sun lamps.

Call your doctor at once if you develop seizures, difficult or rapid breathing, fever and sweating, blood-pressure changes, muscle stiffness, loss of bladder control, or unusual tiredness or weakness. Dry mouth may lead to an increase in dental cavities, gum bleeding, and disease. People taking Protriptyline should pay special attention to maintaining good dental hygiene.

If you miss a dose of Protriptyline, skip it and continue with your regular schedule. Do not take a double dose.

Special Populations

Pregnancy/Breast-feeding

Protriptyline, like other antidepressants, crosses into your developing baby's circulation, and birth defects have been reported if the drug is taken during the first 3 months of pregnancy. There have been reports of newborn infants suffering from heart, breathing, and urinary problems after their mothers had taken an antidepressant of this type immediately before delivery. Avoid taking this medication while pregnant.

Small amounts of tricyclic antidepressants pass into breast milk and sedate the baby. Nursing mothers taking Protriptyline should consider bottle-feeding.

Seniors

Older adults are more sensitive to the effects of this drug, especially abnormal rhythms and other heart side effects, and often require lower doses than younger adults to achieve the same results. Follow your doctor's directions and report any side effects at once.

Proventil

see **Albuterol**, page 30

Provera

see **Medroxyprogesterone Acetate**, page 665

Prozac

see **Fluoxetine Hydrochloride**, page 465

Generic Name

Quazepam

Brand Name

Doral

Type of Drug

Benzodiazepine sedative.

Prescribed for

The short-term treatment of insomnia, difficulty falling asleep, frequent nighttime awakening, and waking too early in the morning.

General Information

Quazepam is a member of the group of drugs known as

benzodiazepines. All have some activity as either antianxiety agents, anticonvulsants, or sedatives. Benzodiazepines work by a direct effect on the brain. Benzodiazepines make it easier to sleep and decrease the number of times you wake up during the night.

The principal differences between these medicines lie in how long they work on your body. They all take about 2 hours to reach maximum blood level, but some remain in your body longer, so they work for a longer period of time. Flurazepam and Quazepam remain in your body and last the longest, thus resulting in the greatest incidence of morning "hangover." Often sleeplessness is a reflection of another disorder that would be untreated by one of these medicines.

Cautions and Warnings

People with respiratory disease may experience **sleep apnea** (intermittent breathing while sleeping) while taking a benzodiazepine sedative.

People with **kidney or liver disease** should be carefully monitored while taking Quazepam. Take the lowest possible dose to help you sleep.

Clinical **depression** may be increased by Quazepam and other drugs with an ability to depress the nervous system. Intentional overdosage is more common among depressed people who take sleeping pills than those who do not.

All benzodiazepine drugs can be **abused** if taken for long periods of time. It is possible for a person taking Quazepam to develop **drug-withdrawal symptoms** if the drug is suddenly discontinued. Withdrawal symptoms include tremors, muscle cramps, insomnia, agitation, diarrhea, vomiting, sweating, and convulsions.

Possible Side Effects

▼ Most common: drowsiness, headache, dizziness, talkativeness, nervousness, apprehension, poor muscle coordination, light-headedness, daytime tiredness, muscle weakness, slowness of movements, hangover, and euphoria (feeling "high").

Possible Side Effects *(continued)*

▼ Less common: nausea, vomiting, rapid heartbeat and abnormal heart rhythms, confusion, temporary memory loss, upset stomach, stomach cramps and pain, depression, blurred or double vision, constipation, changes in taste perception, appetite changes, stuffy nose, nosebleeds, common cold symptoms, asthma, sore throat, cough, breathing problems, diarrhea, dry mouth, allergic reactions, fainting, itching, acne, dry skin, sensitivity to bright light or the sun, rash, nightmares or strange dreams, difficulty sleeping, tingling in the hands or feet, ringing or buzzing in the ears, ear or eye pains, menstrual cramps, frequent or painful urination, blood in the urine, discharge from the penis or vagina, poor control of the urinary function, lower back and joint pains, muscle spasms and pain, fever, swollen breasts, and weight changes.

Drug Interactions

• As with all benzodiazepines, the effects of Quazepam are enhanced if the drug is taken with other nervous-system depressants (including alcoholic beverages, antihistamines, tranquilizers, and barbiturates), anticonvulsant medicines, tricyclic antidepressants, and monoamine oxidase (MAO) inhibitor drugs (most often prescribed for severe depression).

• Oral contraceptives, Cimetidine, Disulfiram, and Isoniazid may increase the effect of Quazepam by interfering with the drug's breakdown in the liver. Probenecid may also increase Quazepam's effect.

• Cigarette smoking, Rifampin, and Theophylline may reduce Quazepam's sedating effect.

• The effect of Levodopa may be decreased by Quazepam.

• Quazepam may increase the amount of Zidovudine, Phenytoin, or Digoxin in your blood, increasing the chances of drug toxicity.

• The combination of Clozapine and benzodiazepines has led to respiratory collapse in a few people. Quazepam should be stopped at least 1 week before starting Clozapine treatment.

Food Interactions

Quazepam may be taken with food if it upsets your stomach.

Usual Dose

Adult (age 18 and older): 7.5 to 15 mg at bedtime. The dose must be individualized for maximum benefit.
Senior: take the lowest effective dose.
Child: not recommended.

Overdosage

The most common symptoms of overdosage are confusion, sleepiness, depression, loss of muscle coordination, and slurred speech. Coma may develop if the overdose is particularly large. Overdose symptoms can develop if a single dose of only 4 times the maximum daily dose is taken. Overdose victims must be made to vomit with Syrup of Ipecac (available at any pharmacy) to remove any remaining drug from the stomach. Call your doctor or a poison control center before doing this. If 30 minutes have passed since the overdose was taken or symptoms have begun to develop, the victim must be taken immediately to a hospital emergency room for treatment. ALWAYS bring the medicine bottle.

Special Information

Never take more of this medication than your doctor has prescribed.

Avoid alcoholic beverages and other nervous-system depressants while taking this medicine.

People taking this drug must be careful when performing tasks requiring concentration and coordination because it may make them tired, dizzy, or light-headed.

If you take Quazepam daily for 3 or more weeks, you may experience some withdrawal symptoms after you stop taking it. Talk with your doctor about how to discontinue the drug.

If you forget to take a dose of Quazepam, and remember within about an hour of your regular time, take it as soon as you remember. If you do not remember until later, skip the forgotten dose and go back to your regular schedule. Do not take a double dose.

Special Populations

Pregnancy/Breast-feeding

Quazepam must absolutely not be used by pregnant women

or women who may become pregnant. Animal studies have shown that this drug passes easily into the fetal blood system and can affect fetal development.

Benzodiazepines pass into breast milk and can affect a nursing infant. Quazepam should not be taken by nursing mothers.

Seniors

Older adults are more susceptible to the effects of Quazepam and should take the lowest possible dosage.

Generic Name

Quinapril Hydrochloride

Brand Name

Accupril

Type of Drug

Angiotensin-converting-enzyme (ACE) inhibitor.

Prescribed for

High blood pressure and congestive heart failure.

General Information

ACE inhibitors work by preventing the conversion of a hormone called *angiotensin I* to another hormone called *angiotensin II*, a potent blood vessel constrictor. Preventing this conversion relaxes blood vessels and helps to reduce blood pressure and relieve the symptoms of heart failure by making it easier for a failing heart to pump blood around your body. The production of other hormones and enzymes that participate in the regulation of blood vessel dilation is also affected by the ACE inhibitors and probably plays a role in the effectiveness of these medicines. Quinapril begins working about an hour after you take it and lasts for a full 24 hours.

Some people who start taking an ACE inhibitor after they are already on a diuretic experience a rapid blood-pressure drop after their first dose or when the dose is increased. To prevent this from happening, you may be told to stop taking the diuretic 2 or 3 days before starting the ACE inhibitor or increase your salt intake during that time. The diuretic may then be restarted gradually. Heart failure patients generally have been on Digoxin and a diuretic before beginning treatment with an ACE inhibitor.

Cautions and Warnings

Do not take Quinapril if you have had an **allergic reaction** to it in the past. It can, rarely, cause very **low blood pressure,** and it can affect your **kidneys,** especially if you have congestive heart failure. It is advisable for your doctor to check your urine for changes during the first few months of treatment.

Dosage adjustment of Quinapril is necessary if you have **reduced kidney function,** since it is eliminated from the body mainly by your kidneys. Ironically, ACE inhibitors may cause a decline in kidney function on their own.

Rarely, Quinapril affects white-blood-cell count, possibly increasing your **susceptibility to infection.** Blood counts should be monitored periodically.

Possible Side Effects

▼ Most common: dizziness, tiredness, headache, and chronic cough. The cough usually goes away a few days after you stop taking the medicine.

▼ Less common: nausea, vomiting, and abdominal pains.

▼ Rare: heart palpitations, rapid heartbeat, chest pain, angina, heart attack, stroke, abdominal pain, fainting, dizziness when rising from a sitting or lying position, sleepiness, feelings of ill health, depression, nervousness, constipation, dry mouth, inflammation of the pancreas, sweating, skin rash or peeling, itching, sun sensitivity, kidney failure, reduced white-blood-cell or blood-platelet counts, stomach or intestinal bleeding, high blood pressure, shock, flushing or redness, back pain, visual disturbances, sore throat, and viral infections.

Drug Interactions

• The blood-pressure-lowering effect of Quinapril is additive with diuretic drugs and beta blockers. Any other drug that causes a rapid blood-pressure drop should be used with caution if you are taking ACE Inhibitors.

• Quinapril may increase potassium levels in your blood, especially when taken with Dyazide or other potassium-sparing diuretics.

• Quinapril may increase the effects of Lithium; this combination should be used with caution.

• Antacids may reduce the amount of Quinapril absorbed into the blood. Separate doses of these two medicines by at least 2 hours.

• Quinapril decreases the absorption of Tetracycline by about ⅓, possibly because of the high Magnesium content of Quinapril tablets.

• Quinapril may increase blood levels of Digoxin, possibly increasing the chance of Digoxin-related side effects.

• Capsaicin may cause or aggravate the cough associated with Quinapril therapy.

• Indomethacin may reduce the blood-pressure-lowering effects of Quinapril.

• Phenothiazine tranquilizers and antiemetics may increase the effects of Quinapril.

• The combination of Allopurinol and Quinapril increases the chance of a drug reaction.

Food Interactions

Quinapril is affected by high-fat food in the stomach and should be taken on an empty stomach or at least 1 hour before or 2 hours after a meal.

Usual Dose

Adult: 10 to 80 mg, once a day. People with kidney disease may require less medicine.

Overdosage

The principal effect of Quinapril overdose is a rapid drop in blood pressure, as evidenced by dizziness or fainting. Take the overdose victim to a hospital emergency room at once. ALWAYS bring the medicine bottle.

Special Information

Call your doctor at once if you develop swelling of the face or throat, if you have sudden difficulty breathing, or if you develop a sore throat, mouth sores, abnormal heartbeat, chest pain, a persistent rash, or loss of taste perception.

ACE inhibitors can cause unexplained swelling of the face, lips, hands and feet. This swelling can also affect the larynx (throat) and tongue and interfere with breathing. If this happens, the victim should be taken to a hospital emergency room at once for treatment.

You may get dizzy if you rise to your feet too quickly from a sitting or lying position.

Avoid strenuous exercise and/or very hot weather because heavy sweating or dehydration can cause a rapid blood-pressure drop.

Avoid nonprescription diet pills, decongestants, and stimulants that can raise blood pressure.

If you forget to take a dose of Quinapril, take it as soon as you remember. If it is within 8 hours of your next dose, skip the one you forgot and continue with your regular schedule. Do not take a double dose.

Special Populations

Pregnancy/Breast-feeding

ACE inhibitors have caused low blood pressure, kidney failure, slow formation of the skull, and death in developing fetuses when taken during the last 6 months of pregnancy. Women who are pregnant should not take Quinapril. Women who may become pregnant while taking Quinapril should use an effective contraceptive method and stop taking the medicine if they do become pregnant.

Relatively small amounts of Quinapril pass into breast milk, and the effect on a nursing infant is likely to be minimal. However, nursing mothers who must take this drug should consider an alternative feeding method since infants, especially newborns, are more susceptible to the effects of these medicines than adults.

Seniors

Older adults may be more sensitive to the effects of Quinapril than younger adults because of the possibility of kidney impairment and should begin at 10 mg daily. Your Quinapril dosage must be individualized to your needs.

Generic Name

Quinidine

Brand Names

Quinidine Sulfate

Quinora*
Quinidex Extentabs (sustained-release)

(*Also available in generic form)

Quinidine Gluconate

Quinaglute Dura-Tabs (sustained-release)
Quinalan (sustained-release)

(Also available in generic form)

Quinidine Polygalacturonate

Cardioquin

Type of Drug

Antiarrhythmic.

Prescribed for

Abnormal heart rhythms.

General Information

Derived from the bark of the cinchona tree (which gives us
Quinine), this drug works by affecting the flow of potassium
into and out of cells of the myocardium (heart muscle). This
function helps it to affect the flow of nervous impulses
throughout the heart muscle. Its basic action is to slow down
the pulse, which allows control mechanisms in the heart to
take over and keep the heart beating at a normal, even rate.

The 3 kinds of Quinidine provide different amounts of
active drug, so they cannot be interchanged without your
doctor making dosage adjustments. Quinidine Sulfate provides the most active drug.

Some of the different brands come in sustained-release form so that fewer pills are required throughout the day.

Cautions and Warnings

Do not take Quinidine if you are **allergic** to it, Quinine, or a related drug. Quinidine sensitivity may be masked if you have **asthma, muscle weakness,** or an **infection** when you start taking the medicine.

Liver toxicity related to Quinidine sensitivity is rare but has occurred. Unexplained fever or liver inflammation may be an indication of this effect. People with **kidney or liver disease** should take this medicine with caution; lower doses may be necessary.

Like other antiarrhythmic drugs, Quinidine can cause its own abnormal heart rhythms. If this happens, you will be told to stop taking the drug and may be hospitalized for further evaluation.

People taking Quinidine for long periods may experience **sudden fainting** and/or an **abnormal heart rhythm.** These may end on their own or respond to medical treatment. Occasionally, these episodes may be fatal.

Possible Side Effects

▼ Most common: nausea, vomiting, abdominal pain, diarrhea, and appetite loss. These may be accompanied by fever.

▼ Less common: Quinidine may cause unusual heart rhythms, but such effects are generally found by your doctor during routine examination or electrocardiogram. It may also cause irritation of the esophagus, affect components of the blood system, and can cause headache, dizziness, feelings of apprehension or excitement, confusion, delirium, muscle aches or joint pains, ringing or buzzing in the ears, mild hearing loss, blurred vision, changes in color perception, sensitivity to bright light, double vision, difficulty seeing at night, flushing of the skin, itching, sensitivity to the sun, cramps, an unusual urge to defecate or urinate, and cold sweat.

▼ Rare: allergic reactions to Quinidine can include

Possible Side Effects *(continued)*

asthma; swelling of the face, hands, and feet; respiratory collapse; and liver problems.

High doses of Quinidine can cause rash, hearing loss, dizziness, ringing in the ears, headache, nausea, or disturbed vision. This group of symptoms, called *cinchonism*, is usually related to taking a large amount of Quinidine (but may appear after a single dose of the medicine) and is not necessarily a toxic reaction. Report any sign of cinchonism to your doctor immediately. Do not stop taking this drug unless instructed to do so by your doctor.

Drug Interactions

• Quinidine increases the effect of Warfarin and other oral anticoagulants (blood thinners). The anticoagulant dose may have to be adjusted.

• Quinidine may increase the effects of Metoprolol, Procainamide, Propafenone, Propranolol and other beta blockers; Benztropine, Oxybutynin, Atropine, Trihexyphenidyl, and other anticholinergic drugs; and tricyclic antidepressants.

• The effect of Quinidine may be decreased by the following medicines: Phenobarbital or other barbiturates, Phenytoin or other hydantoins, Nifedipine, Rifampin, Sucralfate, and cholinergic drugs (such as Bethanechol).

• The effect (and toxicity) of Quinidine may be increased by taking Amiodarone, some antacids, Cimetidine, anything that decreases urine acid levels, and Verapamil.

• Quinidine can dramatically increase the amount of Digoxin in the blood, causing possible Digoxin toxicity. This combination should be monitored closely by your doctor.

• The combination of Disopyramide and Quinidine can result in increased Disopyramide levels and possible drug side effects and/or reduced Quinidine activity.

• Avoid over-the-counter cough, cold, allergy, or diet preparations. These medications may contain drugs that will stimulate your heart and can be dangerous while you are taking Quinidine. Ask your pharmacist if you have any questions about the contents of a particular cough, cold, or allergy remedy.

Food Interactions

You may take Quinidine with food if it upsets your stomach. Quinidine is also available in forms that are less irritating to the stomach. Contact your doctor if upset stomach persists.

Usual Dose

Extremely variable, depending on your disease and response. Most doses are 600 to 1200 mg a day.

Sustained-Release

Most doses are 600 to 1800 mg a day.

Overdosage

Overdose produces depressed mental function, including lethargy, decreased breathing, seizures, and coma. Other symptoms are abdominal pain and diarrhea, abnormal heart rhythms, and symptoms of cinchonism (see *Possible Side Effects*). The victim should be taken to a hospital emergency room. ALWAYS bring the medicine bottle with you.

Special Information

Call your doctor if you develop ringing or buzzing in the ears, hearing or visual disturbances, dizziness, headache, nausea, skin rash, difficulty breathing, or any intolerable side effect (see *Possible Side Effects*).

Do not crush or chew the sustained-release products.

Some side effects of Quinidine may lead to oral discomfort (dry mouth), cavities, periodontal disease, and oral *Candida* infections. See your dentist regularly while taking this drug.

If you forget to take a dose of Quinidine, and you remember within about 2 hours of your regular time, take it right away. If you do not remember until later, skip the forgotten dose and go back to your regular schedule. Do not take a double dose.

Special Populations

Pregnancy/Breast-feeding

This drug passes into the fetal blood circulation and may cause birth defects or interfere with your baby's development. Check with your doctor before taking it if you are, or might be, pregnant.

Quinidine passes into breast milk but is considered acceptable for use while breast-feeding. Consult your doctor.

Seniors

Older adults may be more sensitive to the effects of this medicine because of the likelihood of decreased kidney function. Follow your doctor's directions, and report any side effects at once.

Generic Name

Ramipril

Brand Name

Altace

Type of Drug

Angiotensin-converting-enzyme (ACE) inhibitor.

Prescribed for

High blood pressure and congestive heart failure.

General Information

ACE inhibitors work by preventing the conversion of a hormone called *angiotensin I* to another hormone called *angiotensin II*, a potent blood-vessel constrictor. Preventing this conversion relaxes blood vessels and helps to reduce blood pressure and relieve the symptoms of heart failure by making it easier for a failing heart to pump blood around your body. The production of other hormones and enzymes that participate in the regulation of blood-vessel dilation is also affected by the ACE inhibitors and probably plays a role in the effectiveness of these medicines. Ramipril begins working about an hour after you take it and lasts for a full 24 hours.

Some people who start taking an ACE inhibitor after they are already on a diuretic experience a rapid blood-pressure drop after their first dose or when the dose is increased. To prevent this from happening, you may be told to stop taking the diuretic 2 or 3 days before starting Ramipril or increase your salt intake during that time. The diuretic may then be restarted gradually. Heart failure patients generally have been on Digoxin and a diuretic before beginning treatment with an ACE inhibitor.

Cautions and Warnings

Do not take any ACE inhibitor if you have had an **allergic reaction** to it in the past. Occasionally, severe allergic reactions have occurred in people undergoing desensitization treatments or certain kinds of kidney dialysis. ACE inhibitors can, rarely, cause very low blood pressure, and can affect your **kidneys**, especially if you have congestive heart failure. It is advisable for your doctor to check your urine for changes during the first few months of treatment.

People with **liver disease** who are taking Ramipril may require a lower dosage because they have more drug in their blood and are more likely to develop drug side effects.

ACE inhibitors can affect white-blood-cell count, possibly increasing your susceptibility to **infection**. Blood counts should be monitored periodically.

Possible Side Effects

▼ Most common: chronic cough. The cough is more common in women than men and usually goes away a few days after you stop taking the medicine.

▼ Less common: dizziness, tiredness, headache, nausea, and fatigue.

▼ Other: itching, fever, chest pain, angina, heart attack, stroke, abdominal pain, low blood pressure, dizziness when rising from a sitting or lying position, abnormal heart rhythms, heart palpitations, sleeping difficulty, tingling in the hands or feet, vomiting, appetite loss, abnormal tastes, hepatitis and jaundice, blood in the stool, swollen tongue, hair loss, rash, unusual sensitivity to the sun, flushing, anxiety, sleeplessness, nervousness, reduced sex drive, muscle cramps or weakness, impotence, arthritis, muscle aches, asthma, bronchitis, respiratory infection, sinus irritation, breathing difficulty, weakness, confusion, depression, feelings of ill health, sweating, kidney problems, urinary infection, anemia, blurred vision, and swelling of the arms, legs, lips, face, and throat.

Possible Side Effects *(continued)*

These side effects occur very infrequently but can be bothersome.

Drug Interactions

• The blood-pressure-lowering effect of Ramipril is additive with diuretic drugs and beta blockers. Any other drug that can reduce blood pressure should be used with caution if you are taking Ramipril.

• Ramipril may increase potassium levels in your blood, especially when taken with Dyazide or other potassium-sparing diuretics.

• Ramipril may increase the effects of Lithium; this combination should be used with caution.

• Antacids may reduce the amount of Ramipril absorbed into the blood. Separate doses of the two medicines by at least 2 hours.

• Capsaicin may cause or aggravate the cough associated with Ramipril therapy.

• Indomethacin may reduce the blood-pressure-lowering effects of Ramipril.

• Phenothiazine tranquilizers and antiemetics may increase the effects of Ramipril.

• The combination of Allopurinol and Ramipril increases the chance of a drug reaction.

• Ramipril increases blood levels of Digoxin, possibly increasing the chance of Digoxin-related side effects.

• Cough associated with Ramipril may be reduced by Sulindac, Diclofenlac, Indomethacin, Nifedipine, Cromolyn Sodium, or nebulized Bupivacaine. More study is needed to confirm these interactions.

Food Interactions

Ramipril is affected by larger amounts of food in the stomach and should be taken on an empty stomach or at least 1 hour before or 2 hours after a meal. However, the contents of Ramipril capsules may be mixed with a small amount (about 4 ounces) of applesauce or some apple juice or water and stored for up to 2 days in the refrigerator before you take it.

Usual Dose

2.5 to 20 mg a day. People with moderate to severe kidney disease should begin with 1.25 mg per day and can be increased up to 5 mg a day.

Overdosage

The principal effect of Ramipril overdose is a rapid drop in blood pressure, as evidenced by dizziness or fainting. Take the overdose victim to a hospital emergency room immediately. ALWAYS remember to bring the medicine bottle.

Special Information

Call your doctor if you develop swelling of the face or throat, if you have sudden difficulty breathing, or if you develop a sore throat, mouth sores, abnormal heartbeat, chest pain, a persistent rash, or loss of taste perception.

Ramipril can cause unexplained swelling of the face, lips, hands, and feet, which can also affect the larynx (throat) and tongue and interfere with breathing. If this happens, the victim should be taken to a hospital emergency room at once for treatment.

You may get dizzy if you rise to your feet too quickly from a sitting or lying position.

Avoid strenuous exercise and/or very hot weather because heavy sweating or dehydration can cause a rapid blood-pressure drop.

Avoid nonprescription diet pills, decongestants, and stimulants that can raise blood pressure.

If you forget to take a dose of Ramipril, take it as soon as you remember. If it is within 8 hours of your next dose, skip the one you forgot and continue with your regular schedule. Do not take a double dose.

Special Populations

Pregnancy/Breast-feeding

ACE inhibitors have caused low blood pressure, kidney failure, slow formation of the skull, and death in developing fetuses when taken during the last 6 months of pregnancy. Women who are pregnant should not take Ramipril. Women who may become pregnant while taking Ramipril should use an effective contraceptive method and stop taking the medicine if they do become pregnant.

It is not known if Ramipril passes into breast milk. However, nursing mothers who must take this drug should consider an alternative feeding method since infants, especially newborns, are more susceptible to the effects of these medicines than adults.

Seniors

Older adults may be more sensitive to the effects of Ramipril than younger adults because of the possibility of normal reductions in kidney function. Your dosage must be individualized to your needs.

Generic Name

Ranitidine

Brand Name

Zantac Tablets/EFFERdose/GELdose
Zantac 75 (nonprescription)

Type of Drug

Antiulcer; histamine H_2 antagonist.

Prescribed for

Short-term and maintenance therapy for duodenal (intestinal) and gastric (stomach) ulcers. It is also prescribed for gastroesophageal reflux disease (GERD); for other conditions characterized by the secretions of large amounts of gastric fluids; to prevent bleeding in the stomach and upper intestines; to prevent stress ulcers; and to prevent stomach damage caused by nonsteroidal anti-inflammatory drugs (NSAIDs) prescribed for arthritis and pain relief. A surgeon may prescribe Ranitidine for a patient under anesthesia when it is desirable for the production of stomach acid to be stopped completely.

General Information

Ranitidine and other H_2 antagonists work by actually turning off the system that produces stomach acid and other secretions. Ranitidine starts working within 1 hour and reaches its peak effect in 1 to 3 hours. Its effect lasts for up to 15 hours.

Ranitidine is effective in treating ulcer symptoms and preventing complications of the disease. Since all histamine H_2 antagonists work in the exact same way, ulcers that do not respond to one will probably not respond to another. The only difference among the H_2 antagonists is their potency. Cimetidine is the least potent, with 1000 mg roughly equal to 300 mg of Ranitidine and Nizatidine and 40 mg of Famotidine. The ulcer-healing rates of all of these drugs are roughly equivalent, as is the chance of drug side effects.

Cautions and Warnings

Do not take Ranitidine if you have had an **allergic** reaction to it or another H_2 antagonist in the past. Caution must be exercised by people with **kidney or liver disease** who take Ranitidine because the drug is partly broken down in the liver and passes out of the body through the kidneys. Occasionally, reversible **hepatitis** or other liver abnormality can occur, with or without jaundice (yellowing of the skin, eyeballs, etc.). Reducing acid levels in the stomach of a person with compromised immune functions can lead to a greater chance of some **intestinal worm infections**.

Possible Side Effects

Side effects with Ranitidine are rare.

▼ Most common: dizziness, confusion, hallucinations, depression, sleeplessness, hair loss, inflammation of the pancreas, joint pains, and drug reactions.

▼ Less common: headache, blurred vision (reversible), agitation or anxiety, nausea, vomiting, constipation, diarrhea, abdominal discomfort, rash, painful breast swelling, impotence, loss of sex drive, and rashes.

▼ Rare: reversible reduction in the levels of either white blood cells or blood platelets; hepatitis.

Drug Interactions

• The effects of Ranitidine may be reduced if it is taken together with antacids. This minor interaction may be avoided by separating doses of these medicines by about 2 to 3 hours.

• Ranitidine may interfere with the absorption of Diazepam tablets into the blood. This interaction is considered of only minor importance and is unlikely to affect most people.

• Ranitidine may increase blood concentrations of Glipizide, Glyburide (rare), theophylline drugs (rare), and Procainamide, increasing the chances for drug side effects.

• Ranitidine may interact with Warfarin, an anticoagulant (blood thinner). Persons taking both medicines may need to have their Warfarin doses adjusted by their doctor.

Food Interactions

You may take Ranitidine without regard to food or meals.

Usual Dose

150 to 300 mg per day. People with severe conditions may require up to 600 mg per day. People with severe kidney disease need less medicine.

Overdosage

There is very little experience with Ranitidine overdose. Overdose victims may be expected to show exaggerated side-effect symptoms, but little else is known. Overdose victims must be made to vomit with Syrup of Ipecac (available at any pharmacy) to remove any remaining drug from the stomach. Call your doctor or a poison control center before doing this. If you must go to the emergency room, ALWAYS bring the medicine bottle.

Special Information

It may take several days for Ranitidine to begin to relieve stomach pains. You must take this medicine exactly as directed and follow your doctor's instructions for diet and other treatments to get the maximum benefit from it.

Call your doctor at once if any unusual side effects develop. Especially important are unusual bleeding or bruising, unusual tiredness, diarrhea, dizziness, rash, or hallucinations. Black, tarry stools or vomiting "coffee-ground"-like material may indicate that your ulcer is bleeding.

If you forget to take a dose of Ranitidine, take it as soon as you remember. If it is almost time for your next dose, skip the one you forgot and continue with your regular schedule. Do not take a double dose.

Special Populations

Pregnancy/Breast-feeding
Studies with laboratory animals have revealed no damage to a developing fetus. However, Ranitidine should be avoided by pregnant women and those who might become pregnant while using it. When Ranitidine use is essential, its possible benefits must be carefully weighed against its possible risks.

Large amounts of Ranitidine pass into breast milk, but no problems have been found in nursing infants. Nursing mothers must consider a possible drug effect while nursing their infants.

Seniors
Older adults respond well to Ranitidine but may need less medication than a younger adult to achieve the desired response, because the drug is eliminated through the kidneys, and kidney function tends to decline with age. Older adults may be more susceptible to some side effects of this drug, especially confusion.

Relafen
─────────────────────────────

see **Nabumetone**, page 761

Retin-A
─────────────────────────────

see **Tretinoin**, page 1131

Generic Name
Rifampin
─────────────────────────────

Brand Names
Rifadin
Rimactane

(*Note:* Rifampin is also available under the brand name Rifater in combination with Isonazid and Pyrazinamide.)

Type of Drug

Antitubercular.

Prescribed for

Tuberculosis and many other infections.

General Information

Rifampin is an important agent in the treatment of tuberculosis. It is always used in combination with at least one other tuberculosis drug because it is not effective alone. It is also used to eradicate the organism that causes meningitis in people who are carriers; although these individuals are not infected themselves, they carry the organism and can spread it to others. Rifampin may also be prescribed for staphylococcal infections of the skin, bones, or prostate; for Legionnaire's disease (when Erythromycin does not work); for leprosy; and to prevent meningitis caused by *Haemophilus influenzae*, common among children in day care.

Cautions and Warnings

Do not take this drug if you are **allergic** to it or to Rifabutin (prescribed for *Mycobacterium avium* complex [MAC], an infection commonly associated with advanced cases of AIDS). **Liver damage** and **death** have been reported in people taking this drug; people taking other drugs that may cause liver damage should also avoid Rifampin. People with liver disease need to be carefully monitored by their doctors and should take a reduced dosage of Rifampin.

Bacterial resistance develops very quickly if Rifampin is used for meningococcus infection. It should not be used for this purpose.

A few cases of accelerated **lung cancer** growth have been reported, but a link to Rifampin use is not established. This drug has the potential to **suppress the immune system** in people and animals.

Possible Side Effects

▼ Most common: flu-like symptoms, heartburn, upset stomach, appetite loss, nausea, vomiting, stomach gas, cramps, diarrhea, headache, drowsiness, tiredness, men-

---

Possible Side Effects *(continued)*

strual disturbances, dizziness, fever, pains in the arms and legs, confusion, visual disturbances, numbness, and hypersensitivity to the drug.

▼ Less common: effects on the blood, kidneys, or liver.

Drug Interactions

• Severe liver damage may develop when Rifampin is mixed with other drugs that cause liver toxicity.

• Rifampin may increase your need for oral anticoagulant (blood-thinning) drugs and may also affect angiotensin-converting-enzyme (ACE) inhibitor drugs (especially Enalapril), Acetaminophen, oral antidiabetes drugs, barbiturates, benzodiazepine tranquilizers, beta blockers, Chloramphenicol, Clofibrate, corticosteroids, Cyclosporine, digitalis drugs, Disopyramide, Estrogens, Phenytoin, Methadone, Mexiletine, Quinidine, sulfa drugs, theophylline drugs, Tocainide, and Verapamil.

• Women taking birth control pills should use another contraceptive method while taking Rifampin.

Food Interactions

Take this medicine 1 hour before or 2 hours after a meal, at the same time every day.

Usual Dose

Adult: 600 mg once daily.

Child: 4.5 to 9 mg per pound of body weight, up to 600 mg per day.

Overdosage

Signs of overdosage are nausea, vomiting, and tiredness; with severe liver damage, unconsciousness may develop. Brown-red or orange skin discoloration may develop. Rifampin overdose victims must be taken to a hospital emergency room at once. ALWAYS take the medicine bottle.

Special Information

This drug may cause a red-brown or orange discoloration of

the urine, stool, saliva, sweat, and tears; this is not harmful. Soft contact lenses may become permanently stained.

Call your doctor if you develop flu-like symptoms, fever, chills, muscle pains, headache, tiredness or weakness, loss of appetite, nausea, vomiting, sore throat, unusual bleeding or bruising, yellow discoloration of the skin or eyes, or skin rash or itching.

If you take Rifampin once a day and miss a dose, take it as soon as you remember. If it is almost time for your next dose, skip the missed dose and continue with your regular schedule. Do not take a double dose. Regularly skipping doses of Rifampin increases your chances for drug side effects.

Special Populations

Pregnancy/Breast-feeding
Animal studies indicate that Rifampin may cause cleft palate and spina bifida (backbone problems) in the fetus. Pregnant women should use this drug only if absolutely necessary.

Nursing mothers taking Rifampin should bottle-feed their babies.

Seniors
Older adults with severe liver disease may be more sensitive to the effects of this drug. Report any side effects at once.

Generic Name

Riluzole

Brand Name
Rilutek

Type of Drug
Glutamate-release blocker.

Prescribed for
Amyotrophic lateral sclerosis (also known as ALS or Lou Gehrig's disease).

General Information
ALS is a chronic disease of the nervous system for which

there has been no effective drug treatment until now. Riluzole, the first medicine ever proven to affect ALS, has a number of different actions, though nobody knows exactly how it works. The drug slows the release of glutamate, which is thought to damage important nerve centers in the brains of people with ALS, and protects other aspects of nerve function both inside and outside the nerve cell.

In studies up to 5 years done primarily with people with ALS, Riluzole improved survival during 18 months of treatment, though muscle strength and nerve function were not improved by the drug. Still, death rates at the end of the studies were the same whether people took Riluzole or not. In one study, the average survival improvement for people taking Riluzole was 60 days. Riluzole doses larger than 100 mg a day only increase the chances for drug side effects; they are not more effective.

Animals bred to mimic the nervous-system defects of ALS lived longer when given Riluzole. It also protected nerves from damage in laboratory experiments.

About 90 percent of each Riluzole tablet is absorbed into the blood, but food interferes with this absorption process. Riluzole is broken down in the liver and passes out of the body through the kidneys. Cigarette smoking is likely to increase the rate at which Riluzole is broken down, but there is no indication as yet that cigarette smokers need higher doses than nonsmokers.

Cautions and Warnings

Do not take Riluzole if you are **allergic** to it or any of the tablet ingredients.

Riluzole causes **liver inflammation**, and people with **severe liver disease** should use this drug with caution. Liver function tests should be done for everyone taking Riluzole. People with **kidney disease** should also use Riluzole with caution.

Women break down this drug more slowly than men and tend to have more medicine in their blood than men, but this does not affect drug dosage.

Possible Side Effects

About 14 percent of people who took Riluzole in preapproval studies stopped taking it because of side effects.

Possible Side Effects *(continued)*

▼ Most common: weakness, nausea, dizziness (twice as common in women than men), diarrhea, a tingling sensation around the mouth, appetite loss, fainting, and tiredness. These effects increase as the dose is raised.

▼ Common: poor lung function, abdominal pain, pneumonia, and vomiting.

▼ Less common: back pain, headache, upset stomach (at high doses), stomach gas, stuffed and runny nose, cough, high blood pressure, joint aches, swelling in the arms and legs, urinary infection and painful urination (both at high doses), and dizziness when rising from a lying or sitting position (at high doses).

▼ Rare: aggravation, not feeling well, mouth infections, eczema, rapid heartbeat, and vein irritation.

In studies in which the same number of people took Riluzole as took an inactive pill (placebo), side effects experienced by people taking Riluzole were weight loss, depression, muscle spasticity, dry mouth, itching, bronchitis, sinus irritation, accidental injury, constipation, swallowing and breathing problems, flu symptoms, increased sputum production, pneumonia, and breathing disorders.

Other Riluzole side effects can affect virtually every body system. Report anything unusual to your doctor at once.

Drug Interactions

• Drugs that are toxic to the liver, such as Allopurinol, Methyldopa, and Sulfasalazine, may interact with Riluzole. Combinations of such drugs should be taken with caution.

• Caffeine, Theophylline, Phenacetin, Amitriptytline, and quinolone antibacterials may slow the rate at which Riluzole is eliminated from your body.

• Cigarette smoke, charcoal-broiled foods, Rifampicin, and Omeprazole could increase the rate at which Riluzole is eliminated from your body.

• Riluzole can potentially increase the breakdown of Caffeine, Theophylline, and Tacrine, but these effects have not actually been seen in people.

Food Interactions

Take Riluzole on an empty stomach, 1 hour before or 2 hours after meals.

Usual Dose

Adult: 50 mg every 12 hours.
Child: not recommended.

Overdosage

There have been no reports of Riluzole overdose. Overdose victims should be taken to a hospital emergency room for treatment at once. ALWAYS bring the medicine bottle with you.

Special Information

Doses higher than 50 mg twice a day do not improve your condition and may increase your chances for drug side effects.

Call your doctor at once if you become feverish or ill. This could be a sign of a very low white-blood-cell count.

Riluzole should be taken at the same time each day (morning and evening) to get maximum benefit and keep steady levels of the drug in your blood.

Riluzole can make you dizzy, tired, or faint. Don't drive or do anything that requires intense concentration until you can judge how Riluzole affects you.

People taking this medicine should not drink to excess.

Studies of Japanese natives showed they took twice as long to clear the drug from their bodies as Caucasians. It is possible that genetic factors or environmental factors such as cigarette smoking, alcohol, coffee, or diet could be responsible, but the exact reasons are not known.

Store your Riluzole tablets between 68° and 77° F and protect them from bright light.

If you forget a dose of Riluzole, take it as soon as you remember. If it is almost time for your next dose, skip the forgotten dose and continue with your regular schedule.

Special Populations

Pregnancy/Breast-feeding

Riluzole was toxic to pregnant lab animals at doses up to 11 times larger than the maximum human dose. There are no studies of Riluzole in pregnant women. It should be used during pregnancy only if its possible benefits outweigh its risks.

It is not known if Riluzole passes into breast milk. Nursing mothers who must take this drug should bottle-feed their babies.

Seniors

Older adults with kidney or liver disease should use Riluzole with caution.

Generic Name

Rimantadine

Brand Name

Flumadine

Type of Drug

Antiviral.

Prescribed for

Preventing and treating influenza A viral infections.

General Information

Rimantadine is a synthetic antiviral agent that appears to interfere with the reproduction of various strains of the influenza A virus, a common cause of viral illness. Annual vaccination against the influenza virus is recommended as the best way of preventing the flu, but it takes 2 to 4 weeks to develop immunity; Rimantadine may be taken during that time to prevent viral infection in certain high-risk people or those whose exposure to the virus might be more dangerous.

Cautions and Warnings

People with **severe liver or kidney disease** clear this drug from their bodies only half as fast as those with normal organ function; they will need to have their dosage adjusted based on those factors.

People with a history of **seizures** are likely to suffer another one while taking this medicine. Call your doctor if this happens.

The influenza virus may become resistant to Rimantadine in up to 30 percent of people taking the drug. If this happens, the **resistant influenza virus** could infect others who may not have been vaccinated.

Possible Side Effects

▼ Most common: sleeplessness, nervousness, loss of concentration, headache, fatigue, weakness, nausea, vomiting, loss of appetite, dry mouth, and abdominal pains.

▼ Less common: diarrhea, upset stomach, dizziness, depression, euphoria (feeling "high"), changes in the way you walk, tremors, hallucinations, convulsions, fainting, ringing or buzzing in the ears, changes or loss in the senses of taste or smell, breathing difficulty, skin pallor, rash, heart palpitations, rapid heartbeat, high blood pressure, heart failure, swelling of the ankles or feet, and heart block.

▼ Rare: constipation, swallowing difficulty, mouth sores, agitation, sweating, diminished sense of touch, eye pain or tearing, cough, bronchospasm, increased urination, fever, and fluid oozing from the nipples (women only).

Drug Interactions

• The importance of Rimantadine's interactions is not known because there is no established relationship between the amount of drug in the blood and its antiviral effect. Aspirin and Acetaminophen may reduce the amount of Rimantadine in the blood by about 10 percent. Cimetidine increases the rate at which Rimantadine is broken down by the liver.

Food Interactions

Rimantadine is best taken on an empty stomach, or at least 1 hour before or 2 hours after meals. You may take it with food if it upsets your stomach.

Usual Dose

Adult and Child (age 10 and older): 100 mg twice per day.
Child (under age 10): 2.25 mg per pound of body weight, up to 150 mg, taken once a day.
People with severe liver or kidney disease: up to 100 mg per day.

Overdosage

Symptoms of overdosage are likely to be reflected in nervous-system (agitation, hallucination) and cardiac (abnormal heart rhythms) side effects. Overdose victims should be given Syrup of Ipecac (available at any pharmacy) as soon as possible to remove any remaining drug from their stomach. Follow package directions and give Ipecac only to conscious overdose victims. Call your local poison control center or hospital emergency room before giving Ipecac. ALWAYS bring the medicine bottle if you go to a hospital for treatment.

Special Information

Rimantadine may be given to children to prevent influenza infection, but it is not recommended for treatment of their flu symptoms.

Call your doctor if you develop seizures, convulsions, or any other serious or unusual side effects.

If you forget a dose of Rimantadine, take it as soon as you remember. If it is almost time for your next dose, skip the missed dose and continue with your regular schedule. Do not take a double dose.

Special Populations

Pregnancy/Breast-feeding

In animal studies, Rimantadine was found to be toxic to developing fetuses; pregnant animals given 11 times the human dose experienced drug side effects. Pregnant women should take Rimantadine only after fully discussing its risks and benefits with their doctor.

Animal studies of Rimantadine showed breast milk levels **twice** the blood level within 2 to 3 hours. Nursing mothers taking Rimantadine should bottle-feed their babies.

Seniors

Older adults are more likely to suffer from Rimantadine side effects of the nervous system, stomach, or intestines. Elderly nursing-home patients should receive no more than 100 mg of Rimantadine per day because of the likelihood that they have liver or kidney dysfunction. Otherwise healthy seniors may take this drug without special restriction.

Generic Name

Risperidone

Brand Name

Risperdal

Type of Drug

Antipsychotic.

Prescribed for

Managing psychotic disorders and schizophrenia.

General Information

No one knows exactly how Risperidone works, but it affects different brain receptors for serotonin and dopamine, two important neurohormones. Risperidone is broken down in the liver. Between 6 and 8 percent of Caucasians and a very small number of Asians have very little of the liver enzyme that breaks this drug down and are considered "poor metabolizers" of the drug. Because these people break down Risperidone very slowly, the drug takes about 5 days to reach a steady dose in their blood. People with normal amounts of the enzyme reach a steady dose in about 1 day. People with moderate to severe kidney disease and those with liver disease have trouble releasing Risperidone from their bodies and must take a lower daily dose.

Cautions and Warnings

Don't take this drug if you are **sensitive** or **allergic** to it. Because Risperidone has not been studied for more than 6- to 8-week periods, people taking it for longer periods must be **reevaluated at least every 2 months.**

A serious set of side effects known as **neuroleptic malignant syndrome (NMS)** has been associated with some antipsychotic medicines. The symptoms that make up NMS include high fever, muscle rigidity, mental changes, irregular pulse or blood pressure, sweating, and abnormal heart rhythms. **NMS is potentially fatal** and requires **immediate** medical attention.

Risperidone can produce **uncontrolled movements,** including spasm of the neck muscles, rolling back of the eyes, convulsions, difficulty in swallowing, and symptoms associated with Parkinson's disease. These effects look very serious but usually disappear after the drug has been withdrawn. Face, tongue, and jaw symptoms may persist, especially in older women, though they can appear at any age. Contact your doctor immediately if you experience any of these symptoms.

Risperidone can cause a **life-threatening abnormal heart rhythm** called *torsade de pointes*. It should be used with caution in people with heart disease. Slow heart rate, electrolyte imbalance, and taking other drugs that carry a risk of torsade de pointes can increase the chances of developing this heart rhythm.

Risperidone, like other dopamine antagonists, raises levels of a hormone called *prolactin*. Increased prolactin has been associated with an increase in tumors of the pituitary gland, breast, and pancreas, but no specific problems have been noted with this drug.

Possible Side Effects

▼ Most common: sleepiness, sleeplessness, agitation, anxiety, uncontrolled movements, headache, and nasal stuffiness and irritation.

▼ Less common: dizziness, constipation, nausea, vomiting, upset stomach, abdominal pains, increased saliva, toothache, coughing, upper respiratory infection, sinus infection, sore throat, breathing difficulty, rapid heartbeat, joint or back pains, chest pains, fever, abnormal vision, skin rash, dry skin, and dandruff.

Other side effects have occurred in almost every body system. Be sure to report anything unusual to your doctor.

Drug Interactions

• Risperidone may antagonize the effects of Levodopa.

• Carbamazepine and Clozapine can both increase the rate at which Risperidone is released from the body, possibly reducing its effect.

Food Interactions

Risperidone may be taken without regard to food or meals.

Usual Dose

Adult: starting dose is 1 mg twice a day, increasing gradually up to 6 mg a day if needed. For long-term treatment, your doctor will prescribe the lowest effective dose of Risperidone.

Child: not recommended.

Senior: start with 0.5 mg twice a day and increase gradually if needed.

Overdosage

In general, overdose symptoms are exaggerations of Risperidone's expected effects, including drowsiness, rapid heartbeat, low blood pressure, and abnormal and uncontrolled muscle movements. In 8 reports of overdoses up to 300 mg, no fatalities occurred. Overdose victims should be taken to a hospital emergency room for treatment. ALWAYS bring the medicine bottle with you.

Special Information

Risperidone can make you tired and affect your judgment, an effect that increases with increasing dosage. People taking it should be careful about driving or doing anything that requires concentration or clear thinking. Avoid alcoholic beverages.

Some antipsychotic medicines can interfere with the body's normal temperature-regulating mechanisms. Take care to avoid extreme heat while you are taking this medicine.

Some people will develop a rapid heartbeat and can get dizzy or faint when first taking Risperidone. This risk can be minimized by starting at a low dose—for example, 2 mg a day in adults and 1 mg in older adults or those with kidney or liver disease.

Risperidone can make you unusually sensitive to the sun. Be sure to wear protective clothes and make generous use of a sunscreen before going out in the sun.

Because of the possibility of drug interaction, make sure your doctor knows about any prescription or over-the-counter medicines before you start taking them. Drugs that affect the liver can interfere with Risperidone's breakdown.

If you forget to take a dose of Risperidone, take it as soon as you remember. If it is almost time for your next dose, skip the forgotten dose and continue with your regular schedule. Call your doctor if you forget two doses in a row.

Special Populations

Pregnancy/Breast-feeding
Animal studies with Risperidone showed an increase in birth defects and stillborns. There are no studies of this drug in pregnant women, but there is one report of an infant whose brain developed abnormally after Risperidone. Women taking this drug should be extremely careful about becoming pregnant. It should not be taken unless the possible risk is weighed against the benefit it can produce.

It is not known if Risperidone passes into breast milk. Women who must take this medicine should bottle-feed their babies.

Seniors
Older adults have reduced kidney function and cannot release Risperidone as efficiently from their bodies as younger adults. Your doctor will reduce your daily dose accordingly. Older adults may be more sensitive to the side effects of Risperidone.

Roxicet

see **Percocet**, page 877

Generic Name

Salmeterol

Brand Name
Serevent

Type of Drug
Bronchodilator.

Prescribed for

Prevention of asthma symptoms and bronchial spasms. Salmeterol does not provide immediate symptom relief.

General Information

Salmeterol differs from other bronchodilators in that it does not provide immediate symptom relief. It is used for longer-term symptom prevention. When you first start Salmeterol treatment, you may need to continue your other asthma inhalers for symptom relief. However, after a while, you should need the latter drugs less. Salmeterol works like other bronchodilator drugs, such as Albuterol, Terbutaline, and Metaproterenol, but it has a weaker effect on nerve receptors in the heart and blood vessels; for this reason, it is somewhat safer for people with heart conditions. Still, very large doses of Salmeterol can lead to abnormal heart rhythms.

Salmeterol begins working within 20 minutes and continues for 12 hours. Other drugs in this group do not work this long.

Cautions and Warnings

Salmeterol should be used with caution by people with a history of **angina, heart disease, high blood pressure, stroke or seizure, thyroid disease, prostate disease,** or **glaucoma.**

Used in excess, Salmeterol can actually lead to more difficulty in breathing, instead of relief. In the most extreme cases, people have had **heart attacks** after using excessive amounts of inhalant bronchodilators.

Long-term use of Salmeterol (and similar medicines) can lead to increases in certain ovarian tumors.

Possible Side Effects

Salmeterol's side effects are similar to those of other bronchodilators, except that its effects on the heart and blood vessels are not as pronounced.

▼ Most common: heart palpitations, rapid heartbeat, tremors, dizziness and fainting, shakiness, nervousness, tension, headache, diarrhea, heartburn or upset stomach,

---

Possible Side Effects *(continued)*

dry/sore/irritated throat, respiratory infections, and nasal or sinus conditions.

▼ Less common: nausea and vomiting, joint or back pain, muscle cramps, muscle soreness, aches or pains, giddiness, viral stomach infections, itching, dental pain, feeling ill, rash, and menstrual irregularity.

Drug Interactions

• Monoamine oxidase (MAO) inhibitor drugs, tricyclic antidepressants, thyroid drugs, other bronchodilator drugs, and some antihistamines may increase the effects of Salmeterol.

• The chances of cardiotoxicity may be increased in people taking Salmeterol and Theophylline.

• Salmeterol may antagonize (disrupt) the effects of blood-pressure-lowering drugs, especially Reserpine, Methyldopa, and Guanethidine.

Food Interactions

Do not inhale Salmeterol if you have food or anything else in your mouth.

Usual Dose

Adult and Adolescent (age 12 and over): 2 puffs every 12 hours (each puff delivers 42 micrograms of Salmeterol).

Child (under age 12): not recommended.

Overdosage

Overdose of Salmeterol inhalation usually results in exaggerated side effects, including heart pains and high blood pressure, although blood pressure may drop to a low level after a short period of elevation. People who inhale too much Salmeterol should see a doctor. ALWAYS bring the medicine bottle with you.

Special Information

Be sure to follow the inhalation instructions that come with the product. Salmeterol should be inhaled during the second half of your inhalation, since this will allow it to reach deeper into your lungs. Wait at least 1 minute between puffs.

Call your doctor immediately if you develop chest pains, palpitations, rapid heartbeat, muscle tremors, dizziness, headache, facial flushing, or urinary difficulty, or if you continue to experience difficulty in breathing after using the medicine.

If you forget a dose of Salmeterol, take it as soon as you remember. If it is almost time for your next dose, skip the forgotten one, and go back to your regular schedule. Do not take a double dose.

Special Populations

Pregnancy/Breast-feeding
When used during labor and delivery, Salmeterol may slow or delay natural labor. It can cause rapid heartbeat and high blood sugar in the mother and rapid heartbeat and low blood sugar in the fetus.

It is not known whether Salmeterol causes birth defects in humans, but it has caused defects in pregnant animals. When the drug is deemed essential, the potential risk of taking Salmeterol must be carefully weighed against any benefit it might produce.

Salmeterol may pass into breast milk. Nursing mothers who must take Salmeterol should be monitored closely by their doctor, and must observe for any possible drug effect on their infants.

Seniors
Older adults should use the same dose of Salmeterol as younger adults. Closely follow your doctor's directions, and report any side effects at once.

Generic Name

Saquinavir Mesylate

Brand Name
Invirase

Type of Drug
Protease inhibitor.

Prescribed for

Advanced HIV infection.

General Information

Saquinavir is the first of a new class of anti-HIV drugs that works by a unique method of action: protease inhibition. It is always used together with one of the older nucleoside drugs, such as AZT, ddI, or ddC. When the HIV virus attacks a cell, it must be converted into viral DNA. The older drugs work to prevent this step and are also known as *reverse transcriptase inhibitors.* Saquinavir works at the end of the process of HIV reproduction, when proteins are cut into strands of exactly the correct size. The protein is cut by an enzyme known as *protease*, and Saquinavir prevents the mature virus from being formed through prevention or inhibition of this cutting process. Improperly or uncut proteins are inactive.

Studies have shown that combining the two types of drugs is more effective than taking either one alone (as judged by CD4 cell levels), but there is no conclusive evidence that taking Saquinavir slows disease progression or improves survival.

Cautions and Warnings

Do not take this drug if you are **sensitive** or **allergic** to the drug.

If a serious toxicity occurs while taking Saquinavir, the drug should be stopped so that your doctor can determine the reason for the toxic event or until it resolves. Then, treatment can be restarted.

Caution must be exercised if you have moderate to severe **liver disease.**

There is a chance that strains of the HIV virus may become **resistant** to Saquinavir and that other protease inhibitors under development will also be rendered ineffective, but this effect will have to be studied as other protease inhibitor drugs become available.

Possible Side Effects

Most Saquinavir side effects are mild.

Possible Side Effects *(continued)*

▼ Most common: diarrhea, nausea, and abdominal discomfort. When Saquinavir is taken together with one of the older antiretroviral drugs, other side effects become more prominent, including weakness, muscle pain, and mouth ulcers.

▼ Less common: upset stomach, abdominal pain, mouth ulcers, headache, tingling in the hands or feet, numbness in the hands or feet, dizziness, nerve damage, appetite disturbances, and rash.

▼ Other: side effects of Saquinavir can affect almost any body system. Report anything unusual to your doctor.

Drug Interactions

• Rifampin and Rifabutin increase the rate at which Saquinavir is broken down in the liver and drastically reduce the amount of Saquinavir (by 80 percent and 40 percent, respectively) in the blood. Do not mix these drugs. Other drugs that can reduce Saquinavir blood levels are Phenobarbital, Phenytoin, Carbamazepine, and Dexamethasone.

• Blood levels of Saquinavir may be elevated by Terfenidine, Astemizole, Ketoconazole, Itraconazole, calcium channel blockers, Clindamycin, Dapsone, Quinidine, and Triazolam. Taking these drugs with Saquinavir may lead to drug side effects.

Food Interactions

Take Saquinavir within 2 hours of a full meal. The amount of Saquinavir absorbed into the blood is vastly reduced when it is taken on an empty stomach. You will not get any antiviral activity unless it is taken with food.

Usual Dose

Adult (age 16 and older): 600 mg 3 times a day within 2 hours of a full meal.

Child (under age 16): not recommended.

Overdosage

No acute problems developed in one person who took 8000

mg of Saquinavir at once after the victim was made to vomit. In a study of people taking up to 7200 mg a day for 25 weeks, no unusual effects were seen. Call your local poison center for more information. Overdose victims should be taken to a hospital emergency room for treatment. ALWAYS bring the medicine bottle with you.

Special Information

Saquinavir does not cure HIV infection or AIDS. You may develop opportunistic infections or other illnesses associated with advanced HIV disease. Saquinavir has not been shown to reduce the possibility of transmitting the HIV virus to another person. The long-term effects of this drug are not known.

Saquinavir should be taken at the same time as you take your nucleoside antiviral drug. If you forget a dose of Saquinavir, take it as soon as you remember. If it is almost time for your next dose, skip the forgotten dose and continue with your regular schedule. Do not take a double dose of Saquinavir.

Special Populations

Pregnancy/Breast-feeding

Animal studies with pregnant animals have shown no negative effects of Saquinavir on the developing fetus. There are no reports of pregnant women receiving this drug, but it should be used with caution if you are pregnant.

It is not known if this drug passes into breast milk. Nursing mothers who must take Saquinavir should bottle-feed their babies.

Seniors

Older adults can take this drug without special precaution.

Seldane

see **Terfenadine**, page 1077

Generic Name

Selegiline

Brand Name

Eldepryl

Type of Drug

Antiparkinsonian; selective monoamine oxidase inhibitor.

Prescribed for

Parkinson's disease.

General Information

Selegiline is often combined with Levodopa or Carbidopa to control Parkinson's disease. Most people who take Selegiline find that their doctor can reduce their Levodopa or Carbidopa dose within a few days.

The exact way that Selegiline works is not known. It is a very strong inhibitor of one form of the enzyme monoamine oxidase (MAO) that is found almost exclusively in the brain. Other MAO inhibitor drugs used as antidepressants work on both forms of MAO and affect the entire body. Selegiline also stimulates dopamine receptors in the brain, possibly by making the dopamine that is available in the brain last longer by interfering with its being reabsorbed into brain nerve endings. In order for any drug to work in Parkinson's disease, it must somehow increase the activity of dopamine in the brain.

Some of Selegiline's side effects may be caused by Methamphetamine and Amphetamine, 2 products of the body's breakdown of the drug that are extremely potent stimulants.

Cautions and Warnings

People who have had a **reaction to Selegiline** in the past should be very cautious about using it again.

People already taking Sinemet (which contains Levodopa and Carbidopa) who start on Selegiline may experience an increase in Levodopa side effects. Your doctor can deal with this by reducing your Sinemet dosage.

More than 10 mg of Selegiline per day may inhibit both kinds of MAO, causing unexpected reactions, including **severe and possibly fatal high blood pressure.**

Selegiline should not be used with **Meperidine** or other **narcotic drugs** because of the chance of severe, possibly fatal, reactions such as those seen with other MAO inhibitors.

Possible Side Effects

When Selegiline dosage is less than 10 mg per day, most of the side effects experienced are not caused by the drug itself; rather, Selegiline increases the side effects of Levodopa. That's why it is important for your doctor to reduce your Levodopa dosage as much as possible.

▼ Most common: nausea, vomiting, dizziness, light-headedness or fainting, and abdominal pains.

▼ Less common: tremors or uncontrolled muscle movements, loss of balance, inability to move, increasingly slow movements (associated with Parkinson's disease), facial grimacing, falling down due to loss of balance, stiff neck, muscle cramps, hallucinations, overstimulation, confusion, anxiety, depression, drowsiness, changes in mood or behavior, nightmares or unusual dreams, tiredness, delusions, disorientation, feelings of ill health, apathy, sleep disturbances, restlessness, weakness, irritability, generalized aches and pains, migraine or other headaches, muscle pains in the back or legs, ringing or buzzing in the ears, eye pain, finger or toe numbness, changes in sense of taste, dizziness when rising from a sitting or lying position, blood-pressure changes, abnormal heart rhythms, heart palpitations, chest pains, rapid heartbeat, swelling in the arms or legs, constipation, appetite loss, weight loss, difficulty swallowing, diarrhea, heartburn, rectal bleeding, urinary difficulties, impotence, prostate swelling, increased sweating, increased facial hair, hair loss, rash, unusual skin sensitivity to the sun, bruising or black-and-blue marks, asthma, blurred or double vision, shortness of breath, speech problems, and dry mouth.

At doses above 10 mg per day, Selegiline may cause muscle twitching or spasms, memory loss, increased

Possible Side Effects *(continued)*

energy, a transient "high," grinding of the teeth, decreased feeling in the penis, and inability to achieve orgasm (male).

Drug Interactions

• Selegiline should not be used with Meperidine or other narcotics because of the chance of severe, and possibly fatal, reactions similar to those with other MAO inhibitor drugs.

• Combining Fluoxetine with MAO inhibitors other than Selegiline has been deadly. This effect has **not** been seen with Selegiline, but the combination should be avoided. If you are taking Fluoxetine, allow 5 weeks between the time you stop taking it and start on any MAO inhibitor. If you are already taking an MAO inhibitor, allow at least 2 weeks between stopping it and starting Selegiline.

Food Interactions

Take with food to avoid nausea or stomach upset, but avoid the following: Chianti and red wine, vermouth, unpasteurized or imported beer, beef or chicken liver, fermented sausages, tenderized or prepared meats, caviar, dried fish, pickled herring, cheese (American, Brie, cheddar, Camembert, Emmentaler, Boursault, Stilton, and others), avocados, yeast extracts, bananas, figs, raisins, soy sauce, miso soup, bean curd, fava beans, caffeine, and chocolate. These foods (and others) can cause severe, sudden high blood pressure to occur with Selegiline. Your doctor or pharmacist can give you more information on foods to avoid.

Usual Dose

5 mg with breakfast and lunch.

Overdosage

Selegiline overdose symptoms may include excitement, irritability, anxiety, low blood pressure, sleeplessness, restlessness, dizziness, weakness, drowsiness, flushing, sweating, heart palpitations, and unusual movements (including grimacing and muscle twitching). Serious overdoses may lead to convulsions, incoherence or confusion, severe headache, high fever, heart attack, shock, or coma. Overdose victims should be taken to a hospital emergency room for treatment. ALWAYS bring the medicine bottle.

Special Information

After you have taken Selegiline for 2 or 3 days, your doctor will probably reduce your Carbidopa or Levodopa dose by 10 to 30 percent. If the disease is still under control, your dose may be further reduced to find the lowest effective dose of medication to control your condition.

It is important to maintain regular contact with your doctor while taking Selegiline to allow for observation of drug effects and side effects. Headache, unusual body movements or muscle spasms, mood changes, or other unusual, persistent, or intolerable side effects should be reported to your doctor at once. Do not stop taking Selegiline or change your dose without your doctor's knowledge.

Selegiline reduces saliva flow in the mouth and may increase the chance for cavities, gum disease, and oral infections. Use candy, ice, sugarless gum, or a saliva substitute to avoid dry mouth.

If you forget to take a dose of Selegiline, take it as soon as you remember. If it is almost time for your next dose, take 1 dose right away and another in 5 or 6 hours, then go back to your regular schedule. Do not take a double dose.

Special Populations

Pregnancy/Breast-feeding

Pregnant women and those who might become pregnant should not use Selegiline unless its possible benefits have been carefully weighed against its risks.

It is not known if Selegiline passes into breast milk. Nursing mothers who use this drug should watch their babies for unusual reactions. Report anything unusual to your doctor at once.

Seniors

Older adults may take Selegiline without special restriction. Use the lowest effective dose to minimize side effects.

Brand Name

Septra

Ingredients

Sulfamethoxazole + Trimethoprim

Other Brand Names

Bactrim	Septra DS
Bactrim DS	Septra Pediatric
Bactrim Pediatric	Sulfatrim DS
Cotrim	TMP-SMZ
Cotrim DS	Uroplus
Cotrim Pediatric	Uroplus DS
Co-trimoxazole	

(Also available in generic form)

Type of Drug

Anti-infective.

Prescribed for

A wide variety of infections caused by susceptible organisms in many parts of the body, including urinary tract infections, bronchitis, and ear infections in children. It is also used to treat traveler's diarrhea, *Pneumocystis carinii* infections in AIDS and leukemia patients, and prostate infections. Septra may be used to prevent urinary tract infections in women by taking the medicine immediately after intercourse. It may also be prescribed for cholera, nocardiosis, and *Salmonella* infections.

General Information

Septra is one of many combination products used to treat infections. It is unique because it interferes with the infecting micro-organism's normal use of folic acid in two ways, making it more efficient than other antibacterial drugs. It is effective in many situations where other drugs are not. Bacterial resistance to Septra develops more slowly than to either Sulfamethoxazole or Trimethoprim used alone.

Cautions and Warnings

Do not take Septra if you have a **folic acid deficiency** or are **allergic** to either ingredient or to any sulfa drug, antidiabetes drug, or thiazide-type diuretic. Septra should be used with caution by people with **liver or kidney disease**. Be sure to drink at least 1 full glass of water with each dose of Septra. **Infants under 2 months** of age should not be given this combination product.

Symptoms such as unusual bleeding or bruising, extreme tiredness, rash, sore throat, fever, pallor, or yellowing of the skin or eyes may be early indications of a serious **blood disorder.** If any of these effects occur, contact your doctor immediately, and stop taking the drug. People taking Septra for **Pneumocystis carinii infection** also have compromised immune function. They may not respond to Septra and are more likely to develop less common drug side effects. Side effects are less severe in those taking Septra to prevent PCP.

Septra should **not be used for strep throat,** because of a greater chance of treatment failure than with Penicillin.

Possible Side Effects

▼ Most common: nausea, vomiting, upset stomach, loss of appetite, and skin rash or itching.

▼ Less common: reduced levels of blood cells (red and white) and blood platelets (for blood clotting); allergic reactions (breathing difficulty, hives, etc.); drug fever; swelling around the eyes; arthritis-like pains; diarrhea; coating of the tongue; headache; tingling in the arms or legs; depression; convulsions; hallucinations; ringing in the ears; dizziness; difficulty sleeping; and feelings of apathy, tiredness, weakness, and nervousness. Septra may also affect your kidneys and cause you to produce less urine.

Drug Interactions

• Septra may prolong the effects of anticoagulant (blood-thinning) agents (such as Warfarin) and oral antidiabetes drugs.

• The Trimethoprim in Septra may increase the kidney toxicity and reduce the effectiveness of Cyclosporine.

• The Sulfamethoxazole in Septra can increase the amount of Phenytoin and Methotrexate in the bloodstream, increasing the chance of drug-related side effects. Dosage reduction of the Phenytoin or Methotrexate may be needed to adjust for the presence of Septra.

• Older adults taking a thiazide diuretic and Septra are more likely to develop reduced levels of blood platelets and an increased chance of bleeding under the skin.

• Taking Septra together with Dapsone can result in increased blood levels of both drugs. Septra can interfere with the elimination of Zidovudine (AZT) through the kidneys, increasing the amount of AZT in the blood.

Food Interactions

Take each dose with a full glass of water. Continue to drink plenty of fluids throughout the day to decrease the risk of kidney-stone formation.

Usual Dose

Adult: 2 regular tablets or 1 Septra DS tablet every 12 hours for 5 to 14 days, depending on the condition being treated.
Child (2 months and older):
    up to 22 pounds: 1 teaspoonful every 12 hours
    23 to 44 pounds: 2 teaspoonfuls (or 1 tablet) every 12 hours
    45 to 66 pounds: 3 teaspoonfuls (or 1½ tablets) every 12 hours
    67 to 88 pounds: 4 teaspoonfuls (or 2 tablets) every 12 hours

Overdosage

Small overdoses are not likely to cause harm. Larger overdoses can cause exaggerated drug side effects. Call your local poison control center or hospital emergency room for more information. ALWAYS bring the medicine bottle with you if you go for treatment.

Special Information

Take Septra exactly as prescribed for the full length of the prescription. Do not stop taking it just because you are beginning to feel better. Take each dose with a full glass of water, and drink plenty of fluids all day to lower the risk of kidney-stone formation.

Call your doctor if you develop sore throat, skin rash, or unusual bleeding or bruising, or any other persistent or intolerable drug side effect.

You may develop unusual sensitivity to bright light, particularly sunlight. If you have a history of light sensitivity or if you have sensitive skin, avoid prolonged exposure to sunlight while using Septra.

If you miss a dose of Septra, take it as soon as possible. If you take the medicine twice a day and it is almost time for your next dose, take 1 dose as soon as you remember and another in 5 to 6 hours, then go back to your regular schedule. If you take the medicine 3 or more times a day and it is almost time for your next dose, take 1 dose as soon as you remember and another in 2 to 4 hours, then continue with your regular schedule. Do not take any double doses.

Special Populations

Pregnancy/Breast-feeding

Septra may affect folic acid in the developing fetus throughout pregnancy and should be used with caution. It should never be taken near the time you are ready to deliver because of the direct effect of one of the ingredients, Sulfamethoxazole, on the newborn, including yellowing of the skin or eyes. Talk to your doctor about Septra's risks versus its benefits if the drug is to be used during pregnancy.

Premature infants, infants with too much bilirubin in their blood, and those who are deficient in the enzyme known as G-6-PD are more likely to develop problems with Septra. Septra is not recommended for use if you are nursing because of possible effects on the newborn infant.

Seniors

Older adults are more likely to be sensitive to the effects of this drug, especially if they have liver or kidney problems. Severe skin reactions and decreased levels of blood platelets and red and white blood cells are the most common, especially when a thiazide diuretic is also being taken. Your doctor will reduce your Septra dose if you have kidney disease.

Generic Name

Sertraline Hydrochloride

Brand Name

Zoloft

Type of Drug

Selective serotonin reuptake inhibitor (SSRI) antidepressant.

Prescribed for

Depression. Sertraline has also been prescribed for obsessive-compulsive disorder.

General Information

Sertraline Hydrochloride and the other SSRIs (Fluvoxamine, Paroxetine, and Fluoxetine) are chemically unrelated to the older tricyclic and tetracyclic antidepressant medicines. They work by preventing the movement of a neurohormone, *serotonin*, into nerve endings. This forces the serotonin to remain in the spaces surrounding nerve endings, where it works. Sertraline is effective in treating common symptoms of depression. It can help improve your mood and mental alertness, increase physical activity, and improve sleep patterns. The drug takes about 4 weeks to work and stays in the body for several weeks, even after you stop taking it. This may be important when your doctor starts or stops treatment.

Sertraline Hydrochloride can cause a small (1–2 pounds) weight loss in people taking the drug, but significant weight loss is uncommon with this drug.

Cautions and Warnings

Do not take Sertraline Hydrochloride if you are **allergic** to it. Allergies to other antidepressants should not prevent you from taking Sertraline Hydrochloride because the drug is chemically different from other antidepressants.

A 2-week drug-free period should be allowed between the use of Sertraline and the use of a monoamine oxidase (MAO) inhibitor antidepressant.

Sertraline is broken down by your liver; therefore, people

with **severe liver disease** should be cautious about taking this drug and should be treated with doses that are lower than normal.

People with **reduced kidney function** should take this drug with caution.

Studies in animals receiving doses 10–20 times the maximum human dose revealed an increase in certain liver tumors and reduced fertility. The significance of this information to humans is not known.

A small number of **manic or hypomanic patients** may experience an activation of their condition while taking Sertraline.

Sertraline should be given with caution to patients who suffer from **seizure disorders**.

Sertraline causes a reduction of blood level of uric acid but has not caused kidney failure.

The possibility of suicide exists in severely depressed patients and may be present until the condition is significantly improved. Depressed patients should be allowed to carry only small quantities of Sertraline with them to reduce the chances of overdose.

Possible Side Effects

▼ Most common: dry mouth, sweating, heart palpitations, chest pain, headache, dizziness, tremors, tingling or numbness in the hands or feet, twitching, muscle spasms, confusion, rash, nausea, diarrhea or loose stools, constipation, upset stomach, stomach gas, appetite changes, abdominal pains, muscle aches, sleeplessness or sleepiness, male (15 percent) or female (1.7 percent) sexual dysfunction, agitation, nervousness, anxiety, yawning, loss of concentration, menstrual disorders, sore throat, runny nose, vision changes, ringing or buzzing in the ears, urinary frequency or disorders, fatigue, hot flushes, fever, back pain, thirst, and weakness.

▼ Less common: flushing, pinpoint pupils, increased saliva, cold and clammy skin, dizziness when rising quickly from a sitting or standing position, blood pressure changes, swelling around the eyes and in the arms or legs, coldness in the hands or feet, fainting and dizziness,

Possible Side Effects *(continued)*

rapid heartbeat, weakness, loss of coordination, unusual walk, changes in the general level of activity, migraines, droopy eyelids, acne, hair loss, dry skin, difficulty swallowing, stomach gas, joint pains, muscle pains, cramps and weakness, aggressiveness, abnormal dreaming or thinking, memory loss, apathy, delusions, a feeling of detachment, worsened depression, emotional instability, a "high" feeling, hallucinations, neurosis, paranoia, suicide attempts, teeth grinding, menstrual cramps or pain, bleeding between periods, coughing, bronchospasm, nosebleeds, breathing difficulty, conjunctivitis, double vision, difficulty accommodating to bright lights, eye pain, earaches, painful urination, facial swelling, frequent urination, nighttime urination, loss of urinary control, generalized swelling, a feeling of ill health, weight changes, and lymph swelling.

▼ Other: many other side effects affecting virtually every body system have been reported by people taking this medicine. They are too numerous to mention here but are considered infrequent or rare and affect only a small number of people. Be sure to report anything unusual to your doctor at once.

Drug Interactions

• Sertraline Hydrochloride may prolong the effects of Diazepam and other benzodiazepine-type drugs in your body.

• Serious, sometimes fatal reactions may occur if Sertraline and an MAO inhibitor are taken together (see *Cautions and Warnings*).

• People taking the oral anticoagulant (blood-thinning) agent Warfarin may experience an increase in that drug's effect if they start taking Sertraline Hydrochloride. Your doctor will have to reevaluate your Warfarin dosage.

• Sertraline may affect blood levels of Lithium in patients taking both drugs together.

• Sertraline may decrease the rate at which Tolbutamide (for diabetes) is released from your body.

• Alcohol may increase tiredness and other nervous-system-depressant effects of sertraline.

Food Interactions

Food increases the rate at which Sertraline Hydrochloride is absorbed into the blood and may slightly increase the amount of drug absorbed. For consistent blood levels of this drug, it should be taken on an empty stomach or at least 1 hour before or 2 hours after meals.

Usual Dose

50 to 200 mg once a day in the morning or at night. Seniors, people with kidney or liver disease, and those taking several different medicines should remain at the lowest possible dosage for their condition.

Overdosage

In the 3 cases of Sertraline Hydrochloride overdose reported, all recovered completely without special treatment. Symptoms of overdose are likely to be the most frequent drug side effects. There is no specific antidote for Sertraline Hydrochloride overdose.

Any person suspected of having taken a Sertraline Hydrochloride overdose should be taken to a hospital emergency room for treatment at once, or you may call your local poison control center for information and directions. If you go to an emergency room, ALWAYS take the medicine bottle with you.

Special Information

Sertraline Hydrochloride can make you dizzy or drowsy. Take care when driving or doing other tasks that require alertness and concentration.

Do not drink alcoholic beverages if you are taking Sertraline Hydrochloride.

Be sure your doctor knows if you are pregnant, breast-feeding, or taking other prescription or nonprescription medications while taking Sertraline Hydrochloride. Notify your doctor of any unexpected drug effects.

If you forget a dose of Sertraline Hydrochloride, take it as soon as you remember. If it is almost time for your next dose, skip the forgotten dose and continue with your regular schedule. Do not take a double dose of Sertraline Hydrochloride.

Special Populations

Pregnancy/Breast-feeding

Animal studies using 2½ to 10 times the maximum human dose of Sertraline Hydrochloride have shown some effect on a developing fetus. Do not take this drug if you are, or might become, pregnant without first seeing your doctor and reviewing the benefits of therapy against the risk of taking Sertraline Hydrochloride.

It is not known if Sertraline passes into breast milk. Nursing mothers should use caution if they must take this medicine.

Seniors

Older adults tend to clear this drug more slowly from their bodies, but side-effect patterns are unaffected. Any person with liver or kidney disease, problems that are more common among seniors, should receive a lower dose. Be sure to report any unusual side effects to your doctor.

Generic Name

Simvastatin

Brand Name

Zocor

Type of Drug

Cholesterol-lowering agent (HMG-CoA reductase inhibitor).

Prescribed for

High blood-cholesterol, LDL cholesterol, and triglyceride levels, in conjunction with a low-cholesterol-diet program.

General Information

The HMG-CoA reductase inhibitors work by interfering with the natural body process for manufacturing cholesterol, converting the process to produce a harmless by-product. The value of drugs that reduce blood cholesterol lies in the assumption that reducing levels of blood fats reduces the chance of heart disease. Studies conducted by the National

Heart, Lung, and Blood Institute have closely related high blood-fat levels (total cholesterol, LDL cholesterol, and triglycerides) to heart and blood-vessel disease. Drugs that can reduce the amounts of any of these blood fats and increase HDL cholesterol (the so-called "good" cholesterol) reduce the risk of death and heart attacks.

The drugs in this group (Fluvastatin, Lovastatin, Pravastatin, and Simvastatin) reduce total triglyceride, cholesterol, and LDL-cholesterol counts while raising HDL cholesterol. These drugs have similar profiles in that a very small amount of the drug you swallow actually reaches the body circulation; most is broken down in the liver. Ten to 20 percent of the drug is released from the body through your kidneys, the rest is eliminated by the liver. Blood-fat levels start dropping after 1 to 2 weeks of treatment and reach their lowest levels within 4 to 6 weeks after you start taking Simvastatin. Levels remain low so long as you continue to take the medicine.

Simvastatin generally doesn't benefit anyone under age 30, so it is not generally recommended for children, although it may, under special circumstances, be prescribed for teenagers in the same doses as adults.

Cautions and Warnings

Do not take Simvastatin if you are **allergic** to it or to any other member of this group.

People with a history of **liver disease** and those who drink **large amounts of alcohol** should avoid these medications because of the possibility that the drug can aggravate or cause liver disease. Your doctor should take a blood sample to test your liver function every month or so during the first year of treatment to be sure that the drug is not adversely affecting you.

These medicines cause **muscle aches and/or muscle weakness** in a small number of people, which can be a sign of a more serious condition.

At doses between 50 and more than 100 times the maximum human dose, the HMG-CoA reductase inhibitors have caused central-nervous-system lesions, liver tumors, and male infertility in lab animals. The importance of this information for people is not known.

Possible Side Effects

Most people who take Simvastatin tolerate it quite well. Simvastatin has a lower incidence of side effects than other drugs in this group.

▼ Most common: headache, constipation, diarrhea, heartburn, stomach gas, and abdominal pain or cramps.

▼ Less common: muscle aches, upset stomach, nausea, and vomiting.

▼ Rare: dizziness, rash and itching, hepatitis, inflammation of the pancreas, yellowing of the skin or eyes, appetite loss, blurred vision, changes in taste perception, respiratory infections, common cold symptoms, fatigue, urinary abnormalities, changes in the lens of your eye, reduced sex drive, male impotence and/or breast pain, anxiety, tingling in the hands or feet, hair loss, swelling, and blood-cell changes.

Drug Interactions

• The cholesterol-lowering effects of Simvastatin and Colestipol or Cholestyramine are additive when the drugs are taken together.

• The anticoagulant (blood-thinning) effect of Warfarin may be increased by these medicines. People taking both drugs should be periodically monitored by their doctor.

• The combination of Cyclosporine, Erythromycin, Gemfibrozil, or Niacin with any HMG-CoA reductase inhibitor may cause severe muscle aches or degeneration or other muscle problems. These combinations should be avoided.

• Simvastatin may slightly increase blood levels of Digoxin.

Food Interactions

Simvastatin may be taken without regard to food or meals. Continue your low-cholesterol diet while taking this medicine.

Usual Dose

Adult: 5 to 40 mg a day, taken in the evening.

Senior: 5 to 20 mg a day, taken in the evening.

Your daily dosage of Simvastatin should be adjusted monthly, based on your doctor's assessment of how well the drug is working to reduce your blood cholesterol.

Overdosage

Of the few reports of Simvastatin poisoning (including one 450-mg overdose), all those taking an overdose recovered. Persons suspected of having taken an overdose of Simvastatin should be taken to a hospital emergency room for evaluation and treatment. The effects of overdose are not well understood.

Special Information

Call your doctor if you develop blurred vision or muscle aches, pain, tenderness, or weakness, especially if you are also feverish or feel sick.

These medicines are always prescribed in combination with a low-fat diet. Be sure to follow your doctor's dietary instructions, since both the diet and medicine are necessary to treat your condition.

Do not take more cholesterol-lowering medicine than your doctor has prescribed or stop taking the medicine without your doctor's knowledge.

If you forget to take a dose of Simvastatin, take it as soon as you remember. If it is almost time for your next regularly scheduled dose, skip the one you forgot and continue with your regular schedule. Do not take a double dose.

Special Populations

Pregnancy/Breast-feeding

Pregnant women and those who might become pregnant absolutely must not take Simvastatin. Since hardening of the arteries is a long-term process, you should be able to stop this medication during pregnancy with no serious problems. If you become pregnant while taking any of these medicines, stop the drug immediately and call your doctor.

Simvastatin may pass into breast milk. Women taking it should bottle-feed their infants to avoid possible interference with the baby's development.

Seniors

Seniors may be more sensitive to the effects of Simvastatin and are likely to require less medication than a younger adult. Be sure to report any side effects to your doctor.

Brand Name

Sinemet

Ingredients

Carbidopa + Levodopa

(Also available in generic form)

Other Brand Name

Sinemet CR

Type of Drug

Antiparkinsonian.

Prescribed for

Parkinson's disease.

General Information

The 2 ingredients in Sinemet—Levodopa and Carbidopa—work together to produce a beneficial drug interaction. Levodopa is the active ingredient that affects Parkinson's disease. Vitamin B_6 (Pyridoxine) destroys Levodopa, but Carbidopa slows this process, making more Levodopa available to get into the brain, where it actually works.

This combination is so effective that your dose of Levodopa can be reduced by about 75 percent, which results in fewer side effects and, generally, safer drug treatment. Unfortunately, Sinemet is not the ultimate in Parkinson's disease treatment. People still become resistant to the effects of Levodopa, even under the improved circumstances offered by this combination. Carbidopa is available under the brand name **Lodosyn** for people who need individual doses of both Carbidopa and Levodopa; most people can be maintained on Sinemet.

Cautions and Warnings

Do not take this drug if you are **allergic** to either of its ingredients. If you are being **switched from Levodopa to Sinemet,** you should stop taking Levodopa 8 hours before your first dose of Sinemet. The nervous-system side effects of Sinemet can occur at much lower dosages than with Levodopa because of the added effect of Carbidopa.

Possible Side Effects

▼ Most common: uncontrolled muscle movements, loss of appetite, nausea, vomiting, stomach pain, dry mouth, difficulty swallowing, drooling, shaky hands, headache, dizziness, numbness, weakness, feeling faint, grinding of the teeth, confusion, sleeplessness, nightmares, hallucinations, anxiety, agitation, tiredness, feelings of ill health, and euphoria (feeling "high").

▼ Less common: heart palpitations, dizziness when rising quickly from a sitting or lying position, sudden extreme slowness of movement ("on-off" phenomenon), and mental changes (including paranoia, psychosis, depression, and a slowdown of mental functioning).

▼ Other: difficult urination, muscle twitching, eyelid spasms, lockjaw, burning sensation on the tongue, bitter taste, diarrhea, constipation, stomach gas, flushing of the skin, rash, sweating, unusual breathing, blurred or double vision, pupil dilation, hot flashes, changes in body weight, and darkening of the urine or sweat.

Occasionally, Sinemet may cause stomach bleeding or ulcer development, high blood pressure, adverse effects on blood components, blood-vessel irritation, convulsions, inability to control eye-muscle movements, hiccups, feeling of being stimulated, retention of body fluid, hair loss, hoarseness of the voice, and persistent penile erection. The drug may affect blood tests for kidney and liver function. Tell your doctor if you are taking it.

Drug Interactions

• Sinemet's effectiveness may be increased by taking drugs with an anticholinergic effect (such as Trihexyphenidyl).

• Methyldopa, an antihypertensive drug, has the same effect on Levodopa as Carbidopa. It can increase the amount of Levodopa available in the central nervous system, and it may have a slight effect on Sinemet as well.

• People taking Guanethidine or a diuretic to treat high

blood pressure may find they need less of either of those medications to control their pressure.

• Reserpine, benzodiazepine tranquilizers, antipsychotic medicines, Phenytoin, and Papaverine may interfere with the effects of Sinemet. Vitamin B_6 will interfere with Levodopa but not with Sinemet.

• Diabetics who start taking Sinemet may need adjustments in their antidiabetic drugs.

• People taking Sinemet together with a monoamine oxidase (MAO) inhibitor drug may experience a rapid increase in blood pressure. MAO inhibitors should be stopped 2 weeks before starting on Sinemet.

• Sinemet may increase the effects of Ephedrine, amphetamines, Epinephrine, and Isoproterenol. These interactions can result in adverse effects on the heart. This reaction may also occur with some antidepressants when taken concurrently with Sinemet.

Food Interactions

Regular Sinemet may be taken with food to reduce stomach upset. Sinemet CR, the sustained-release form of this product, should be taken on an empty stomach because food can increase Levodopa levels by 25 percent.

Usual Dose

Three different Sinemet strengths are available to allow for individual variation: Sinemet 10/100, 25/100, and 25/250. The first number represents Carbidopa content and the second the Levodopa content, both in mg.

Dosage must be tailored by your doctor to your individual needs based on previous drug treatment. Dosage adjustments are made by adding or omitting ½ to 1 tablet per day. Maximum dose is 8 25/250 tablets per day.

Sinemet CR is started at an amount roughly equal to 10 percent more Levodopa per day than was being taken previously. Dosage adjustments are then tailored to your specific needs.

If needed, extra Carbidopa (Lodosyn) is added to an existing Sinemet dosage in increments of no more than 25 mg (1 tablet) per day until an effect is realized.

Overdosage

Overdose symptoms are exaggerated side effects. Take the

victim to a hospital emergency room. ALWAYS bring the medicine bottle.

Special Information

Sinemet can cause tiredness or lack of concentration: Take care while driving or operating hazardous machinery.

Call your doctor if you experience dizziness, light-headedness or fainting spells, mood or mental changes, abnormal heart rhythm or heart palpitations, difficult urination, persistent nausea or vomiting (or other stomach complaints), or any uncontrollable movements of the face, eyelids, mouth, tongue, neck, arms, hands, or legs. This drug may cause darkening of the urine or sweat. This effect is not harmful but may interfere with urine tests for diabetes. Make sure all your doctors know you are taking this medicine.

Take as prescribed, and call your doctor before making any adjustments in your treatment.

If you forget to take a dose of Sinemet, take it as soon as you remember. If it is within 2 hours of your next dose, skip the one you forgot and continue with your regular schedule. Do not take a double dose.

Special Populations

Pregnancy/Breast-feeding

Sinemet is known to cause birth defects in laboratory animals; the effect in humans is not known. Women who are pregnant or breast-feeding should use this drug only if it is absolutely necessary.

Seniors

Older adults may require smaller doses because they are less tolerant of the drug's effects. Also, the body enzyme that breaks down Levodopa (and against which Carbidopa protects) decreases with age, reducing the overall dosage requirement. Seniors, especially those with heart disease, are more likely to develop abnormal heart rhythms or other cardiac side effects of this drug.

Seniors who respond to this treatment, especially those with osteoporosis, should resume activity gradually. Sudden increases in activity and mobility lead to a greater chance of broken bones than a gradual return to physical activity.

Generic Name

Sotalol

Brand Name

Betapace

Type of Drug

Beta-adrenergic-blocking agent.

Prescribed for

Abnormal heart rhythms.

General Information

Sotalol is one of 14 beta-adrenergic-blocking drugs that interfere with the action of a specific part of the nervous system. Beta receptors are found all over the body and affect many body functions. This accounts for the usefulness of beta blockers against a wide variety of conditions. The first member of this group, *Propranolol,* was found to affect the entire beta-adrenergic portion of the nervous system. Newer beta blockers have been refined to affect only a portion of that system, making them more useful in the treatment of cardio-vascular disorders and less useful for other purposes. Other beta blockers are mild stimulants to the heart or have other characteristics that make them more useful for a specific purpose or better for certain people.

Cautions and Warnings

You should be **cautious about taking Sotalol** if you have **asthma, severe heart failure,** a **very slow heart rate,** or **heart block** because this drug may aggravate these conditions.

People with **angina** who take Sotalol for high blood pressure should have their **drug dosage reduced gradually** over 1 to 2 weeks rather than suddenly discontinued to avoid possible aggravation of the angina.

Sotalol should be used with caution if you have **liver or kidney disease,** because your ability to eliminate this drug from your body may be impaired.

Sotalol reduces the amount of blood pumped by the heart

with each beat. This reduction in blood flow can aggravate or worsen the condition of people with **poor circulation** or **circulatory disease**.

If you are undergoing **major surgery**, your doctor may want you to stop taking Sotalol at least 2 days before surgery to permit the heart to respond more acutely to things that happen during the surgery. This is still controversial and may not hold true for all people preparing for surgery.

Possible Side Effects

Side effects are usually mild, relatively uncommon, develop early in the course of treatment, and are rarely a reason to stop taking Sotalol.

▼ Most common: male impotence.

▼ Less common: unusual tiredness or weakness, slow heartbeat, heart failure (swelling of the legs, ankles, or feet), dizziness, breathing difficulty, bronchospasm, mental depression, confusion, anxiety, nervousness, sleeplessness, disorientation, short-term memory loss, emotional instability, cold hands and feet, constipation, diarrhea, nausea, vomiting, upset stomach, increased sweating, urinary difficulty, cramps, blurred vision, skin rash, hair loss, stuffy nose, facial swelling, aggravation of lupus erythematosus (a disease of the body's connective tissues), itching, chest pains, back or joint pains, colitis, drug allergy (fever, sore throat), and liver toxicity.

Drug Interactions

• Sotalol may interact with surgical anesthetics to increase the risk of heart problems during surgery. Some anesthesiologists recommend gradually stopping your medicine 2 days before surgery.

• Sotalol may interfere with the signs of low blood sugar and can interfere with the action of oral antidiabetes medicines.

• Sotalol enhances the blood-pressure-lowering effects of other blood-pressure-reducing agents (including Clonidine, Guanabenz, and Reserpine) and calcium-channel-blocking drugs (such as Nifedipine).

• Aspirin-containing drugs, Indomethacin, Sulfinpyrazone, and estrogen drugs can interfere with the blood-pressure-lowering effect of Sotalol.

• Cocaine may reduce the effects of all beta-blocking drugs.

• Sotalol may increase the cold hands and feet associated with taking ergot alkaloids (for migraine headaches). Gangrene is a possibility in people taking an ergot and Sotalol.

• Sotalol will counteract the effects of thyroid hormone replacement medicines.

• Calcium channel blockers, Flecainide, Hydralazine, oral contraceptives, Propafenone, Haloperidol, phenothiazine tranquilizers (Molindone and others), quinolone antibacterials, and Quinidine may increase the amount of Sotalol in the bloodstream and the effect of that drug on the body.

• Sotalol should not be taken within 2 weeks of taking a monoamine oxidase (MAO) inhibitor antidepressant drug.

• Cimetidine increases the amount of Sotalol absorbed into the bloodstream from oral tablets.

• Sotalol may interfere with the effectiveness of Theophylline, Aminophylline, and some antiasthma drugs (especially Ephedrine and Isoproterenol).

• The combination of Sotalol and Phenytoin or digitalis drugs can result in excessive slowing of the heart, possibly causing heart block.

• Your Sotalol dose may be reduced if you stop smoking, because your liver will break down the drug more slowly after you stop.

Food Interactions

Food reduces the amount of Sotalol that is absorbed into the blood; it should be taken on an empty stomach.

Usual Dose

160 to 320 mg per day. Some people may need up to 640 mg per day. Dosage must be adjusted for those with poor kidney function.

Overdosage

Symptoms of overdosage are changes in heartbeat (unusually slow, unusually fast, or irregular), severe dizziness or fainting, difficulty breathing, bluish-colored fingernails or palms, and seizures. The overdose victim should be taken to a hospital emergency room where proper therapy can be given. ALWAYS bring the medicine bottle.

Special Information

Sotalol is meant to be taken continuously. Do not stop taking it unless directed to do so by your doctor; abrupt withdrawal may cause chest pain, difficulty breathing, increased sweating, and unusually fast or irregular heartbeat. The dose should be lowered gradually over a period of about 2 weeks.

Call your doctor at once if any of the following symptoms develop: back or joint pains, difficulty breathing, cold hands or feet, depression, skin rash, or changes in heartbeat. Sotalol may produce an undesirable lowering of blood pressure, leading to dizziness or fainting. Call your doctor if this happens to you. Call your doctor about the following side effects only if they persist or are bothersome: anxiety, diarrhea, constipation, sexual impotence, headache, itching, nausea or vomiting, nightmares or vivid dreams, upset stomach, trouble sleeping, stuffy nose, frequent urination, unusual tiredness, or weakness.

Sotalol can cause drowsiness, dizziness, light-headedness, or blurred vision. Be careful when driving or performing complex tasks.

It is best to take your medicine at the same time each day. If you forget a dose of Sotalol tablets, take it as soon as you remember. If you take your medicine once a day and it is within 8 hours of your next dose, skip the forgotten tablet and continue with your regular schedule. If you take Sotalol twice a day and it is within 4 hours of your next dose, skip the forgotten dose and continue with your regular schedule. Do not take a double dose.

Special Populations

Pregnancy/Breast-feeding

Infants born to women who took a beta blocker weighed less at birth and had low blood pressure and reduced heart rate. Sotalol should be avoided by pregnant women and those who might become pregnant while taking it. When the drug is considered essential by your doctor, its potential benefits must be carefully weighed against its risks.

Sotalol passes into breast milk, but problems are rare. Still, nursing mothers taking Sotalol should bottle-feed their babies.

Seniors

Older adults may absorb and retain more Sotalol in their bodies, thus requiring less medicine. Your doctor will need to adjust your dosage to meet your individual needs. Seniors taking this medicine may be more likely to suffer from cold hands and feet, reduced body temperature, chest pains, general feelings of ill health, sudden breathing difficulty, increased sweating, or changes in heartbeat.

Generic Name

Stavudine

Brand Name

Zerit

Type of Drug

Antiviral.

Prescribed for

Advanced HIV infection.

General Information

Stavudine is a synthetic nucleoside-type antiviral drug that inhibits the reproduction of the HIV virus in human cells by interfering with viral DNA duplication. Stavudine can also interfere with DNA in human cells and can affect the duplication of some cells. Stavudine is rapidly absorbed into the blood after it is swallowed. The drug is eliminated primarily through your kidneys, and people with reduced kidney function should have their daily dose of Stavudine adjusted. Stavudine is approved only for adults with AIDS, though the drug has been studied in children for as long as 3 years. In the children who were studied, the drug acted similarly to the way it acts in adults.

Cautions and Warnings

Stavudine should be taken only by adults with **advanced HIV infection** who cannot take or tolerate other AIDS treatments or whose disease has progressed despite receiving other antiviral drugs. There is no proof that Stavudine can prolong the lives of people with AIDS. Zidovudine (AZT) does lengthen the lives of people with AIDS and should be used as first-line treatment.

People taking Stavudine or any other anti-HIV treatment may continue to develop **opportunistic infections** and other complications of the disease and should remain under the direct care of a doctor while taking this medicine.

Peripheral neuropathy is the most common side effect of Stavudine (see *Special Information*). People who have had these symptoms before are more likely to have this problem with Stavudine.

Pancreas inflammation occurred in 1 percent of people taking Stavudine and was associated with 14 deaths among people taking the drug.

Possible Side Effects

▼ Most common: peripheral neuropathy, which can produce tingling, burning, numbness, or pain in your hands, arms, feet, or legs; diarrhea, nausea, and vomiting; headache, fever, and chills; weakness; abdominal pains; back pains; muscle or joint aches; generalized pain; a feeling of ill health; sleeplessness; anxiety; depression; nervousness; difficulty breathing; appetite and weight loss; rash; itching; and sweating.

▼ Common: allergic reactions, flu-like symptoms, swollen lymph glands (usually under your arms or in your neck), chest pain, constipation, upset stomach, and dizziness.

▼ Less common: pelvic pain, tumors, high blood pressure, swelling or flushing, stomach ulcers, confusion, migraine headaches, sleepiness, tremors, nerve pain, asthma, pneumonia, skin tumors, conjunctivitis, visual disturbances, painful urination, genital pains, painful menstruation, and vaginitis.

▼ Rare: frequent urination, blood in the urine, male

> **Possible Side Effects** *(continued)*
>
> impotence, fainting, inflammation of the pancreas, nerve pain, and skin peeling.

Drug Interactions

None known.

Food Interactions

Stavudine can be taken without regard to food or meals.

Usual Dose

Adult: 30 mg to 40 mg every 12 hours.
Senior: dosage reduction may be needed.
Child: not recommended.

Overdosage

Adults given 12 to 14 times the usual daily dose experienced no acute effects. Chronic overdosage, however, can produce peripheral neuropathy (see *Special Information* for details) and liver toxicity. Call your local poison center for more information. Overdose victims should be taken to a hospital emergency room for treatment. ALWAYS bring the medicine bottle with you.

Special Information

Peripheral neuropathy (tingling, pain, or numbness in the hands, arms, legs, or feet) appears in 15 percent to 20 percent of people who take Stavudine. If the drug is stopped, symptoms may disappear, but they can actually worsen for a time after you stop taking Stavudine. If the symptoms do go away, your doctor may restart Stavudine at a lower daily dosage.

Your Stavudine dosage will be reduced if you develop symptoms of neuropathy or if you have reduced kidney function.

This drug does not cure AIDS, nor does it decrease the chance of your transmitting the virus to another person. Stavudine may not prevent some illnesses associated with AIDS from continuing to develop. The long-term effects of Stavudine are not known.

It is very important to take Stavudine according to your doctor's directions. If you forget a dose, take it as soon as you remember. If it is almost time for your next dose, take the dose you forgot, take the next 2 doses 8 hours apart, then go back to your regular schedule. Do not take a double dose of Stavudine. Call your doctor if you skip more than 2 consecutive doses.

Special Populations

Pregnancy/Breast-feeding

Animal studies showed that Stavudine passed into the developing fetus and caused birth defects, but there is no direct information on what happens in humans. Stavudine should be taken during pregnancy only if it is absolutely necessary.

Animal studies show that Stavudine passes into mother's milk, but it is not known if this occurs in humans. Because of the possibility of drug side effects in a nursing infant, mothers who must take this medicine should bottle-feed their babies.

Seniors

Older adults are likely to have reduced kidney function and may need to have their daily dose adjusted to account for this fact.

Generic Name

Sucralfate

Brand Name

Carafate

Type of Drug

Antiulcer therapy.

Prescribed for

Short-term (up to 8 weeks) treatment of duodenal (intestinal) ulcer. This drug has also been used for stomach ulcers, stomach irritation caused by Aspirin and nonsteroidal anti-inflammatory drugs (NSAIDs), stomach bleeding, treatment of gastroesophageal reflux disease (GERD), irritations of the

oin. The dosage of these drugs may have to be reduced by your doctor.

• The amount of Cyclosporine in your blood may be reduced by sulfa drugs, possibly increasing kidney toxicity.

• Erythromycin increases the effect of sulfa drugs against infections caused by *Haemophilus influenzae*, a common cause of middle-ear infections.

• The effects of Folic Acid and Digoxin may be antagonized by Sulfasalazine. Dosage increases may be needed.

Food Interactions

Sulfa drugs should be taken on an empty stomach with a full glass of water. Sulfasalazine may be taken with food if it upsets your stomach.

Usual Dose

Sulfacytine

Adult and Adolescent (age 14 and older): 500 to 1000 mg per day for 10 days.

Child (under 14 years of age): not recommended.

Sulfadiazine

Adult: 2 to 4 grams per day.

Child (2 months of age and older): 34 to 68 mg per pound of body weight daily.

Child (under 2 months of age): do not use, except in the treatment of certain infections present at birth. Then, the dose is 11.3 mg per pound of body weight, 4 times per day.

Sulfamethizole

Adult: 1.5 to 4 grams per day.

Child (over 2 months of age): 13 to 20 mg per pound of body weight per day.

Sulfamethoxazole

Adult: 2 to 3 grams per day.

Child (over 2 months of age): 23 to 27 mg per pound of body weight per day.

Sulfasalazine

Adult: 2 to 4 grams per day in evenly divided doses.

Child (age 2 years and older): 9 to 27 mg per pound of body weight per day in evenly divided doses.

Child (under 2 years): not recommended.

Sulfisoxazole
Adult: 2 to 8 grams per day.
Child (over 2 months of age): 34 to 68 mg per pound of body weight per day.

Trisulfapyrimidines
Adult: 3 to 4 grams per day in divided doses.
Child (2 months of age and older): 34 to 68 mg per pound of body weight every day in divided doses; no more than 6 grams per day.
Child (under 2 months of age): not recommended.

Overdosage

Overdose symptoms include appetite loss, nausea, vomiting and colic, dizziness, headache, drowsiness, unconsciousness, and high fever. Individuals suspected of having taken a sulfa drug overdose should be taken to a hospital emergency room at once. ALWAYS take the medicine bottle.

Special Information

Sulfa drugs often cause unusual skin sensitivity to the sun. Be sure to use a sunscreen or wear protective clothing until you see how sulfas affect you.

Sore throat, fever, chills, unusual bleeding or bruising, rash, and drowsiness are signs of serious blood disorders and should be reported to your doctor at once. Also call your doctor if you experience ringing in the ears, blood in the urine, or difficulty breathing.

Be sure to take the full course of medicine your doctor has prescribed, even if you notice an improvement in your health.

Sulfasalazine may turn your urine orange-yellow. This is a harmless reaction. Skin discoloration has also occurred. This drug may permanently stain soft contact lenses.

Sulfa drugs may interfere with some tests for sugar in the urine.

If you forget to take a dose of sulfa medicine, take it as soon as you remember. If you take the medicine 2 times per day and it is almost time for your next dose, take 1 dose as soon as you remember and another after 5 to 6 hours, then go back to your regular schedule. If you take the medicine 3 or more times per day and it is almost time for your next dose, take 1 dose as soon as you remember and another after 2 to 4 hours, then go back to your regular schedule.

Special Populations

Pregnancy/Breast-feeding

Sulfa drugs pass into the fetal circulation and can affect a developing fetus if taken near delivery: Malformations have been seen in animals given these drugs but not in humans. Pregnant women should not take any sulfa drugs unless directed to do so by their doctors. When a sulfa drug is considered essential by your doctor, its potential benefits should be carefully weighed against its risks.

Small amounts of sulfa drugs pass into breast milk, but this rarely causes problems in healthy, full-term babies. The notable exceptions are premature infants, infants deficient in the enzyme known as *G-6-PD*, or those with hyperbilirubinemia (too much bilirubin in the blood). A nursing infant may also develop diarrhea, rashes, and other problems. Talk to your doctor about taking a sulfa drug while nursing.

Seniors

Older adults who suffer from kidney or liver problems should take sulfa drugs with caution. Other seniors may take these drugs without special restriction. Follow your doctor's directions, and report any side effects at once.

Generic Name

Sulindac

Brand Name

Clinoril

(Also available in generic form)

Type of Drug

Nonsteroidal anti-inflammatory drug (NSAID).

Prescribed for

Rheumatoid arthritis, juvenile rheumatoid arthritis, osteoarthritis, ankylosing spondylitis, tendinitis, bursitis, painful shoulder, gout, and sunburn treatment.

General Information

Sulindac is one of 16 nonsteroidal anti-inflammatory drugs (NSAIDs) that are used to relieve pain and inflammation. We do not know exactly how NSAIDs work, but part of their action may be due to an ability to inhibit the body's production of a hormone called *prostaglandin* and to inhibit the action of other body chemicals, including cyclo-oxygenase, lipoxygenase, leukotrienes, lysosomal enzymes, and a host of other factors. NSAIDs are generally absorbed into the bloodstream fairly quickly. Pain relief comes within 1 hour after taking the first dose of Sulindac, but its anti-inflammatory effect takes a lot longer (several days to 1 week) to become apparent, and may take 3 weeks to reach its maximum effect. Suldinac must be converted to its active form by the liver before it can have an effect.

Cautions and Warnings

People who are **allergic** to Sulindac (or any other NSAID) and those with a history of **asthma** attacks brought on by another NSAID, by Iodides, or by Aspirin should not take Sulindac.

Sulindac can cause gastrointestinal **(GI) bleeding, ulcers, and stomach perforation.** These can occur at any time, with or without warning, in people who take chronic Sulindac treatment. People with a history of active GI bleeding should be cautious about taking any NSAID. Minor stomach upset, distress, or gas is common during the first few days of treatment with Sulindac. People who develop bleeding or ulcers and continue treatment should be aware of the possibility of developing more serious drug toxicity.

Sulindac can affect platelets and **blood clotting** at high doses, and should be avoided by people with clotting problems and by those taking Warfarin.

People with **heart problems** who use Sulindac may experience swelling in their arms, legs, or feet.

Sulindace can cause **inflammation of the pancreas.**

People taking Sulindac may experience an unusually severe **drug-sensitivity reaction.** Report any unusual symptoms to your doctor at once.

Sulindac can cause severe toxic effects to the **kidney.**

Report any unusual side effects to your doctor, who may need to periodically test your kidney function.

Sulindac can cause **unusual sensitivity to the effects of the sun** (photosensitivity).

Possible Side Effects

▼ Most common: diarrhea, nausea, vomiting, constipation, stomach gas, stomach upset or irritation, and loss of appetite.

▼ Less common: stomach ulcers, gastrointestinal bleeding, hepatitis, gallbladder attacks, painful urination, poor kidney function, kidney inflammation, blood and protein in the urine, dizziness, fainting, nervousness, depression, hallucinations, confusion, disorientation, tingling in the hands or feet, light-headedness, itching, increased sweating, dry nose and mouth, heart palpitations, chest pain, difficulty breathing, and muscle cramps.

▼ Rare: severe allergic reactions, including closing of the throat, fever and chills, changes in liver function, jaundice (yellowing of the skin or eyes), and kidney failure. People who experience such effects must be promptly treated in a hospital emergency room or doctor's office.

NSAIDs have caused severe skin reactions; if this happens to you, see your doctor immediately.

Drug Interactions

• Sulindac can increase the effects of oral anticoagulant (blood-thinning) drugs such as Warfarin. You may take this combination, but your doctor may have to reduce your anticoagulant dose.

• Taking Sulindac with Cyclosporine may increase the toxic kidney effects of both drugs. Methotrexate toxicity may be increased in people also taking Sulindac.

• Sulindac may reduce the blood-pressure-lowering effect of beta blockers and loop diuretics.

• Sulindac may increase blood levels of Phenytoin, leading to increased Phenytoin side effects. Blood-Lithium levels may be decreased or unaffected in people taking Sulindac.

• Sulindac blood levels may be affected by Cimetidine because of that drug's effect on the liver.

• Probenecid may interfere with the elimination of Sulindac from the body, increasing the chances for Sulindac toxicity.

• Aspirin and other salicylates may decrease the amount of Sulindac in your blood. These medicines should never be taken at the same time.

• Suldinac may increase the effects of thiazide diuretics.

Food Interactions

Take Sulindac with food or a magnesium/aluminum antacid if it upsets your stomach.

Usual Dose

200 to 300 mg twice per day. Take each dose with a full glass of water, and don't lie down for 15 to 30 minutes after you take the medicine. Do not crush or chew any delayed- or long-acting NSAID tablet.

Overdosage

People have died from NSAID overdoses. The most common signs of overdose are drowsiness, nausea, vomiting, diarrhea, abdominal pain, rapid breathing, rapid heartbeat, sweating, ringing or buzzing in the ears, confusion, disorientation, stupor, and coma. Take the victim to a hospital emergency room at once. ALWAYS bring the medicine bottle with you.

Special Information

Check with your pharmacist if you are unsure about whether you may or may not crush or chew a particular product.

Sulindac can make you drowsy and/or tired: Be careful when driving or operating hazardous equipment. Do not take any nonprescription products with Acetaminophen or Aspirin while taking this drug; also, avoid alcoholic beverages.

Contact your doctor if you develop skin rash or itching, visual disturbances, weight gain, breathing difficulty, fluid retention, hallucinations, black or tarry stools, persistent headache, or any unusual or intolerable side effects.

If you forget to take a dose of Sulindac, take it as soon as you remember. If you take several doses a day and it is within 4 hours of your next dose, skip the one you forgot and continue with your schedule. Do not take a double dose.

Special Populations

Pregnancy/Breast-feeding

NSAIDs may cross into the fetal blood circulation. They have not been found to cause birth defects but may affect a developing fetal heart during the second half of pregnancy; animal studies indicate a possible effect. Women who are or who might become pregnant should not take Sulindac without their doctor's approval; pregnant women should be particularly cautious about using this drug during the last 3 months of their pregnancy. When the drug is considered essential by your doctor, its potential benefits must be carefully weighed against its risks.

NSAIDs may pass into breast milk but have caused no problems among breast-fed infants, except for seizures in a baby whose mother was taking Indomethacin. Other NSAIDs have caused problems in animal studies. There is a possibility that a nursing mother taking Sulindac could affect her baby's heart or cardiovascular system. If you must take Sulindac, bottle-feed your baby.

Seniors

Seniors may be more susceptible to Sulindac's side effects, especially ulcer disease.

Generic Name

Sumatriptan

Brand Name

Imitrex Injection/Tablets

Type of Drug

Antimigraine.

Prescribed for

Treatment of migraine attacks.

General Information

Sumatriptan may work by slowing the activity of certain serotonin-controlled nerves in the brain. Specifically, it is thought that Sumatriptan relieves the pain of migraine headaches by slowing the firing of a very specific serotonin receptor ($5-HT_{1D}$). Sumatriptan does not affect other serotonin receptors.

Sumatriptan should not be used until other pain-relieving alternatives have been tried (including Aspirin, Acetaminophen and other nonsteroidal anti-inflammatory drugs [NSAIDs], etc.). Sumatriptan also relieves the nausea, vomiting, and light and sound sensitivity that generally accompany migraines.

If serious, incapacitating migraines occur more often than twice a month, your doctor may have you take medications other than Sumatriptan on a regular basis to reduce the number and severity of migraine attacks. Some of the medicines that may be used in this way are beta-adrenergic blockers, calcium channel blockers, tricyclic antidepressants, monoamine oxidase (MAO) inhibitors, Methysergide, and Cyproheptadine (especially in children). Other measures that may reduce your need for medication are the identification and avoidance of those factors that trigger headaches, and relaxation or biofeedback techniques.

Sumatriptan is poorly absorbed (only 15 percent) from oral tablets but is 97 percent absorbed after subcutaneous (under the skin) injection. It starts relieving migraine pain within 10 minutes after injection. Migraine symptoms (nausea, vomiting, and light and sound sensitivity) begin resolving within 20 minutes of injection. Sumatriptan's maximum effect occurs in about 2 hours. The drug is broken down by the liver and eliminated from the body through the kidneys. People with liver disease may absorb more medication than those with normal liver function and may require less medicine.

Cautions and Warnings

Do not use this drug if you have had an **allergic reaction** to it in the past.

Sumatriptan should not be used if you have **angina or poor blood supply to the heart muscle, uncontrolled high blood pressure, or a previous heart attack**. It may be used with caution if you have **abnormal heart rhythms, rapid heartbeat,**

coronary artery disease, liver or kidney disease, or controlled high blood pressure, or if you have had a **previous stroke**.

Possible Side Effects

▼ Common: most Sumatriptan side effects are mild, last for less than 1 hour after injection, and resolve on their own. Some side effects reported for Sumatriptan (nausea, vomiting, dizziness, fainting, a feeling of ill health, drowsiness, and sedation) may also be associated with migraines, and it is not clear how much more, if any, Sumatriptan adds to the problem.

▼ Less common: abnormal heart rhythms, cardiogram changes, low blood pressure, slow heart rate, fainting, angina pain, chest pressure, flushing and dizziness, painful blood vessel spasms in the legs, kidney failure, seizures, stroke, swallowing difficulty, unusual thirst, dehydration, vomiting, breathing difficulty, skin redness, rash, stomach ulcers, gallstones, swelling of the arms or legs, transient paralysis, loss of muscle control or muscle tone, muscle spasms, hysterical reactions, depression, an intoxicated feeling, painful urination, frequent urination, and kidney stones.

▼ Rare: coronary artery spasm can be caused by Sumatriptan, usually in people with a history of coronary artery disease. Numerous other rare side effects have been reported, but their relationship to the drug is not known.

Drug Interactions

• Lithium, MAO inhibitor drugs, and selective serotonin reuptake inhibitor (SSRI) antidepressants (those that affect serotonin) may lead to a dangerous condition in which there is too much serotonin in the brain. Don't use these medicines with Sumatriptan.

• Ergotamine and Dihydroergotamine may add to the effects of Sumatriptan. Allow at least 24 hours between taking either of these drugs and taking Sumatriptan.

Food Interactions

Sumatriptan may be taken with food.

Usual Dose

Tablets

Adult (age 18 and older): take 1 tablet as soon as migraine symptoms begin or at any time during the attack. If the symptoms don't go away, you may take another tablet after checking with your doctor. You should not take another tablet less than 2 hours after taking the first. Don't take more than 300 mg a day. People with liver disease should take the lowest possible dose of Sumatriptan.

Child: not recommended.

Injection

Adult (age 18 and older): 6 mg as a subcutaneous injection; dose may be repeated if headache pain returns at the same or a worse level; no more than 12 mg every 1 or 2 days. Single doses larger than 6 mg are no more effective and are not recommended.

Child: not recommended.

Overdosage

Overdose symptoms could be convulsions or tremors, tiredness, swelling of the arms or legs, abnormal breathing, bluish discoloration of the skin under the fingernails or lips, weakness, dilated pupils, inflammation, hair loss, and paralysis. The injection may cause scabs and other reactions.

Special Information

Notify your doctor if you have other medical conditions that could be a problem with Sumatriptan (see *Cautions and Warnings*).

Be sure to take your Sumatriptan at the first sign of a migraine (pain or aura). You may get a greater effect from the drug if you lie down in a quiet, dark room.

Avoid alcoholic beverages because they can worsen your headaches.

Sumatriptan can cause dizziness or drowsiness. Take care if you have to drive or do anything else that requires intense concentration while taking Sumatriptan.

Read and follow instructions for use that come with the medicine.

Call your doctor if the usual dose does not relieve 3 consecutive headaches, if your headaches become more frequent or worse, or if you develop chest pain; difficulty swallowing; chest pressure, tightness, or heaviness; injection site reactions; nausea; vomiting; or other side effects that are particularly bothersome.

If you are taking Sumatriptan tablets and develop tightness in the chest or throat; shortness of breath; heart throbbing; swollen eyelids, face, or lips; skin rash; or lumps or hives, contact your doctor. Call your doctor **at once** if chest pain does not go away.

Sumatriptan causes clouding of the cornea of the eye in dogs; this effect could be seen in people taking Sumatriptan over a long period, although it has never actually been reported. People taking this drug regularly should have their eyes checked periodically.

If the first dose (up to 2 tablets) doesn't work, don't take a second one. You should take other medicines prescribed by your doctor to relieve migraine attacks. If you get some relief and the migraine returns, you may take a second dose at least 1 hour after the first one.

Special Populations

Pregnancy/Breast-feeding
Animal studies have shown possible toxic effects of Sumatriptan on a developing fetus at varying dosage levels. It should be used by pregnant women only after they have fully discussed the possible benefits and the potential risks of taking Sumatriptan with their doctors.

Sumatriptan may pass into breast milk and should be used with caution by nursing mothers.

Seniors
Most published studies of Sumatriptan exclude people over age 65, but small studies in people between 65 and 86 years revealed no special differences between older and younger adults in how Sumatriptan affected them. Nevertheless, seniors may be more sensitive to the effects of Sumatriptan because of the chance of reduced kidney and/or liver function.

Suprax

see **Cephalosporin Antibiotics**, page 171

Synthroid

see **Thyroid Hormone Replacements**, page 1099

Generic Name

Tacrine Hydrochloride

Brand Name

Cognex

Type of Drug

Cholinesterase inhibitor.

Prescribed for

Alzheimer's disease.

General Information

Tacrine is the first and only pill proven to raise levels of acetylcholine in the brain. People with Alzheimer's disease, a degenerative condition of the nervous system, develop a shortage of this important neurohormone early in their disease. As Alzheimer's progresses, many other brain systems are affected, but Tacrine does not help those problems. The acetylcholine shortage in the brain is believed to account for some Alzheimer's symptoms: gradual loss of memory, judgment, and the ability to think and reason.

    Studies of Tacrine show that between 10 and 25 percent of people who start taking it will be helped by the drug. One problem is that not everyone can tolerate it; about 12 percent of people who start on Tacrine stop permanently because of drug side effects. Many others who stop because of drug side effects may try again and can continue on Tacrine. Another problem is that people with Alzheimer's disease continue to worsen as time passes. It is difficult to estimate the drug's effect on any individual because nobody knows how one person's condition would have changed without Tacrine. Age, sex, and other variables do not affect individual response to Tacrine.

Larger doses of Tacrine are definitely more effective. In a 30-week study, those people who took 120 and 160 mg of Tacrine continued to get better for the first 24 weeks. After that, their condition slowly reversed itself. People taking 80 mg improved for the first 18 weeks, then declined toward their starting point for the rest of the study. Alzheimer's disease patients who took a placebo (inactive drug) showed some minor improvement for a short time, then steadily declined for the rest of the study period.

Cautions and Warnings

People who are **sensitive** or **allergic** to Tacrine or similar drugs and those who have developed Tacrine-related **jaundice** (yellowing of the skin or eyes) in the past should not take this drug.

Tacrine may **slow heart rate**, a problem that can adversely affect some people with preexisting heart disease.

Tacrine will increase the amount of stomach acid you make. People with a history of **ulcers** and those taking **nonsteroidal anti-inflammatory drugs** (NSAIDs) should be aware of the possibility that Tacrine may increase your chances of stomach or intestinal bleeding.

People with **asthma, bladder disease, seizure disorders,** or current or past **liver disease** should take this drug with caution, because it is likely to worsen (or cause a reappearance of) these conditions.

Women who take Tacrine have about 1 ½ times as much of it in their blood as men and may be more likely to develop drug side effects, especially liver inflammation.

Possible Side Effects

▼ Most common: liver inflammation, headache, nausea or vomiting, diarrhea, and dizziness; also, chills, fever,

Possible Side Effects *(continued)*

feelings of ill health, swelling in the legs or feet, blood-pressure changes, broken bones, joint pain and/or inflammation, spasticity, fainting, convulsions, hyperactivity, tingling in the hands or feet, nervousness, sore throat, sinus inflammation, bronchitis, pneumonia, breathing difficulty, sweating, and conjunctivitis ("pink-eye").

▼ Less common: facial swelling, dehydration, weight gain, a sickly appearance, swelling, heart failure, heart attack, angina pains, stroke, vein irritation, cardiac insufficiency, heart palpitation, abnormal heart rhythms, migraine headache, slow heart rate, blood clot in the lung, elevated blood cholesterol, inflamed tongue, swollen gums, dry mouth or throat, sores in the mouth, upset stomach, increased saliva, difficulty swallowing, irritation of the esophagus or stomach, stomach or intestinal bleeding or ulcers, hemorrhoids, hiatal hernia, bloody stools, diverticulitis, loss of bowel control, impacted colon, gallbladder irritation and/or stones, increased appetite, diabetes, anemia, osteoporosis, tendinitis, bursitis, abnormal dreams, difficulty speaking, memory loss, wandering, twitching, delirium, paralysis, slow muscle movements, nerve inflammation or disease, movement disorders and unusual movements usually associated with Parkinson's disease, apathy, increased sex drive, paranoid feelings, neurosis, nosebleeds, chest congestion, asthma, rapid breathing, respiratory infection, acne, hair loss, skin rash, eczema, dry skin, shingles, psoriasis, skin inflammation, cysts, furuncles, cold sores, herpes infections of the skin, blood in the urine, kidney stones, kidney infections, sugar in the urine, painful urination, frequent urination, nighttime urination, puss in the urine, cystitis, urinary urgency, difficulty urinating, vaginal bleeding, genital itching, breast pain, impotence, prostate cancer, cataracts, dry eyes, eye pain, styes, double vision or other visual defects, glaucoma, earache, ringing or buzzing in the ears, deafness, middle or inner ear infections, and unusual taste sensations.

▼ Rare: heat exhaustion, blood infection, severely abnormal heart rhythms, bowel obstruction, duodenal ulcer,

Possible Side Effects *(continued)*

changes in thyroid status, reduced white-blood- cell and platelet counts, muscle disease, some sensory loss (especially the sense of touch), tortuous movements (of the tongue, eyes, or face), loss of muscle tone, inflammation of the brain or central nervous system, Bell's palsy, suicidal thoughts, hysteria, psychosis, vomiting blood, fluid in the lungs, lung cancer, sudden choking, skin peeling, oily skin, skin ulcers, skin cancer, melanoma, tumors of the bladder or kidney, kidney failure, urinary obstruction, breast cancer, ovarian cancer, inflammation of the male reproductive tract, blindness, droopy or inflamed eyelids, and inner ear disturbances or inflammation.

Drug Interactions

• Tacrine is a cholinesterase inhibitor and is likely to increase the effects of some muscle relaxants used during surgery. Be sure your surgeon knows you are taking it.

• Tacrine increases Theophylline concentrations twofold, requiring a Theophylline dose reduction to avoid side effects.

• Cimetidine increases the amount of Tacrine absorbed into the blood by 50 percent. Your doctor should take this interaction into account when determining the final Tacrine dose.

• Tacrine will interfere with the effect of all anticholinergic medicines.

• Cigarette smoking will increase the speed at which Tacrine is broken down by the liver.

Food Interactions

Food reduces the amount of Tacrine absorbed into the blood by 30 to 40 percent. Take it at least 1 hour before or 2 hours after meals.

Usual Dose

40 to 160 mg per day, divided into 4 doses.

Overdosage

Tacrine overdose can cause salivation, severe nausea and

vomiting, increased sweating, slow heartbeat, low blood pressure, collapse, and convulsions. Muscles may become increasingly weak; this can lead to death if the respiratory muscles are involved. Overdose victims should be taken to an emergency room for treatment. ALWAYS bring the medicine bottle.

Special Information

Call your doctor if you develop very light-colored or black and tarry stools, or if you vomit a "coffee-ground"-like material. Report yellowing of the eyes or skin, rash, or other side effects that are bothersome or persistent. Your doctor may have to stop your treatment if you develop liver inflammation; your doctor will need to take blood samples for at least the first 18 weeks of treatment to watch for signs of this problem.

Abruptly stopping this medicine or reducing the dose by 80 mg or more at a time is likely to cause changes in behavior and a noticeable worsening of the Alzheimer's disease. Do not change doses or stop taking Tacrine without your doctor's knowledge.

For consistent results, this drug should be taken at the same time each day. If you forget a dose, take it as soon as possible. If it is almost time for the next dose, space the remaining doses over the rest of the day, and then go back to your regular schedule. Call your doctor if you miss more than one dose.

Special Populations

Pregnancy/Breast-feeding

The effect of Tacrine on pregnant women is not known. Discuss the possible risks with your doctor if you are or may become pregnant and must take this drug.

It is not known if Tacrine passes into breast milk, although it is unlikely. Still, nursing mothers taking Tacrine should bottle-feed their infants.

Seniors

Seniors may take this drug without special restriction, except for those with liver disease, who are more likely to experience toxic side effects.

Generic Name

Tacrolimus

Brand Name

Prograf

Type of Drug

Immunosuppressant.

Prescribed for

Preventing the rejection of transplanted organs.

General Information

Tacrolimus, formerly known as *FK506*, is derived from a bacterium. It has been shown to prolong the survival of transplanted liver, kidney, heart, bone marrow, small bowel and pancreas, lungs and trachea, skin, cornea, and limbs in animal studies. In people, the drug is used in liver transplants and has been studied in kidney, bone marrow, heart, pancreas, and small bowel transplants, among others.

Tacrolimus works by inhibiting the activation of T-cells, an essential element of the body's immune response, producing immune-system suppression.

Cautions and Warnings

Transplant patients who are **sensitive** or **allergic** to Tacrolimus should be given another drug. Some people may also be allergic to chemically modified castor oil, which is used in Tacrolimus injection.

Tacrolimus can cause **kidney damage,** especially when taken in high doses. This effect has been noted in 33 to 40 percent of liver transplant patients. To avoid excess kidney damage, this drug should not be taken together with Cyclosporine, another organ transplant drug. These drugs should be separated by at least 24 hours.

Mild elevations of blood potassium were noted in 10 to 44 percent of liver transplant patients.

Tremors, headaches, muscle function changes, changes in mental state and sense perception, or other nervous-system

problems occur in about half of people receiving a liver transplant. **Seizures** have also occurred. In some cases, these side effects may be associated with large amounts of Tacrolimus in the blood.

As with other immune suppressants, people taking Tacrolimus have a better chance of **developing a lymphoma or other malignancy.** The chance increases with the degree of immune suppression and the length of time that the drug is taken. A disorder related to **Epstein-Barr virus (EBV) infection** has also been reported.

People with **kidney disease** should receive lower doses of Tacrolimus. People who experience post-transplant reduction in liver function can develop kidney damage.

Mild to moderate **high blood pressure** is a common side effect of Tacrolimus and can be a sign of kidney damage. People taking this drug should measure their blood pressure regularly.

Possible Side Effects

▼ Most common: headache, tremors, sleeplessness, tingling in hands or feet, diarrhea, nausea, constipation, loss of appetite, vomiting, liver or kidney abnormalities, high blood pressure, urinary infection, infrequent urination, anemia, increased white-blood-cell counts, reduced blood-platelet counts, changes in blood-potassium level, reduced blood-magnesium, high blood-sugar, fluid in the lungs and other lung problems, difficulty breathing, itching, rash, abdominal pains, pain, fever, weakness, back pains, abdominal fluid buildup, and retention of fluid.

▼ Less common: abnormal dreaming, anxiety, confusion, depression, dizziness, instability, hallucination, poor coordination, muscle spasms, psychosis, tiredness, unusual thoughts, double vision or other visual disturbances, ringing or buzzing in the ears, upset stomach, yellow discoloration of skin or whites of the eyes, trouble swallowing, stomach gas, stomach bleeding, fungus infection of the mouth, bloody urine, chest pain, rapid heartbeat, low blood pressure, diabetes, black-and-blue marks, muscle and joint aches, leg cramps, muscle weakness, asthma, bronchitis, coughing, sore throat, pneumonia,

---

Possible Side Effects *(continued)*

stuffy and runny nose, sinus irritation, voice changes, sweating, skin rashes, and herpes infections.

Drug Interactions

• Tacrolimus should not be taken at the same time as other immune suppressants so as to avoid excessive suppression of the immune system.

• Tacrolimus may cause more kidney damage when taken together with other drugs that also cause kidney problems, including aminoglycoside antibiotics, Amphotericin B, Cisplatin, and Cyclosporine.

• Antifungal drugs, Bromocriptine, calcium channel blockers, Cimetidine, Clarithromycin, Danazol, Diltiazem, Erythromycin, Methylprednisolone, and Metoclopramide can increase Tacrolimus blood levels and possible drug side effects.

• Carbamazepine, Phenobarbital, Phenytoin, Rifampin, and Rifampicin can reduce the amount of Tacrolimus in the blood.

• Vaccination may be less effective during Tacrolimus use. Live vaccines (measles, mumps, rubella, oral polio, BCG, yellow fever, and TY 21 typhoid) should be avoided.

Food Interactions

Food interferes with the absorption of Tacrolimus into the blood. Take this drug either 1 hour before or 2 hours after meals.

Usual Dose

Adult and Child: 0.075 to 0.15 mg per pound per day divided into 2 doses. Your dosage will be reduced to the lowest effective dose. Children may require larger doses than adults. Dosing is usually started at the high end of the recommended dose and then reduced to the lowest effective level.

Overdosage

Tacrolimus overdose can be expected to produce exaggerated drug side effects. Overdose victims should be taken to a hospital emergency room for treatment. ALWAYS bring the medicine bottle with you.

Special Information

It is extremely important for you to take this medicine exactly as prescribed. If you do forget a dose of Tacrolimus, take it as soon as you remember. If it is almost time for your next dose, skip the forgotten dose and continue with your regular schedule. Do not take a double dose, and call your doctor if you forget 2 or more doses in a row.

People taking Tacrolimus require regular testing to monitor their progress.

Call your doctor at the first sign of fever; sore throat; tiredness; weakness; nervousness; unusual bleeding or bruising; tender or swollen gums; convulsions; irregular heartbeat; confusion; numbness or tingling of your hands, feet, or lips; difficulty breathing; severe stomach pains with nausea; or bloody urine. Other drug effects are less serious but should be brought to your doctor's attention, particularly if they are unusually bothersome or persistent.

It is important to maintain good dental hygiene while taking Tacrolimus and to use extra care when using your toothbrush or dental floss because the drug may make you more susceptible to dental infections. Tacrolimus suppresses the normal body systems that fight infection. See your dentist regularly while taking this medicine.

This medicine should be continued as long as prescribed by your doctor. Do not stop taking it because of side effects or other problems. If you cannot tolerate the oral form, this drug can be given by injection, though the oral capsules are preferable.

Special Populations

Pregnancy/Breast-feeding

In animal studies using half the human dose, this drug was lethal to embryos and affected the ability of females to become pregnant. Malformations were seen at higher doses. The drug passes into the blood of the developing fetus and should be used during pregnancy only if absolutely necessary. Babies born to mothers taking this drug have had high blood potassium and poor kidney function.

Tacrolimus passes into breast milk. Nursing mothers who must take this drug should bottle-feed their babies.

Seniors
Older adults may take this drug, but their dose may have to be reduced to accommodate normal loss of kidney function.

Generic Name

Tamoxifen Citrate

Brand Name
Nolvadex

Type of Drug
Antiestrogen.

Prescribed for
Breast cancer in women. When used together with chemotherapy after mastectomy surgery, Tamoxifen is effective in delaying the recurrence of surgically curable cancers in postmenopausal women or women over age 50. It has been used in the prevention of breast cancer among high-risk women who have no current signs of the disease. Tamoxifen has also been prescribed to treat painful breasts and to decrease swollen painful breasts in men. It may also be used in the treatment of male breast cancer and in pancreatic cancer.

General Information
Tamoxifen is effective against breast cancer in women whose tumors are tested and found to be estrogen-positive. It works by competing with the sites in tissues to which estrogens attach. Once Tamoxifen binds to an estrogen receptor, it disrupts the cell in the same way that an estrogen would and prevents the cancer cell from dividing. Of those women whose breast cancer has spread to other parts of their bodies, 50 to 60 percent may benefit from taking Tamoxifen.

Another medicine, Anastrozole (Arimidex) can be given to postmenopausal women with advanced breast cancer who don't respond to Tamoxifen. Anastrozole is the first of a new drug type (aromatase inhibitors) that reduces estrogen production in your body.

Cautions and Warnings

Visual difficulty has occurred in patients taking Tamoxifen for 1 year or more in doses at least 4 times above the maximum recommended dosage. A few cases of decreased visual clarity and other eye side effects have been reported at normal doses.

People taking Tamoxifen have experienced **liver inflammation** and, rarely, **other more serious liver abnormalities**.

Animal studies have shown that very high doses of this drug (15 mg per pound of body weight) may cause liver cancer.

Possible Side Effects

Side effects are usually mild.

▼ Most common: hot flashes, nausea, and vomiting (up to 25 percent of all patients).

▼ Less common: vaginal bleeding or discharge, irregular periods, and skin rash.

▼ Rare: high blood-calcium levels, swelling of the arms or legs, changes in sense of taste, vaginal itch, depression, dizziness, light-headedness, headache, visual difficulty, and reduced white-blood-cell count or reduced platelet count. Ovarian cysts have occurred in premenopausal women with advanced breast cancer who have taken Tamoxifen. Increases in tumor pain and local disease sometimes follow a good response with Tamoxifen.

Drug Interactions

• The effects of Warfarin and other anticoagulant (blood-thinning) drugs may be increased by Tamoxifen. Tamoxifen may increase blood-calcium levels.

• Bromocriptine may increase the amount of Tamoxifen in the bloodstream.

Food Interactions

Tamoxifen is best taken on an empty stomach but may be taken with food or milk if it upsets your stomach.

Usual Dose

10 to 20 mg morning and evening.

Overdosage

Overdose may lead to breathing difficulty or convulsions. Other symptoms are tremors, overactive reflexes, dizziness, and unsteadiness. Overdose victims should be taken to a hospital emergency room for treatment. ALWAYS bring the prescription bottle.

Special Information

Take this medicine according to your doctor's directions. Tell your doctor if you become very weak or sleepy, or if you experience confusion, pain, or swelling of your legs, difficulty breathing, blurred vision, bone pain, hot flashes, nausea, vomiting, weight gain, irregular periods, dizziness, headache, or loss of appetite while taking this drug. If you vomit shortly after taking a dose of Tamoxifen, your doctor may tell you to take another dose or wait until the next dose.

Women taking Tamoxifen should use effective contraception until treatment is complete.

If you forget to take a dose of Tamoxifen, skip the forgotten dose, call your doctor, and continue your regular dosing schedule. Do not take a double dose.

Special Populations

Pregnancy/Breast-feeding

Because of its antiestrogen effects, Tamoxifen can harm a developing fetus. Although there are no specific studies of its effects in pregnant women, Tamoxifen should be avoided by women who are pregnant.

It is not known if Tamoxifen passes into breast milk. Nursing mothers should bottle-feed their babies.

Seniors

Seniors may take Tamoxifen without special restriction.

Tegretol

*see **Carbamazepine**, page 157*

Generic Name

Temazepam

Brand Name

Restoril

(Also available in generic form)

Type of Drug

Benzodiazepine sedative.

Prescribed for

Short-term treatment of insomnia, difficulty falling asleep, frequent nighttime awakening, and waking too early in the morning.

General Information

Temazepam is one of the group of drugs known as *benzodiazepines*. All have some activity as either antianxiety agents, anticonvulsants, or sedatives. Benzodiazepines work by a direct effect on the brain. Benzodiazepines make it easier to go to sleep and decrease the number of times you wake up during the night.

These medicines differ primarily in how long they work on your body. They all take about 2 hours to reach maximum blood level, but some remain in your body longer, so they work for a longer period of time. Temazepam is considered to be an intermediate-acting sedative and generally remains long enough to give you a good night's sleep with minimal "hangover."

Often sleeplessness is a reflection of another disorder that would be untreated by one of these medicines.

Cautions and Warnings

People with **respiratory disease** may experience sleep apnea (intermittent breathing while asleep) while taking Temazepam.

People with **kidney or liver disease** should be carefully monitored while taking this medicine. Take the lowest possible dose to help you sleep.

Clinical depression may be increased by the benzodiazepines and other drugs that depress the nervous system. Intentional overdosage is more common among depressed people who take sleeping pills than among those who do not.

All benzodiazepine drugs can be **abused** if taken for long periods of time, and it is possible for a person taking a benzodiazepine drug to develop **drug-withdrawal symptoms** if the drug is suddenly discontinued. Withdrawal symptoms include tremors, muscle cramps, insomnia, agitation, diarrhea, vomiting, increased sweating, and convulsions.

Possible Side Effects

▼ Most common: drowsiness, headache, dizziness, talkativeness, nervousness, apprehension, poor muscle coordination, light-headedness, daytime tiredness, muscle weakness, slowness of movements, hangover, and euphoria (feeling "high").

▼ Less common: nausea, vomiting, rapid heartbeat, confusion, temporary memory loss, upset stomach, cramps and pain, depression, blurred or double vision, constipation, changes in taste perception, appetite changes, stuffy nose, nosebleeds, common cold symptoms, asthma, sore throat, cough, breathing problems, diarrhea, dry mouth, allergic reactions, fainting, abnormal heart rhythms, itching, acne, dry skin, sensitivity to bright light or the sun, rash, nightmares or strange dreams, difficulty sleeping, tingling in the hands or feet, ringing or buzzing in the ears, ear or eye pain, menstrual cramps, frequent or painful urination, blood in the urine, discharge from the penis or vagina, poor control of the urinary function, lower back and joint pain, muscle spasms and pain, fever, swollen breasts, and weight changes.

Drug Interactions

• Temazepam's effects are enhanced if it is taken with other nervous-system depressants, including alcoholic beverages, antihistamines, tranquilizers, barbiturates, anticonvulsants, antidepressants, and monoamine oxidase (MAO) inhibitor drugs (most often prescribed for severe depression).

• Oral contraceptives may increase the effect of Temazepam by interfering with the drug's breakdown in the liver. Probenecid also increases Temazepam's effects.

• Cigarette smoking, Rifampin, and Theophylline may reduce Temazepam's effect on your body.

• Temazepam may decrease Levodopa's effectiveness.

• Temazepam may increase the amount of Zidovudine (AZT), Phenytoin, or Digoxin in your blood, increasing the chances of drug toxicity.

• The combination of Clozapine and a benzodiazepine has led to respiratory collapse in a few people. Temazepam should be stopped at least 1 week before starting Clozapine treatment.

• Temazepam blood levels may be increased when taken with one of the macrolide antibiotics (Azithromycin, Erythromycin, or Clarithromycin).

Food Interactions

Temazepam may be taken with food if it upsets your stomach.

Usual Dose

Adult (age 18 and older): 15 to 30 mg at bedtime. The dose must be individualized for maximum benefit.

Senior: begin treatment with 15 mg at bedtime. Dosage may be increased if needed.

Child: not recommended.

Overdosage

The most common symptoms of overdosage are confusion, sleepiness, depression, loss of muscle coordination, and slurred speech. Coma may develop if the overdose is particularly large. Overdose symptoms can develop if a single dose of only 4 times the maximum daily dose is taken. Overdose victims must be made to vomit with Syrup of Ipecac (available at any pharmacy) to remove any remaining drug from the stomach. Call your doctor or a poison control center before doing this. If 30 minutes have passed since the overdose was taken or symptoms have begun to develop, the victim must be taken immediately to a hospital emergency room for treatment. ALWAYS bring the medicine bottle.

Special Information

Never take more of this medication than prescribed. Avoid

alcoholic beverages and other nervous-system depressants while taking this medicine.

Be careful when performing tasks requiring concentration and coordination because this drug may make you drowsy, dizzy, or light-headed.

If you take Temazepam daily for 3 or more weeks, you may experience some withdrawal symptoms when you stop taking it. Talk with your doctor about the best way to discontinue the drug.

If you forget to take a dose of Temazepam and remember within about an hour of your regular time, take it as soon as you remember. If you do not remember until later, skip the forgotten dose and go back to your regular schedule. Do not take a double dose.

Special Populations

Pregnancy/Breast-feeding
Temazepam should absolutely **not** be used by pregnant women or women who may become pregnant. Animal studies have shown that the drug passes easily into the fetal blood system and can affect fetal development.

Benzodiazepines pass into breast milk and can affect an infant. Temazepam should not be taken by nursing mothers.

Seniors
Seniors are more susceptible to the effects of Temazepam and should take the lowest possible dosage.

Generic Name

Terazosin

Brand Name

Hytrin

Type of Drug

Alpha blocker.

Prescribed for

High blood pressure; urinary symptoms of benign prostatic hypertrophy (BPH) in men.

General Information

Terazosin lowers blood pressure by opening blood vessels and reducing pressure within them. Terazosin and similar drugs block nerve endings known as *alpha₁ receptors.* Other blood-pressure-lowering drugs block beta receptors, interfere with the movement of calcium in blood-vessel muscle cells, affect salt and electrolyte balance in the body, or interfere with the process for manufacturing norepinephrine. The maximum blood-pressure-lowering effect of Terazosin is seen between 2 and 6 hours after taking a single dose. Terazosin's effect lasts for 24 hours. In BPH, Terazosin works by relaxing smooth muscles in the prostate and neck of the bladder. Here, too, this effect is produced by blockade of alpha receptors in the affected muscles. Despite the fact that Terazosin reduces the symptoms of BPH, the drug's long-term effect on complications of BPH or the need for urinary surgery is not known. Age and race have no effect on response. Alpha blockers are broken down in the liver and/or pass out of the body through the feces. About 40 percent of Terazosin passes out of the body via the kidneys.

Cautions and Warnings

Terazosin can cause **dizziness** and **fainting**, especially with the first few doses. This is known as the *first-dose effect.* This effect can be minimized by limiting the first dose to 1 mg at bedtime. The first-dose effect occurs in about 1 percent of people taking an alpha blocker and can recur if the drug is stopped for a few days and then restarted.

People who are **allergic** or **sensitive** to any of the alpha blockers should avoid the others because of the chance that they will react to them as well.

Terazosin may slightly reduce cholesterol levels and increase the HDL/LDL (important blood fats) ratio, a positive step for people with a blood-cholesterol problem. People with an already **high blood-cholesterol level** should discuss this situation with their doctors.

Red- and white-blood-cell counts may be slightly decreased in people taking Terazosin.

People taking Terazosin may gain a small amount of weight (about 2 pounds).

Possible Side Effects

▼ Most common: dizziness, weakness, and headache.

▼ Less common: dizziness when rising from a sitting or lying position; low blood pressure; rapid heartbeat; abnormal heart rhythms; chest pain; flushing in the face, arms, or legs; fainting; vomiting; dry mouth; diarrhea; constipation; abdominal pain or discomfort; stomach gas; breathing difficulty; stuffy nose; sinus inflammation; cold or flu symptoms; cough; bronchitis; worsening of asthma; nosebleeds; sore throat; runny nose; shoulder, neck, or back pain; pain in the arms or legs; joint pains; arthritis; muscle pain, blurring or other visual disturbances; conjunctivitis ("pink-eye"); eye pain; nervousness; tingling in the hands or feet; tiredness; anxiety; trouble sleeping; frequent urination; urinary infection; itching; rash; sweating; swelling of the face, arms, or legs; and fever.

▼ Rare: depression, reduced sex drive or abnormal sexual function, fluid retention, and weight gain.

Drug Interactions

• Terazosin may interact with beta-blocking drugs to produce a higher rate of dizziness or fainting after taking the first dose of Terazosin.

• The blood-pressure-lowering effect of Terazosin may be reduced by Indomethacin.

• When taken with other blood-pressure-lowering drugs, Terazosin produces an exaggerated reduction of blood pressure.

• The blood-pressure-lowering effect of Clonidine may be reduced by Terazosin.

• This drug does not affect the results of the prostate-specific antigen (PSA) test often used to monitor the progress of BPH.

Food Interactions

Terazosin may be taken without regard to food or meals.

Usual Dose

The usual starting dose of Terazosin is 1 mg at bedtime. The dosage may be increased in 1- to 5-mg increments to a total of 20 to 40 mg per day. Terazosin may be taken once or twice a day. Doses of 10 mg once a day are generally needed to control the symptoms of BPH.

Overdosage

Terazosin overdose may produce drowsiness, poor reflexes, and very low blood pressure. Overdose victims should be taken to a hospital emergency room at once. ALWAYS bring the prescription bottle.

Special Information

Take this drug exactly as prescribed, and do not stop taking it unless directed to do so by your doctor. Avoid nonprescription drugs that contain stimulants because they can increase your blood pressure. Your pharmacist will be able to tell you what you can and cannot take.

Terazosin can cause dizziness, headache, and drowsiness, especially 2 to 6 hours after you take your first drug dose, although these effects can persist after the first few doses.

Call your doctor if you develop severe dizziness, heart palpitations, or other bothersome or persistent side effects.

Wait 12 to 24 hours after taking the first dose before driving or doing anything that requires intense concentration. You should take it at bedtime to minimize this problem.

If you forget to take a dose of Terazosin and you take it once a day, take it as soon as you remember. If you take it twice a day and it is almost time for your next dose, skip the forgotten dose and continue with your regular medication schedule. Taking your medicine at the same time each day will help you to remember your medicine.

Special Populations

Pregnancy/Breast-feeding

Animal studies of large doses of Terazosin in animals showed an effect on developing fetuses, but the effect of Terazosin in pregnant women is not known. It should be used only when its benefits clearly outweigh its potential dangers.

It is not known if Terazosin passes into breast milk. Nursing mothers who must take this medication should bottle-feed their babies.

Seniors

Older adults may be more sensitive to the effects and side effects of Terazosin. Report any unusual side effects to your doctor.

Generic Name

Terbinafine

Brand Name

Lamisil Cream

Type of Drug

Antifungal.

Prescribed for

Fungal infections of the skin.

General Information

Terbinafine is a general-purpose antifungal product. It can cure common athlete's foot, jock itch, and ringworm faster than other medicines of this type. It is also effective against *Candida* and other fungal infections of the skin. Terbinafine is unique because it accumulates in the skin after application and continues to kill fungus organisms even after you stop using it. Most other antifungals applied to the skin do not kill the fungus; they only stop it from growing. Because of its strength, Terbinafine may be prescribed for fungal infections of the skin that do not respond to nonprescription products.

Cautions and Warnings

Do not take this product if you are **allergic** to Terbinafine or any other ingredient in Lamisil Cream.

Terbinafine is **meant to be applied only to the skin**. Do not put it into your eyes, swallow it, or use it for a vaginal infection.

Laboratory animals fed almost 400 times the daily human

dose of Terbinafine for 2 years developed tumors. Terbinafine
should be used only for specific fungal infections and only on
your doctor's prescription.

Possible Side Effects

▼ Most common: itching and irritation of the skin
immediately after application.

▼ Less common: burning, irritation, and dryness of the
skin.

Drug and Food Interactions

None known.

Usual Dose

Apply Terbinafine to affected areas morning and night for 1 to
4 weeks. Use this medicine exactly as prescribed.

Overdosage

Overdosage of Terbinafine is a problem only if the cream is
swallowed. Overdosage can lead to tiredness, poor muscle
coordination, breathing difficulty, and bulging of the eyes.
Overdose victims should be taken to a hospital emergency
room. ALWAYS bring the prescription package.

Special Information

Do not put Terbinafine cream into your eyes, nose, mouth, or
any other mucous membrane tissues.

Do not stop using Terbinafine before your prescription is
completely finished, even if your rash clears up. The full
prescription may be necessary to eliminate the offending
fungus.

Do not cover the cream with plastic wrap or anything that
restricts ventilation after application unless so instructed by
your doctor.

Call your doctor if your skin becomes red, burns, itches,
blisters, or swells, or if oozing develops.

If you forget to apply a dose, take it as soon as you
remember. If it is almost time for your next dose, skip the
forgotten dose and continue with your treatment.

Special Populations

Pregnancy/Breast-feeding

There is no information on the effect of Terbinafine on a developing fetus. Pregnant women and those who might become pregnant should use Terbinafine only if it is absolutely necessary.

Very small amounts of Terbinafine may pass into breast milk after application. Nursing mothers should not apply this cream to the breast and should carefully consider its use on other parts of the body.

Seniors

Older adults can use Terbinafine without special restriction.

Generic Name

Terbutaline Sulfate

Brand Names

Brethine
Bricanyl

Type of Drug

Bronchodilator.

Prescribed for

Asthma, bronchial spasms, premature labor.

General Information

Terbutaline Sulfate is similar to other bronchodilator drugs such as Metaproterenol and Isoetharine, but it has a weaker effect on nerve receptors in the heart and blood vessels; for this reason, it is somewhat safer for people with heart conditions.

Terbutaline Sulfate tablets begin to work within 30 minutes and continue working for 4 to 8 hours. Terbutaline Sulfate inhalation begins working within 5 to 30 minutes and continues for 3 to 6 hours. Terbutaline injection starts working in 5 to 15 minutes and lasts for 1½ to 4 hours.

Cautions and Warnings

Terbutaline Sulfate should be used with caution by people with a history of **angina, heart disease, high blood pressure, stroke or seizure, thyroid disease, prostate disease,** or **glaucoma.**

Using excessive amounts of Terbutaline Sulfate can lead to **increased difficulty breathing,** instead of providing breathing relief. In the most extreme cases, people have had heart attacks after using excessive amounts of inhalant.

Animal studies with Terbutaline Sulfate have revealed a significant increase in certain kinds of tumors.

Possible Side Effects

Terbutaline Sulfate's side effects are similar to those of other bronchodilators, except that its effects on the heart and blood vessels are not as pronounced.

▼ Most common: heart palpitations, abnormal heart rhythms, tremors, dizziness and fainting, shakiness, nervousness, tension, drowsiness, headache, nausea and vomiting, and heartburn or upset stomach.

▼ Less common: rapid heartbeat, chest pains and discomfort, angina, weakness, sleeplessness, wheezing, bronchial spasms and difficulty breathing, dry throat, sore or irritated throat, flushing, sweating, and changes in your sense of smell and taste.

Drug Interactions

• Terbutaline Sulfate's effects may be increased by monoamine oxidase (MAO) inhibitor drugs, tricyclic antidepressants, thyroid drugs, other bronchodilator drugs, and some antihistamines.

• The chances of cardiac toxicity may be increased in people taking Terbutaline Sulfate and Theophylline.

• Terbutaline Sulfate is antagonized by the beta-blocking drugs (Propranolol and others).

• Terbutaline Sulfate may antagonize the effects of blood-pressure-lowering drugs, especially Reserpine, Methyldopa, and Guanethidine.

Food Interactions

Terbutaline Sulfate tablets are more effective taken on an empty stomach, 1 hour before or 2 hours after meals, but can be taken with food or meals if they upset your stomach. Do not inhale Terbutaline Sulfate if you have food or anything else in your mouth.

Usual Dose

Inhalation
Adult and child (age 12 and over): 1 or 2 puffs every 4 to 6 hours (each puff delivers 0.2 mg of Terbutaline Sulfate).

Tablets
Adult and child (age 15 and over): 2½ to 5 mg every 6 hours 3 times a day; no more than 15 mg a day.

Child (age 12 to 15 years): 2½ mg 3 times a day; no more than 7½ mg a day.

Child (under age 12): not recommended.

Overdosage

Overdose of Terbutaline Sulfate inhalation usually results in exaggerated side effects, including heart pains and high blood pressure, although the pressure may drop to a low level after a short period of elevation. People who inhale too much Terbutaline Sulfate should see a doctor, who may prescribe a beta-blocking drug such as Metoprolol or Atenolol to counteract the overdose effect.

Overdose of Terbutaline Sulfate tablets is more likely to lead to side effects of changes in heart rate, palpitations, unusual heart rhythms, heart pains, high blood pressure, fever, chills, cold sweats, nausea, vomiting, and dilation of the pupils. Convulsions, sleeplessness, anxiety, and tremors may also develop, and the victim may collapse.

If the overdose was taken within the past half hour, give the victim Syrup of Ipecac (available at any pharmacy) to induce vomiting and remove any remaining medicine from the stomach. DO NOT GIVE SYRUP OF IPECAC IF THE VICTIM IS UNCONSCIOUS OR CONVULSING. If symptoms have already begun to develop, the victim may have to be taken to a hospital emergency room for treatment. ALWAYS bring the prescription bottle with you.

Special Information

If you are inhaling Terbutaline Sulfate, be sure to follow the inhalation instructions that come with the product. The drug should be inhaled during the second half of your breath, since this will allow it to reach deeper down into your lungs. Wait at least 1 minute between puffs if you use more than 1 puff per dose.

Do not take more Terbutaline Sulfate than prescribed by your doctor. Taking more than you need could actually result in worsening of your symptoms. If your condition worsens instead of improving after using your medicine, stop taking it and call your doctor at once.

Call your doctor immediately if you develop chest pains, palpitations, rapid heartbeat, muscle tremors, dizziness, headache, facial flushing, or urinary difficulty, or if you continue to experience difficulty in breathing after using the medicine.

If you forget a dose of Terbutaline Sulfate, take it as soon as you remember. If it is almost time for your next dose, skip the forgotten one. Do not take a double dose.

Special Populations

Pregnancy/Breast-feeding

When used during labor and delivery, Terbutaline Sulfate can slow or delay natural labor. It should not be taken after the first 3 months of pregancy. It can cause rapid heartbeat and high blood sugar in the mother and rapid heartbeat and low blood sugar in the fetus.

It is not known if Terbutaline Sulfate causes birth defects in humans, but it has caused defects in pregnant-animal studies. When it is deemed essential, the potential risk of taking Terbutaline Sulfate must be carefully weighed against any benefit it might produce.

Terbutaline Sulfate passes into breast milk. Nursing mothers must observe their infants for any possible drug effect while taking Terbutaline Sulfate. You may want to consider using an alternate feeding method.

Seniors

Older adults are more sensitive to the effects of Terbutaline Sulfate. Closely follow your doctor's directions, and report any side effects at once.

Generic Name

Terconazole

Brand Names

Terazol 3 Vaginal Suppositories
Terazol 7 Vaginal Cream 0.4%
Terazol 3 Vaginal Cream 0.8%

Type of Drug

Antifungal.

Prescribed for

Fungal infections of the vagina.

General Information

Terconazole is available as a vaginal cream and as vaginal suppositories. It may also be applied to the skin to treat common fungal infections. The exact mechanism by which Terconazole exerts its effect is not known.

Cautions and Warnings

Do not use Terconazole if you are **allergic** to it. **Proper diagnosis** is essential for effective treatment. Do not use this product without first consulting your doctor.

Possible Side Effects

▼ Most common: headache, which affects 1 in 4 women who use it.
▼ Other: painful menstruation, genital pain, body pain, abdominal pain, fever, chills, vaginal burning or irritation, and itching. Application of Terconazole cream to the skin can cause unusual sensitivity to the sun.

Drug and Food Interactions

None known.

Usual Dose

Vaginal Suppository or Cream

One applicatorful or suppository into the vagina at bedtime for 3 or 7 days, depending on formulation.

Topical

Apply to affected areas of skin twice a day for up to 1 month.

Overdosage

Terconazole overdose may cause irritation or, if swallowed, upset stomach. Call your local poison control center or hospital emergency room for more information.

Special Information

When using the vaginal cream, insert the whole applicatorful of cream high into the vagina. Be sure to complete the full course of treatment prescribed. Call your doctor if you develop burning or itching.

Refrain from sexual intercourse or use a condom while using this product to avoid reinfection. Use of sanitary napkins may prevent Terconazole from staining your clothing.

If you forget to take a dose of Terconazole, take it as soon as you remember. If it is almost time for your next regularly scheduled dose, skip the forgotten dose and continue with your regular schedule. Do not take a double dose.

Special Populations

Pregnancy/Breast-feeding

Pregnant women should avoid using the vaginal cream during the first 3 months of pregnancy; during the last 6 months, it should be used only if absolutely necessary.

Terconazole may cause problems in breast-fed infants. Women who must use it should bottle-feed their babies.

Seniors

Older adults may take this medication without special restriction. Follow your doctor's directions, and report any side effects at once.

Generic Name

Terfenadine

Brand Name

Seldane

Type of Drug

Antihistamine.

Prescribed for

Relief of seasonal allergy, stuffy and runny nose, itchy eyes, scratchy throat caused by allergies, and other allergic symptoms (such as rash, itching, and hives).

General Information

Terfenadine causes less sedation than most other antihistamines available in the United States. It has been widely used and accepted by people who find other antihistamines unacceptable because of the drowsiness they cause. Terfenadine appears to work in exactly the same way as Chlorpheniramine and other widely used antihistamines.

Cautions and Warnings

Do not take Terfenadine if you have had an **allergic reaction** to it in the past. People with **asthma** or other deep-breathing problems, **glaucoma** (pressure in the eye), **stomach ulcer,** or **other stomach problems** should avoid Terfenadine because its side effects may aggravate these problems.

In rare cases, Terfenadine may cause **serious adverse heart rhythms** or other cardiac events. It should be taken with caution by people with serious liver disease and by those taking Erythromycin, Ketoconazole, or Itraconazole.

Possible Side Effects

The most important side effects of Terfenadine are the rare cardiac consequences that most often occur in

---

Possible Side Effects *(continued)*

people with liver disease and those taking Erythromycin,
Ketoconazole, or Itraconazole. Dizziness or fainting may
be the first sign of a cardiac problem with Terfenadine.

▼ Most common: headache; nervousness; weakness;
upset stomach; nausea; vomiting; dry mouth, nose, or
throat; sore throat; nosebleeds; cough; stuffy nose; and
changes in bowel habits.

▼ Less common: rapid heartbeat, palpitations and
other cardiac abnormalities, hair loss, allergic reactions,
depression, sleeplessness, menstrual irregularities, muscle
aches, sweating, tingling in the hands or feet, frequent
urination, and visual disturbances. A few people taking
this drug have developed liver damage.

In scientific studies, Terfenadine was found to cause the
same amount of drowsiness as a placebo (inactive pill)
and about half that caused by other antihistamines. It is
considered safe for use by people who cannot tolerate
the sedating effects of other antihistamines.

Drug Interactions

• People taking Erythromycin, Ketoconazole, or Itraconazole in combination with Terfenadine have been reported
rarely to develop serious and possibly fatal cardiac side
effects. Do not mix these medicines with Terfenadine.

• Unlike other antihistamines, Terfenadine does not interact with alcohol or other nervous-system depressants to
produce drowsiness or loss of coordination.

Food Interactions

Terfenadine is best taken on an empty stomach, or at least 1
hour before or 2 hours after food or meals. However, it may
be taken with food or milk if it upsets your stomach. Avoid
drinking grapefruit juice if you are taking this medicine.

Usual Dose

Adult and Adolescent (over age 13): 60 mg twice per day.
Child (age 6 to 12): 30 to 60 mg twice per day.
Child (age 3 to 5): 15 mg twice per day.

Overdosage

Terfenadine overdose is likely to cause serious cardiac effects or exaggerated side effects. Overdose victims should be given Syrup of Ipecac (available in any pharmacy) as soon as possible to make them vomit and taken to an emergency room for treatment. ALWAYS bring the prescription bottle.

Special Information

Dizziness or fainting may be the first sign of serious drug side effects: Call your doctor at once if this happens to you. Report sore throat, unusual bleeding, bruising, tiredness or weakness, or any other unusual side effects to your doctor.

If you forget to take a dose of Terfenadine, take it as soon as you remember. If it is almost time for your next regularly scheduled dose, skip the one you forgot and continue with your regular schedule. Do not take a double dose.

Special Populations

Pregnancy/Breast-feeding

Do not take any antihistamine without your doctor's knowledge. Animal studies of Terfenadine have shown that doses several times larger than the human dose lower the baby's weight and increase the risk of the baby's death.

Small amounts of antihistamine pass into breast milk and may affect a nursing infant. Nursing mothers should avoid Terfenadine or use an alternative feeding method.

Seniors

Seniors may be more sensitive to Terfenadine's side effects. Follow your doctor's directions carefully and report any unusual occurrences.

Generic Name

Terpin Hydrate with Codeine

(Available only in generic form)

Type of Drug

Cough suppressant/expectorant combination.

Prescribed for

Relief of coughs due to colds or other respiratory infections.

General Information

Terpin Hydrate thins mucus and other bronchial secretions that can cause coughs. The cough-suppressant effect of this product is due to the Codeine.

The effectiveness of expectorants has been questioned by experts. The most widely used expectorant today is *Guaifenesin*.

Cautions and Warnings

Do not take this drug if you are **allergic** or **sensitive** to Codeine. Use this drug with extreme caution if you suffer from **asthma** or other breathing problems. Long-term use of Codeine may cause **drug dependence or addiction**. Codeine is a respiratory depressant and affects the central nervous system, producing sleepiness, tiredness, and/or inability to concentrate.

Possible Side Effects

▼ Most common: light-headedness, dizziness, sedation or sleepiness, nausea, vomiting, and sweating.

▼ Less common: euphoria (feeling "high"), weakness, sleepiness, headache, agitation, uncoordinated muscle movement, minor hallucinations, disorientation or visual disturbances, dry mouth, loss of appetite, constipation, facial flushing, rapid heartbeat, palpitations, faintness, urinary difficulties or hesitancy, reduced sex drive and/or potency, itching, rashes, anemia, lowered blood sugar, and yellowing of the skin or eyes. Narcotics such as Codeine may aggravate seizure disorders.

Drug Interactions

• Codeine has a depressant effect and a potential effect on breathing, and it should be taken with extreme care in combination with alcohol, sedatives, tranquilizers, antihistamines, or other depressant drugs.

Usual Dose

Take 1 to 2 teaspoons every 3 or 4 hours as needed for cough relief.

Overdosage

Overdose symptoms may include sleepiness, dizziness, or breathing difficulty. Victims should be taken to an emergency room for treatment. ALWAYS bring the medicine bottle.

Special Information

Terpin Hydrate with Codeine elixir contains 40 percent alcohol (80 proof) and is easily abused. Codeine can cause tiredness or difficulty concentrating. Be careful if you are driving or performing other complex tasks.

Try to cough up as much mucus as possible while taking this medication. This will help to reduce your cough.

If you forget to take a dose of Terpin Hydrate with Codeine, take it as soon as you remember. If it is almost time for your next dose, skip the one you forgot and continue with your regular schedule. Do not take a double dose.

Special Populations

Pregnancy/Breast-feeding

Pregnant women taking any product containing alcohol risk fetal-alcohol syndrome and should avoid this product. Narcotics such as Codeine may also cause breathing problems in the infant during delivery.

Alcohol and Codeine may affect your nursing infant. Do not nurse while taking this medicine.

Seniors

Seniors are more sensitive to the effects of this drug. Follow your doctor's directions, and report any side effects at once.

Type of Drug

Tetracycline Antibiotics

Brand Names

Generic Name: Demeclocycline

Declomycin

Generic Name: Doxycycline Hydrochloride*

Doryx	Doxychel Hyclate	Vibra-Tabs
Doxy-Caps	Vibramycin	

Generic Name: Meclocycline Sulfosalicylate

Meclan Cream

Generic Name: Minocycline Hydrochloride

Minocin

Generic Name: Oxytetracycline*

Terramycin	Uri-Tet

Generic Name: Tetracycline Hydrochloride Capsules/Tablets/Suspension*

Achromycin V	Sumycin	Tetracyn
Panmycin	Teline	Tetralan
Robitet Robicaps	Tetracap	Tetram

Generic Name: Tetracycline Eye Ointment/Drops

Achromycin

Generic Name: Tetracycline Topical Solution*

Topicycline

(*Also available in generic form)

Prescribed for

Infections caused by micro-organisms susceptible to these drugs.

General Information

Tetracycline antibiotics are effective against a wide variety of bacterial infections, including gonorrhea; infections of the mouth, gums, and teeth; Rocky Mountain spotted fever and other fevers caused by ticks and lice (including Lyme disease); urinary tract infections; and respiratory system infections (such as pneumonia and bronchitis). Doxycycline has been prescribed to treat and prevent "traveler's diarrhea." Tetracycline Hydrochloride has also been used together with other medicines to treat amebic infections of the intestinal tract, known as *amebic dysentery*.

The Tetracycline antibiotics work by interfering with the normal growth cycle of the invading bacteria, preventing them from reproducing. This allows the body's normal defenses to fight off the infection. This process is referred to as *bacteriostatic action*.

The Tetracycline antibiotics may be used as a substitute for people who are allergic to Penicillin. They have also been successfully used to treat some skin infections but are not considered the first-choice antibiotic for these applications.

Tetracycline Hydrochloride and Meclocycline have been successful in the treatment of adolescent acne, in small doses over a long period of time. Adverse effects and toxicity in this type of therapy are almost unheard of.

Cautions and Warnings

Tetracycline antibiotics should not be given to people with **liver disease** or **kidney or urinary problems.**

If the antibiotic your doctor has prescribed doesn't work, a number of things could have happened. You may not have taken the drug for a long enough time. Or you may be the victim of a *superinfection,* where another organism (usually a fungus), unaffected by the Tetracycline antibiotic, begins to grow in the same area as the bacteria being treated. If this happens, it may seem like a **relapse or a new infection.** Only your doctor can determine which medicine to take for it.

Avoid prolonged exposure to the sun if you are taking high doses of a Tetracycline antibiotic, especially Demeclocycline, because these antibiotics can interfere with your body's normal sun-screening mechanism, making you more prone to severe sunburn.

If you are **allergic** to any Tetracycline antibiotic or any other drug in this category, chances are you're allergic to them all. If this is your situation, avoid taking Tetracycline antibiotics.

Tetracycline antibiotics should **not be used by children under age 8** because they have been shown to interfere with the development of the long bones and may retard growth. Also, **permanent tooth discoloration** can result.

People taking **Demeclocycline** can experience the *diabetes insipidus syndrome:* excessive thirst, urination, and weakness. The severity of this condition depends on the amount of drug taken and is reversible when the medicine is stopped.

Minocycline can cause light-headedness, dizziness, or fainting. People taking this drug must be careful when driving or performing tasks requiring concentration.

Tetracyclines have been associated with *Pseudotumor cerebri*, a condition characterized by **headache and blurred vision**.

Possible Side Effects

▼ Most common: stomach upset, nausea, vomiting, diarrhea, and rash.

▼ Less common: hairy tongue, and itching and irritation of the anal and/or vaginal region. If these symptoms appear, call your doctor immediately. Periodic physical examinations and laboratory tests should be given to those who are on long-term Tetracycline antibiotic treatment.

▼ Rare: loss of appetite, peeling of the skin, sensitivity to the sun, fever, chills, anemia, possible brown spotting of the skin, decrease in kidney function, and damage to the liver.

Drug Interactions

• Tetracycline antibiotics, which are bacteriostatic, may interfere with the action of bactericidal (bacteria-killing) agents, such as Penicillin. You should not take both kinds of antibiotics for the same infection.

• Antacids, mineral supplements, and multivitamins containing Bismuth, Calcium, Zinc, Magnesium, and Iron can reduce the effectiveness of Tetracycline antibiotics (except Doxycycline and Minocycline) by interfering with their absorption into the bloodstream. Sodium Bicarbonate powder can also be a problem if used as an antacid. Separate doses of your antacid, mineral supplement, vitamin with minerals, or Sodium Bicarbonate and your antibiotic by at least 2 hours.

• Tetracycline antibiotics may increase the effect of anticoagulant (blood-thinning) drugs, such as Warfarin. Consult your doctor, because an adjustment in the anticoagulant dosage may be required.

• Barbiturates, Carbamazepine, and the hydantoin antiseizure medicines may increase the rate at which Doxycycline is broken down by the liver, reducing its effectiveness. More Doxycycline, or a different antibiotic, may be needed.

• Cimetidine, Ranitidine, and other H_2 antagonists may reduce the amount of Tetracycline antibiotic absorbed into the bloodstream, thereby decreasing its effectiveness.

• Tetracycline antibiotics may increase blood levels of Digoxin in a small number of people, leading to possible Digoxin side effects. This effect can last for months after the Tetracycline antibiotic has been stopped, in susceptible people. If you are taking this combination, watch carefully for Digoxin side effects and call your doctor if they develop.

• Tetracycline antibiotics may reduce Insulin requirements for diabetics. If you are using this combination, be sure to carefully monitor your blood-sugar level.

• Tetracycline antibiotics may increase or decrease blood-Lithium levels. These drugs may reduce the effectiveness of oral contraceptives. Breakthrough bleeding or pregnancy is possible; you should use backup contraception while you are taking one of these antibiotics.

Food Interactions

Take all Tetracycline antibiotics, except for Doxycycline and Minocycline, on an empty stomach 1 hour before or 2 hours after meals and with 8 ounces of water. The antibacterial effect of these antibiotics may be neutralized when they are taken with food, some dairy products (such as milk or cheese), or antacids.

Doxycycline and Minocycline may be taken with food or milk.

Usual Dose

Demeclocycline
Adult: 600 mg per day.
Child (age 9 and older): 3 to 6 mg per pound per day.
Child (age 8 and younger): do not use.

Doxycycline Hydrochloride
Adult and Child (age 9 and older, and over 100 pounds): first day, 200 mg given in 2 100-mg doses 12 hours apart. Maintenance, 100 mg per day in 1 to 2 doses.

Child (age 9 and older, and under 100 pounds): first day, 2 mg per pound of body weight divided in 2 doses. Maintenance, 1 mg per pound as a single daily dose.

Your doctor may double the maintenance dose for severe infections.

For gonorrhea: 300 mg in 1 dose and then a second 300-mg dose in 1 hour.

For syphilis: 300 mg per day for not less than 10 days.

An increased incidence of side effects is observed with doses over 200 mg per day.

Meclocycline Sulfosalicylate
Apply to affected areas morning and night.

Minocycline Hydrochloride
Adult: first dose, 200 mg, followed by 100 mg every 12 hours. Or 100 to 200 mg may be given to start, followed by 50 mg 4 times per day.

Child (age 9 and older): approximately 2 mg per pound of body weight at first, followed by 1 mg per pound every 12 hours.

Child (up to age 8): do not use.

Oxytetracycline and Tetracycline Hydrochloride
Adult: 250 to 500 mg 4 times per day.

Child (age 9 and older): 10 to 20 mg per pound of body weight per day in 4 equal doses.

Child (up to age 8): do not use.

Tetracycline Ointment/Solution
Apply to affected area morning and night.

Overdosage

Overdose is most likely to affect the stomach and digestive system. Call your local poison control center or hospital emergency room for more information. ALWAYS take the medicine bottle with you if you go for treatment.

Special Information

Do not take any antibiotic after the expiration date on the label. Decomposed Tetracycline antibiotics produce a highly toxic substance that can cause serious kidney damage.

Since the action of this antibiotic depends on its concentration within the invading bacteria, it is imperative that you completely follow the doctor's directions and complete the full course of treatment prescribed by your doctor.

Call your doctor if you develop excessive thirst, urination, and weakness; unusual discoloration of the skin or mucous membranes (with Minocycline); appetite loss; headache; vomiting; visual changes; abdominal pain with nausea and vomiting; yellowing of the skin or eyes; or any other persistent or intolerable side effects, including dizziness, light-headedness, or unsteadiness; burning or cramps in the stomach; diarrhea with nausea and vomiting; or itching of the mouth, rectal, or vaginal areas (may show a superinfection). Call the doctor if your child develops tooth discoloration.

Avoid excessive exposure to the sun while taking any Tetracycline antibiotic, especially Demeclocycline, because these drugs can make you more sensitive to sunburn.

Tetracycline antibiotics can cause dizziness, light-headedness, or fainting. Be careful when doing anything requiring concentration.

If you are using Tetracycline Hydrochloride topical solution or Meclocycline Sulfosalicylate for acne, apply the product generously to your skin until the area to be treated is completely wet. Stinging or burning may occur, but this will last for only a few minutes. Tetracycline Hydrochloride solution may stain your skin yellow, but the stain can usually just be washed away. Do not apply the solution or cream inside your eyes, nose, or mouth.

If you miss a dose of your Tetracycline antibiotic, take it as soon as possible. If you take the medicine once a day and it is almost time for your next dose, space the missed dose and your next dose 10 to 12 hours apart, then go back to your regular schedule.

If you take your Tetracycline antibiotic twice a day and it is almost time for your next dose, space the missed dose and your next dose by 5 to 6 hours, then go back to your regular schedule.

If you take your medicine 3 or more times a day and it is almost time for your next dose, space the missed dose and your next dose by 2 to 4 hours, then go back to your regular schedule.

Special Populations

Pregnancy/Breast-feeding

Tetracycline antibiotics should not be taken if you are pregnant, especially during the last half of pregnancy. They interfere with the formation of normal skull and bone structures in the baby.

Tetracycline antibiotics pass into breast milk and should never be taken if you are breast-feeding, because they interfere with the healthy development of your child's skull, bones, and teeth.

Seniors

Older adults, especially those with poor kidney function, may be more likely to suffer from less common drug side effects.

Type of Drug

Thiazide Diuretics

Brand Names

Generic Name: Bendroflumethiazide

Naturetin

Generic Name: Benzthiazide

Exna

Generic Name: Chlorothiazide*

Diuril

Generic Name: Chlorthalidone*

Hygroton
Thalitone

Generic Name: Hydrochlorothiazide*

| Esidrix | HyroDIURIL | Oretic |
| Ezide | Hydro-Par | |

Generic Name: Hydroflumethiazide*

Diucardin
Saluron

Generic Name: Indapamide*

Lozol

Generic Name: Methyclothiazide*

Aquatensen
Enduron

Generic Name: Metolazone

Mykrox
Zaroxolyn

Note: Switching between the two brands of Metolazone is not recommended because they are not equivalent and may not have the same effects.

Generic Name: Polythiazide

Renese

Generic Name: Quinethazone

Hydromox

Generic Name: Trichlormethiazide*

Diurese
Metahydrin
Naqua

(*Also available in generic form)

Prescribed for

Congestive heart failure, cirrhosis of the liver, kidney malfunction, high blood pressure, and other conditions where it is necessary to rid the body of excess water.

General Information

Thiazide diuretics act on the kidneys to stimulate the production of large amounts of urine. They also cause you to lose sodium, magnesium, bicarbonate, chloride, and potassium ions from the body. Calcium elimination is moderated and uric acid is retained as a result of thiazide treatment. Thiazide diuretics may also raise blood sugar. These medicines are used as part of the treatment of any disease where it is desirable to eliminate large quantities of water from the body. Thiazide diuretics are often taken together with other medicines to treat high blood pressure and other conditions. The exact way in which they reduce blood pressure is not known. The drugs in this group all begin to work within about 2 hours and produce their effect in 2 to 6 hours. The differences lie in the duration of their effect (6 to 12 hours for some and as long as 48 to 72 hours for others) and how much of each dose is actually absorbed into the body. Thiazide diuretic doses must be adjusted until maximum therapeutic response at minimum effective dose is reached. Some of these drugs also can be given by injection.

Cautions and Warnings

Do not take a thiazide diuretic if you are **allergic or sensitive** to any of the drugs in this group or to sulfa drugs. If you have a history of **allergy** or **bronchial asthma,** you may also have a sensitivity or allergy to thiazide diuretics. Thiazide diuretics can aggravate **lupus erythematosus,** a disease of the connective tissue.

Thiazides may raise total cholesterol, LDL cholesterol, and total triglycerides. They should be used with caution by people with **moderate to high blood-cholesterol or triglyceride levels.** Thiazides should be used with caution if you have **severe kidney disease** because they may precipitate kidney failure; only Metolazone and Indapamide can be safely given in this group. Diuretics should be used with care in people with **severe liver disease** because minor changes in electrolyte (salt) balance can throw them into hepatic coma.

Possible Side Effects

▼ Common: Thiazide diuretics cause loss of body potassium. Signs of low potassium are dryness of the mouth, thirst, weakness, lethargy, drowsiness, restlessness, muscle pains or cramps, muscular tiredness, low

---

Possible Side Effects *(continued)*

blood pressure, decreased frequency of urination and decreased amount of urine produced, abnormal heart rate, and stomach upset including nausea and vomiting. This problem can be prevented by taking potassium supplements in the form of tablets, liquids, or powders, or by increasing the consumption of foods such as bananas, citrus fruits, melons, and tomatoes.

▼ Less common: loss of appetite, stomach upset, nausea, vomiting, cramping, abdominal pains, bloating, diarrhea, constipation, dizziness, yellowing of the skin or eyes, headache, tingling of the toes and fingers, restlessness, changes in blood composition, unusual sensitivity to the sun, rash, itching, fever, difficulty in breathing, allergic reactions, dizziness when rising quickly from a sitting or lying position, muscle spasms, impotence and reduced sex drive, weakness, and blurred vision.

Drug Interactions

• Thiazide diuretics increase the action of other blood-pressure-lowering drugs. Consequently, people with high blood pressure often take such drugs in combination.

• The possibility of developing imbalances in body fluids (electrolytes) is increased if you take medications such as digitalis drugs, Amphotericin B, and adrenal corticosteroids while you take a thiazide diuretic.

• If you are taking Insulin or an oral antidiabetic drug and begin taking a thiazide diuretic, the Insulin or antidiabetic dose may have to be modified.

• Concurrent use of a thiazide diuretic and Allopurinol may increase the chances of experiencing Allopurinol side effects.

• Thiazides may decrease the effects of oral anticoagulant (blood-thinning) drugs such as Warfarin.

• Antigout drug dosage may have to be modified since thiazide diuretics raise blood-uric-acid levels.

• Thiazide diuretics may prolong the white-blood-cell reducing effects of chemotherapy drugs.

• Thiazides may increase the effects of Diazoxide, leading to symptoms of diabetes.

• Thiazides should not be taken together with loop diuretics because the combination can lead to an extreme diuretic effect and an extreme effect on blood electrolyte levels.

• Thiazides can increase the biological actions of Vitamin D, leading to a possibility of high blood-calcium levels.

• Propantheline and other anticholinergics taken with a thiazide diuretic may increase diuretic effect by increasing the amount of drug absorbed into the body.

• When Lithium Carbonate is taken with a thiazide diuretic, the patient should be monitored carefully by a doctor because there may be an increased risk of Lithium toxicity.

• Cholestyramine and Colestipol bind thiazide diuretics and basically prevent them from being absorbed into the blood. Thiazide diuretics should be taken more than 2 hours before the Cholestyramine or Colestipol.

• Methenamine and other urinary agents may reduce the effect of thiazides by reducing urinary acidity.

• Some of the nonsteroidal anti-inflammatory drugs (NSAIDs), particularly Indomethacin, may reduce the effectiveness of thiazide diuretics. Sulindac, another NSAID, may increase the effect of thiazide diuretic drugs.

Food Interactions

Thiazide diuretics may be taken with food if they upset your stomach. Your doctor may recommend high-potassium foods like bananas and orange juice to offset the potassium-lowering effect of these medicines.

Usual Dose

Bendroflumethiazide

Initial dose: up to 20 mg, 1 to 2 times per day. *Maintenance dose:* 2.5 to 5 mg per day. It is recommended that you take this drug in the morning to avoid the possibility of sleep disturbance by the need to urinate.

Benzthiazide

Initial dose: 50 to 200 mg per day. Daily dosages over 100 mg should be divided into 2 doses, to be taken after morning and evening meals. *Maintenance dose:* 50 to 150 mg per day.

Chlorothiazide

Adult: 0.5 to 1 gram, 1 to 2 times per day. Often people respond to intermittent therapy, that is, taking the drug on alternate days or 3 to 5 days per week. This reduces the drug's side effects.

Child: 10 mg per pound of body weight each day in 2 equal doses.

Infant (under age 6 months): up to 15 mg per pound of body weight per day in 2 equal doses.

Chlorthalidone
50 to 100 mg per day, or 100 mg on alternate days or 3 days per week. Some people may require 150 or 200 mg per day; doses of more than 200 mg per day generally do not produce greater response. A single dose is taken with food in the morning.

Hydrochlorothiazide
Adult: 25 to 200 mg per day, depending on condition treated. Maintenance dose, 25 to 100 mg per day; some people may require up to 200 mg per day. It is recommended that you take this drug early in the morning to avoid the possibility of your sleep being disturbed by the need to urinate.

Child (age 6 months and older): 1 mg per pound of body weight per day in 2 doses.

Infant (under age 6 months): 1.5 mg per pound of body weight per day in 2 doses.

Hydroflumethiazide
Initial dose: 50 mg, 1 or 2 times per day. *Maintenance dose:* 25 to 200 mg per day. Daily dosages of more than 100 mg should be divided into separate doses.

Indapamide
1.25 to 2.5 mg every morning. Depending on the condition under treatment and your response, dosage may be increased to 5 mg per day.

Methyclothiazide
2.5 to 10 mg per day, in the morning.

Metolazone
Dosage is individualized.

Zaroxolyn: 2.5 to 20 mg once per day, depending on condition treated.

Mykrox: 0.5 mg once per day, taken in the morning. Dosage may be increased to 1 mg per day.

Polythiazide
1 to 4 mg per day.

Quinethazone
50 to 100 mg per day. Occasionally, dosages of 100 mg are divided into 2 doses. Some patients may require 150 to 200 mg per day.

Trichlormethiazide
2 to 4 mg per day.

Overdosage

Signs include tingling in the arms or legs, weakness, fatigue, fainting, dizziness, changes in your heartbeat, a sickly feeling, dry mouth, restlessness, muscle pains or cramps, urinary difficulty, nausea, or vomiting. Take the victim to a hospital emergency room for treatment at once. ALWAYS bring the prescription bottle and any remaining medicine.

Special Information

Thiazide diuretics will cause excess urination at first, but that effect will subside after several weeks. Ordinarily, diuretics are taken early in the day to prevent excessive nighttime urination from interfering with your sleep.

Call your doctor if you develop muscle pain, sudden joint pain, weakness, cramps, nausea, vomiting, restlessness, excessive thirst, tiredness, drowsiness, increased heart or pulse rate, diarrhea, or dizziness. Diabetic patients may experience an increased blood-sugar level and a need for dosage adjustments of their antidiabetic medicines.

Avoid drinking alcohol or taking other medicines (unless directed by your doctor) while taking a thiazide diuretic.

If you are taking a thiazide diuretic for the treatment of high blood pressure or congestive heart failure, avoid over-the-counter medicines for the treatment of coughs, colds, and allergies: Such medicines may contain stimulants. If you are unsure about them, ask your pharmacist.

If you forget to take a dose of a thiazide diuretic, take it as soon as you remember. If it is almost time for your next regularly scheduled dose, skip the one you forgot and continue with your regular schedule. Do not take a double dose.

Special Populations

Pregnancy/Breast-feeding

Although these drugs have been used to treat specific conditions in pregnancy, their routine use during normal pregnancy is improper, and unsupervised use by pregnant patients should be avoided. Thiazide diuretics cross the placenta and can cause side effects in the newborn infant, such as jaundice, blood problems, and low potassium. Birth defects have not been seen in animal studies.

Thiazide diuretics pass into breast milk. No problems have been reported in nursing infants, but nursing mothers who must take diuretics should bottle-feed their babies.

Seniors

Older adults are more sensitive to the effects of these drugs, especially dizziness. They should closely follow their doctor's directions and report any side effects at once.

Generic Name

Thiothixene

Brand Name

Navane Capsules/Concentrate
Thiothixene Intensol Solution

(Also available in generic form)

Type of Drug

Thioxanthene antipsychotic.

Prescribed for

Psychotic disorders.

General Information

Thiothixene acts on a portion of the brain called the *hypothalamus*, which controls metabolism, body temperature, alertness, muscle tone, hormone balance, and vomiting. This drug may be used to treat problems related to any of these functions. Thiothixene is available in liquid form for those who have trouble swallowing tablets.

Cautions and Warnings

Do not take Thiothixene if you are **allergic** to it or to Chlorprothixene. Avoid using this drug if you have **very low blood pressure, Parkinson's disease**, or **any blood, liver, kidney, or heart disease**. If you have **glaucoma, epilepsy, ulcers**, or **difficulty passing urine,** Thiothixene should be used with caution and under strict supervision of your doctor.

Avoid exposure to **extreme heat,** because this drug can upset your body's normal temperature-control mechanism.

Possible Side Effects

▼ Most common: drowsiness, especially during the first or second week of therapy. If the drowsiness becomes troublesome, contact your doctor. Do not allow the liquid forms of this medicine to come in contact with your skin because they can cause contact reactions.

Thiothixene can cause jaundice (yellowing of the eyes or skin), usually within the first 2 to 4 weeks. The jaundice usually goes away when the drug is discontinued, but there have been cases where it did not. If you notice this effect, or if you develop symptoms such as fever and general feelings of ill health, contact your doctor immediately.

▼ Less common: changes in blood components, including anemias; raised or lowered blood pressure; abnormal heart rates; heart attack; and faintness or dizziness.

▼ Other: Thiothixene can produce extrapyramidal effects, such as spasm of the neck muscles, rolling back of the eyes, convulsions, difficulty in swallowing, and symptoms associated with Parkinson's disease. These effects seem very serious but usually disappear after the drug has been withdrawn; however, symptoms affecting the face, tongue, or jaw may persist for as long as several years, especially in older adults with a history of brain

Possible Side Effects *(continued)*

damage. If you experience extrapyramidal effects, contact your doctor immediately.

Thiothixene may cause an unusual increase in psychotic symptoms or may cause paranoid reactions, tiredness, lethargy, restlessness, hyperactivity, confusion at night, bizarre dreams, inability to sleep, depression, and euphoria (feeling "high"). Other reactions are itching, swelling, unusual sensitivity to bright light, red skin or rash, stuffy nose, headache, nausea, vomiting, loss of appetite, change in body temperature, loss of facial color, excessive salivation or perspiration, constipation, diarrhea, changes in urine and stool habits, worsening of glaucoma, blurred vision, weakening of eyelid muscles, spasms in bronchial or other muscles, increased appetite, excessive thirst, and skin discoloration (particularly in exposed areas). There have been cases of breast enlargement, false-positive pregnancy tests, and changes in menstrual flow in females, and impotence and changes in sex drive in males.

Drug Interactions

• Be cautious about taking Thiothixene with barbiturates, sleeping pills, narcotics or tranquilizers, alcohol, or any other medication that may produce a depressive effect.

• Aluminum antacids may interfere with the absorption of Thioxanthene drugs into the bloodstream, reducing their effectiveness.

• Thiothixene can reduce the effects of Bromocriptine and appetite suppressants.

• Anticholinergic drugs can reduce the effectiveness of Thiothixene and increase the chance of drug side effects.

• The blood-pressure-lowering effect of Guanethidine may be counteracted by Thiothixene.

• Taking Lithium together with Thiothixene may lead to disorientation, loss of consciousness, and uncontrolled muscle movements.

• Mixing Propranolol and Thiothixene may lead to unusually low blood pressure.

• Blood concentrations of tricyclic antidepressant drugs

may increase if they are taken together with Thiothixene. This can lead to antidepressant side effects.

Food Interactions

You may take this drug with food if it upsets your stomach.

Usual Dose

Adult and Adolescent (age 12 and older): 2 mg 3 times per day, to start. Your doctor may increase the dose up to 60 mg a day depending on your requirements and response.

Child (under age 12): not recommended.

Overdosage

Symptoms of overdosage are depression, extreme weakness, tiredness, coma, lowered blood pressure, uncontrolled muscle spasms, agitation, restlessness, convulsions, fever, dry mouth, and abnormal heart rhythms. The victim should be taken to a hospital emergency room immediately. ALWAYS bring the medicine bottle.

Special Information

This medication may cause drowsiness. Use caution when driving or operating hazardous equipment, and avoid alcoholic beverages.

The drug may also cause unusual sensitivity to the sun and can turn your urine reddish-brown to pink.

If dizziness occurs, avoid sudden changes in posture and climbing stairs. Use caution in hot weather because this medicine may make you more prone to heat stroke.

If you forget to take a dose of Thiothixene, take it as soon as you remember. If you take 1 dose per day and forget to take a dose, skip the missed dose and continue your regular dose schedule the next day. If you take more than 1 dose per day, skip the missed dose and continue with your regular schedule. Do not take a double dose.

Special Populations

Pregnancy/Breast-feeding

Infants born to women taking this medication have experienced drug side effects (liver jaundice, nervous-system effects) just after birth. Check with your doctor about taking this medicine if you are, or might become, pregnant.

This drug may pass into breast milk and affect a nursing infant. Consider bottle-feeding your baby.

Seniors

Older adults are more sensitive to Thiothixene's effects and usually require a lower dosage to achieve the desired results. Also, seniors are more likely to develop drug side effects, and some experts feel they should be treated with ¼ to ½ the usual adult dose.

Type of Drug

Thyroid Hormone Replacements

Brand Names

Generic Name: Levothyroxine Sodium*

| Levothroid | Levoxyl | Synthroid |
| Levoxine | | |

Generic Name: Liothyronine Sodium*

Cytomel

Generic Name: Liotrix*

Euthroid
Thyrolar

Generic Name: Thyroglobulin

Proloid

Generic Name: Thyroid Hormone*

| Armour Thyroid | Thyroid Strong | Thyrar |
| SPT | | |

(*Also available in generic form)

Prescribed for

Hypothyroidism (when the thyroid gland is producing insufficient amounts of natural thyroid hormones).

General Information

The major differences between the various thyroid hormone products are their source and hormone content. The first thyroid replacement products (Thyroid Hormone) were, and still are, made from beef and pork thyroid. These were effective but lacked standardization, which made it difficult for some doctors to control their patients' thyroid condition. Synthetic thyroid hormone replacement products are more desirable because their tablet-to-tablet content is easily standardized, ensuring that you are receiving the amount you and your doctor think you are getting. Basically, there are two important thyroid hormones: Levothyroxine and Liothyronine. Levothyroxine is converted in the blood to Liothyronine by the removal of 1 Iodine atom. This slows the absorption of Levothyroxine and lowers the chances for drug side effects. Liothyronine's potency and its potential for side effects make it less desirable for older adults. Thyroglobulin contains both Liothyronine and Levothyroxine in a proportion of about 2.5:1 (they are normally found in the body in a ratio of 4:1). Because Thyroglobulin is a natural product (more difficult to standardize) and Levothyroxine is converted naturally to Liothyronine, there is no advantage to this product. Liotrix contains both Levothyroxine and Liothyronine in the same proportions they are found in the body. Since Levothyroxine is converted naturally to Liothyronine, there is no advantage to taking both hormones. **These considerations make Levothyroxine the treatment of choice for thyroid hormone replacement.**

Although generic versions of virtually all thyroid replacement products are sold, the bioequivalence of these drugs has not been established; you **should not switch between brands of thyroid replacement hormones,** especially Levothyroxine, without your doctor's knowledge.

Cautions and Warnings

If you have **hyperthyroid disease** or **high output of thyroid hormone,** you should not use a thyroid replacement product. Symptoms of hyperthyroid disease include headache, nervousness, sweating, rapid heartbeat, chest pains, and other signs of central-nervous-system stimulation.

If you have **heart disease** or **high blood pressure,** thyroid replacement therapy should not be used unless it is clearly indicated and supervised by your physician. If you develop chest pains or other signs of heart disease while taking this drug, contact your doctor immediately.

Thyroid hormone replacement therapy should not be used to treat **infertility**, unless the person also has an underactive thyroid gland.

Thyroid hormone replacement products have been prescribed for **weight loss.** Thyroid treatments don't work in people with a normal thyroid status unless large doses are used. Large doses of thyroid replacement products can produce serious or fatal drug side effects, especially when taken together with appetite-suppressing drugs.

Thyroid hormone replacement treatments increase metabolism and can worsen the symptoms of other endocrine system (hormone-related) diseases, including **diabetes and Addison's disease.** Adjustments in the levels of treatment for these other diseases may be needed when you begin treatment with a thyroid replacement product.

Possible Side Effects

Thyroid hormone side effects are rare except during the initial treatment period, when the proper dosage is being established, or at a time when your dosage is being adjusted.

▼ Most common: heart palpitations, rapid heartbeat, abnormal heart rhythms, weight loss, chest pains, hand tremors, headache, diarrhea, nervousness, menstrual irregularity, inability to sleep, sweating, and intolerance to heat. These symptoms may be controlled by adjusting the hormone dosage. If you develop any side effects, contact your doctor at once so that your dosage can be adjusted.

Drug Interactions

• Colestipol and Cholestyramine can reduce the effect of thyroid hormone replacements by preventing their passage into the bloodstream. Take your thyroid hormone and either Colestipol or Cholestryamine 4 to 5 hours apart.

• The combination of Maprotiline and a thyroid hormone

may increase the chances for abnormal heart rhythms. Your doctor may have to adjust the dose of your thyroid hormone.

• Aspirin and other salicylate products may increase the effectiveness of your thyroid hormone by releasing more drug into the blood from body storage sites.

• Estrogen drugs may increase your need for thyroid hormones.

• Avoid taking over-the-counter products that contain stimulants (such as many of the drugs used to treat coughs, colds, or allergies) that will affect your heart and may cause symptoms of overdosage.

• Thyroid replacement therapy may increase the effect of anticoagulant (blood-thinning) drugs like Warfarin. Be sure your doctor knows if you are taking an anticoagulant because your anticoagulant dosage will have to be cut by about one-third when you begin thyroid therapy (to avoid hemorrhage). More adjustments may be made after your doctor reviews your blood tests.

• Diabetics may need to have their doctor increase their Insulin or oral antidiabetic drug dosages when they start taking a thyroid replacement product.

• Thyroid replacement therapy may reduce the effectiveness of some beta-blocking drugs when people with an underactive thyroid are converted to a normal thyroid status. The beta-blocker dose may need to be increased.

• Theophylline drugs are eliminated from the body more slowly in people with an underactive thyroid gland. Taking a thyroid hormone replacement product increases your body metabolism, including the way in which it processes theophylline drugs. Dosage adjustment of the theophylline product may be required after your thyroid function is normalized.

Food Interactions

Thyroid replacement products should be taken as a single dose, preferably before breakfast. More Levothyroxine is absorbed into the bloodstream when it is taken on an empty stomach. It is essential to take Levothyroxine at the same time each day.

Usual Dose

Levothyroxine

Initial dose, as little as 25 micrograms per day; then

increased in steps of 25 micrograms once every 3 to 4 weeks, depending upon response, with final dose of 100 to 400 micrograms per day.

Liothyronine

Adult: 5 to 100 micrograms per day, depending on the condition being treated and response to therapy.

Child and Senior: begin at the low end of the dosage range and increase slowly until the desired effect has been achieved.

Liotrix

Adult: a single "1/4" to "2" tablet each day (see explanation below), depending on the condition being treated and your response to therapy.

Child and Senior: begin at the low end of the dosage range and increase slowly until the desired effect has been achieved.

Liotrix tablets are rated according to their approximate equivalent to thyroid hormone. A "1/2" tablet is roughly equal to 30 mg of thyroid hormone, a "1" tablet to 60 mg, a "2" tablet to 120 mg, and so on.

Thyroglobulin and Thyroid Hormone

Initial dose, 15 to 30 mg (1/4 to 1/2 grain) per day, then increase in 15-mg steps every 1 to 2 weeks until response is satisfactory. Maintenance dose, 30 to 180 mg per day.

Overdosage

Symptoms of overdosage are headache, irritability, nervousness, sweating, rapid heartbeat with unusual stomach rumbling (with or without cramps), chest pains, heart failure, and shock. The patient should be taken to a hospital emergency room immediately. ALWAYS bring the medicine bottle.

Special Information

Thyroid replacement therapy is usually a lifelong treatment. Be sure you always have a fresh supply of medication on hand, and remember to follow your doctor's directions. Do not stop taking the medicine unless instructed to do so by your doctor.

Do not switch brands of your thyroid replacement product, especially Levothyroxine, without your doctor's and/or pharmacist's knowledge. Different brands of the same thyroid hormone replacement drug are not always equivalent to each other.

Call your doctor if you develop nervousness, diarrhea, excessive sweating, chest pains, increased pulse rate, heart palpitations, intolerance to heat, or any other unusual occurrence.

Children beginning thyroid treatment may lose some hair during the first few months, but this is only temporary, and the hair generally grows back.

If you forget to take a dose of a thyroid hormone replacement, take it as soon as you remember. If it is almost time for your next regular dose, skip the one you forgot and continue with your regular schedule. Do not take a double dose. Call your doctor if you miss 2 or more consecutive doses.

Special Populations

Pregnancy/Breast-feeding
Very small amounts of the thyroid hormones will find their way into the fetal bloodstream, but these drugs have not been associated with any problems when used to maintain normal thyroid function in the mother. Pregnant women who have been taking a thyroid hormone replacement product should continue their treatment, under their doctor's supervision.

Small amounts of the thyroid hormones pass into breast milk but have not been associated with problems in nursing infants. Nursing mothers should observe their infants for possible thyroid-associated side effects.

Seniors
Older adults may be more sensitive to the effects of the thyroid hormones. Thyroid hormone replacement needs are generally about 25 percent less in people over age 60.

Generic Name

Ticlopidine

Brand Name

Ticlid

Type of Drug

Anticoagulant.

Prescribed for

Ticlopidine is used to reduce stroke risk in people who have already had a stroke or those who are considered at high risk for one. Ticlopidine has also been prescribed for intermittent claudication (leg pains when walking, especially in cold weather), for chronic circulatory occlusion, in stroke patients (to reduce the damage caused by the stroke), before open heart surgery to reduce the expected drop in platelet count, during coronary artery bypass surgery to improve the chances of the graft taking, in some forms of kidney disease to help improve the kidney function, and in sickle cell disease to reduce the number and severity of sickle cell attacks.

General Information

Ticlopidine reduces the stickiness of blood platelets, reducing the chances for blood clotting and the possible consequences of clot formation. It interferes with the functioning of the platelet cell membrane, changing platelet cells irreversibly, until they are replaced by new ones. Maximum effect (60 to 70 percent reduction in platelet function) is seen 8 to 11 days after 250 mg of Ticlopidine twice a day. In clinical studies of the drug, patients taking Ticlopidine regularly for 2 to 5 years experienced a 24 percent reduction in stroke.

Cautions and Warnings

Ticlopidine can cause severe reductions in white-blood-cell counts, making you much more **susceptible to infection**. Some cases have been fatal. Your doctor should take white-blood-cell counts starting 2 weeks after you begin taking Ticlopidine and continuing every 2 weeks for the first 3 months of treatment. Then, only people showing signs of infection need to be tested. Blood counts usually return to normal 1 to 3 weeks after you stop taking the drug.

Blood-platelet counts can also be depressed, leading to spontaneous **bruising** or **bleeding**. Gastrointestinal bleeding can also be worsened.

Do not take this medication if you are **allergic** to it or if you have an **active bleeding site** (ulcer, etc.), **reduced blood-cell counts,** or **severe liver disease**.

Ticlopidine causes an **increase in blood-cholesterol** of 8 to 10 percent within a month after you start taking the drug.

Ticlopidine patients being switched from another anti-coagulant or a thrombolytic should stop taking the other drug and allow it to clear the system before starting Ticlopidine.

People with **severe kidney disease** may need less Ticlopidine. People with **severe liver disease** should avoid this drug.

Possible Side Effects

▼ Most common: diarrhea, nausea, upset stomach, rash, stomach pain. Of all patients who take this drug, 60 percent experience some side effect; about 13 percent stop taking Ticlopidine because of stomach side effects.

▼ Less common: reduced white-blood-cell counts, vomiting, bruising, stomach gas, itching, dizziness, loss of appetite, and liver function changes.

Drug Interactions

• Antacids reduce the amount of Ticlopidine absorbed into the blood by about 20 percent when the 2 drugs are taken together; to avoid this, separate doses by at least 1 hour.

• Taking Cimetidine on a regular basis can reduce the clearance of Ticlopidine from the body by 50 percent, increasing the chances for drug toxicities and side effects.

• Aspirin has an effect similar to Ticlopidine on the platelets and may increase the chances of bleeding due to loss of platelet effectiveness when taken with Ticlopidine. Do not take these drugs at the same time.

• Ticlopidine may slightly reduce blood levels of Digoxin. This is not a problem for most people but should be watched by your doctor in case some dose adjustment is needed.

• Ticlopidine reduces the body's clearance of Theophylline and may force the need for a Theophylline dosage reduction.

Food Interactions

Ticlopidine should be taken with meals to reduce possible stomach upset and maximize the absorption of the drug. To gain maximum benefit from Ticlopidine, do not vary the way in which you take it.

Usual Dose

250 mg taken twice a day with food.

Overdosage

Ticlopidine overdose may lead to increased bleeding and some liver inflammation. Other possible effects include stomach bleeding, convulsions, breathing difficulty, and low body temperature. Take the victim to a hospital emergency room. ALWAYS bring the medicine bottle.

Special Information

Call your doctor if you develop fever, chills, sore throat, or any other indication of infection; severe or persistent diarrhea; skin rashes or bleeding under the skin; yellowing of the skin or eyes; or dark urine or light-colored stools; or if you develop any other unusual, persistent, or severe side effects.

Bleeding may be more difficult to stop if you are taking this medicine. Be sure all doctors, dentists, and other health professionals know you are taking this medicine.

If you miss a dose of Ticlopidine, take it as soon as you can. If it is 4 hours or less until your next regular dose, skip the missed dose and go back to your regular dose schedule. Do not take a double dose.

Special Populations

Pregnancy/Breast-feeding

The effect of Ticlopidine on a developing fetus is not known. When the drug is considered essential by your doctor, its potential benefits must be carefully weighed against its risks.

Ticlopidine may pass into breast milk. Nursing mothers should bottle-feed their infants if they must take this drug.

Seniors

Older adults may be more sensitive to the effects of this drug since it is cleared more slowly as you age. Follow your doctor's directions, and report any side effects at once.

Generic Name

Timolol

Brand Names

Blocadren*
Timoptic Eye Drops
Timoptic Ocudose
Timoptic XC

(*Also available in generic form)

Type of Drug

Beta-adrenergic-blocking agent.

Prescribed for

High blood pressure, abnormal heart rhythms, preventing second heart attack, preventing migraine headaches, tremors, and stage fright and other anxieties. The eyedrops are used to treat glaucoma.

General Information

Timolol is one of 14 beta-adrenergic-blocking drugs that interfere with the action of a specific part of the nervous system. Beta receptors are found all over the body and affect many body functions. This accounts for the usefulness of beta blockers against a wide variety of conditions. The first member of this group, *Propranolol*, was found to affect the entire beta-adrenergic portion of the nervous system. Newer beta blockers have been refined to affect only a portion of that system, making them more useful in the treatment of cardiovascular disorders and less useful for other purposes. Other beta blockers are mild stimulants to the heart or have other characteristics that make them more useful for a specific purpose or better for certain people.

When applied to the eye, Timolol reduces fluid pressure inside the eye by reducing the production of eye fluids and slightly increasing the rate at which fluids flow through and leave the eye. People who cannot tolerate Timolol eyedrops because of its effect on the heart may receive Betaxolol, another beta-blocker eyedrop. Beta blockers produce a greater drop in eye pressure than either Pilocarpine or Epinephrine but may be combined with these or other drugs to produce a more pronounced drop in eye pressure.

Cautions and Warnings

You should be **cautious about taking Timolol** if you have **asthma, severe heart failure**, a **very slow heart rate**, or **heart block** because this drug may aggravate these conditions.

People with **angina** who take Timolol for high blood pressure should have their **drug dosage reduced gradually** over 1 to 2 weeks rather than suddenly discontinued to avoid possible aggravation of the angina.

Timolol should be used with caution if you have **liver or kidney disease**, because your ability to eliminate this drug from your body may be impaired.

Timolol reduces the amount of blood pumped by the heart with each beat. This reduction in blood flow can aggravate or worsen the condition of people with **poor circulation** or **circulatory disease**.

If you are undergoing **major surgery**, your doctor may want you to stop taking Timolol at least 2 days before surgery to permit the heart to respond more acutely to things that happen during the surgery. This is still controversial and may not hold true for all people preparing for surgery.

Timolol eyedrops should not be used by people who cannot tolerate oral beta-blocking drugs (such as Propranolol).

Possible Side Effects

Side effects are usually mild, relatively uncommon, develop early in the course of treatment, and are rarely a reason to stop taking Timolol.

▼ Most common: male impotence.

▼ Less common: unusual tiredness or weakness, slow heartbeat, heart failure (swelling of the legs, ankles, or feet), dizziness, breathing difficulty, bronchospasm, mental depression, confusion, anxiety, nervousness, sleeplessness, disorientation, short-term memory loss, emotional instability, cold hands and feet, constipation, diarrhea, nausea, vomiting, upset stomach, increased sweating, urinary

---

Possible Side Effects *(continued)*

difficulty, cramps, blurred vision, skin rash, hair loss, stuffy nose, facial swelling, aggravation of lupus erythematosus (a disease of the body's connective tissues), itching, chest pains, back or joint pains, colitis, drug allergy (fever, sore throat), and liver toxicity.

Drug Interactions

• Timolol may interact with surgical anesthetics to increase the risk of heart problems during surgery. Some anesthesiologists recommend gradually stopping your medicine 2 days before surgery.

• Timolol may interfere with the signs of low blood sugar and can interfere with the action of oral antidiabetes drugs.

• Timolol enhances the blood-pressure-lowering effects of other blood-pressure-reducing agents (including Clonidine, Guanabenz, and Reserpine) and calcium-channel-blocking drugs (such as Nifedipine).

• Aspirin-containing drugs, Indomethacin, Sulfinpyrazone, and estrogen drugs can interfere with the blood-pressure-lowering effect of Timolol.

• Cocaine may reduce the effects of all beta-blocking drugs.

• Timolol may increase the cold hands and feet associated with taking ergot alkaloids (for migraine headaches). Gangrene is a possibility in people taking an ergot and Timolol.

• Timolol will counteract the effects of thyroid hormone replacement medicines.

• Calcium channel blockers, Flecainide, Hydralazine, oral contraceptives, Propafenone, Haloperidol, phenothiazine tranquilizers (Molindone and others), quinolone antibacterials, and Quinidine may increase the amount of Timolol in the bloodstream and the effect of that drug on the body.

• Timolol should not be taken within 2 weeks of taking a monoamine oxidase (MAO) inhibitor antidepressant drug.

• Cimetidine increases the amount of Timolol absorbed into the bloodstream from oral tablets.

• Timolol may interfere with the effectiveness of Theophylline, Aminophylline, and some antiasthma drugs (especially Ephedrine and Isoproterenol).

• The combination of Timolol and Phenytoin or Digitalis drugs can result in excessive slowing of the heart, possibly causing heart block.

• If you stop smoking while taking Timolol, your dose may have to be reduced because your liver will break down the drug more slowly after you stop.

• If you take other glaucoma eye medicines, separate them to avoid physically mixing them. Small amounts of Timolol eyedrops are absorbed into the general circulation and may interact with some of the same drugs as do beta blockers taken by mouth, but this is unlikely.

Food Interactions

Timolol may be taken without regard to food or meals.

Usual Dose

Tablets
10 to 60 mg per day divided into 2 doses.

Eyedrops
1 drop twice per day.

Overdosage

Symptoms of overdosage are changes in heartbeat (unusually slow, unusually fast, or irregular), severe dizziness or fainting, difficulty breathing, bluish-colored fingernails or palms, and seizures. The overdose victim should be taken to a hospital emergency room where proper therapy can be given. ALWAYS bring the medicine bottle with you.

Special Information

Timolol is meant to be taken continuously. Do not stop taking it unless directed to do so by your doctor; abrupt withdrawal may cause chest pain, difficulty breathing, increased sweating, and unusually fast or irregular heartbeat. The dose should be lowered gradually over a period of about 2 weeks.

Call your doctor at once if any of the following symptoms develop: back or joint pains, difficulty breathing, cold hands or feet, depression, skin rash, or changes in heartbeat. Timolol may produce an undesirable lowering of blood pressure, leading to dizziness or fainting. Call your doctor if this happens to you. Call your doctor about the following side effects only if they persist or are bothersome: anxiety, diarrhea, constipation, sexual impotence, headache, itching, nausea or vomiting, nightmares or vivid dreams, upset stomach, trouble sleeping, stuffy nose, frequent urination, unusual tiredness, or weakness.

Timolol can cause drowsiness, dizziness, light-headedness, or blurred vision. Be careful when driving or performing complex tasks.

It is best to take your medicine at the same time each day. If you forget a dose of Timolol tablets, take it as soon as you remember. If you take Timolol twice a day and it is within 4 hours of your next dose, skip the forgotten dose and continue with your regular schedule. Do not double the dose.

To administer Timolol eyedrops, lie down or tilt your head backward and look at the ceiling. Hold the dropper above your eye and drop the medicine inside your lower lid while looking up. To prevent possible infection, don't allow the dropper to touch your fingers, eyelids, or any surface. Release the lower lid and keep your eye open. Don't blink for about 30 seconds. Press gently on the bridge of your nose at the inside corner of your eye for about 1 minute. This will help circulate the medicine around your eye. You should wait at least 5 minutes before using any other eyedrops.

If you forget to take a dose of Timolol eyedrops, take it as soon as you remember. If it is almost time for your next dose, skip the missed dose and continue with your regular schedule. Do not take a double dose.

Special Populations

Pregnancy/Breast-feeding
Infants born to women who took a beta blocker weighed less at birth and had low blood pressure and reduced heart rate. Timolol should be avoided by pregnant women and those who might become pregnant while taking it. When the drug is considered essential by your doctor, its potential benefits must be carefully weighed against its risks.

Timolol passes into breast milk, but problems are rare. Still, nursing mothers taking Timolol should bottle-feed their babies.

Seniors
Older adults may absorb and retain more Timolol in their bodies, thus requiring less medicine to achieve the same

results. Your doctor will need to adjust your dosage to meet your individual needs. Seniors taking this medicine may be more likely to suffer from cold hands and feet, reduced body temperature, chest pains, general feelings of ill health, sudden breathing difficulty, sweating, or changes in heartbeat.

Timoptic

see Timolol, page 1108

Generic Name

Tioconazole

Brand Name

Vagistat-1

Type of Drug

Antifungal.

Prescribed for

Treatment of fungal infections in the vagina.

General Information

Tioconazole is used as a vaginal cream. It may also be applied to the skin to treat common fungal infections. The exact mechanism by which Tioconazole exerts its effect is not known.

Cautions and Warnings

Do not use Tioconazole if you are **allergic** to it. **Proper diagnosis** is essential for effective treatment. Do not use this product without first consulting your doctor.

Possible Side Effects

▼ Most common: vaginal burning, itching, or irritation.

Possible Side Effects *(continued)*

▼ Less common: vaginal discharge, swelling of the vulva, vaginal pain, painful urination, nighttime urination, vaginal dryness, and pain during intercourse.

Drug and Food Interactions

None known.

Usual Dose

One applicatorful into the vagina at bedtime for 3 to 7 days.

Special Information

When using the vaginal cream, insert the whole applicatorful of cream high into the vagina. Be sure to complete the full course of treatment prescribed. Call your doctor if you develop burning or itching.

Refrain from intercourse or use a condom while using this product to avoid reinfection. Use of sanitary napkins may prevent Tioconazole from staining of your clothing.

If you forget to take a dose of Tioconazole, take it as soon as you remember. If it is almost time for your next dose, skip the missed dose and continue with your regular schedule. Do not take a double dose.

Special Populations

Pregnancy/Breast-feeding

Pregnant women should avoid using this product during pregnancy because the use of a vaginal applicator may cause problems. Also, the effect of Tioconazole on the developing fetus is not known.

It is not known if Tioconazole passes into breast milk. Nursing mothers should watch their babies for possible drug-related side effects.

Seniors

Older adults may take this medication without special restriction. Follow your doctor's directions, and report any side effects at once.

Generic Name

Tiopronin

Brand Name

Thiola

Type of Drug

Kidney-stone preventive.

Prescribed for

Preventing kidney stones.

General Information

Tiopronin prevents the formation of kidney stones by forming a complex with *cysteine*, a key component of kidney stones. People with kidney stones normally have very high urine-cysteine levels. Each dose of Tiopronin causes a long-lasting reduction in the urine-cysteine level, which lasts until the drug is stopped.

Cautions and Warnings

Do not take Tiopronin if you are **allergic** to it. People with a history of **agranulocytosis** or **thrombocytopenia** (blood problems) caused by drug treatment should avoid Tiopronin.

Tiopronin can cause excessive protein loss through the urine.

Possible Side Effects

▼ Common: drug fever, especially during the first month of treatment. The drug may be restarted once the fever has gone down and gradually increased to the usual dose.

▼ Less common: loss of the sense of taste, vitamin B_6 (Pyridoxine) deficiency, and skin rash and itching (itching can be controlled with antihistamines and clears up when the drug is stopped). Skin becomes thin and wrinkled after long-term treatment because of the drug's effect on skin connective tissue. Fever, joint pain or swelling, and

---

> **Possible Side Effects** *(continued)*
>
> swollen lymph glands may be signs of serious drug side effects.

Drug Interactions

• Tiopronin should not be taken with other medicines that are toxic to the kidney or liver or those that reduce white blood cells or platelets.

Food Interactions

You may take this drug with food if it upsets your stomach. Be sure to follow your doctor's advice about diet restriction.

Usual Dose

Tiopronin doses are adjusted based on urine cysteine level.
  Adult: 800 to 1000 mg per day.
  Child (age 9 and older): 6.75 mg per pound.
  Child (less than age 9): not recommended.

Overdosage

Tiopronin overdose results in exaggerated side effects. Overdose victims should be taken to a hospital emergency room for treatment. ALWAYS bring the medicine bottle.

Special Information

Stop taking Tiopronin and call your doctor at once if you develop fever, joint pain, swelling, swollen lymph glands, changes in urinary function, unusual skin reactions, or muscle weakness, or if you begin to vomit blood or have difficulty breathing. These can be signs of severe side effects.

If you forget a dose of Tiopronin, take it as soon as you remember. If it is almost time for your next dose, skip the missed dose and continue with your regular schedule.

Special Populations

Pregnancy/Breast-feeding
Tiopronin has caused birth defects in laboratory animals.

Women who are or who might become pregnant should avoid this drug.

Tiopronin may pass into breast milk. Mothers who must take Tiopronin should bottle-feed their babies.

Seniors
Seniors may be more sensitive to the side effects of this drug and should report any problems to their doctor at once.

Generic Name

Tocainide Hydrochloride

Brand Name

Tonocard

Type of Drug

Antiarrhythmic.

Prescribed for

Abnormal heart rhythms. Tocainide has also been used for muscular dystrophy and trigeminal neuralgia (tic douloureux).

General Information

Tocainide works in the same way as Lidocaine (one of the most widely used injectable antiarrhythmic drugs). Tocainide slows the speed at which nerve impulses are carried through the heart's ventricle, helping the heart to maintain a stable rhythm by making heart muscle cells less easily excited. Tocainide affects different areas of the heart than many other widely used oral antiarrhythmic drugs. Tocainide is usually prescribed as a follow-up to intravenous Lidocaine for people with life-threatening arrhythmias.

Cautions and Warnings

People taking this drug may develop **bone-marrow depression,** a drastic drop in white-blood-cell count, low platelet count, or other abnormalities of blood components. Physically, these can be represented by **fever, chills, sore throat, mouth sores, bruising, or bleeding.** Call your doctor if any of these occur. Because these abnormalities happen most often in the first 3 months on Procainamide, you should be checked with weekly blood counts during your first 3 months of taking this medicine.

This drug should not be used by people who are **allergic** to it, or to Lidocaine or local anesthetics.

Some people using Tocainide may develop **respiratory difficulties,** including fluid buildup in the lungs, pneumonia, and irritation of the lungs. Report any **cough, wheezing, shortness of breath,** or **trouble breathing** to your doctor immediately. Tocainide should not be used by people with **heart failure,** because the drug can actually worsen their condition.

Like other antiarrhythmic drugs, Tocainide may occasionally **worsen heart rhythm problems** and has not been proven to actually help people live longer.

Possible Side Effects

▼ Most common: nausea, dizziness, fainting, tingling in the hands or feet, and tremors. These reactions are generally mild and short-lived, and usually go away when dosage is reduced or when you take Tocainide with food.

▼ Less common: vomiting, reduced appetite, light-headedness, confusion, disorientation, hallucinations, nervousness, mood or self-awareness changes, poor muscle coordination, blurred or double vision, increased sweating, giddiness, restlessness, anxiety, low blood pressure, slowing of the heart rate, heart palpitations, chest pains, cold sweats, headache, drowsiness, lethargy, ringing or buzzing in the ears, visual disturbances, rolling of the eyes, diarrhea, unusual feelings of heat or cold, joint inflammation and pain, and muscle aches.

▼ Rare: seizures, depression, psychosis, mental changes, alterations of taste (including a metallic taste) and/or smell, agitation, slurred speech, difficulty concentrating, memory loss, difficulty sleeping, nightmares, unusual thirst, weakness, upset stomach or abdominal pains and discomfort, difficulty swallowing, breathing difficulty (see *Cautions and Warnings*), changes in white-blood-cell counts, anemia, urinary difficulty, hair loss, cold hands or

Possible Side Effects *(continued)*

feet, leg pains after minor exercise, dry mouth, earache, fever, hiccups, aching, feelings of ill health, muscle twitches or spasms, neck or shoulder pains, facial flushing or pallor, and yawning.

Drug Interactions

• Tocainide taken with Metoprolol or other beta-blocking drugs (for high blood pressure) can cause too rapid a drop in blood pressure and slow the heart.

• Tocainide may produce an additive cardiac side effect if taken with other antiarrhythmic drugs.

• Tocainide may increase the effects of other drugs that depress bone-marrow function, leading to reduced levels of white blood cells and blood platelets.

• Cimetidine and Rifampin reduce the amount of Tocainide absorbed into the bloodstream. Ranitidine (which can be used instead of Cimetidine) does not have this effect.

Food Interactions

You may take Tocainide without regard to food or meals.

Usual Dose

Adults: 1200 to 1800 mg per day, in 2 or 3 divided doses.

Seniors and people with kidney or liver disease: lower doses usually required.

Overdosage

The first symptoms of Tocainide overdose are usually tremors or other nervous-system effects. Other more serious Tocainide side effects may follow. At least 1 person has died of a Tocainide overdose. Victims should be taken to a hospital emergency room for treatment. ALWAYS bring the medicine bottle.

Special Information

Be sure to report any side effects to your doctor, particularly difficulty breathing after exertion, cough, wheezing, tremors, palpitations, rash, easy bruising or bleeding, fever, chills, sore throat or mouth, or mouth sores. Most of these side effects are minor or will respond to minimal dosage adjustments.

Tocainide can make you dizzy or drowsy. Be careful while driving or doing anything else that requires concentration.

Do not take more or less of this drug than prescribed. If you forget to take a dose of Tocainide Hydrochloride and you remember within about 4 hours of your regular time, take it as soon as you remember. If you do not remember until later, skip the missed dose and go back to your regular schedule. Do not take a double dose.

Special Populations

Pregnancy/Breast-feeding
Animal studies of Tocainide doses 1 to 4 times larger than the human equivalent revealed an increase in spontaneous abortions and stillbirths. When Tocainide is considered essential by your doctor, its potential benefits must be carefully weighed against its risks.

This drug passes into breast milk in amounts as high as or higher than those in the blood, increasing the risk of possible side effects in the nursing infant. Nursing mothers who must take this drug should bottle-feed their babies.

Seniors
Older adults are more sensitive to the side effects of this drug, especially dizziness and low blood pressure. Follow your doctor's directions, and report any side effects at once.

Generic Name

Tolmetin Sodium

Brand Names
Tolectin
Tolectin DS

Type of Drug
Nonsteroidal anti-inflammatory drug (NSAID).

Prescribed for

Rheumatoid arthritis, juvenile rheumatoid arthritis, osteo-arthritis, and sunburn treatment.

General Information

Tolmetin Sodium is one of 16 nonsteroidal anti-inflammatory drugs (NSAIDs) used to relieve pain and inflammation. We do not know exactly how NSAIDs work, but part of their action may be due to an ability to inhibit the body's production of a hormone called *prostaglandin* and to inhibit the action of other body chemicals, including cyclo-oxygenase, lipoxyge-nase, leukotrienes, lysosomal enzymes, and a host of other factors. NSAIDs are generally absorbed into the bloodstream fairly quickly. Pain relief comes within an hour after taking the first dose of Tolmetin, but its anti-inflammatory effect takes a lot longer (several days to 1 week) to become apparent, and may take 2 weeks to reach its maximum effect. Tolmetin is broken down in the liver and eliminated through the kidneys.

Cautions and Warnings

People who are **allergic** to Tolmetin (or to any other NSAID) and those with a history of **asthma** attacks brought on by another NSAID, by iodides, or by Aspirin should not take Tolmetin.

Tolmetin can cause **gastrointestinal (GI) bleeding, ulcers,** and **stomach perforation.** This can occur at any time, with or without warning, in people who take chronic Tolmetin treatment. People with a history of active GI bleeding should be cautious about taking any NSAID. Minor stomach upset, distress, or gas is common during the first few days of treatment with Tolmetin. People who develop **bleeding** or **ulcers** and continue treatment should be aware of the possibility of developing more serious drug toxicity.

Tolmetin can affect platelets and **blood clotting** at high doses, and should be avoided by people with clotting problems and by those taking Warfarin.

People with **heart problems** who use Tolmetin may experience swelling in their arms, legs, or feet.

Tolmetin can cause severe **toxic effects to the kidney.** Report any unusual side effects to your doctor, who may need to periodically test your kidney function.

Tolmetin can make you unusually **sensitive to the effects of the sun** (photosensitivity).

Possible Side Effects

▼ Most common: diarrhea, nausea, vomiting, constipation, stomach gas, stomach upset or irritation, and loss of appetite.

▼ Less common: stomach ulcers, GI bleeding, hepatitis, gallbladder attacks, painful urination, poor kidney function, kidney inflammation, blood and protein in the urine, dizziness, fainting, nervousness, depression, hallucinations, confusion, disorientation, tingling in the hands or feet, light-headedness, itching, sweating, dry nose or mouth, heart palpitations, chest pain, difficulty breathing, and muscle cramps.

▼ Rare: severe allergic reactions, including closing of the throat, fever and chills, changes in liver function, jaundice (yellowing of the skin or eyes), and kidney failure. People who experience such effects must be promptly treated in a hospital emergency room or doctor's office.

NSAIDs have caused severe skin reactions; if this happens to you, see your doctor immediately.

Drug Interactions

• Tolmetin can increase the effects of oral anticoagulant (blood-thinning) drugs such as Warfarin. You may take this combination, but your doctor may have to reduce your anticoagulant dose.

• Taking Tolmetin with Cyclosporine may increase the toxic kidney effects of both drugs. Methotrexate toxicity may be increased in people also taking Tolmetin.

• Tolmetin may reduce the blood-pressure-lowering effect of beta blockers and loop diuretic drugs.

• Tolmetin may increase blood levels of Phenytoin, leading to increased Phenytoin side effects. Blood-Lithium levels may be increased in people taking Tolmetin.

• Tolmetin blood levels may be affected by Cimetidine because of that drug's effect on the liver.

• Probenecid may interfere with the elimination of Tolmetin from the body, increasing the chances for Tolmetin toxic reactions.

• Aspirin and other salicylates may decrease the amount of Tolmetin in your blood. These medicines should never be taken at the same time.

Food Interactions

Take Tolmetin with food or a magnesium/aluminum antacid if it upsets your stomach.

Usual Dose

Adult: 400 mg 3 times a day to start. Dosage must then be adjusted to individual need. Do not take more than 2000 mg per day.

Child: (age 2 and over): 9 mg per pound of body weight given in divided doses 3 to 4 times a day, to start. Adjust dose to individual need. Do not give more than 13.5 mg per pound of body weight to a child.

Child (under age 2): not recommended.

Take each dose with a full glass of water, and don't lie down for 15 to 30 minutes.

Overdosage

People have died from NSAID overdoses. The most common signs of overdose are drowsiness, nausea, vomiting, diarrhea, abdominal pain, rapid breathing, rapid heartbeat, sweating, ringing or buzzing in the ears, confusion, disorientation, stupor, and coma. Take the victim to a hospital emergency room at once. ALWAYS bring the medicine bottle.

Special Information

Tolmetin can make you drowsy and/or tired: Be careful when driving or operating hazardous equipment. Do not take any nonprescription products with Acetaminophen or Aspirin while taking this drug; also, avoid alcoholic beverages.

Contact your doctor if you develop skin rash or itching, visual disturbances, weight gain, breathing difficulty, fluid retention, hallucinations, black or tarry stools, persistent headache, or any unusual or intolerable side effects.

If you forget to take a dose of Tolmetin Sodium, take it as

soon as you remember. If you take several doses a day and it is within 4 hours of your next dose, skip the one you forgot and continue with your regular schedule. Do not take a double dose.

Special Populations

Pregnancy/Breast-feeding

NSAIDs may cross into the fetal blood circulation. They have not been found to cause birth defects but may affect a developing fetal heart during the second half of pregnancy; animal studies indicate a possible effect. Women who are or who might become pregnant should not take Tolmetin without their doctor's approval; pregnant women should be particularly cautious about using this drug during the last 3 months of their pregnancy. When the drug is considered essential by your doctor, its potential benefits must be carefully weighed against its risks.

NSAIDs may pass into breast milk but have caused no problems among breast-fed infants, except for seizures in a baby whose mother was taking Indomethacin. Other NSAIDs have caused problems in animal studies. There is a possibility that a nursing mother taking Tolmetin could affect her baby's heart or cardiovascular system. If you must take Tolmetin, consider bottle-feeding your baby.

Seniors

Older adults may be more susceptible to Tolmetin side effects, especially ulcer disease.

Toradol

see Ketorolac, page 571

Generic Name

Tramadol Hydrochloride

Brand Name

Ultram

Type of Drug

Nonnarcotic pain reliever.

Prescribed for

Mild to moderate pain.

General Information

Tramadol is a synthetic compound that works in the central nervous system to relieve pain. No one knows the exact way in which this drug works, but it binds to natural opioid receptors and reduces the uptake of two important neurohormones, *serotonin* and *norepinephrine*, into nerves. Pain relief begins about an hour after you take a dose and reaches its maximum effect in 2 to 3 hours. Like the narcotic pain relievers, Tramadol can cause dizziness, tiredness, nausea, constipation, sweating, and itching. Unlike the narcotics, this drug causes little interference with breathing and does not cause histamine reactions. It has no effect on heart function.

Cautions and Warnings

Do not take this drug if you are **sensitive** or **allergic** to it or if you are intoxicated with drugs, alcohol, or narcotics. People who must take **tranquilizers, sedatives,** or **other nervous-system depressants** should take reduced doses of Tramadol.

Large doses of Tramadol can interfere with **your ability to breathe,** especially if you take alcohol at the same time.

Tramadol use should be avoided in people who have had **abdominal conditions** or a **head injury** because the drug can interfere with diagnosing the injury or understanding its severity.

This drug causes **seizures** in test animals; similar reactions have been seen in people taking excessive oral doses (700 mg) or large intravenous doses (300 mg).

People who are **dependent on narcotics** and who take Tramadol may experience drug withdrawal symptoms.

People with **reduced kidney function** or **liver disease** should receive reduced doses of Tramadol because excessive quantities will remain in the blood if usual doses are taken.

Possible Side Effects

▼ Most common: dizziness or fainting, nausea, constipation, headache, tiredness, vomiting, itching, weakness, sweating, upset stomach, dry mouth, and diarrhea.

▼ Less common: feelings of ill health, warmth and flushing, nervousness, anxiety, agitation, euphoria (feeling "high"), emotional instability, trouble sleeping, abdominal pain, appetite loss, stomach gas, rash, visual disturbances, urinary problems, and symptoms of menopause in women.

▼ Rare: allergies, accidents, weight loss, suicidal thoughts, dizziness when rising from a sitting or lying position, rapid heartbeat, heart palpitations, heart pains, seizures, tingling in the hands or feet, difficulty learning or understanding, tremors, hallucinations, memory loss, difficulty concentrating, migraines, unusual walk, stomach bleeding, hepatitis, mouth lesions, itching, taste changes, cataracts, deafness or ringing or buzzing in the ears, painful urination, and menstrual difficulties.

Drug Interactions

• Taking Carbamazepine at the same time as Tramadol increases the rate at which Tramadol is broken down in the body, reducing its effectiveness. People taking this combination may need twice the usual dose of Tramadol.

• The combination of Tramadol with a monoamine oxidase (MAO) inhibitor drug should be used with caution and can cause severe reactions.

• Quinidine may slow the breakdown of Tramadol because it affects the liver enzyme that breaks down Tramadol. The full impact of this interaction is not known.

Food Interactions

Tramadol may be taken without regard to food or meals.

Usual Dose

Adult and adolescent (over age 16): 50 to 100 mg every 4 to 6 hours, up to 400 mg a day.

Child (under age 16): not recommended.

Senior: up to 300 mg a day.

Other: people with cirrhosis should receive 50 mg every 12 hours. People with severe kidney disease should receive no more than 100 mg every 12 hours.

Overdosage

The most serious effects of Tramadol are usually difficulty breathing and seizures. Some people have died from Tramadol overdose; it is estimated that they took between 3000 and 5000 mg (3 to 5 grams) of the drug. The lowest fatal dose was thought to be between 500 and 1000 mg in an 88-pound woman. Tramadol overdose victims should be taken to a hospital emergency room for treatment at once. ALWAYS bring the medicine bottle with you.

Special Information

Drowsiness may occur: Be careful when driving or operating complicated or hazardous machinery.

Do not drink alcoholic beverages or use illegal drugs while taking Tramadol.

If you forget a dose of Tramadol, take it as soon as you remember. If it is almost time for your next dose, skip the one you forgot and continue with your regular schedule. Do not take a double dose.

Special Populations

Pregnancy/Breast-feeding

Tramadol is toxic to animal fetuses at doses only 3 to 15 times the maximum adult dose. In people, Tramadol passes into the blood circulation of the developing fetus. Pregnant women should not take this drug unless it is absolutely necessary.

This drug should not be taken by nursing mothers.

Seniors

In people age 75 and older, blood concentrations are somewhat higher than in younger adults. Older adults can also be expected to be more sensitive to the side effects of this drug. Older adults should not take more than 300 mg a day.

Generic Name

Trazodone

Brand Names

Desyrel Tablets
Desyrel Dividose Tablets

(Also available in generic form)

Type of Drug

Antidepressant.

Prescribed for

Depression (with or without anxiety), Cocaine withdrawal, panic disorder, agoraphobia (fear of open spaces), and aggressive behaviors.

General Information

Trazodone is as effective in treating the symptoms of depression as other antidepressant tablets. It is chemically different from the other antidepressants and may be less likely to cause side effects.

For many people, symptoms will be relieved as early as 2 weeks after starting the medicine, but 4 weeks or more may be required to achieve maximum benefit.

Cautions and Warnings

Do not use Trazodone if you are **allergic** to it. It is not recommended during the initial stages of recovery from a **heart attack**. People with a previous history of heart disease should not use Trazodone because **it may cause abnormal heart rhythms.**

Rarely, **painful and sustained erections** have occurred in men taking Trazodone. If this happens, stop taking it and call your doctor. One-third of these men may need surgery or could permanently lose their ability to gain an erection.

Possible Side Effects

▼ Most common: upset stomach; constipation; abdominal pains; a bad taste in the mouth; nausea, vomiting; diarrhea; palpitations; rapid heartbeat; rashes; swelling of the arms or legs; blood pressure changes; difficulty breathing; dizziness; anger; hostility; nightmares and/or vivid dreams; confusion; disorientation; loss of memory or concentration; drowsiness; fatigue; light-headedness; difficulty sleeping; nervousness; excitement; headache; loss of coordination; tingling in the hands or feet; tremor of the hands or arms; ringing or buzzing in the ears; blurred vision; red, tired, and itchy eyes; stuffy nose or sinuses; loss of sex drive; muscle aches and pains; loss of appetite; changes in body weight (up or down); increased sweating; clamminess; and feelings of ill health.

▼ Less common: drug allergy, chest pain, heart attack, delusions, hallucinations, agitation, difficulty speaking, restlessness, numbness, weakness, seizures, increased sex drive, reverse ejaculation, impotence, missed or early menstrual periods, stomach gas, increased salivation, anemia, reduced levels of some white blood cells, muscle twitches, blood in the urine, reduced urine flow, increased urinary frequency, increased appetite. Trazodone may cause elevations in levels of body enzymes, which are used to measure liver function.

Drug Interactions

• Trazodone, when taken together with Digoxin or Phenytoin, may increase the amount of those drugs in your blood, leading to a greater possibility of drug side effects.

• Trazodone may make you more sensitive to drugs that work by depressing the nervous system, including sedatives, tranquilizers, and alcohol.

• This medicine may cause a slight reduction in blood pressure. If you are taking medicine for high blood pressure and begin to take Trazodone, you may find that a minor reduction in the dosage of your blood-pressure medicine is required. On the other hand, the action of Clonidine (for high blood pressure) can be inhibited by Trazodone. These interactions must be evaluated by your doctor. Do not change any blood-pressure medicines on your own.

• Little is known about the potential interaction between Trazodone and the monoamine oxidase (MAO) inhibitor drugs. With most antidepressants, it is suggested that one drug be discontinued for 2 weeks before the other is begun. If used together, they should be used cautiously.

Food Interactions

Take each dose of Trazodone with food to increase the amount of drug absorbed into your bloodstream and to reduce the chances of upset stomach, dizziness, or light-headedness.

Usual Dose

Adult: 150 mg per day with food, to start. This dose may be increased by 50 mg per day every 3 to 4 days, to a maximum of 400 mg per day. Severely depressed people may be given as much as 600 mg per day.

Overdosage

Drowsiness and vomiting are the most frequent signs of Trazodone overdose. The other signs are simply more severe side effects, especially those affecting the heart and mood. Fever may develop at first, but body temperature will drop below normal as time passes. ALL victims of antidepressant overdosage, especially children, must be taken to an emergency room immediately. ALWAYS bring the medicine bottle.

Special Information

Use care while driving or doing anything else requiring concentration or alertness, and avoid alcohol or any other depressant while taking Trazodone.

Call your doctor if any side effects develop, especially blood in the urine, dizziness, or light-headedness. Trazodone may cause dry mouth, irregular heartbeat, nausea, vomiting, or difficulty breathing. Call your doctor if these symptoms become severe.

If you forget to take a dose of Trazodone, take it as soon as possible. However, if it is within 4 hours of your next dose, skip the forgotten dose and go back to your regular schedule. Do not take a double dose.

Special Populations

Pregnancy/Breast-feeding
This drug may damage a developing fetus and should not be taken by women who are pregnant or who may become pregnant.

Trazodone passes into breast milk. When it is deemed essential, the potential risk of taking Trazodone must be carefully weighed against the benefit it might produce.

Seniors
Seniors are likely to be more sensitive to the effects and side effects of usual doses of Trazodone than younger adults. Medical experts recommend starting with lower doses and then slowly increasing the dosage.

Trental

see Pentoxifylline, page 874

Generic Name
Tretinoin

Other Names
Retinoic Acid
Vitamin A Acid

Brand Name
Retin-A Cream/Gel/Liquid
Renova

Type of Drug
Antiacne; antiwrinkling.

Prescribed for
Acne, other skin conditions, and several forms of skin cancer

(Retin-A). Skin aged by excess sun exposure (wrinkling and liver spots) appears to improve when treated with Tretinoin (Renova).

General Information

This drug (as Retin-A) works in acne by decreasing the cohesiveness of skin cells, causing the skin to peel. Because it is a skin irritant, any other irritant (such as extreme weather or wind, cosmetics, and some soaps) can cause severe irritation. Excessive application of Tretinoin will cause more peeling and irritation but will not give better results. This drug is usually not effective in treating severe acne.

Regular application of Tretinoin cream in a moisturizing base (Renova) to aging skin prevents wrinkling and could even reverse the wrinkling process for some people. Tretinoin causes a temporary "plumping" of the skin when it is applied to peel the outer layer of skin. This gives the overall appearance of improved skin health and reduced wrinkling. Some Tretinoin (about 5 percent) is absorbed after it is applied to the skin.

Cautions and Warnings

Do not use this drug if you are **allergic** to it or any of its components. This drug may **increase the skin-cancer-causing effects of ultraviolet light**. Therefore, people using this drug should allow their skin to "rest" before using other skin irritants or peeling agents. Also, they must **limit sun exposure** and **avoid sunlamps**. If you can't avoid sun exposure, use a sunscreen and protective covering. Do not apply Tretinoin close to your eyes, to the sides of the nose, or to mucous membrane tissue.

Possible Side Effects

▼ Common: skin redness, swelling, blistering, or formation of crusts on the skin near the application site. Temporary over- or undercoloration of the skin and greater sensitivity to the sun also occur. All side effects disappear after the drug has been stopped.

Drug Interactions

• Other skin irritants will cause excessive sensitivity, irritation, and side effects. Among the substances that cause this interaction are medications that contain Sulfur (topical), Resorcinol, Benzoyl Peroxide, or Salicylic Acid; abrasive soaps or skin cleansers; cosmetics or other creams, ointments, etc., with a severe drying effect; and products with a high alcohol, astringent, spice, or lime content.

• Tretinoin increases the absorption of Minoxidil into the bloodstream when they are applied together, leading to blood-pressure reduction.

Food Interactions

None known.

Usual Dose

Apply a small amount of Tretinoin to the affected area when you go to bed, after thoroughly cleansing the area.

Overdosage

Applying too much Tretinoin will cause skin irritation and peeling. Swallowing this product is like taking vitamin A; this can be extremely dangerous in pregnant women, who should not take more vitamin A than is contained in their prenatal vitamins, and infants, who should be taken to a hospital emergency room for treatment.

Special Information

You may experience an increase in acne lesions during the first few weeks of treatment, because the drug is acting on deeper lesions. This is beneficial and is not a reason to stop using the drug. Results should be seen in 2 to 6 weeks; normal cosmetics can be used during this time.

Keep this drug away from your eyes, nose, mouth, and mucous membranes. Avoid exposure to sunlight or sunlamps.

You may feel warmth and slight stinging when you apply Tretinoin. If you develop an extreme skin reaction (such as burning, peeling, or redness) or are uncomfortable, stop using this product for a short time.

If you forget a dose of Tretinoin, do not apply the forgotten dose. Skip it and go back to your regular schedule. Do not apply a double dose.

Special Populations

Pregnancy/Breast-feeding

Tretinoin has been shown to cause abnormal skull formation and other birth defects in animal fetuses at doses 500 to 1000 times the human dose. No human studies have been done, but the drug is rapidly broken down by the skin. Pregnant women should use Tretinoin only after possible risks and benefits have been discussed.

It is not known if this drug passes into breast milk. Nursing mothers should be cautious if using this drug.

Seniors

Older adults may use this product without special restriction.

Tri-Levlen

see **Contraceptives**, page 262

Triamterene/Hydrochlorothiazide

see **Dyazide**, page 380

Generic Name

Triazolam

Brand Name

Halcion

Type of Drug

Benzodiazepine sedative.

Prescribed for

Short-term treatment of insomnia or sleeplessness; difficulty falling asleep; frequent nighttime awakening; waking too early in the morning.

General Information

Triazolam is a member of the group of drugs known as *benzodiazepines*. All have some activity as either antianxiety agents, anticonvulsants, or sedatives. Benzodiazepines work by a direct effect on the brain. Benzodiazepines make it easier to go to sleep and decrease the number of times you wake up during the night.

The principal differences between these medicines lie in how long they work in your body. They all take about 2 hours to reach maximum blood level, but some remain in your body longer, so they work for a longer period of time. Triazolam has the shortest action. While this virtually eliminates hangover, it raises the possibility for some people that they will get up earlier in the morning than they wanted to because the drug has stopped working. Often sleeplessness is a reflection of another disorder that would be untreated by this medicine.

Cautions and Warnings

Triazolam has been associated with **memory loss,** especially when higher doses are taken. This is more common among travelers (traveler's amnesia) who take this medicine. The problem may also be associated with drinking alcoholic beverages and trying to start daily activity too soon after waking up.

If you abruptly stop taking Triazolam, you may experience a **rebound effect** where sleeplessness is worse during the first 1 to 3 nights after you stop the drug than it was before you started it.

People with respiratory disease may experience **sleep apnea** (intermittent breathing while asleep) while taking it.

People with **kidney or liver disease** should be carefully monitored while taking Triazolam. Take the lowest possible dose to help you sleep.

Clinical depression may be increased by Triazolam, which can depress the nervous system. Intentional overdosage is more common among depressed people who take sleeping pills than those who do not.

All benzodiazepines can be **abused** if taken for long periods of time. It is possible for a person taking a benzodiazepine to develop **drug-withdrawal symptoms** if the drug is suddenly discontinued. Withdrawal symptoms include tremors, muscle cramps, insomnia, agitation, diarrhea, vomiting, sweating, and convulsions.

Possible Side Effects

▼ Common: drowsiness, headache, dizziness, talkativeness, nervousness, apprehension, poor muscle coordination, light-headedness, daytime tiredness, muscle weakness, slowness of movements, hangover, and euphoria (feeling "high").

▼ Other: nausea, vomiting, rapid heartbeat, confusion, temporary memory loss, upset stomach, stomach cramps and pain, depression, blurred or double vision and other visual disturbances, constipation, changes in taste perception, appetite changes, stuffy nose, nosebleeds, common cold symptoms, asthma, sore throat, cough, breathing problems, diarrhea, dry mouth, allergic reactions, fainting, abnormal heart rhythms, itching, acne, dry skin, sensitivity to the sun, rash, nightmares or strange dreams, difficulty sleeping, tingling in the hands or feet, ringing or buzzing in the ears, ear or eye pains, menstrual cramps, frequent urination and other urinary difficulties, blood in the urine, discharge from the penis or vagina, lower back and other pains, muscle spasms and pain, fever, swollen breasts, and weight changes.

Drug Interactions

• As with all benzodiazepines, the effects of Triazolam are enhanced if it is taken with an alcoholic beverage, antihistamine, tranquilizer, barbiturate, anticonvulsant medicine, tricyclic antidepressant, or monoamine oxidase (MAO) inhibitor drug (most often prescribed for severe depression).

• Oral contraceptives, Cimetidine, Disulfiram, and Isoniazid may increase the effect of Triazolam by interfering with the drug's breakdown in the liver. Probenecid may also increase Triazolam's effect.

• Cigarette smoking, Rifampin, and Theophylline may reduce the effect of Triazolam.

• The drug decreases the effectiveness of Levodopa.

• Triazolam may increase the amount of Zidovudine (AZT),

Phenytoin, or Digoxin in your blood, increasing the chances of drug toxicity.

• The combination of Clozapine and benzodiazapines has led to respiratory collapse in a few people. Triazolam should be stopped at least 1 week before starting Clozapine treatment.

• The effects of Triazolam may be increased by the macrolide antibiotics (Azithromycin, Erythromycin, and Clarithromycin).

Food Interactions

Triazolam may be taken with food if it upsets your stomach.

Usual Dose

Adult (age 18 and older): 0.125 to 0.5 mg about 30 minutes before you want to go to sleep.

Senior: 0.125 mg to start, then increase by 0.125-mg increments until the desired effect is achieved.

Child: not recommended.

Overdosage

The most common symptoms of overdose are confusion, sleepiness, depression, loss of muscle coordination, and slurred speech. Coma may develop if the overdose is particularly large. Overdose symptoms can develop if a single dose of only 4 times the maximum daily dose is taken. Overdose victims must be made to vomit with Syrup of Ipecac (available at any pharmacy) to remove any remaining drug from the stomach. Call your doctor or a poison control center before doing this. If 30 minutes have passed since the overdose was taken or symptoms have begun to develop, the victim must be taken immediately to a hospital emergency room for treatment. ALWAYS bring the medicine bottle with you.

Special Information

Never take more Triazolam than your doctor has prescribed.

Avoid alcoholic beverages and other nervous-system depressants while taking Triazolam.

People taking this drug must be careful when performing tasks requiring concentration and coordination because of the chance that the drug will make them tired, dizzy, or light-headed.

If you take Triazolam daily for 3 or more weeks, you may experience some withdrawal symptoms when you stop taking the drug. Talk with your doctor about the best way to discontinue the drug.

Do not take Triazolam unless circumstances will allow for a full night's sleep and time for the drug to clear your body after you awaken and before you need to be alert and active. The total time necessary varies among people, and you may have to determine your own reaction to this drug.

If you forget to take a dose of Triazolam and remember within 1 hour of your regular time, take it as soon as you remember. If you do not remember until later, skip the forgotten dose and go back to your regular schedule. Do not take a double dose.

Special Populations

Pregnancy/Breast-feeding

Triazolam should absolutely **not** be used by pregnant women or women who may become pregnant. Animal studies have shown that Triazolam passes easily into the fetal blood system and can affect fetal development.

Triazolam passes into breast milk and can affect a nursing infant. The drug should not be taken by nursing mothers.

Seniors

Older adults are more susceptible to the effects of Triazolam and should take the lowest possible dosage.

Generic Name

Trimethobenzamide Hydrochloride

Brand Names

Tebamide Suppositories
T-Gen Suppositories
Tigan Capsules/Suppositories
Trimazide Capsules/Suppositories

(Also available in generic form)

Type of Drug

Antiemetic.

Prescribed for

Controlling nausea and vomiting.

General Information

Trimethobenzamide Hydrochloride works in the same way as Scopolamine and other anticholinergic drugs on the brain's *chemoreceptor trigger zone*, where impulses are carried to the vomiting center. It can help control nausea and vomiting. Once a mainstay of antiemetic therapy, this drug has largely been replaced by other medicines, especially Ondansetron and Granisetron.

Cautions and Warnings

Do not use this drug if you are **allergic** or **sensitive** to it. Trimethobenzamide Hydrochloride rectal suppositories contain a local anesthetic and should **not be used in newborn infants** or by people who are allergic to local anesthetics.

Trimethobenzamide should **not be used for vomiting children who have no other complications**. Trimethobenzamide and other antiemetics that act in the brain may worsen **Reye's syndrome;** they should not be used in children with signs of this condition. Reye's syndrome is an acute, possibly fatal, childhood disease, characterized by sudden, persistent, or severe vomiting; tiredness; and irrational behavior. It can progress to convulsions, coma, and death—usually following a nonspecific illness associated with a high fever.

Trimethobenzamide can obscure the signs of drug overdose or disease because it controls nausea and vomiting.

Possible Side Effects

▼ Most common: drowsiness.

▼ Less common: blurred vision, diarrhea, dizziness, muscle cramps, and tremors.

▼ Rare: sore throat, fever, unusual tiredness, headache, yellowing of the skin or eyes, depression, body spasms, and shakiness or tremors. If you develop a rash or breathing difficulty while on Trimethobenzamide, stop taking it and tell your doctor. Usually these symptoms will disappear by themselves, but additional treatment may be necessary.

Drug Interactions

• Trimethobenzamide may increase the depressant effects of barbiturates, sleeping pills, tranquilizers, alcohol, and antihistamines.

Food Interactions

Take this drug with food if it upsets your stomach.

Usual Dose

Capsules
Adult: 250 mg 3 to 4 times per day.
Child (30 to 90 pounds): 100 to 200 mg 3 or 4 times daily.

Rectal Suppositories
Adult: 200 mg 3 to 4 times per day.
Child (30 to 90 pounds): 100 to 200 mg 3 or 4 times daily.
Child (under 30 pounds): 100 mg 3 or 4 times daily.
Dose is adjusted according to disease severity and individual response.

Overdosage

Overdose symptoms are likely to be exaggerated drug side effects. Take the victim to a hospital emergency room for treatment. ALWAYS bring the prescription bottle.

Special Information

Severe vomiting should not be treated with just an antiemetic drug; the cause of your vomiting should be established and treated. Antiemetic drugs may delay diagnosis of why you are vomiting and mask the toxic signs of other drugs. The most important part of treatment for emesis is reestablishing body fluid and electrolyte balance, relieving fever (if present), and treating the causative disease process.

Use care when driving or performing other complex tasks because of this drug's sedating effects.

If you forget to take a dose of Trimethobenzamide Hydrochloride, take it as soon as you remember. If it is almost time for your next dose, skip the one you forgot and continue with your regular schedule. Do not take a double dose.

Special Populations

Pregnancy/Breast-feeding
Animal studies with this drug show an increased number of

stillbirths. Trimethobenzamide should not be taken during pregnancy unless its possible benefits outweigh its risks.

Nursing mothers who take this drug should watch their infants for Trimethobenzamide side effects.

Seniors
Seniors may take this medication without special restriction. Follow your doctor's directions, and report any side effects.

Generic Name

Trimethoprim

Brand Names
Proloprim
Trimpex

(Also available in generic form)

Type of Drug
Anti-infective.

Prescribed for
Urinary tract infections.

General Information
Trimethoprim works by blocking the utilization of folic acid by micro-organisms that may infect the urinary tract. It is often used in combination with a sulfa drug, and was first made available in the United States only as part of a combination product known as *Septra* or *Bactrim*. However, Trimethoprim by itself is effective for some uncomplicated urinary infections. Your doctor should take a sample of urine to test it against this and other anti-infectives to determine the best drug for the infection that is affecting you.

Cautions and Warnings
Do not take Trimethoprim if you are **allergic** to it or if you are **folic-acid deficient**.

Large doses of Trimethoprim can interfere with your ability

to make blood cells. **Sore throat, paleness, fever,** or **black-and-blue marks** can be **early signs** of a **dangerous blood disorder**. Report these to your doctor.

This drug should be used with care in people with **liver or kidney disease**.

Possible Side Effects

▼ Most common: itching, rash, and peeling of the skin.

▼ Less common: stomach upset, nausea, vomiting, inflammation of the tongue, fever, reductions in blood-cell counts (red and white) and platelet counts, and elevation of liver and kidney enzymes.

Drug Interactions

• Trimethoprim may increase the effects of the anticonvulsant Phenytoin by interfering with its breakdown in the liver.

• Trimethoprim may increase the toxicity and reduce the effectiveness of Cyclosporine.

Food Interactions

This medicine is best taken on an empty stomach, but you may take it with food if it upsets your stomach.

Usual Dose

Adult and Child (age 12 and older): 200 mg a day for 10 days. People with kidney disease should take less.

Child (under age 12): do not use.

Overdosage

Signs of overdosage may appear after taking as little as 1000 mg. They include nausea, vomiting, dizziness, headache, depression, confusion, and adverse effects on the blood system. People taking high doses of Trimethoprim or those taking it for long periods of time may develop abnormalities in their blood system. Overdose victims should be taken to a hospital emergency room at once for treatment. ALWAYS bring the medicine bottle with you.

Special Information

Take this medication exactly as directed. Call your doctor if you develop sore throat, fever, black-and-blue marks, or very pale (sickly) skin.

Be sure to complete the full treatment your doctor has prescribed.

If you miss a dose of Trimethoprim, take it as soon as possible. If you take your medication once a day, and it is almost time for your next dose, space the missed dose and your next dose 10 to 12 hours apart, then go back to your regular schedule. If you take it twice a day, and it is almost time for your next dose, space the missed dose and your next dose by 5 to 6 hours, then go back to your regular schedule.

Special Populations

Pregnancy/Breast-feeding

This drug crosses into the blood circulation of a developing fetus. Animal studies have shown that very large doses of Trimethoprim can affect fetal development. Since Trimethoprim can interfere with the metabolism of folic acid—vital to normal functioning and fetal development—it generally should be avoided during pregnancy.

This drug passes into breast milk but has not caused problems among breast-fed infants. Still, nursing mothers taking Trimethoprim should bottle-feed their babies because of the drug's possible effects.

Seniors

Older adults with poor liver or kidney function are more sensitive to the effects of this drug; your doctor will tailor your dose as needed. Otherwise-healthy seniors may not require dose adjustment. Follow your doctor's directions, and report any side effects at once.

Trimethoprim/Sulfamethoxazole

see Septra, page 1011

Generic Name

Trimipramine

Brand Name

Surmontil

Type of Drug

Tricyclic antidepressant.

Prescribed for

Depression (with or without anxiety); sleep disturbance; peptic ulcer disease.

General Information

Trimipramine and other tricyclic antidepressants block the movement of certain stimulant chemicals (norepinephrine or serotonin) in and out of nerve endings, have a sedative effect, and counteract the effects of a hormone called *acetylcholine* (making them anticholinergic drugs).

Theory says that people with depression have a chemical imbalance in their brains and that drugs such as Trimipramine work to reestablish a proper balance. Although Trimipramine and similar antidepressants immediately block neurohormones, it takes 2 to 4 weeks for their clinical antidepressant effect to come into play. They can also elevate mood, increase physical activity and mental alertness, and improve appetite and sleep patterns in a depressed patient. These drugs are mild sedatives and therefore useful in treating mild forms of depression associated with anxiety. If your don't improve after 6 to 8 weeks, contact your doctor. Trimipramine is broken down in the liver.

Cautions and Warnings

Do not take Trimipramine if you are **allergic** or **sensitive** to it or other tricyclic antidepressants. Trimipramine should not be used if you are **recovering from a heart attack**.

Trimipramine may be taken with caution if you have a **history of epilepsy** or other seizure disorders, **difficulty in urination, glaucoma, heart disease, liver disease,** or **hyper-**

thyroidism. People who are **schizophrenic** or **paranoid** may get worse if given a tricyclic antidepressant, and manic-depressive people may switch phase. This can also happen if they are changing or stopping antidepressants. Suicide is always a possibility in severely depressed people, who should be allowed to keep only small amounts of medication in their possession.

Possible Side Effects

▼ Most common: sedation and anticholinergic effects (blurred vision, disorientation, confusion, hallucinations, muscle spasms or tremors, seizures and/or convulsions, dry mouth, constipation [especially in older adults], difficult urination, worsening glaucoma, sensitivity to bright light or sunlight).

▼ Less common: blood-pressure changes, abnormal heart rates, heart attack, anxiety, restlessness, excitement, numbness and tingling in the extremities, poor coordination, rash, itching, retention of fluids, fever, allergy, changes in composition of blood, nausea, vomiting, loss of appetite, stomach upset, diarrhea, breast enlargement (both sexes), changes in sex drive, and blood-sugar changes.

▼ Infrequent: agitation, inability to sleep, nightmares, feeling of panic, a peculiar taste in the mouth, stomach cramps, black coloration of the tongue, yellowing eyes and/or skin, changes in liver function, increased or decreased weight, excessive perspiration, flushing, frequent urination, drowsiness, dizziness, weakness, headache, loss of hair, nausea, and feelings of ill health.

Drug Interactions

• Interaction with monoamine oxidase (MAO) inhibitors can cause high fevers, convulsions, and occasionally death. Don't take any MAO inhibitor until at least 2 weeks after Trimipramine has been discontinued. Patients who must take Trimipramine and an MAO inhibitor require close medical observation.

• Trimipramine interacts with Guanethidine and Clonidine. If Trimipramine is being considered, be sure your doctor knows if you are taking **any** high-blood-pressure medicine.

- Trimipramine increases the effects of barbiturates, tranquilizers, other sedative drugs, and alcohol. Also, barbiturates may decrease the effectiveness of Trimipramine
- Taking Trimipramine and thyroid medicine together will enhance the effects of both medicines, possibly causing abnormal heart rhythms.
- The combination of Trimipramine and Reserpine may cause overstimulation.
- Oral contraceptives can reduce the effect of Trimipramine, as can smoking.
- Charcoal tablets can prevent Trimipramine absorption into the bloodstream.
- Estrogens can increase or decrease the effect of Trimipramine.
- Drugs such as Bicarbonate of Soda, Acetazolamide, Quinidine, or Procainamide will increase the effect of Trimipramine.
- Cimetidine, Methylphenidate, and phenothiazine drugs (such as Thorazine and Compazine) block the liver metabolism of Trimipramine, causing it to stay in the body longer, which can lead to severe drug side effects.

Food Interactions

Take Trimipramine with food if it upsets your stomach.

Usual Dose

Adult: 75 mg a day in divided doses to start, then increased as necessary to 150 or 200 mg. The entire dose may be given at bedtime or in divided doses several times per day. Hospitalized adults may receive up to 300 mg a day.

Adolescent and Senior: 50 mg a day to start. Maintenance dose up to 100 mg daily.

Child: not recommended.

Overdosage

Symptoms are confusion, inability to concentrate, hallucinations, drowsiness, lowered body temperature, abnormal heart rate, heart failure, enlarged pupils, convulsions, severely lowered blood pressure, stupor, and coma. Agitation, stiffening of body muscles, vomiting, and high fever can also occur. The victim should be taken to an emergency room immediately. ALWAYS bring the medicine bottle with you.

Special Information

Avoid alcohol and other depressants while taking this drug. Do not stop taking this medicine unless your doctor has specifically told you to do so. Abruptly stopping this medicine may cause nausea, headache, and a sickly feeling.

This medicine can cause drowsiness, dizziness, and blurred vision. Be careful when driving or operating hazardous machinery. Avoid prolonged exposure to the sun or sunlamps.

Call your doctor at once if you develop seizures, difficult or rapid breathing, fever and sweating, blood-pressure changes, muscle stiffness, loss of bladder control, or unusual tiredness or weakness. Dry mouth may lead to an increase in dental cavities or gum bleeding and disease. People taking Trimipramine should pay special attention to dental hygiene.

If you forget to take a dose of Trimipramine, skip it and go back to your regular schedule. Do not take a double dose.

Special Populations

Pregnancy/Breast-feeding

Trimipramine, like other antidepressants, crosses into the fetal circulation. There have been reports of newborn infants suffering from heart, breathing, and urinary problems after their mothers had taken an antidepressant of this type immediately before delivery. Avoid taking this medication while pregnant.

Small amounts of Trimipramine pass into breast milk and can sedate the baby. Nursing mothers taking Trimipramine should consider bottle-feeding.

Seniors

Older adults are more sensitive to the effects of this drug, especially abnormal rhythms and other heart side effects, and often require less medicine. Follow your doctor's directions, and report any side effects at once.

Trimox

see Penicillin Antibiotics, page 868

Triphasil

see **Contraceptives**, page 262

Brand Name

Tussionex Pennkinetic Suspension

Ingredients

Hydrocodone + Chlorpheniramine

Type of Drug

Cough suppressant/antihistamine combination.

Prescribed for

Relief of cough and other symptoms of a cold or other respiratory condition.

General Information

This drug is one of many cough suppressant/antihistamine combinations that may be prescribed to treat a cough or congestion that has not responded to other medication. The narcotic cough-suppressant ingredient (Hydrocodone) in this combination is more potent than Codeine.

Cautions and Warnings

Do not use Tussionex if you are **allergic** to any of its ingredients. Those **allergic to Codeine** may also be allergic to Tussionex. **Long-term use** of this or any other narcotic-containing drug can lead to **drug dependence** or **addiction**. Tussionex can cause **drowsiness, tiredness,** or **loss of concentration**. Use with caution if you have a **history of convulsions, glaucoma, stomach ulcer, high blood pressure, thyroid disease, heart disease,** or **diabetes**.

Possible Side Effects

▼ Most common: light-headedness, dizziness, sleepiness, nausea, vomiting, increased sweating, itching, rash, sensitivity to bright light, chills, and dryness of the mouth, nose, or throat.

▼ Less common: euphoria (feeling "high"), weakness, agitation, uncoordinated muscle movement, disorientation and visual disturbances, minor hallucinations, loss of appetite, constipation, flushing of the face, rapid heartbeat, palpitations, faintness, difficult urination, reduced sexual potency, low blood sugar, anemia, yellowing of the skin or eyes, blurred or double vision, ringing or buzzing in the ears, wheezing, and nasal stuffiness.

Drug Interactions

• Do not use alcohol or other depressant drugs because they will increase the depressant effect of the Tussionex.

• This drug should not be combined with monoamine oxidase (MAO) inhibitor drugs.

Food Interactions

Take Tussionex with food if it upsets your stomach.

Usual Dose

1 teaspoon every 12 hours.

Overdosage

Signs of overdosage are depression, slowed breathing, flushing of the skin, and upset stomach. Overdose victims should be taken to an emergency room for treatment. ALWAYS bring the medicine bottle.

Special Information

Because of the sedating effects of Tussionex, use caution while driving or operating hazardous equipment.

If you forget to take a dose of Tussionex, take it as soon as you remember. If it is almost time for your next dose, skip the one you forgot and continue with your regular schedule. Do not take a double dose.

Special Populations

Pregnancy/Breast-feeding

Narcotics such as Hydrocodone, one of the ingredients in Tussionex, have not been associated with birth defects, but taking too much of any narcotic during pregnancy can lead to the birth of a drug-dependent infant and drug-withdrawal symptoms in the baby. All narcotics, including Hydrocodone, can cause breathing problems in the newborn if taken just before delivery. Antihistamines may pass into your developing baby's circulation but have not been the source of birth defects.

Nursing mothers should bottle-feed their babies while taking this medication.

Seniors

Seniors are more likely to be sensitive to both ingredients in Tussionex; it may produce more of a depressant effect; dizziness, light-headedness, or fainting when rising suddenly from a sitting or lying position; confusion; difficult or painful urination; feelings of faintness; dry mouth, nose, or throat; nightmares; or excitement, nervousness, restlessness, or irritability.

Brand Name

Tussi-Organidin DM NR Liquid

Ingredients

Dextromethorphan Hydrobromide + Guaifenesin

Other Brand Names

Cheracol D Cough Liquid
Diabetic Tussin DM Ⓢ Ⓐ
Extra Action Cough Syrup
Genatuss DM Liquid Ⓐ
Glycotuss-dM Tablets
Guiatuss-DM Liquid Ⓐ
Guiatussin with
    Dextromethorphan Liquid
Halotussin-DM Liquid Ⓐ

Halotussin-DM Sugar
    Free Liquid Ⓢ Ⓐ
Humibid DM Tablets/Sprinkle
    Capsules
Kolephrin GG/DM Liquid Ⓐ
Mytussin DM Liquid
Naldecon Senior
    DX Liquid Ⓢ Ⓐ
Rhinosyn-DMX Syrup

Robafen DM Syrup   Tolu-Sed DM Syrup   Ⓢ
Robitussin DM Liquid   Tuss-DM Tablets
Safe Tussin 30 Liquid Ⓐ   Unitussin DM Syrup   Ⓐ

(Also available in generic form)

Type of Drug

Cough suppressant/expectorant combination.

Prescribed for

Relief of coughs due to colds or other respiratory infections.

General Information

Most of the combination products in this profile may be purchased without a prescription. The cough-suppressant effect of Tussi-Organidin DM NR is due to the presence of Dextromethorphan, the most effective of all nonnarcotic cough suppressants. Guaifenesin, an expectorant, is supposed to increase the production of mucus and other bronchial secretions. Once these thick secretions are loosened up, they should be easier for the body to deal with, thus relieving the cough. Expectorants do not suppress a cough. Many experts question whether Guaifenesin has any real effect, especially in removing the mucus that accumulates in serious respiratory conditions such as bronchitis, bronchial asthma, emphysema, cystic fibrosis, or chronic sinusitis. Drinking plenty of fluids will work as well as any expectorant for the average cold or upper-respiratory cough.

Cautions and Warnings

Do not take Tussi-Organidin DM NR if you are **allergic** or **sensitive** to either of its ingredients.

Possible Side Effects

▼ Common: nausea, vomiting, diarrhea, and stomach pains.

Drug Interactions

• Hallucinations have occurred when people have taken

Fluoxetine together with Dextromethorphan, the most common nonprescription cough-suppressant ingredient. Don't take this combination.

Food Interactions

Tussi-Organidin DM NR should be taken with a full glass of water or other fluid for best results.

Usual Dose

2 teaspoons every 3 or 4 hours as needed for cough relief.

Overdosage

There have been no reports of any serious problems caused by Tussi-Organidin DM NR overdose. Call your local poison control center or emergency room for more information.

Special Information

Report any persistent or intolerable side effects to your doctor.

If you take Tussi-Organidin DM NR 3 or more times per day and forget a dose, take it as soon as you remember. If it is almost time for your next dose, take 1 dose as soon as you remember and another in 3 or 4 hours, then go back to your regular schedule. Do not take a double dose.

Special Populations

Pregnancy/Breast-feeding

Tussi-Organidin DM NR may be taken by women who are pregnant or nursing.

Seniors

Older adults may take Tussi-Organidin DM NR without special restriction. Follow your doctor's directions, and report any side effects at once.

Brand Name

Tussi-Organidin NR Liquid

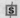

Ingredients

Codeine Phosphate + Guaifenesin

Other Brand Names

Cheracol Cough Syrup	Mytussin AC Cough Syrup
Guiatuss AC Syrup	Robafen AC Cough Syrup
Guiatussin with Codeine	Robitussin A-C Syrup $\boxed{\$}$

(Also available in generic form)

Type of Drug

Cough suppressant/expectorant combination.

Prescribed for

Relief of coughs due to colds or other upper respiratory infections.

General Information

The cough-suppressant effect of Tussi-Organidin is due to the Codeine present in the mixture. Guaifenesin, an expectorant, increases the production of mucus and other bronchial secretions. Once these thick secretions become diluted, it should be easier for the body to deal with them, thus relieving the cough. Many experts question the effectiveness of Guaifenesin, especially for removing the mucus that accumulates in serious respiratory conditions such as bronchitis, bronchial asthma, emphysema, cystic fibrosis, or chronic sinusitis. Drinking plenty of fluids will work as well as any expectorant for the average cold or upper-respiratory cough. Expectorants do not suppress your cough.

Cautions and Warnings

Do not take Tussi-Organidin if you are **allergic** or **sensitive** to it or its Codeine ingredient. **Long-term use** of Codeine may lead to **drug dependence** or **addiction**.

Possible Side Effects

▼ Most common: light-headedness, dizziness, sedation or sleepiness, nausea, vomiting, diarrhea, stomach pains, and sweating.

Possible Side Effects *(continued)*

▼ Less common: euphoria (feeling "high"), weakness, headache, agitation, uncoordinated muscle movement, minor hallucinations, disorientation and visual disturbances, dry mouth, loss of appetite, constipation, facial flushing, rapid heartbeat, palpitations, faintness, urinary difficulties or hesitancy, reduced sex drive and/or potency, itching, rash, anemia, lowered blood sugar, and yellowing of the skin or eyes. Narcotic analgesics such as Codeine may aggravate convulsions in those who have had convulsions in the past.

Drug Interactions

• Codeine, one of the ingredients in these combination drugs, has a general depressant effect and can affect breathing. Tussi-Organidin should be taken with extreme care in combination with alcohol, sedatives, tranquilizers, antihistamines, or other depressant drugs.

Food Interactions

Tussi-Organidin should be taken with a full glass of water or other fluid for best results.

Usual Dose

2 teaspoons every 4 hours as needed for cough relief.

Overdosage

Symptoms are breathing difficulty, pinpointed pupils, lack of response to pain stimulation (for example, a pin prick), cold or clammy skin, slow heartbeat, low blood pressure, convulsions, heart attack, or extreme tiredness progressing to stupor and then coma. The victim should be taken to an emergency room immediately. ALWAYS bring the medicine bottle.

Special Information

Codeine is a respiratory depressant and affects the central nervous system, producing sleepiness, tiredness, and/or inability to concentrate. Be careful if you are driving or performing other functions requiring concentration. Report any persistent or intolerable side effects to your doctor.

If you take Tussi-Organidin 3 or more times per day and forget a dose, take it as soon as you remember. If it is almost time for your next dose, take 1 dose as soon as you remember and another in 3 or 4 hours, then go back to your regular schedule. Do not take a double dose.

Special Populations

Pregnancy/Breast-feeding
Tussi-Organidin should be avoided by pregnant women. Codeine may cause breathing problems in infants during delivery.

Nursing mothers should not take products containing Codeine because they pass into breast milk and can affect the infant's breathing and general respiratory function.

Seniors
Older adults are more sensitive to the effects of the Codeine in this drug. Follow your doctor's directions, and report any side effects at once.

Generic Name

Ursodiol

Brand Name

Actigall

Type of Drug

Gallstone dissolver.

Prescribed for

People with cholesterol gallstones readily identifiable by x-ray examination who refuse gallstone surgery or for whom surgery might be risky.

General Information

Ursodiol is a natural bile acid that suppresses the production of cholesterol in the liver and interferes with the absorption of dietary cholesterol through the intestine. It will not dissolve gallstones that are encased in calcium, stones that are not visible on x-ray, or noncholesterol stones. Your doctor should examine your gallbladder every 6 months to see if the drug is working. Most people who show progress at the first 6-month evaluation are likely to lose their gallstones. No change in the stones at 12 months is a sign that the treatment is not likely to work at all. An alternative to taking Ursodiol is watchful waiting to see if anything happens before taking action; it may be that no treatment will ever be needed. Only 7 to 27 percent of people with silent or mild gallstone problems will experience moderate to severe symptoms or a complication within 5 years.

Cautions and Warnings

Before taking this drug, it is important that your doctor perform a **complete gallstone examination,** including x-ray tests, to be sure your **bile duct** is functioning normally. Bile acids (including Ursodiol) may be weakly linked to the development of colon cancer among people who have had **gallbladder surgery.**

People with **chronic liver disease** or who are **allergic** to bile acids should not take this product.

Possible Side Effects

▼ Most common: diarrhea.

▼ Less common: nausea; vomiting; upset stomach; abdominal pain; bile pain; gallstone pain; a metallic taste; constipation; stomach gas; itching; rash; dry skin; sweating; hair thinning; headache; fatigue; anxiety; depression; sleep disturbances; joint, muscle, and back pains; cough; and runny nose.

Drug Interactions

• Aluminum-based antacids, Cholestyramine, and Colestipol interfere with the absorption of Ursodiol.

• Blood-cholesterol-lowering drugs (especially Clofibrate), Neomycin, estrogens, and progestins may reduce Ursodiol's ability to dissolve cholesterol gallstones.

Food Interactions

Follow your doctor's dietary instructions while being treated for gallstones. For best results, take Ursodiol with meals.

Usual Dose

3.5 to 4.5 mg per pound of body weight per day, divided into 2 or 3 doses.

Overdosage

The most likely result of overdose is diarrhea. Call your local poison control center for more information.

Special Information

You must take this medicine for the full course of treatment, even if you begin to feel better. If you stop treatment, your gallstones may not dissolve as quickly as possible, or they may not dissolve at all. Months of Ursodiol treatment are required to dissolve most gallstones, and some may never be dissolved. Success with this drug depends on the size of the stones and their cholesterol content. Age, weight, and sex do not influence the dissolving of gallstones.

Half of all people who use this drug to dissolve their gallstones may have another gallstone attack within 5 years.

People with severe, uncontrollable gallstone attacks, bile duct obstruction, inflammation of the pancreas, or other serious problems should not depend on this drug to dissolve their stones; surgery is more appropriate. Your doctor will determine which is the proper course of action for you.

Report diarrhea and any severe side effects to your doctor, especially pain in the abdomen, nausea, vomiting, and severe right-upper-abdominal pain that travels to your shoulder.

If you take Ursodiol twice a day and forget a dose until it is almost time for your next dose, take 1 dose right away and another in 5 or 6 hours, then go back to your regular schedule. If you take Ursodiol 3 times a day and miss a dose, and it is almost time for your next dose, take 1 dose then and another in 3 or 4 hours, and go back to your regular schedule.

Special Populations

Pregnancy/Breast-feeding

Four women who accidentally took Ursodiol during the first 3 months of pregnancy all delivered normal babies. Still, the drug's effect on the developing fetus is not known. Ursodiol should not be used by pregnant women.

It is not known if Ursodiol passes into breast milk. Nursing mothers must be cautious when taking this drug.

Seniors
Seniors may take this medicine without special restriction.

Generic Name

Valacyclovir

Brand Name

Valtrex

Type of Drug

Antiviral.

Prescribed for

Herpes zoster infections.

General Information

Valacyclovir is rapidly converted to Acyclovir in the liver and intestine after it is absorbed into the blood. Although it is effective and approved for use against the two types of herpes virus infection (herpes zoster, which causes shingles, and varicella zoster, which causes chickenpox), studies of this drug have been mostly in shingles. Valacyclovir works by inhibiting and inactivating an enzyme that is key to viral reproduction and by affecting the growing viral DNA chain.

Cautions and Warnings

Do not take Valacyclovir if you are **allergic** to it, Acyclovir, or any component of the tablet.

Some people with **advanced HIV disease** or who have had a **bone marrow transplant** or an **organ transplant** developed a potentially fatal condition known as TTP while taking Valacyclovir. This drug should not be taken by anyone with **AIDS** or others with a **compromised immune system**.

High doses of Acyclovir taken over long periods of time have caused reduced sperm count in lab animals, but this effect has not yet been reported in humans.

Possible Side Effects

▼ Most common: headache, diarrhea, dizziness, weakness, constipation, abdominal pain, appetite loss, nausea, and vomiting. These effects are comparable to those seen with Acyclovir.

▼ Less common: aching joints, tingling in the hands or feet, stomach gas, fatigue, rash, feelings of ill health, leg pains, sore throat, a bad taste in the mouth, sleeplessness, and fever.

Drug Interactions

• Cimetidine and Probenecid slow the rate at which Valacyclovir is converted to Acyclovir, but this does not change the drug's effectiveness. Valacyclovir dosage does not need to be changed if you are also taking those drugs.

• Cimetidine and Probenecid may decrease Acyclovir elimination from your body and increase drug blood levels, raising the chance of drug side effects.

• Taking Valacyclovir and Zidovudine (AZT) together may lead to severe drowsiness or lethargy.

Food Interactions

Valacyclovir may be taken without regard to food or meals.

Usual Dose

Adult: 1,000 mg 3 times a day for 7 days. The dose is lowered in people with kidney disease.

Overdosage

There have been no cases of Valacyclovir overdose. Acyclovir overdose, though, is likely to lead to kidney damage caused by the deposit of drug crystals in the kidney. Up to 4.8 grams of Acyclovir a day for 5 days has been taken without serious adverse effects.

Special Information

Treatment with Valacyclovir must be started as soon as possible after your shingles is diagnosed. All of the information on the effectiveness of this medicine was gathered from people who started treatment no more than 72 hours after diagnosis.

Women with genital herpes have an increased risk of cervical cancer. Check with your doctor about the need for an annual Pap smear.

Herpes can be transmitted even if you don't have symptoms of active disease. To avoid transmitting the condition to a sex partner, do not have intercourse while visible herpes lesions are present. A condom should protect against transmission of the virus, but spermicidal products or diaphragms won't. Acyclovir alone also does not protect against spreading the herpes virus.

Call your doctor if the drug does not relieve your condition, if side effects become severe or intolerable, or if you become pregnant or want to begin breast-feeding.

Check with your dentist or doctor about how to take care of your teeth if you notice swelling or tenderness of the gums.

Special Populations

Pregnancy/Breast-feeding

Acyclovir crosses into the circulation of a developing fetus. Animal studies of Acyclovir have shown that large doses (up to 125 times the human dose) caused damage to both mother and developing fetus. While there is no information to indicate that Acyclovir affects a developing baby, you should not use it during pregnancy unless it is specifically prescribed by your doctor and the benefit outweighs the possible risk of taking it. The manufacturer of this drug maintains a registry for pregnant women taking this drug to keep track of how it affects birth outcomes.

Nothing is known about the effects of Valacyclovir in nursing mothers, but Acyclovir passes into breast milk at concentrations up to 4 times the concentration in blood, and it has been found in the urine of a nursing infant. No drug side effects have been found in nursing babies, but mothers who must take Valacyclovir should consider bottle-feeding their infants.

```
Possible Side Effects (continued)
```
before the eyes, loss of muscle control or coordination,
and tremors.
   Side effects worsen as your Valproic Acid dose increases.

Drug Interactions

• Valproic Acid may increase the depressive effects of
alcohol, sleeping pills, tranquilizers, Phenobarbital, Primidone, and other depressant drugs.

• Dosages of Carbamazepine, Clonazepam, Ethosuximide,
or Phenytoin may have to be adjusted when you begin
Valproic Acid treatment.

• Valproic Acid may affect oral anticoagulant (blood-
thinning) drugs, such as Warfarin; your anticoagulant dose
may have to be adjusted.

• Aspirin, Cimetidine, and Chlorpromazine may increase
the chances of Valproic Acid side effects.

• Valproic Acid may increase the need for Levocarnitine.

• Valproic Acid may increase the risk of bleeding or bruising
if taken together with other drugs that affect platelet stickiness.
Some of these are Aspirin (also increases Valproic Acid side
effects), Dipyridamole, nonsteroidal anti-inflammatory drugs
(NSAIDs), Sulfinpyrazone, and Ticlopidine.

• Valproic Acid may cause false-positive reactions in ketone-
urine tests (used in diabetes).

Food Interactions

Food slightly prolongs the time it takes for Valproic Acid to be
absorbed into the bloodstream. Nevertheless, you may take it
with food if it upsets your stomach. Do not take Divalproex
(Depakote) with milk.

   Depakote Sprinkle Capsules can be taken whole or mixed
with a small amount (teaspoonful) of pudding, applesauce, or
other soft food. The food/drug mixture should be swallowed,
and not chewed, as soon as it is mixed.

   Mix Valproic Acid syrup with food to make it taste better.

Usual Dose

7 to 27 mg per pound per day. Valproic Acid is best taken in 1

dose at bedtime to minimize any sedation that might occur. Daily doses greater than 250 mg should be split into 2 or more doses per day.

Overdosage

Valproic Acid overdose can result in restlessness, hallucinations, flapping tremors of the hands, deep coma, or death. Call your doctor or take the victim to a hospital emergency room at once. ALWAYS bring the medicine bottle with you.

Special Information

This medicine may cause drowsiness: Be careful while driving or operating hazardous machinery.

Do not chew or crush Valproic Acid capsules or tablets.

Do not switch brands of Valproic Acid without your doctor's knowledge. In at least 1 case, seizures resulted when a person was switched to a new product after 3 seizure-free years on another brand of Valproic Acid.

Valproic Acid can cause mouth, gum, and throat irritation or bleeding, and carries an increased risk of mouth infections. People taking this medicine should pay special attention to caring for their mouth and gums. Dental work should be delayed if your blood counts are low.

People with a seizure disorder should carry special identification indicating their condition and the drug being taken.

If you take Valproic Acid once a day and forget a dose, take it as soon as possible. If you don't remember until the next day, skip the forgotten dose and continue with your regular schedule.

If you take the medicine 2 or more times per day and forget a dose, and you remember within 6 hours of your regular time, take it as soon as possible. Take the rest of that day's doses at regularly spaced time intervals. Go back to your regular schedule the next day. Do not take a double dose.

Special Populations

Pregnancy/Breast-feeding

Valproic Acid crosses into the fetal blood circulation and has caused birth defects in 1 to 2 percent of all women who take this drug during the first 3 months of pregnancy. However, most pregnant women who take Valproic Acid (as with most anticonvulsants) deliver healthy, normal babies. Anticonvulsants should be used only to control maternal seizures.

Valproic Acid passes into breast milk and may affect a nursing infant. Women who must take this drug should consider bottle-feeding their babies.

Seniors
Valproic Acid is broken down by the liver and passes out of the body through the kidneys. Because older adults tend to have reduced kidney and liver function, they often have more Valproic Acid in the bloodstream and are more likely to develop drug side effects; seniors should be treated with smaller doses of Valproic Acid.

Vancenase AQ

see **Corticosteroids, Nasal**, page 284

Vasotec

see **Enalapril**, page 389

Generic Name
Venlafaxine

Brand Name
Effexor

Type of Drug
Antidepressant.

Prescribed for
Depression.

General Information
Venlafaxine is chemically different from other antidepres-

sants. It is believed to work by affecting the ability of nerve endings in the brain to absorb serotonin, norepinephrine, and dopamine; it does not affect monoamine oxidase (MAO). Venlafaxine is well absorbed into the bloodstream and passes out of the body primarily via the urine.

Cautions and Warnings

People with **severe liver** or **kidney disease** may require smaller than usual doses of Venlafaxine because these conditions can cause blood levels of the drug to increase by 30 to 50 percent.

Venlafaxine **raises blood pressure**. If this happens, your dosage of Venlafaxine may have to be reduced. Venlafaxine has not been studied in people with a recent heart attack or unstable heart disease, though a small study of the cardiograms of such patients revealed no unusual changes.

Possible Side Effects

Many drug side effects increase as you increase the dosage of Venlafaxine.

▼ Most common: sleepiness, dry mouth, dizziness, sleeplessness, nervousness, tremors, weakness, sweating, nausea, constipation, loss of appetite, anorexia, vomiting, and impotence or abnormal ejaculation.

▼ Less common: changes in taste perception, ringing in the ears, dilated pupils, blurred vision, high blood pressure, rapid heartbeat, anxiety, reduced sex drive, agitation, chills, yawning, orgasm disturbance, dizziness when rising from a sitting or lying position, unusual dreams, muscle stiffness, tingling in the hands or feet, confusion, abnormal thinking, depression, urinary difficulties, twitching, chest pain, trauma, weight loss, itching, rash, diarrhea, upset stomach, gas, menstrual disturbances, and urinary difficulty.

▼ Rare: swelling, weight gain, a hangover-type reaction, hernia, unusual sensitivity to the sun, suicide attempts, appendicitis, thyroid changes, migraines, angina pains, heart rhythm changes, increased pulse rate, swallowing difficulty, stomach irritation, irritated or bleeding

---

Possible Side Effects *(continued)*

gums, salivation, soft stools, tongue discoloration, ulcers, reduced blood-cell counts, abnormal vision, ear pain, acne, hair loss, brittle nails, dry skin, herpes, and hairiness.

Drug Interactions

• People who take Venlafaxine within 2 weeks after taking an MAO inhibitor antidepressant may experience severe reactions, including high fever, muscle rigidity or spasm, mental changes, and fluctuations in pulse, temperature, or breathing rate. People stopping an MAO inhibitor should wait at least 2 weeks before starting Venlafaxine. People stopping Venlafaxine should wait at least 1 week before starting an MAO inhibitor drug.

• Cimetidine reduces the rate at which Venlafaxine is broken down in the body, and thus may increase drug levels in the blood, although the effect on your body may be minimal.

Food Interactions

Take each dose of Venlafaxine with food.

Usual Dose

Adult: 75 to 350 mg per day, divided into 2 or 3 doses. People with severe kidney or liver disease should receive half the usual daily dose. Those with moderate kidney disease may have their daily dose reduced by only 25 percent.

Child: not recommended for children under age 18.

Overdosage

Most people taking overdoses of Venlafaxine reported no symptoms, although some experienced fatigue. One person experienced mild convulsions and cardiac effects—contact your doctor or emergency room if you experience similar effects. People who take an overdose of Venlafaxine should be taken to a hospital emergency room for treatment. ALWAYS bring the medicine bottle with you.

Special Information

Call your doctor if you develop rash, hives, or any other allergic reaction.

Venlafaxine can make you tired. Avoid alcoholic beverages while taking Venlafaxine, and take care while performing complicated functions, driving, or operating complex equipment.

Contact your doctor or pharmacist if you are taking any other medicines, because of possible adverse drug interactions. If you forget to take a dose of Venlafaxine, take it as soon as you remember. If it is almost time for your next dose, skip the forgotten dose and continue with your regular schedule.

Do not suddenly discontinue this medicine. It is recommended that the dosage of Venlafaxine be gradually reduced over a 2-week period.

Special Populations

Pregnancy/Breast-feeding

Animal studies of Venlafaxine in doses 10 times larger than the maximum human dose caused low birth weight and deaths. No information is available on the effect of Venlafaxine on human pregnancy; it should be taken during pregnancy only if it is clearly needed.

It is not known if Venlafaxine or its breakdown products pass into breast milk; therefore, risks to the infant should be carefully weighed against the benefits to the mother. Nursing mothers should consider bottle-feeding with formula.

Seniors

Some older adults may be more sensitive to Venlafaxine's side effects.

Ventolin

see **Albuterol**, page 30

Possible Side Effects *(continued)*

weakness; swelling of the ankles, feet, or legs; headache; dizziness; light-headedness; constipation; and nausea.

▼ Rare: chest pain, rapid or irregular heartbeat, unusual production of breast milk, bleeding or tender gums, fainting, flushing or feeling warm.

Other rare side effects have affected a variety of body systems. Report anything unusual to your doctor.

In addition, some patients taking Verapamil have experienced heart attack and abnormal heart rhythms, but the occurrence of these effects has not been directly linked to Verapamil.

Drug Interactions

• Long-term Verapamil use will cause the levels of Digoxin and Digitoxin drugs in the blood to increase by 50 to 70 percent. The dose of these drugs will have to be drastically lowered if Verapamil is added.

• Disopyramide should not be taken within 48 hours of taking Verapamil, because of possible interaction.

• Patients taking Verapamil together with Quinidine may experience very low blood pressure, slow heartbeat, and fluid in the lungs.

• Verapamil's effectiveness and its side effects may be reversed by taking calcium products (including antacids).

• Verapamil may interact with beta-blocking drugs to cause heart failure, very low blood pressure, or increased angina pain. However, in many cases these drugs have been taken together with no problem. Low blood pressure can also result from taking Verapamil with Fentanyl, a narcotic pain reliever.

• Through interaction with other antihypertensive drugs, Verapamil may cause unexpected blood pressure reduction in patients already taking medicine to control their high blood pressure.

• Cimetidine and Ranitidine increase the amount of Verapamil in the blood and may account for a slight increase in its effect.

• The combination of Dantrolene and Verapamil can lead to high blood-calcium levels and heart muscle depression. If you are taking Dantrolene, a calcium channel blocker other than Verapamil should be precribed by your doctor.

• Verapamil can increase the effects of Carbamazepine, Cyclosporine, and Theophylline products, increasing the chance of side effects with those drugs.

• Verapamil may decrease the amount of Lithium in your body, leading to a possible loss of antimanic control, Lithium toxicity, and psychotic symptoms.

• Rifampin, barbiturates, Phenytoin and similar antiseizure medicines, vitamin D, and Sulfinpyrazone may decrease the amount of Verapamil in your blood and its effect on your body.

Food Interactions

Take regular Verapamil tablets at least 1 hour before or 2 hours after meals.

Sustained-release Verapamil products may be taken without regard to food or meals. Take them with food if they upset your stomach.

Usual Dose

120 to 480 mg a day, individualized to patient need.

Overdosage

Overdosage of Verapamil can cause low blood pressure. Symptoms are dizziness, weakness, and (possibly) slowed heartbeat. If you have taken an overdose of Verapamil, call your doctor or go to a hospital emergency room. ALWAYS bring the medicine bottle with you.

Special Information

Call your doctor if you develop abnormal heart rhythm, swelling in the arms or legs, difficulty breathing, increased heart pains, dizziness, light-headedness, or low blood pressure. Do not stop taking Verapamil abruptly.

If you forget to take a dose of Verapamil, take it as soon as you remember. If it is almost time for your next regularly scheduled dose, skip the one you forgot and continue with your regular schedule. Do not take a double dose.

Special Populations

Pregnancy/Breast-feeding

Verapamil may cause birth defects or interfere with your

baby's development. Check with your doctor before taking it if you are, or might be, pregnant.

Verapamil passes into breast milk. Taking Verapamil during nursing may cause problems; nursing mothers should take the drug only if absolutely necessary.

Seniors

Older adults are more sensitive to the side effects of Verapamil and are more likely to develop low blood pressure while taking it. Follow your doctor's directions and report any side effects at once.

Voltaren

see **Diclofenac**, page 321

Generic Name

Warfarin Sodium

Brand Names

Coumadin   Panwarfin   Sofarin

(Also available in generic form)

Type of Drug

Oral anticoagulant.

Prescribed for

Preventing the formation of blood clots or coagulation. Warfarin may also be prescribed to reduce the risk of recurring heart attack or stroke. It may be of benefit in preventing recurrent transient ischemic attacks (TIAs), in which blood flow to the brain is temporarily interrupted.

General Information

Anticoagulation (thinning of the blood) is generally a secondary way of preventing other diseases—including blood clots in the arms and legs, pulmonary embolism, heart attack, or abnormal heart rhythms—in which the formation of blood clots may cause serious problems. Anticoagulants work by suppressing the body's normal production of various factors that are essential to the coagulation mechanism. If you are taking Warfarin, you must take it exactly as prescribed. Notify your doctor at the earliest sign of unusual bleeding or bruising, passage of blood in your urine or stool, and/or passage of black tarry stool. Anticoagulant drug interactions are extremely important (see *Drug Interactions*).

Warfarin can be extremely dangerous if not used properly. Periodic blood tests to monitor clotting time or the time it takes to begin the clotting process are required for proper control of Warfarin therapy.

Cautions and Warnings

Warfarin must be taken with care if you have any **blood-clotting disease**. Other conditions in which the use of Warfarin should be discussed with your doctor are **threatened abortion, recent surgery, protein C deficiency** (a hereditary condition), **liver inflammation, kidney disease, infection, active tuberculosis, severe or prolonged dietary deficiencies, stomach ulcers, bleeding from the genital or urinary areas, moderate to severe high blood pressure, severe diabetes, vein irritation, disease of the large bowel** (such as diverticulitis or ulcerative colitis), and **subacute bacterial endocarditis**.

People taking Warfarin must be extremely careful to **avoid cuts or bruises**, or other injuries that might cause **internal or external bleeding.**

Possible Side Effects

▼ Most common: bleeding, which may occur within therapeutic dosage ranges and even when blood tests normally used to monitor anticoagulant therapy are within normal limits. If you bleed abnormally while you are taking anticoagulants and have eliminated the possibility of drug interactions, discuss this matter immediately with your doctor. Another underlying problem may be present.

Possible Side Effects *(continued)*

▼ Less common: abdominal cramps, nausea, vomiting, diarrhea, fever, anemia, adverse effects on blood components, hepatitis, jaundice (yellowing of the skin or eyes), itching, rash, hair loss, sore throat or mouth, red-orange urine, painful or persistent erection in males, and "purple-toes" syndrome.

Drug Interactions

• Warfarin and other oral anticoagulant drugs are probably involved in more drug interactions than any other kind of drug. Your doctor and pharmacist should have records of all medications you are taking in order to review for possible negative drug interactions.

• Drugs that may increase the effect of Warfarin include the following: Acetaminophen, aminoglycoside antibiotics, Amiodarone, androgens, Aspirin and other salicylate drugs, beta blockers, cephalosporin antibiotics, Chloral Hydrate, Chloramphenicol, Cimetidine, Clofibrate, corticosteroids, Cyclophosphamide, Dextrothyroxine, Diflunisal, Disulfiram, Erythromycin, Fluconazole, Gemfibrozil, Glucagon, hydantoin antiseizure drugs (blood levels of the hydantoins may also be increased in this interaction), Ifosfamide, influenza virus vaccine, Isoniazid, Ketoconazole, loop diuretics, Lovastatin, Metronidazole, Miconazole, mineral oil, Moricizine, Nalidixic Acid, nonsteroidal anti-inflammatory drugs (NSAIDs), Omeprazole, penicillins, Phenylbutazone, Propafenone, Propoxyphene, Quinidine, Quinine, quinolone antibacterials, Septra, sulfa drugs, Sulfinpyrazone, Tamoxifen, tetracycline antibiotics, Thioamines, thyroid hormones, and vitamin E.

• Some drugs decrease the effect of Warfarin, and the interaction can be just as dangerous. Some examples are alcohol (chronic alcoholism), Aminoglutethimide, Ascorbic Acid, barbiturates, Carbamazepine, Cholestyramine, Dicloxacillin, Glutethimide, Ethchlorvynol, Meprobamate, Griseofulvin, estrogens, oral contraceptives, Chlorthalidone, Nafcillin, Rifampin, Spironolactone, Sucralfate, thiazide diuretics, Trazodone, and vitamin K.

• No matter what the interaction, it is essential that your doctor and pharmacist know every medicine you are taking, including nonprescription drugs containing Aspirin. Consult your physician or pharmacist before buying any over-the-counter drugs.

Food Interactions

This medicine is best taken on an empty stomach because food slows the rate at which it is absorbed into the blood.

Vitamin K counteracts Warfarin. You should avoid eating large quantities of foods rich in vitamin K, such as green leafy vegetables. Also, any change in dietary habits or alcohol intake can affect Warfarin's action in your body.

Usual Dose

2 to 15 (or more) mg a day; dosage is variable and must be individualized by your doctor.

Overdosage

The primary symptom of overdosage is bleeding. Bleeding can make itself known by appearance of blood in the urine or stool, an unusual number of black-and-blue marks, oozing of blood from minor cuts, or bleeding from the gums after brushing the teeth. If bleeding does not stop within 10 to 15 minutes, call your doctor, who may tell you to skip a dose of anticoagulant or to go to a hospital or doctor's office where blood evaluations can be made; or your doctor may give you a prescription for vitamin K, which antagonizes the effect of Warfarin. This approach has some dangers because it can complicate subsequent anticoagulant therapy, but this is a decision that your doctor must make.

Special Information

Do not change Warfarin brands without your doctor's knowledge. Different brands of Warfarin may not be equivalent to each other and may not produce the same effect on your blood.

Do not stop taking your Warfarin unless directed to do so by your doctor. Be sure you have enough medicine when you travel or at other times when you might not have access to your regular pharmacy.

Do not stop or start any other medicine without your doctor's and/or pharmacist's knowledge. Avoid alcohol, Aspirin (and other salicylates), and drastic changes in your diet, since all of these can affect your response to Warfarin.

Call your doctor if you develop unusual bleeding or bruising; red or black tarry stool; or red or dark-brown urine. Warfarin can turn your urine a red-orange color. This is different from blood in the urine (red to brownish color) and generally happens only if your urine has less acid in it than normal.

If you forget to take a dose of Warfarin, take it as soon as you remember, then go back to your regular schedule. If you don't remember until the next day, skip the missed dose and continue with your regular schedule. Do not take a double dose. Doubling the dose may cause bleeding. Be sure to tell your doctor if you miss any doses.

Special Populations

Pregnancy/Breast-feeding

Warfarin should not be taken by pregnant women. If you are taking Warfarin and become pregnant, see your doctor immediately. Warfarin passes into the fetus and cause bleeding, brain and other abnormalities, and stilbirth in 30 percent of fetuses exposed to the drug.

In some pregnant women, the benefits to be gained from taking Warfarin (or another anticoagulant) may outweigh its possible negative effects, but the drug should not be taken during the first 3 months of pregnancy. The decision to use an anticoagulant is an important one that should be made by you and your doctor together. Often, pregnant women who need anticoagulant treatment are given Heparin (which must be injected) because it does not cross into the fetal blood system.

Warfarin passes into breast milk in an inactive form. Full-term babies are not affected, but the effect on premature babies is not known. You should bottle-feed your baby until you stop taking this drug.

Seniors

Older adults may be more sensitive to the effects of Warfarin and other anticoagulant drugs. The reasons for this are not clear but may have to do with a reduced ability to clear the drug from their bodies. Seniors generally require lower doses to achieve the same results.

Xanax

see **Alprazolam**, page 41

Type of Drug

Xanthine Bronchodilators

Brand Names

Generic Name: Aminophylline*
_____
Phyllocontin Controlled Release Tablets
Truphylline Suppositories

Generic Name: Dyphylline*
_____
Dilor Liquid/Tablets   Lufyllin Elixir/Tablets
Dyflex Tablets   Neothylline Tablets

Generic Name: Oxtriphylline*
_____
Choledyl Tablets/Elixir
Choledyl Syrup   🅐
Choledyl SA

Generic Name: Theophylline*
_____
Aquaphyllin   🅐   Slo-Phyllin   🅐
Asmalix   Theoclear   🅐
Bronkodyl   Theolair   🅐
Elixomin   Theostat
Elixophyllin

Timed-Release Products
_____
Aerolate Capsules   Theobid Jr.   Theophylline S.R.
Quibron-T/SR   Duracaps   Theo-Sav
  Dividose   Theochron   Theospan-SR
Respbid   Theoclear L.A.   Theo-X
Slo-bid   Theo-Dur   Theovent
  Gyrocaps   Theo-Dur Sprinkle   T-Phyl
Sustaire   Theolair-SR   Uniphyl
Theobid Duracaps

(*Also available in generic form)

Prescribed for

Relief of bronchial asthma and spasms of bronchial muscles

associated with emphysema, bronchitis, and other diseases. May also be prescribed to treat essential tremors and chronic obstructive pulmonary disease (COPD).

General Information

Xanthine bronchodilators are a mainstay of therapy for bronchial asthma and similar diseases. Although the dose of each of these drugs is different, they all work by relaxing bronchial muscles and helping reverse spasms in these muscles, though the exact way in which they work is not known.

Timed-release products allow the xanthine bronchodilators to act throughout the day, minimizing possible drug side effects by avoiding peaks and valleys associated with short-acting xanthine drugs. This also allows you to reduce the total number of daily doses.

The initial treatment with a xanthine bronchodilator requires your doctor to take blood samples to assess how much of the drug is in your blood. For Theophylline, the standard against which all other members of the group are compared, a level of between 10 and 20 micrograms per milliliter (quantity per blood volume) is generally considered desirable. For Dyphylline, the minimum effective level is 12 micrograms per milliliter. Dosage adjustments may be required based on these blood tests and your response to the therapy.

Because Dyphylline is not eliminated by the liver, it is not subject to many of the drug interactions or limitations placed on the other xanthine bronchodilators. However, dosage must be altered in the presence of kidney failure.

Cautions and Warnings

Do not use a xanthine bronchodilator if you are **allergic** or **sensitive** to any of these medicines. If you have a **stomach ulcer, congestive heart failure, heart disease, liver disease, low blood-oxygen levels,** or **high blood pressure,** or are an **alcoholic,** you should use this drug with caution. People with **seizure disorders** should not take a xanthine bronchodilator unless they are receiving appropriate anticonvulsant medicines. **Theophylline** may cause or worsen preexisting abnormal heart rhythms. Any **change in heart rate or rhythm** warrants your doctor's immediate attention.

Status asthmaticus, a medical condition in which the breathing passages are virtually completely closed, does not respond to oral bronchodilators. Victims of this condition must be taken to a hospital emergency room at once for treatment. Serious side effects, including **convulsions, serious arrhythmias,** and **death,** may be among the initial signs of drug toxicity. Periodic monitoring by your physician is mandatory if you are taking one of these medicines.

Possible Side Effects

Drug side effects are directly related to the amount of drug in your blood. As long as you stay in the proper range (below 20 micrograms per milliliter of blood), you should experience few, if any, problems.

The first side effects you may experience when you exceed this level are nausea, vomiting, stomach pain, diarrhea, irritability, restlessness, and difficulty sleeping. Other possible drug side effects include rectal irritation or bleeding (especially with suppositories) and rapid breathing.

As drug levels increase (over 35 micrograms per milliliter), you may experience excitability, high blood sugar, muscle twitching or spasms, heart palpitations, seizures, brain damage, or death.

▼ Rare: vomiting blood, regurgitating stomach contents while lying down, fever, headache, rash, hair loss, and dehydration.

Drug Interactions

- Taking two xanthine bronchodilators together may increase side effects.
- Xanthine bronchodilators are often given in combination with a stimulant drug, such as Ephedrine. Such combinations can cause excessive stimulation and should be used only as specifically directed by your doctor.
- Reports have indicated that combining Erythromycin, flu vaccine, Allopurinol, beta blockers, calcium channel blockers, Cimetidine (and, rarely, Ranitidine), oral contraceptives, corticosteroids, Disulfiram, Ephedrine, Interferon, Mexiletine, quinolone antibacterials, or Thiabendazole with a xanthine bronchodilator will increase blood levels of the xanthine

bronchodilator. Higher blood levels mean the possibility of more side effects. Tetracycline may also increase the chances for xanthine bronchodilator side effects.

• The following drugs may decrease Theophylline levels: Aminoglutethimide, barbiturates, charcoal, Phenytoin and other hydantoin anticonvulsants (the hydantoin level may also be reduced), Ketoconazole, Rifampin, Sulfinpyrazone, and sympathomimetic drugs.

• Smoking cigarettes or marijuana makes xanthine bronchodilators (except Dyphylline) less effective by increasing the rate at which your liver breaks them down.

• Drugs that may either increase or decrease xanthine bronchodilator levels include Carbamazepine, Isoniazid, and Furosemide and other loop diuretics. Persons combining a xanthine bronchodilator with one of these drugs must be evaluated individually. Again, consult your doctor when combining xanthine bronchodilators with any of these drugs.

• People with an overactive thyroid clear xanthine bronchodilators faster and may require a larger dose. People with an underactive thyroid have the opposite reaction. Normalizing thyroid function through medical or surgical treatment will normalize your response to a xanthine bronchodilator.

• A xanthine bronchodilator may counteract the sedative effect of Valium and other benzodiazepine tranquilizers.

• Xanthine bronchodilators may interfere with or interact with a number of different drugs used during anesthesia. Your doctor may temporarily alter your bronchodilator dose or change drugs to avoid this problem.

• Blood-lithium levels may be lowered by xanthine bronchodilators.

• Probenecid may increase the effects of Dyphylline by interfering with its removal from the body through the kidneys.

• Xanthine bronchodilators may counteract the sedative effects of Propofol.

Food Interactions

To obtain a consistent effect from your medicine, take it at the same time each day on an empty stomach (at least 1 hour before or 2 hours after meals).

Theophylline is eliminated from the body faster if your diet is high in protein and low in carbohydrates. Eating charcoal-broiled beef also has this effect. On the other hand, the rate at which your body eliminates Theophylline is reduced by a high-carbohydrate, low-protein diet. You may take some food with a liquid or non–sustained-release xanthine bronchodilator if it upsets your stomach. Dyphylline is not affected in this way.

Caffeine (a xanthine derivative) may add to the side effects of the xanthine bronchodilators, except Dyphylline. Avoid large amounts of caffeine-containing products such as coffee, tea, cola, cocoa, and chocolate, while taking one of these drugs.

Usual Dose

Aminophylline
Each 100 mg of Aminophylline is equal in potency to 79 mg of Theophylline. Aminophylline dosage is calculated on the basis of Theophylline equivalents and must be tailored to your specific condition. The best dose for you is the lowest dose that will control your symptoms.

Adult: 100 to 200 mg every 6 hours.

Child (up to age 16): 50 to 100 mg every 6 hours, or 1 to 2.5 mg per pound of body weight every 6 hours.

Timed-Release Products
1 to 3 times per day, based on your symptoms and response to treatment. Usual dose is 200 to 500 mg per day.

Dyphylline
There is no established Theophylline equivalent dosage for Dyphylline. The usual dose is up to 7 mg per pound of body weight 4 times per day. Dosage must be reduced in the presence of kidney failure. Dyphylline dosage must be tailored to your specific condition. The best dose is the lowest that will control your symptoms.

Oxtriphylline
Each 100 mg of Oxtriphylline is roughly equal to 64 mg of Theophylline. Oxtriphylline dosage is calculated on the basis of Theophylline equivalents and must be tailored to your specific condition.

Adult: about 2 mg per pound of body weight, 3 times per day. Sustained Action (SA): 400 to 600 mg every 12 hours.

Child (age 1 to 9): 2.8 mg for every pound of body weight taken 4 times per day.

Theophylline

These dosage guidelines may seem backward because children (1 year and older) require more drug per pound of body weight than adults. This is because children metabolize (chemically change) xanthine bronchodilators faster than adults do.

Adult: up to 6 mg per pound of body weight per day, to a maximum daily dose of 900 mg.

Adolescent (age 12 to 16): up to 8.1 mg per pound of body weight per day.

Child (age 9 to 11): up to 9 mg per pound of body weight per day.

Child (age 1 to 9): up to 10.9 mg per pound of body weight per day.

Infant (6 to 52 weeks): The total daily dose in mg is calculated by the following: 0.2 times age in weeks + 5. Up to 6 months, give ⅓ the total dose every 8 hours. From age 26 weeks to 1 year, divide the daily total into 4 doses.

Premature Infant (25 days or older): 0.68 mg per pound of body weight every 12 hours.

Premature Infant (24 days or younger): 0.45 mg per pound of body weight every 12 hours.

Timed-release products are usually taken 1 to 3 times per day at the same dose, depending on your response.

The best dose of xanthine bronchodilators is that which is tailored to your condition and is the lowest dose that will produce maximum control of your symptoms.

Overdosage

The first symptoms of overdosage are loss of appetite, nausea, vomiting, nervousness, difficulty sleeping, headache, and restlessness, followed by rapid or abnormal heart rhythms, unusual behavior patterns, extreme thirst, delirium, convulsions, very high temperature, and collapse. These serious toxic symptoms are rarely experienced after overdose by mouth, which produces loss of appetite, nausea, vomiting, and stimulation. The overdose victim should be taken to a hospital emergency room immediately. ALWAYS bring the medicine bottle with you.

Special Information

Do not chew or crush coated or sustained-release capsules or tablets before you take them. This could result in the immediate release of large amounts of medicine, which can cause serious drug side effects.

To ensure consistent effectiveness, take your medicine at the same time and in the same way each day (with or without food).

Call your doctor if you develop nausea, vomiting, heartburn or vomiting, sleeplessness, jitteriness, restlessness, headache, rash, severe stomach pain, convulsions, or a rapid or irregular heartbeat. Serious side effects, including convulsions, serious arrhythmias, and death, may be the first signs of drug toxicity. Periodic monitoring by your physician is mandatory if you are taking one of these medicines.

Do not change bronchodilator drug brands without notifying your doctor or pharmacist. Different brands of the same xanthine bronchodilator may not be identical in their effect on your body.

If you forget to take a dose of your xanthine bronchodilator, take it as soon as you remember. If it is almost time for your next dose, skip the one you forgot and continue with your regular schedule. Do not take a double dose.

Special Populations

Pregnancy/Breast-feeding

Xanthine bronchodilators pass into the circulation of the developing baby. They do not cause birth defects but may result in dangerous drug levels in the infant's bloodstream. Babies born to mothers taking this medication may be nervous, jittery, and irritable, and may gag or vomit when fed. Women who must use this medication to control asthma or other conditions should talk with their doctor about the relative risks of using this medication versus its benefits.

These drugs pass into breast milk and it may cause a nursing infant to be nervous or irritable, or to have difficulty sleeping. Nursing mothers who must use one of these drugs should bottle-feed their babies.

Seniors

Older adults (especially men age 55 and older) may take longer to clear the xanthine bronchodilators from their bodies

People taking Zalcitabine should take care of their teeth and gums to minimize the possibility of oral infections.

Call your doctor if you develop any of the following symptoms of Zalcitabine drug toxicity: numbness and burning pain in the hands and feet, sharp shooting pains or a severe and continuous burning pain, nausea, vomiting, or abdominal pain.

If you forget to take a dose of Zalcitabine, take it as soon as you remember. If it is almost time for your next dose, space the missed dose and your next dose by 2 to 4 hours, then continue your regular schedule. Call your doctor for more specific advice if you forget to take several doses.

Special Populations

Pregnancy/Breast-feeding

In animal studies, Zalcitabine caused the development of malformed fetuses. There are no studies of pregnant women taking this medication. Women who are, or might become, pregnant should use effective contraception while taking this medicine.

It is not known if Zalcitabine passes into breast milk. HIV-infected women who must take this medication should bottle-feed their babies.

Seniors

People with reduced kidney function, including older adults, should receive smaller doses of Zalcitabine than those with normal kidneys.

Zantac

see **Ranitidine**, page 984

Zestril

see **Lisinopril**, page 599

Generic Name

Zidovudine

Brand Name

Retrovir
(Also known as AZT, Azidothymidine, and Compound S)

(Also available in generic form)

Type of Drug

Antiviral.

Prescribed for

HIV infection.

General Information

Zidovudine was the first drug approved for use in the United States under a special government program for drugs considered essential for the treatment of specific diseases. Drugs in this program are released to the public before they have been completely tested for safety and effectiveness because of the concern for the severity of the disease they are designed to treat. Zidovudine inhibits the production of several viruses, including the AIDS virus. It works by interfering with specific enzymes within the virus that are responsible for essential steps in the virus' reproduction process. It has been generally recognized that Zidovudine helps people with AIDS to live longer, but an international study of AIDS patients questions this claim. Treatment recommendations emphasize that Zidovudine be used to fight the HIV virus only in the later stages of the illness, when symptoms develop and CD4 cell counts are below 500. CD4 cells are an important part of the immune system, and the numbers of such cells in the blood are widely regarded as an indication of the severity of the disease; fewer cells usually indicate a more serious disease. Early treatment of HIV-positive patients who do not have symptoms of the disease are now focused on general health measures and supportive therapies. The true safety and effectiveness of this drug after prolonged use, and in people with less-advanced disease, are not known.

Cautions and Warnings

Zidovudine can cause severe **reductions in white- and red-blood-cell counts** and should be taken with caution by people with **bone-marrow disease** or those whose bone marrow has already been compromised by other treatments. Your doctor should take a blood count every 2 weeks; if problems develop, the dosage should be reduced.

In rare instances, people taking Zidovudine or other nucleoside-type antivirals have developed a possibly fatal condition known as *lactic acidosis,* a disorder of metabolism. Possible signs of this are **unexplained rapid breathing, breathing difficulty,** and **reduced blood bicarbonate level** (your doctor can tell this with a routine blood test).

People with **impaired kidney** or **liver function** should use this drug with caution.

Prolonged use of Zidovudine can cause **muscle irritation** and **abnormalities** similar to those caused by HIV infection.

Possible Side Effects

In adults
▼ Most common: anemia, reduced white-blood-cell count, headache, nausea, sleeplessness, and muscle aches.

▼ Less common: body odor, chills, flu-like symptoms, greater susceptibility to feeling pain, back pains, chest pains, swelling of the lymph nodes, flushing and warmth, constipation, difficulty swallowing, swelling of the lips and tongue, bleeding gums, mouth sores, stomach gas, flatulence, bleeding from the rectum, joint pains, muscle spasms, tremors, twitching, anxiety, confusion, depression, emotional flare-ups, dizziness, fainting, loss of mental sharpness, cough, nosebleeds, runny nose, sinus inflammation, hoarseness, acne, itching, rash, double vision, sensitivity to bright lights, hearing loss, painful or difficult urination, and frequent urination.

In children
▼ Most common: anemia, reduced white-blood-cell counts, vomiting, abdominal pains, fever, and sleeplessness.

Possible Side Effects *(continued)*

▼ Less common: headache, blood infection, nervousness, and irritability.

▼ Rare: nausea, diarrhea, weight loss, seizures, heart failure and other cardiac abnormalities, blood in the urine, and bladder infections.

Drug Interactions

• Combining Zidovudine with other drugs that can damage your kidneys (Pentamidine, Dapsone, Amphotericin B, Flucytosine, Vincristine, Vinblastine, Adriamycin, and Alpha- and Beta-Interferon) will increase the chance of loss of some kidney function.

• Probenecid may reduce the rate at which your body eliminates this drug, increasing the amount of drug in your blood and the chances for drug side effects. Other drugs that can reduce the liver's ability to break down Zidovudine are Acetaminophen, Aspirin, Indomethacin, and Trimethoprim; any of these combinations can lead to increased drug toxicity.

• Acyclovir, often used in combination with Zidovudine to combat opportunistic infections in AIDS victims, may cause lethargy or seizure when taken together with Zidovudine.

• Other drugs that can cause anemia, including Ganciclovir or Zalcitabine, should be used carefully in combination with Zidovudine because of the chance of worsening any drug-related anemia.

• Taking Zidovudine together with Rifampin or Rifampicin can reduce the amount of Zidovudine absorbed into the blood.

• Taking Phenytoin and Zidovudine together can affect the amounts of both drugs in the blood, usually increasing the amount of Zidovudine. But the effect on Phenytoin is variable. People have had both too much Phenytoin (leading to side effects) and too little Phenytoin (possibly increasing the number of seizures). Your doctor should check Phenytoin levels if you are also taking Zidovudine.

Food Interactions

This medicine is best taken on an empty stomach, but you may take it with food if it upsets your stomach.

Usual Dose

Adult: for symptomatic AIDS, 100 mg every 4 hours around the clock, even if sleep is interrupted. Your dosage may be reduced if signs of drug toxicity develop. Asymptomatic AIDS may be treated with 100 mg every 4 hours during waking hours.

When given as combination therapy with Zalcitabine: 200 mg of Zidovudine with 0.8 mg of Zalcitabine every 8 hours.

Pregnant women (to prevent infecting the developing baby with HIV) after 14 weeks of pregnancy: 100 mg 5 times a day until labor starts. During labor and delivery, the drug should be given intravenously until the umbilical cord is clamped.

Child (3 months to 12 years): up to 100 mg every 6 hours.

Infant: about 1 mg per pound every 6 hours by mouth, starting within 12 hours of birth and continuing through 6 weeks of age. The drug can be given intravenously if needed.

Overdosage

The most serious effect of drug overdose is suppression of the bone marrow and its ability to make red and white blood cells. Overdose victims should be taken to a hospital emergency room at once. ALWAYS bring the medicine bottle with you.

Special Information

This drug does not cure AIDS, nor does it decrease the chance of your transmitting the virus to another person. Zidovudine may not prevent some illnesses associated with AIDS or AIDS-related complex (ARC) from continuing to develop.

See your doctor if any significant change in your health occurs. Periodic blood counts are very important while taking Zidovudine to detect possibly serious side effects. Avoid Acetaminophen, Aspirin, and other drugs that can increase Zidovudine toxicity.

Be sure to take this drug exactly as prescribed (around the clock if needed) even though it will interfere with your sleep. Do not take more than your doctor has prescribed.

People taking Zidovudine must take especially good care of their teeth and gums to minimize the chance of developing oral infections.

If you miss a dose of Zidovudine, take it as soon as

possible. If it is almost time for your next dose, space the missed dose and your next dose by 2 to 4 hours, and then continue with your regular schedule.

Protect Zidovudine capsules and liquid from light.

Special Populations

Pregnancy/Breast-feeding

HIV-positive women should be sure to use effective contraception to avoid infecting an unborn child. However, if you are HIV-positive and pregnant, talk to your doctor about taking or continuing your Zidovudine. Treating HIV-infected pregnant women with Zidovudine has been shown to sharply reduce the chances of transmitting the HIV virus to their babies. Treatment should begin by the 14th week of pregnancy and continue through delivery. The baby should also get Zidovudine for the first 6 weeks of life. These studies have also shown that the risk of birth defects is not increased by taking Zidovudine during pregnancy.

It is not known if Zidovudine passes into breast milk. Nursing mothers who are HIV-positive should bottle-feed their babies to avoid transmitting the virus.

Seniors

Older adults may be at a greater risk of Zidovudine side effects because of reduced kidney function.

Zithromax

see **Azithromycin**, page 106

Zocor

see **Simvastatin**, page 1019

Zoloft

see **Sertraline Hydrochloride**, page 1015

Generic Name

Zolpidem

Brand Name

Ambien

Type of Drug

Sedative.

Prescribed for

Insomnia.

General Information

Zolpidem is a nonbenzodiazepine sleeping pill that works in the brain in much the same way as benzodiazepine sleeping pills and tranquilizers. Unlike the benzodiazepines, however, Zolpidem has little muscle-relaxing or antiseizure effect. It is meant for short-term (7 to 10 days) use and should not be taken regularly for longer than that without your doctor's knowledge, although it has been studied for longer periods of time. Unlike the benzodiazepines, Zolpidem causes little or no hangover, nor are there any rebound effects on nights following treatment when you do not take any medication. Zolpidem has only a minimal effect on sleep stages, especially the all-important rapid eye movement (REM) sleep stage, in which many important functions are accomplished, including dreaming. Zolpidem is broken down in the liver.

Cautions and Warnings

Sleeping problems are often part of a physical or psychological illness. Drugs like Zolpidem may treat the symptom (sleeplessness) but do not affect the underlying reason why you can't sleep. They should be taken only with your doctor's knowledge. If you still cannot sleep after 7 to 10 days of taking Zolpidem, it may mean that the basic problem is getting worse and that you should see your doctor for other treatment.

Zolpidem has little effect on memory, unlike some of the short-acting benzodiazepine sleeping pills. It has caused some amnesia (memory loss), but this happens mostly at doses larger than 10 mg a night.

Suddenly stopping Zolpidem after having taken it for some time may produce drug withdrawal symptoms (fatigue, nausea, flushing, light-headedness, crying, vomiting, stomach cramps, panic, nervousness, and general discomfort). Other more serious signs of drug withdrawal (not feeling well, sleeplessness, muscle cramps, abdominal cramps, increased sweating, tremors, and convulsions) have not been seen after sudden withdrawal from Zolpidem. People with a history of substance abuse may be **more** likely to develop drug dependence on Zolpidem.

Zolpidem has all the effects of other nervous-system depressants and can cause loss of coordination and concentration. It should be taken **only before bedtime** and never if you need to do something that requires complete concentration. There is a possibility that activities to be performed on the day following a Zolpidem dose could also be affected, especially if alcohol was taken together with Zolpidem.

People with **liver disease** are much more sensitive to the effects of Zolpidem and need less medicine to produce the same effect as people with normal liver function. People with **severe kidney disease** should be watched for any unusual drug effect, but that has not occurred so far.

Other conditions with which Zolpidem should be avoided are **severe depression**, **severe lung disease**, **sleep apnea** (intermittent breathing while sleeping), and **drunkenness**. In these conditions, the depressive effects of Zolpidem may be increased and/or could be detrimental to your overall condition.

Possible Side Effects

▼ Most common: during short-term use (up to 10 days), drowsiness, dizziness, and diarrhea. With longer-term use (28 to 35 days), the most common side effects are drowsiness and a feeling of being drugged. Other common side effects of long-term use are headache, allergy symptoms, back pain, flulike symptoms, lethargy, sensitivity to light, depression, upset stomach, constipation, abdominal pain, muscle and joint pains, upper respi-

---

Possible Side Effects *(continued)*

ratory infection, sinus irritation, sore throat, rash, urinary infection, heart palpitations, and dry mouth.

▼ Less common: chest pain, fatigue, unusual dreaming, memory loss, anxiety, nervousness, sleeping difficulties, appetite loss, vomiting, and runny nose (long-term).

▼ Rare: numerous, involving almost any part of your body.

Drug Interactions

• Zolpidem is a central-nervous-system depressant. Avoid alcohol because its effects and those of Zolpidem compound each other. Other nervous-system depressants, including tranquilizers, narcotics, barbiturates, monoamine oxidase (MAO) inhibitors, antihistamines, and antidepressants, may have a similar effect. Taking a benzodiazepine, such as Diazepam, with Zolpidem may result in excessive depression, tiredness, sleepiness, difficulty breathing, or similar symptoms.

Food Interactions

For the most rapid and complete effect, take Zolpidem on an empty stomach, at least 2 hours after a meal.

Usual Dose

Adult (age 18 and older): 10 mg immediately before bedtime.

Senior and those with severe liver disease: 5 mg immediately before bedtime.

Child: do not use.

Overdosage

Zolpidem overdose results in excessive nervous-system depression, from unconsciousness to light coma. Combining Zolpidem with alcohol or other nervous-system depressants could be fatal or affect other body organs. Zolpidem overdose victims should be taken to a hospital emergency room at once. ALWAYS bring the medicine bottle.

Special Information

Zolpidem can cause tiredness, drowsiness, and the inability to concentrate. Be careful if you are driving, operating machinery, or performing other activities that require concentration on the day following a Zolpidem dose.

People taking Zolpidem on a regular basis may develop drug-withdrawal reactions if the medication is stopped suddenly (see *Cautions and Warnings*).

If you forget a dose of Zolpidem, take it as soon as you remember. If it is almost time for your next dose, skip the forgotten one and continue with your regular schedule. Do not take a double dose.

Special Populations

Pregnancy/Breast-feeding

Animal studies with large doses show that Zolpidem could affect a developing fetus. Because there is no reliable information about its effect during pregnancy, it should be used only if it is clearly needed.

Small amounts of Zolpidem pass into breast milk, but its effect on a nursing infant is not known. If you must take this medicine, you should bottle-feed your baby.

Seniors

Seniors are likely to be more sensitive to the effects of Zolpidem and its side effects. Seniors should take the lowest effective dose. Report any unusual side effects to your doctor.

Drugs and . . .

DRUGS AND ALCOHOL

Drug interactions with alcohol, itself a potent drug, are an important problem and can be experienced by anyone. Many over-the-counter medicines are alcohol-based and have the potential to interact with prescription drugs. Alcohol may be used to dissolve the active drugs, or to enhance or provide a sedative effect. Alcohol is found in most decongestant cold-suppressing mixtures, although many others are alcohol free. Your pharmacist can tell you which liquid medicines contain alcohol and which are alcohol free, and the symbol Ⓐ will tell you which liquid medicines listed in *The Pill Book* do not contain alcohol.

In the body, alcohol simply functions as a depressant of the central nervous system, and can either increase or decrease the effect of a drug on the nervous system. In some drug/alcohol interactions, the amount of alcohol consumed may not be as important as the chemical reaction it causes in your body. Small amounts of alcohol can cause excess stomach secretions, while larger amounts can *inhibit* stomach secretions, eroding the stomach's lining. For seniors, the use of over-the-counter alcohol-based products is especially dangerous, since their systems may be more sensitive to alcohol. People with stomach disorders, such as peptic or gastric ulcer, should be fully aware of the alcohol levels in products they use.

Alcohol does not interact with every medicine. When it

does, the effects of alcohol on your prescription can be found in the *Drug Interactions* section of each pill profile.

DRUGS AND FOOD

Foods can interfere with the ability of drugs to be absorbed into the blood through the gastrointestinal system. For this reason, most medications are best taken at least 1 hour before or 2 hours after meals, unless specific characteristics of the drug dictate that it should be taken with or immediately following meals. Each pill profile contains a *Food Interactions* section that tells you the best time to take your medicine and what foods, if any, to avoid while taking it. Check with your doctor or pharmacist if you are unsure about how best to take your medicine.

Some drugs should be taken with meals because food reduces the amount of drug-related stomach irritation. However, food can also interfere with a drug by reducing the amount of medication available to be absorbed into the bloodstream. For example, juice or milk taken to help you swallow a drug may interfere with the medicine's passage into the bloodstream. Milk or milk products (like cheese or ice cream) can interfere with the absorption of some drugs because they form a complex with the drug and prevent it from being absorbed into the blood.

Drugs can also affect your appetite. Some medicines that can stimulate your appetite include tricyclic antidepressants and phenothiazine tranquilizers. Drugs that can cause you to lose your appetite include antibiotics (especially Penicillin) and any medication that can cause nausea and/or vomiting.

Many drugs can interfere with the normal absorption of one or more body nutrients, including antacids, anticholinergics, (e.g., Atropine), anticonvulsants, barbiturates, cathartics (laxatives), Chloramphenicol, Clofibrate, Colchicine, Glutethimide, Isoniazid, Methotrexate, Neomycin Sulfate, oral contraceptives, and sulfa drugs.

DRUGS AND SEXUAL ACTIVITY

Sexual activity is usually not limited by drugs; however, some drugs can have an effect on sex drive, and can cause impotence, difficulty in getting or keeping an erection, or retrograde ejaculation (where ejaculation goes in the wrong direction) in men. This is especially true for men taking certain high-blood-pressure drugs, beta blockers, and antidepressants, which affect the central nervous and/or circulatory systems. It's important to discuss such effects with your doctor: A simple reduction in dosage or change to another drug in the same class may help you to deal with the problem. Each pill profile in *The Pill Book* will tell you if the medicine will affect you sexually.

DRUGS AND PREGNANCY

People are acutely aware of the potential damage drugs can cause to a developing fetus. In order for a drug to affect the fetus, it must cross from the mother's bloodstream into the fetal blood circulation. This process is made more difficult by the placenta, but it is possible for drugs to pass into the fetal bloodstream. Once in the fetal bloodstream, a drug may affect any of the normal fetal growth and development processes. Because a fetus grows much more rapidly than a fully developed human, the effects of any drug on these processes are exaggerated. The results of these effects can range from mild physical changes to death.

Most doctors tell pregnant and nursing women to avoid all unnecessary medicine, including simple pain relievers like Aspirin, and suggest that pregnant women use only vitamins or iron supplements, and limit tobacco and caffeine intake. Unfortunately, the chances of damage to a fetus are usually greatest during the first 3 months of pregnancy, when a woman may not even be aware that she is pregnant. If you are considering becoming pregnant, curtail drug use immediately, and discuss it fully with your doctor.

Drinking alcoholic beverages during pregnancy is associated with a set of effects on the newborn called *fetal alcohol syndrome*. Nobody knows how little alcohol a woman must drink before these problems will develop. To be safe, don't drink at all during pregnancy.

The Food and Drug Administration has classified all prescription drugs according to their safety for use during pregnancy. Every profile in *The Pill Book* contains information on drug safety for pregnant and nursing women.

DRUGS AND CHILDREN

Medicine should be given to children only on direct orders from a pediatrician or other doctor. Of course, children suffer from colds and runny noses, and there are many widely used over-the-counter medicines. Parents should be aware of the ingredients in such products (including alcohol, if any) and possible side effects.

Infants and young children are at greater risk than adults for experiencing drug side effects and interactions because their body systems are not fully developed. Some drugs, like the tetracyclines, have been linked to important side effects in young children and should be avoided completely. It's wise to ask your doctor whether side effects, such as fever or rash, are to be expected when a drug is prescribed for a child.

Drug doses for children are usually lower and are often determined by body weight or, in a few cases, by body surface area. In the past several years, the Food and Drug Administration has encouraged drug manufacturers to study the effects of their medicines on children and submit their research for government evaluation. This has resulted in many more medicines being officially approved for use in children, even though they have been widely used in children for years. Be sure you know all there is to know about a drug before you give it to your child. Check with your doctor or pharmacist about over-the-counter medicines unless you've used them before and know they can't interact with any other drugs your child is taking.

DRUGS AND SENIORS

Body changes caused by age or disease make older adults three times as likely to suffer an adverse drug reaction, such as nausea, dizziness, blurred vision, etc, than younger people. Drug interactions are another potential source of danger for seniors. Since many older adults take more than one medicine, their potential for drug interaction is much greater. Older adults often suffer from silent, undetected reactions caused by slowly building amounts of drugs that are not being properly metabolized by older, less efficient systems. Two thirds of people over the age of 65 take prescription drugs regularly; in fact, 30 to 35 percent of all prescriptions are filled for older adults, who make up only 15 percent of the population. Many spend hundreds of dollars each year to obtain an average of 13 prescriptions. The 1.5 million seniors in nursing homes are also at great risk for drug interactions: 54 percent of them take 6 or more pills per day, and some receive as many as 23!

Studies have shown that 70 to 90 percent of seniors take pills and over-the-counter medicines with little knowledge of their dangerous effects. Older adults may develop speech or hearing problems, be absentminded, or experience other symptoms we attribute to aging when they are really suffering from drug reactions. This condition has been called *reversible dementia.*

Seniors are often victims of overdose, and not necessarily because of mistaken dosages. Often body weight fluctuations and normal changes in body composition lead to overdose unless the dosage of a drug is altered accordingly.

It's important to make sure that older adults understand their drugs as completely as possible. Follow the tips for safe drug use found on pages 1211 and 1212 to help an older person manage his or her medicines properly. Develop a simple drug control system that lists the pills prescribed, the sequence in which they should be taken, the time of day, how they should be taken, and a place to indicate what was taken. Every pill profile in *The Pill Book* contains drug information for seniors.

DRUGS AND AIDS

AIDS is the most important infectious disease in the world, with Africa being the hardest hit. About 170,000 people are now living with AIDS in the United States and a million more Americans are infected with the human immunodeficiency virus (HIV). Many patients develop one or more symptoms of AIDS within 7 years of the initial infection, though 10 or more years can pass until the immune system is suppressed so much that problems develop. Despite the progress made in understanding AIDS and the HIV virus, it is estimated that fewer than 15 percent of people with AIDS live for more than 3 years after developing full-blown symptoms.

HIV attaches to white blood cells called helper T cells, which carry a protein known as CD4. The virus also attaches to other important white-blood-cell elements. HIV infects a wide variety of other cells, but CD4 cell counts are important because the number of CD4 cells serves as a direct indicator of the progress of the disease, the patient's condition, and the need for drug treatment. Once diagnosed by a series of skin and blood tests, including CD4 cell counts, treatment for AIDS or one of its many associated diseases or complications may be started.

Anti-HIV Therapy

As of this writing, five drugs are approved for use as anti-HIV agents: Lamivudine (3TC), Zidovudine (AZT), Stavudine (d4T), Zalcitabine (ddC), and Didanosine (ddI). (Information on these antivirals can be found in their individual pill profiles.) A new class of anti-HIV drugs, protease inhibitors, work by a different method than the older agents. The first of these, Saquinavir, has been approved, and others are on the way. The protease inhibitors work very well when taken with Zidovudine or another of the older medicines. It is reasonable to expect that additional agents with anti-HIV effects, including indinavir (Crixivan), ritonavir, AzdU, and others, will also be approved to treat the virus as time passes. Until then, they may be available under research protocols to limited numbers of people with AIDS. The most interesting development in anti-HIV therapy is combining antiviral drugs to obtain an improved effect. Some of the combinations that have been used are Lamivudine plus Zidovudine (probably the best of the combination therapies), Zalcitabine plus Zidovudine, and Zerit plus Lamivudine. Saquinavir is intended for use only in combination with another medicine. Typically, combination therapy is considered if the patient can't tolerate Zidovudine, if his or her T-cell count continues to go down despite therapy, or if his or her viral load increases substantially.

Antiviral agents can affect white- and red-blood-cell production in the body, and are often given together with other drugs intended to raise cell counts and extend the time that the antiviral drug can be taken. Erythropoietin may be given by injection to raise red-blood-cell levels, and drugs known as colony-stimulating factors (G-CSF and GM-CSF) may be given to raise white-blood-cell counts. Ganciclovir and TMP/SMZ, treatments for some complications of AIDS, may interact with Zidovudine to increase its negative effects on red and white blood cells. For this reason, other treatments may be used, or a decision may be made to stop Zidovudine treatment for a time. Foscarnet, another treatment for complications of AIDS, does not worsen the effects of these antiviral drugs on blood cells and may be used with them.

Complications of AIDS

Because of its effect on the human immune system, AIDS exposes patients to a variety of bacterial and fungal infections that non-AIDS patients can easily fight on their own. These are known as *opportunistic conditions:* They flourish because of the opportunity they find in an immune-deficient person.

Pneumocystis *pneumonia*   *Pneumocystis,* one of the first complications associated with the AIDS epidemic, can be deadly. Its presence is considered evidence of HIV infection. Preventive therapy is normally begun for all people with AIDS whose CD4 counts fall to 200 or less. The treatment of choice has, for many years, been Pentamidine, which is inhaled directly into the lungs in doses of about 300 mg monthly. Controversies over this drug's cost and some of its complications have caused physicians to reconsider use of one of the original preventive treatments for *Pneumocystis*, the antibacterial combination of Trimethoprim and Sulfamethoxazole (TMP/SMZ—Bactrim, Septra). The most common preventive dose of TMP/SMZ is one double dose taken three times a week. This drug has the advantages of low cost, the ability to be taken by mouth, and effectiveness equal to Pentamidine. When *Pneumocystis* develops, the same drugs are used for treatment, but in higher doses. Prednisone may also be given, together with an antifungal drug, to control inflammation within the lungs. Other, as yet unapproved, treatments like Trimetrexate or Dapsone may be given if neither Pentamidine nor TMP/SMZ works.

Candida *infection*   *Candida* infections are rarely fatal in AIDS patients, but they can be extremely troublesome. Any number of standard antifungal drugs may be given to treat *Candida* of the mouth (thrush), including Nystatin suspension, Clotrimazole tablets dissolved in the mouth, Ketoconazole, and Fluconazole. Fluconazole is the newest and most effective remedy against fungal infections that are resistant to other drugs.

Sexually transmitted diseases   All sexually transmitted diseases, including syphilis, chlamydia, and gonorrhea, are especially problematic for people with AIDS, but recurrent herpes is a major problem. Herpes can be present together with *Candida* and must be treated. Acyclovir is the drug of choice for treating herpes infections. Many AIDS patients require intravenous doses of the drug to get large quantities of it into their systems. Most people with AIDS take 800 mg of Acyclovir daily to prevent the recurrence of herpes.

Central-nervous-system infections   People with AIDS are particularly susceptible to meningitis and other nervous-system infections caused by fungal organisms that are rarely associated with this kind of infection in people not infected with HIV. This creates the need for suppressive therapy with Flucytosine or Fluconazole, and treatment with large doses of these drugs combined with sulfa drugs. Clindamycin may also be used in these situations.

Sinus infections and pneumonia   People with AIDS are subject to severe respiratory infections that may become chronic as time passes. As in other kinds of infections, the kinds of organisms involved create a more serious situation and require more potent and toxic drug treatment than in non-AIDS patients.

Cytomegalovirus (CMV) infection   CMV infection is one of the most serious complications of AIDS. It affects about one quarter of people with the virus and typically does not strike until the final phase of the illness. CMV, which is a member of the herpes family of viruses, can infect almost any part of the body but is particularly serious when it affects the eye. CMV retinitis, as the eye infection is known, is the leading cause of blindness among people with AIDS and is cited as the leading reason for suicide among people with AIDS. CMV retinitis can be treated with two drugs: Ganciclovir, which has been available for some time, or Foscarnet, which was approved in late 1991 by the FDA. Ganciclovir is available as a capsule or intravenous solution. Foscarnet is available only as an intravenous injection. Of the two, Foscarnet may be a better single therapeutic alternative because it not only is as effective as Ganciclovir in slowing the progression of the infection but also can contribute to life extension in two ways: It does not interact with AZT, allowing the continuation of antiviral treatment, and it has some anti-HIV effects of its own. However, new research has demonstrated that the best alternative may be to combine both drugs. Ganciclovir capsules can also be taken to *prevent* CMV infection.

Diarrhea Diarrhea is common among people with AIDS and can be due to any of a variety of causes. It can become serious and, regardless of the cause, is treated with general-purpose antidiarrheal drugs like Lomotil and Imodium because they provide general relief. Sometimes, more potent antidiarrheal products like Paregoric or Morphine Sulfate may be employed if the other medications don't work. If the exact cause of the diarrhea can be determined, another drug may be added to fight the specific cause of the problem.

Tuberculosis AIDS increases the risk of tuberculosis. People with AIDS who develop tuberculosis usually respond to standard antituberculosis drugs like Ethambutol, Isoniazid, or Rifampin, but these treatments do not cure the infection. For many people, the side effects of drug treatment may be more serious than the tuberculosis infection, so decisions must be made about how aggressively to treat the tuberculosis based on the general condition of the patient. People who show few symptoms related to the tuberculosis should probably not be treated. Those who are losing weight, running a chronic temperature, and feeling sickly should be treated.

Kaposi's sarcoma There is no treatment for Kaposi's sarcoma, which is also considered a diagnostic indicator for the presence of HIV. Interferon and a variety of anticancer drugs have been tried with limited success. Some that have been tried are Adriamycin, Bleomycin, Vincristine, and Vinblastine, but the side effects of these drugs, normally hard for anyone to tolerate, are especially difficult for people with AIDS. The basic problem is that people with AIDS who develop Kaposi's sarcoma have very low CD4 cell counts, reflective of a poorly functioning immune system. Because these drugs depend on a functioning immune system to bolster their effect, many of them just end up making people who are already sick even sicker.

Dental problems   People with AIDS may develop a variety of oral problems, including mouth sores, warts, Kaposi's sarcoma, *Candida* and other fungus infections, and gum disease. These are treated with many of the same drugs used in other parts of the body or to treat oral infections.

Skin problems   People with AIDS can develop a variety of common bacterial and fungal skin infections, including Impetigo and hair follicle infections, or may develop any of a host of rare skin infections requiring extraordinary treatments. Most common infections can be treated with standard antibacterial or antifungal creams, and ointments are used to fight many of these infections. Oral drugs may be needed when these infections become more widespread or unusually severe.

The treatment of AIDS is a complex and difficult problem. Researchers are still struggling to find the best ways to deal with HIV and its many complications. The ultimate treatment for AIDS will likely be a vaccine against the virus or a combination of drug therapies that bolster the immune system. A number of HIV vaccine products are in development, but all of them are years away from being proven effective.

Twenty Questions to Ask Your Doctor and Pharmacist About Your Prescription

1. What is the name of this medicine?

2. What results can be expected from taking it?

3. How long should I wait before reporting if this medicine does not help me?

4. How does the medicine work?

5. What is the exact dose of the medicine?

6. What time of day should I take it?

7. Do alcoholic beverages have an effect on this medicine?

8. Do I have to take special precautions with this medicine in combination with other prescription drugs I am taking?

9. Do I have to take special precautions with this medicine in combination with nonprescription (over-the-counter) drugs?

10. Does food have any effect on this medicine?

11. Are there any special instructions I should have about how to use this medicine?

12. How long should I continue to take this medicine?

13. Is my prescription renewable?

14. For how long a period can my prescription be renewed?

15. Which side effects should I report, and which ones can I disregard?

16. Can I save any unused part of this medicine for future use?

17. How should I store this medicine?

18. How long can I keep this medicine without it losing its strength?

19. What should I do if I miss a dose of this medicine?

20. Does this drug come in a less expensive, generic form?

Other Points to Remember
for Safe Drug Use

- Store your medicines in a sealed, light-resistant container to maintain maximum potency, and be sure to follow any special storage instructions listed on your medicine bottle, such as "refrigerate," "do not freeze," "protect from light," or "keep in a cool place." Protect all medicines from excessive humidity.
- Make sure you tell the doctor everything that is wrong. The more information your doctor has, the more effectively he or she can treat you.
- Make sure each doctor you see knows about all the medicines you use regularly, including prescription and nonprescription drugs.
- Keep a record of any bad reaction you have had to a medicine.
- Fill each prescription you are given. If you don't fill a prescription, make sure your doctor knows you aren't taking the medicine.
- Don't take extra medicine without consulting your doctor or pharmacist.
- Follow the label instructions exactly. If you have any questions, call your doctor or pharmacist.
- Report any unusual symptoms that you develop after taking any medicine.
- Do not save unused medicine for future use unless you have consulted your doctor. Dispose of unused medicine by flushing it down the toilet.

- Never keep medicine where children can see or reach it.
- Always read the label before taking your medicine. Don't trust your memory.
- Consult your pharmacist for guidance on the use of over-the-counter (nonprescription) drugs.
- Don't share your medicine with anyone. Your prescription was written for you and only you.
- Be sure the label stays on the container until the medicine is used or destroyed.
- Keep the label facing up when pouring liquid medicine from the bottle.
- Don't use a prescription medicine unless it has been specifically prescribed for you. Whenever you travel, carry your prescription in its original container.
- If you move to another city, ask your pharmacist to forward your prescription records to your new pharmacy. Carry important medical facts about yourself in your wallet. Such things as drug allergies, chronic diseases (diabetes, etc), and special requirements can be very useful.
- Don't hesitate to discuss the cost of medical care with your doctor or pharmacist.
- Exercise your right to make decisions about purchasing medicines:
  1. If you suffer from a chronic condition, you can probably save money by buying in larger quantities.
  2. Choose your pharmacist as carefully as you choose your doctor.
  3. Remember, the cost of your prescription includes the professional services offered by your pharmacy. If you want more service, you may have to pay for it.

THE TOP 200
PRESCRIPTION DRUGS
IN THE UNITED STATES

**RANKED BY NUMBER OF PRESCRIPTIONS DISPENSED FROM
JANUARY TO MAY 1995**

(Generic products are followed by manufacturer name in
parentheses.)

1. Premarin
2. Amoxil
3. Trimox
4. Zantac
5. Synthroid
6. Lanoxin
7. Procardia XL
8. Vasotec
9. Prozac
10. Proventil
11. Cardizem CD
12. Biaxin
13. Augmentin
14. Coumadin Sodium
15. Zoloft
16. Amoxicillin Trihydrate (Biocraft)
17. Zestril
18. Hydrocodone with APAP (Watson)
19. Cipro
20. Ventolin
21. Triamterene/HCTZ (Geneva)
22. Veetids
23. Prilosec
24. Acetaminophen with Codeine (Purepac)
25. Mevacor
26. Propoxyphen Napsylate with APAP (Mylan)
27. Capoten
28. Norvasc
29. Provera
30. Furosemide (Mylan)
31. Claritin
32. Dilantin
33. Humulin N
34. Ibuprofen (Boots)
35. Alprazolam
36. Ortho-Novum 7/7/7 [28]
37. Acetaminophen with Codeine (Lemmon)
38. Hytrin
39. Pepcid
40. Cephalexin
41. K-Dur
42. Paxil
43. Cefaclor (Mylan)
44. Propacet 100
45. Seldane
46. Relafen
47. Triphasil 28

48. Ceftin
49. Ery-Tab
50. Cefzil
51. Klonopin
52. Vancenase AQ
53. Cephalexin (Apothecon)
54. Trimethoprim/
    Sulfamethoxazole
    (Mutual)
55. Atrovent
56. Zocor
57. Prinivil
58. Axid
59. Estraderm
60. Estrace
61. Amitriptyline HCl
    (Mylan)
62. Calan SR
63. Xanax
64. Hydrocodone with APAP
    (Halsey)
65. Pravachol
66. Lodine
67. Dyazide
68. Deltasone
69. Voltaren
70. Ortho-Cept 26
71. Nitrostat
72. Ambien
73. Duricef
74. Lasix
75. Atenolol (IPR)
76. Levoxyl
77. Ceclor
78. Glyburide
79. Beconase AQ
80. Lorabid
81. Roxicet
82. Propulsid
83. Verapamil SR (Goldline)
84. Daypro
85. Humulin 70/30

86. Lotensin
87. Zithromax 2-Pak
88. Lotrisone
89. Azmacort
90. Buspar
91. Motrin
92. Suprax
93. Methylphenidate (MD)
94. Seldane-D
95. Darvocet-N 100
96. Lorazepam (Mylan)
97. Cimetidine (Mylan)
98. Timoptic
99. Accupril
100. Desogen
101. Trental
102. Trimethoprim/
     Sulfamethoxazole
     (Mutual)
103. Cycrin
104. Toradol
105. Amoxicillin Trihydrate
     (Warner-Chilcott)
106. Claritin D
107. Medroxyprogesterone
     (Greenstone)
108. Albuterol (Lemmon)
109. Atenolol (IPR)
110. Adalat CC
111. Prednisone (Schein)
112. Lo/Ovral-28
113. Glynase Prestab
114. Lorazepam (Purepac)
115. Retin-A
116. Lopressor
117. Naproxen (Mylan)
118. Tegretol
119. DiaBeta
120. Amoxicillin Trihydrate
     (Novopharm)
121. Potassium Chloride
     (Ethex)

122. Metoprolol Tartrate (Geneva)
123. Micronase
124. Glipizide
125. Phenergan
126. Tri-Levlen 28
127. Depakote
128. Hydrochlorothiazide (Zenith)
129. Tenormin
130. Zovirax Capsules
131. Nitro-Dur
132. Theo-Dur
133. Gemfibrozil
134. Cardura
135. Cyclobenzaprine HCl (Mylan)
136. Glucotrol
137. Alprazolam (Greenstone)
138. Doxycycline Hyclate (Zenith)
139. Tylenol with Codeine (McNeil)
140. Lozol
141. Verelan
142. Cephalexin (Biocraft)
143. Macrobid
144. Humulin R
145. Diflucan
146. Glucotrol XL
147. Erythrocin Stearate
148. Nortriptyline HCl (Schein)
149. Altace
150. Lescol
151. Terazol 7
152. Ortho-Novum 1/38 [28]
153. Naproxen (Hamilton)
154. Neomycin/Polymyxin/ HC (Schein)
155. Lorcet Plus
156. Ritalin
157. Dilacor XR
158. Floxin
159. E.E.S.
160. Carafate
161. Diazepam (Mylan)
162. Klor-Con 10
163. Lorcet 10/650
164. Hismanal
165. Promethazine with Codeine
166. Albuterol (Lemmon)
167. Methylprednisolone
168. Bactroban
169. Temazepam (Mylan)
170. Vanceril
171. Sumycin (Apothecon)
172. Ibuprofen (Winsor)
173. Guaifenesin/PPA (Duramed)
174. One Touch
175. Children's Advil
176. Vicodin
177. Dicyclomine HCl (Rugby)
178. Atenolol (Geneva)
179. Penicillin VK
180. Serevent (Mylan)
181. Cyclobenzaprine HCl (Mylan)
182. Metoprolol Tartarzine (Mylan)
183. Nasacort
184. Cotrim DS
185. Vantin
186. Effexor
187. Hydrocodone with APAP (Warner-Chilcot)
188. Hydrocodone with APAP (Rugby Labs)
189. Loestrin-Fe 1.5/30
190. Valium

191. Imitrex
192. Fiorinal with Codeine
193. Compazine
194. Elocon
195. Dumex

196. Zovirax Tablets
197. Entex LA
198. Oruvail
199. Principen
200. Furosemide (Geneva)

Source: NPA *Plus*™, IMS America, Ltd., 1995

Index of Generic and Brand Name Drugs

How to Find Your Drug in *The Pill Book*

- Most generic drugs produce the same therapeutic effects as their brand name equivalents, but are much less expensive. Because of the prominence of many brand name drugs, consumers may not always be aware of generic alternatives. *The Pill Book* lists most drugs in alphabetic order by their generic name because a drug may have many brand names, but can have only one generic name. By listing generic names, *The Pill Book* makes it easier for you to locate your medicine, no matter what the brand name.

- When a drug has 2 or more active ingredients, it is listed by the most widely known major brand name. In a few cases, pill profiles are listed by drug type (antidiabetes drugs, contraceptives).

- *The Pill Book* now includes brand names of the top 100 drugs, with the page numbers they appear on, in alphabetic order with the pill profiles. You can find the most widely used drugs by simply looking for them in alphabetic order throughout the book.

- All brand and generic names are cross-referenced in the Index.

- Sugar-free and alcohol-free brand name drugs are indicated by the Ⓢ and Ⓐ symbols in the beginning of each pill profile.

ABOUT THE EDITOR

Educated at Columbia University, Dr. Harold Silverman has been a hospital pharmacist, author, educator, and pharmaceutical industry consultant. Currently, he is a director at *Interscience*, a global health-care communications consultancy. Professionally, Dr. Silverman seeks to help people understand why medicines are prescribed and how to get the most from them. In addition to *THE PILL BOOK*, Dr. Silverman is coauthor of *THE VITAMIN BOOK: A No-Nonsense Consumer Guide* and *The MED FILE Drug Interactions System.* He is also the author of *THE PILL BOOK GUIDE TO SAFE DRUG USE, THE CONSUMER'S GUIDE TO POISON PROTECTION, THE WOMAN'S DRUG STORE,* and *TRAVEL HEALTHY.* Dr. Silverman's contributions to the professional literature include more than 70 articles, research papers, and textbook chapters. He is a member of many professional organizations and has served as an officer for several, including the New York State Council of Hospital Pharmacists, for which he served as president. He has taught pharmacology and clinical pharmacy at several universities and won numerous awards for his work. Dr. Silverman resides in a Washington suburb with his wife, Judith Brown, and their son, Joshua.